Renal Transport and Diuretics · Renaler Transport und Diuretica

Renal Transport and Diuretics

International Symposium Feldafing, June 21 – 23, 1968

Chairmen

K. KRAMER · H. SCHWIEGK

Editors

K. THURAU · H. JAHRMÄRKER

Sponsors

K. H. BEYER · H. F. HOFMANN
MERCK SHARP & DOHME Research Laboratories, Rahway
and SHARP & DOHME G.m.b.H., München

With 235 Figures and 62 Tables

Springer-Verlag
Berlin · Heidelberg · New York 1969

Renaler Transport und Diuretica

Internationales Symposium Feldafing, 21.–23. Juni 1968

Leitung

K. KRAMER · H. SCHWIEGK

Herausgeber

K. THURAU · H. JAHRMÄRKER

Veranstalter

K. H. BEYER · H. F. HOFMANN

MERCK SHARP & DOHME Research Laboratories, Rahway
und SHARP & DOHME G.m.b.H., München

Mit 235 Abbildungen und 62 Tabellen

Springer-Verlag
Berlin · Heidelberg · New York 1969

ISBN 978-3-642-88091-9 ISBN 978-3-642-88089-6 (eBook)
DOI 10.1007/978-3-642-88089-6

softcover reprint of the hardcover 1st edition 1969

Preface

It is generally appreciated that large congresses are not the optimal means of facilitating communication within specialized areas of medical research. Small symposia, where scientific discussion can be confined to limited groups, have lately become successful vehicles of information transfer. However, such symposia, although eminently suited to the exploration of specific problems, often have the inherent disadvantage of not being able to successfully address themselves to larger themes.

Accordingly, the planners of this symposium have solicited the participation of internationally acclaimed investigators to consider current problems both in the physiological and clinical domains of nephrology. The observant reader will note that the variety of theoretical and experimental approaches used by the physiologists are reflected in the clinical studies, while the clinicians, in turn, have provided the physiologists with useful insights.

The part of the symposium which attempted to correlate metabolic characteristics of kidney cells with their transport functions has proven to be particularly fruitful. For example, the presentations dealing with aldosterone, angiotensin and diuretics have offered a multi-faceted approach that was previously unavailable.

The contributions of investigators from many countries and their enthusiastic participation have led to the success of this symposium. To them we wish to express our deep gratitude.

We also wish to sincerely thank Dr. K. H. Beyer, Senior Vice President of Merck, Sharp & Dohme Research Laboratories, and Dr. H. F. Hofmann, Director of Medical Research of Sharp & Dohme GmbH for their full support and their constant attention to our many requests.

The excellent and efficient assistance of Mrs. Hella Steichele in the organization of the symposium and the administrative duties involved in the publication of the manuscripts is gratefully acknowledged.

Munich, March 1969 K. Kramer · H. Schwiegk

Vorwort

Es ist allgemein bekannt, daß die Kommunikation und Information der Wissenschaftler auf den einzelnen Gebieten der Medizin durch größere Kongreßveranstaltungen nicht mehr befriedigend erreicht werden kann. Symposien, d. h. wissenschaftliche Diskussionen in kleinem und kleinsten Kreis werden als das Mittel der Wahl angesehen. Diese Art der gegenseitigen Unterrichtung und Verständigung hat jedoch oft den Nachteil, daß nur ganz spezielle, zu einem kleinen Gebiet der Forschung gehörende Fragen abgehandelt werden, ohne daß sie Bezug auf ein übergeordnetes Problem nehmen.

Die Planer des Symposiums haben daher den Versuch gemacht, Grundprobleme der theoretischen *und* klinischen Nephrologie in gemeinsamer Arbeit internationaler Wissenschaftler zu behandeln. Dem aufmerksamen Leser wird nicht entgehen, daß die Vielfalt der Denk- und Experimentalmethodik der Theoretiker ihren Niederschlag im klinischen Bereich gefunden hat und daß andererseits auch der Theoretiker für seine Forschungen entscheidende Anregungen von seinen klinischen Kollegen auf diesem Symposium erhalten hat.

Das Thema, das die Verknüpfung von Stoffwechsel der Nierenzellen und ihrer Transportfunktionen anstrebt, hat sich wohl als besonders glücklich erwiesen. So konnte durch das Zusammenführen von Forschern verschiedenster Gebiete ein Gesamtbild entworfen werden, wie dies z. B. in der Endokrinologie der Niere oder in den Beziehungen der Diuretica zu den renalen Transportfunktionen bisher nicht möglich war.

Die Teilnahme zahlreicher Forscher aus aller Welt und ihre Aufgeschlossenheit in der Aussprache hat wesentlich zum Gelingen des Symposiums beigetragen. Dafür sagen wir ihnen unseren herzlichen Dank.

Unser besonderer Dank gilt Herrn Dr. K. H. Beyer, dem Vizepräsidenten der Merck Sharp & Dohme Forschungslaboratorien und Herrn Dr. med. H. F. Hofmann der Sharp & Dohme GmbH München, die das Symposium ermöglichten, für ihre unermüdliche Förderung und ihr großes Verständnis für unser Anliegen. Frau Hella Steichele hat in hervorragender Weise die organisatorische Durchführung des Symposiums und die Herausgabe der vorliegenden Veröffentlichung betreut.

München, März 1969 K. Kramer · H. Schwiegk

Contents – Inhaltsverzeichnis

Renal Metabolism – Nierenstoffwechsel

H. A. Krebs
Renal Carbohydrate and Fatty Acid Metabolism 1
Kohlehydrat- und Fettsäure-Stoffwechsel der Niere 1
Discussion: Deetjen, Krebs, Epstein, Kramer, Ullrich, Leaf, Edelman 9

R. F. Pitts
Renal Metabolism of Amino Acids and Ammonia 11
Aminosäuren- und Ammoniak-Stoffwechsel der Niere 11

H. Oelert, E. Uhlich, A. G. Hills
Transport of Ammonia in the Mammalian Cortical Nephron 25
Ammoniak-Transport im corticalen Nephron der Säugetierniere 25
Discussion: Pitts, Krück 27

K. Kramer, E. Bassenge, H. Brechtelbauer
Remarks on Renal Gaseous Metabolism 29
Bemerkungen zum Gasstoffwechsel der Säugetierniere 29
Discussion: Reubi, Gross, Kramer 36

Renal Transport Processes – Renale Transportvorgänge

W. Thoenes, K. H. Langer
Relationship Between Cell Structures of Renal Tubules and Transport Mechanisms . . 37
Zellstrukturen der Harnkanälchen in Beziehung zum Stofftransport 37
Discussion: Thurau, Thoenes, Hierholzer, Bohle, Mertz, Burg 64

F. Epstein
The Role of Sodium and Potassium ATPase in Renal Sodium Reabsorption 67
Die Rolle der Natrium- und Kalium-ATPase bei der renalen Natriumresorption 67
Discussion: Hierholzer, Ebel, Epstein, Edelman, Bohle 75

J. M. Diamond
The Coupling of Solute and Water Transport in Epithelia 77
Die Verknüpfung von Wasser- und Natriumtransport in Epithelien 77
Discussion: Herms, Diamond, Ullrich, Mertz, Holzgreve, Thurau 97

K. J. Ullrich
Water Permeability of Different Nephron Segments in the Mammalian Kidney 99
Die Wasserpermeabilität verschiedener Tubulusabschnitte der Säugetierniere 99

M. B. Burg

Transport Characteristics of Isolated Perfused Proximal Tubules 109

Transport-Charakteristika des isolierten, perfundierten proximalen Tubulus.. 109

Discussion: Gertz, Burg, Thoenes 121

G. Giebisch, G. Malnic

The Regulation of Distal Tubular Potassium Transport 123

Regulation des Kaliumtransportes im distalen Tubulus 123

Discussion: Burg, Thurau, Giebisch 137

I. S. Edelman

Intracellular Action of Aldosterone on Sodium Transport 139

Intrazellulärer Wirkungsmechanismus von Aldosteron für den Natriumtransport . .. 139

Discussion: Crabbé, Edelman, Gross, Leaf 151

K. Hierholzer

Intrarenal Action of Steroid Hormones on Sodium Transport 153

Intrarenale Wirkung von Steroidhormonen auf den Natriumtransport 153

Discussion: Gross, Hierholzer, Deetjen, Ochwadt, Krück 171

K. Thurau

Intrarenal Action of Angiotensin 173

Intrarenale Wirkung des Angiotensins 173

Discussion: Gross, Thurau, Ochwadt, Bohle, Gessler 182

W. Schoeppe

The Effect of Angiotensin Upon Blood Pressure-Dependent Increases of Na-Excretion in Essential Hypertension 185

Über die Beeinflussung der blutdruckabhängigen Zunahme der Natriumausscheidung bei essentieller Hypertonie durch Angiotensin 185

C. A. Baldamus, E. Uhlich

Countercurrent Considerations Relating to Renal Medullary pCO_2 and Bicarbonate Concentrations 187

Verhalten von CO_2-Druck und Bikarbonat im Gegenstrom-System des Nierenmarks .. 187

J. Eigler J. Crabbé

Effects of Diuretics on Active Sodium Transport in Amphibian Membranes 195

Wirkung von Diuretica auf den aktiven Natriumtransport an Amphibienmembranen .. 195

Discussion: Giebisch, Edelman, Eigler, Crabbé, Baer 207

W. Herms

The Effect of Diuretic Agents and Metabolic Inhibitors on O_2-Consumption and Lactate Production of the Isolated Frog Skin 209

Sauerstoffverbrauch und Laktatproduktion der isolierten Amphibienhaut von rana temporaria unter Einfluß von Diuretica und Stoffwechselhemmern 209

Discussion: Baer 213

P. Deetjen
The Localization of Transport Processes in the Nephron and their Inhibition by Diuretic Agents as Analyzed by Micropuncture Techniques 215
Mikropunktionsmethoden zur Lokalisation der Transportvorgänge in der Niere und ihre Beeinflussung durch Diuretica 215

Discussion: Levine, Husmann, Deetjen, Reubi, Thurau, Heidenreich 226

H. Holzgreve
The Pattern of Inhibition of Proximal Tubular Reabsorption by Diuretics 229
Hemmwirkung der Diuretica auf die proximale, tubuläre Resorption 229

Clinical Application of Diuretics – Klinische Anwendung der Diuretica

K. H. Beyer, Jr.
Present Status of Diuretic Therapy 235
Heutiger Stand der diuretischen Therapie 235

J. E. Baer
Pharmacology of Antikaliuretic Substances 247
Pharmakologie antikaliuretischer Substanzen 247

Discussion: Oelert, Baer 254

W. H. Wilkinson
The Clinical Assessment of Diuretic Agents 255
Die klinische Erprobung von Diuretica 255

Discussion: Gross, Wilkinson, Jahrmärker, Leppla 267

Kh. R. Koczorek, H. Jahrmärker, H. Hofmann, W. Vogt, P. Schmiedek, B. Simon, E. Balde
Effects of Combined Application of Antikaliuretic Agents and Diuretics 269
Kombinierte Anwendung antikaliuretischer Substanzen mit konventionellen Diuretica 269

Discussion: Muller, Koczorek, Heinz, Krück, Jahrmärker, Reubi 298

E. Schmid, G. Fricke
On the Urinary Excretion of a New Antikaliuretic Agent 301
Über die Harnausscheidung einer neuen antikaliuretischen Substanz 301

F. Husmann, P. Suchan
Serum Electrolytes During Combined Administration of Ethacrynic Acid and Amiloride 305
Das Verhalten der Serum-Elektrolyte unter der Verabreichung einer Etacrynsäure-Amilorid-Kombination 305

K. W. Fritz, R. Richter
Clinical Results with Ethacrynic Acid in Combination with MK 870 309
Klinische Ergebnisse mit Etacrynsäure in Kombination mit MK 870 309

N. Heinz
Amiloride in Edematous Patients 313
Amilorid-Anwendung bei der Ödemausschwemmung 313

F. Wessels
The Action of Amiloride on the Sodium Transport at the Erythrocyte Membrane . .. 317
Die Wirkung von Amilorid auf den Natrium-Transport an der Erythrozytenmembran 317

E. Wollheim
Diuretics in the Treatment of Hypertension.. 321
Bedeutung der Diuretica für die Hypertoniebehandlung 321

O. H. Arnold
The Treatment of Hypertension with Diuretics 337
Zur Behandlung der Hypertonie mit Diuretica 337

Discussion: Krecke, Herms, Wollheim, Schwiegk, Reubi, Baethmann, Arnold, Kleinfelder, Holzgreve, Kramer, Baer, Krück 350

H. Kampffmeyer, J. Conway
The Importance of Diuretics for the Treatment of Hypertension 353
Bedeutung der Diuretica für die Hypertoniebehandlung 353

D. P. Mertz, P. Schwoerer
Natriuresis in Arterial Hypertension During Treatment with Saluretics 359
Natriurese bei arterieller Hypertonie unter der Wirkung von Diuretica 359

Sh. Sherlock
Diuretic Therapy in Patients with Cirrhosis 365
Die diuretische Therapie bei Cirrhose-Patienten 365

Discussion: Dölle, Schwiegk, Jahrmärker, Gessler, Reubi, Sherlock, Muller, Leppla, Krück, Koczorek 373

F. Dürr, W. Kaufmann, B. Steiner
The Administration of Diuretics and the Metabolism of Aldosterone in Liver Disease .. 377
Zur Diuretica-Anwendung und zum Aldosteron-Stoffwechsel bei Erkrankungen der Leber 377

F. Reubi
Clinical Application of Diuretics in Renal Disease 381
Klinische Anwendung der Diuretica bei Erkrankungen der Niere 381

Discussion: Holzgreve, Gessler, Oelert, Krecke, Reubi, Scheler 392

A. Heidland, K. Klütsch, H. Hennemann, U. Löwenstein, H. J. Kuschke
The Influence of Diuretics on the Fractional Fluid and Electrolyte-Elimination in Renal Insufficiency 395
Der Einfluß von Diuretica auf die fraktionelle Flüssigkeits- und Elektrolytelimination bei eingeschränkter Nierenfunktion 395

W. Holler
Symptomatic Diuretic Therapy of the Nephrotic Edema with the Fixed Combination Ethacrynic Acid/Amiloride 403
Symptomatische diuretische Behandlung des nephrotischen Ödems mit dem Kombinationspräparat Etacrynsäure/Amilorid 403

E. Buchborn
The Application of Diuretics in Diabetes Insipidus 409
Die Anwendung von Diuretica bei Diabetes insipidus 409

Discussion: Herms, Ullrich, Klaus, Buchborn 412

H. Dobbelstein, H. H. Edel
The Effect of Diuretics on the Extracorporeal Transplanted Kidney . . . 413
Diureticawirkung an der extrakorporal transplantierten Niere . . . 413
Discussion: Reinhardt, Dobbelstein, Reubi, Kramer, Schwiegk . . . 418

A. F. Muller, A. Grandchamp, R. Veyrat
Diuretics in Cardiac Diseases . . . 421
Diuretica bei Herzkrankheiten . . . 421
Discussion: Krück, Muller, Wessels, Kramer, Baethmann, Husmann, Koczorek 430

H. Jahrmärker, Kh. R. Koczorek, H. Avenhaus, H. Grohmann
Clinical Application of Diuretics in Cardiac Diseases . . . 433
Klinische Anwendung der Diuretica bei Erkrankungen des Herzens . . . 433
Discussion: Heidland, Jahrmärker . . . 444

W. Siegenthaler
On the Use of Diuretics in Congestive Heart Failure . . . 445
Zur Anwendung der Diuretica bei Herzinsuffizienz . . . 445

W. Kaufmann, B. Steiner, F. Dürr, K. A. Meurer
The Use of Diuretics in Cardiac Diseases . . . 451
Zur Anwendung der Diuretica bei Erkrankungen des Herzens . . . 451

D. Klaus
The Effect of Various Diuretics on Plasma Renin Activity in the Acute Experiment . . 455
Die Beeinflussung der Plasmareninaktivität durch verschiedene Diuretica in akuten Versuchen . . . 455

H. Oelert, F. Sebening
Clinical Application of Diuretics During and After Heart Surgery . . . 459
Klinische Anwendung von Diuretica während und nach Herzoperationen . . . 459
Discussion: Herms, Oelert, Jahrmärker, Koczorek, Kramer . . . 468

H. J. Reulen, M. Samii, Kh. R. Koczorek, A. Baethmann, K. Schürmann
Diuretics in Cerebral Edema . . . 469
Diuretica beim cerebralen Ödem . . . 469
Discussion: Herms, Reulen, Muller, Baethmann, Kramer, Wessels, Hierholzer 480

Index . . . 483

Contributors – Sprecher

ARNOLD, O. H., Medizinische Klinik der Med. Fakultät Essen
BAER, J. E., Merck Institute for Therapeutic Research, West Point, Pa., U. S. A.
BAETHMANN, A., Chirurgische Universitätsklinik München
BALDAMUS, C. A., Max-Planck-Institut für Biophysik, Frankfurt/M.
BEYER, K. H., Jr., Merck Sharp & Dohme Research Laboratories, West Point, Pa., U.S.A.
BOHLE, A., Pathologisches Institut der Universität Tübingen
BUCHBORN, E., Medizinische Universitätsklinik Köln
BURG, M. B., National Heart Institute, Bethesda, Md., U.S.A.
CRABBÉ, J., Departement de Physiologie, Université de Louvain, Belgien
DEETJEN, P., Physiologisches Institut der Universität München
DIAMOND, J. M., Department of Physiology, UCLA Medical School, Los Angeles, Calif., U.S.A.
DOBBELSTEIN, H., I. Medizinische Universitätsklinik München
DÖLLE, W., Medizinische Universitätsklinik Marburg
DÜRR, F., Medizinische Universitätsklinik Tübingen
EBEL, H., Physiologisches Institut der Freien Universität Berlin
EDELMAN, I. S., University of California Medical Center, San Francisco, Calif., U. S. A.
EIGLER, J., Medizinische Universitätsklinik Köln
EPSTEIN, F., Department of Medicine, Yale University, New Haven, Conn., U.S.A.
FRITZ, K. W., Medizinische Universitätsklinik Bonn
GERTZ, K.-H., Physiologisches Institut der Freien Universität Berlin
GESSLER, U., IV. Medizinische Klinik Nürnberg
GIEBISCH, G., Department of Physiology, Yale University, New Haven, Conn., U.S.A.
GROSS, F., Pharmakologisches Institut der Universität Heidelberg
HEIDENREICH, O., Pharmakologisches Institut der Technischen HochschuleAachen inFreiburg
HEIDLAND, A., Medizinische Universitätsklinik Würzburg
HEINZ, N., Medizinische Universitätsklinik Hamburg-Eppendorf
HERMS, W., I. Medizinische Universitätsklinik Düsseldorf
HIERHOLZER, K., Physiologisches Institut der Freien Universität Berlin
HOLLER, W., Medizinische Universitäts-Poliklinik Freiburg
HOFMANN, H. F., Medizinische Forschung, Sharp & Dohme GmbH., München
HOLZGREVE, H., Medizinische Universitätsklinik Köln
HUSMANN, F., Medizinische Universitäts-Poliklinik Würzburg
JAHRMÄRKER, H., I. Medizinische Universitätsklinik München
KAMPFFMEYER, H., Pharmakologisches Institut der Universität München
KAUFMANN, W., Medizinische Universitätsklinik Tübingen
KLAUS, D., Medizinische Universitäts-Poliklinik Tübingen
KLEINFELDER, H., III. Medizinische Klinik der Städtischen Krankenanstalten Nürnberg
KOCZOREK, KH. R., I. Medizinische Universitätsklinik München
KRAMER, K., Physiologisches Institut der Universität München
KREBS, H. A., Nuffield Department of Clinical Medicine, Oxford, England
KRECKE, H., Medizinische Universitätsklinik Heidelberg
KRÜCK, F., II. Medizinische Universitätsklinik Homburg
LEAF, A., Massachussets General Hospital, Boston, Mass., U. S. A.
LEPPLA, W., I. Medizinische Universitätsklinik Homburg
LEVINE, D., Physiologisches Institut der Universität München
MERTZ, D. P., Medizinische Universitäts-Poliklinik Freiburg

MULLER, A. F., Clinique Universitaire de Médecine Hôpital Cantonal, Genf
OCHWADT, B., Max-Planck-Institut für experimentelle Medizin, Göttingen
OELERT, H., Chirurgische Klinik, Medizinische Hochschule Hannover
PITTS, R. F., Department of Physiology, Cornell University, New York, N.Y., U.S.A.
REINHARDT, H. W., Physiologisches Institut der Universität München
REUBI, F., Medizinische Poliklinik der Universität Bern, Schweiz
REULEN, H. J., Neurochirurgische Universitätsklinik Mainz
RIECKER, G., Medizinische Universitätsklinik Göttingen
SCHELER, F., Medizinische Universitätsklinik Göttingen
SCHMID, E., I. Medizinische Klinik und Poliklinik der Medizinischen Akademie Lübeck
SCHOEPPE, W., II. Medizinische Universitätsklinik Frankfurt
SCHWIEGK, H., I. Medizinische Universitätsklinik München
SHERLOCK, SH., Postgraduate Medical School, London W. C. I., England
SIEGENTHALER, W., Medizinische Universitäts-Poliklinik Zürich, Schweiz
THOENES, W., Pathologisches Institut der Universität Würzburg
THURAU, K., Physiologisches Institut der Universität München
UHLICH, E., Max-Planck-Institut für Biophysik Frankfurt
ULLRICH, K. J., Max-Planck-Institut für Biophysik Frankfurt
WESSELS, F., Medizinische Universitätsklinik Münster
WILKINSON, W. H., Merck Sharp & Dohme Research Laboratories, West Point, Pa., U.S.A.
WOLLHEIM, E., Medizinische Universitätsklinik Würzburg

Renal Carbohydrate and Fatty Acid Metabolism

H. A. KREBS

General Comment

The kidney is not only an excretory organ, it also possesses major metabolic functions. Foremost among the latter, from the quantitative point of view, is gluconeogenesis from amino acids, lactate, intermediates of the tricarboxylic acid cycle, propionate, glycerol, hexoses, hexitols, pentoses and pentitols (1, 2). Other metabolic functions are detoxication reactions [such as the synthesis of hippuric acid (3)], the synthesis of glutamine (4, 5), the synthesis of arginine from citrulline and aspartate (6), and the synthesis of creatine from glycine, arginine and methionine (7, 8). The metabolic processes of the kidney arise from two kinds of functional requirements – those which serve directly the needs of the production of urine and those which lead to the synthesis of substances needed by the organism as a whole.

Another general aspect of renal metabolism concerns the great differences between the cortex and the inner medulla. I will ignore in my discussion the metabolism of the outer medulla because (as far as I am aware) there is no detailed information available on the *special* metabolism, as opposed to the overall energy providing reaction, of this segment. As the outer medulla consists mainly of blood vessels, collecting ducts, distal tubules and loops of Henle, its metabolism is expected to be a mixture of that of vessels, of cortical elements and of the inner medulla.

Metabolic experiments on the *intact* kidney resting essentially on analyses of ingoing and outgoing blood, or of changes in the perfusion fluid used in a closed system do not supply information on the cortex and medulla separately. To obtain quantitative data on these tissues it is necessary to resort to the slice technique or similar procedures utilising tissue fragments, though the micro-puncture technique can also be useful in the study of certain problems.

Table 1. *Comparison of O_2-consumption of perfused rat kidney and slices of rat kidney cortex.* The data for the perfused kidney are taken from (9); those for slices are based on those of KREBS, HEMS & GASCOYNE (10) and KREBS, SPEAKE & HEMS (11).

Substrate added	O_2 used (µmole/g. dry wt./hr.)	
	Perfused kidney	Sliced cortex
None	1390	900
Pyruvate (5 mM)	1940	1470
None	1610	900
Lactate (5 mM)	2230	1200

Whilst the possibility of examining cortex and inner medulla separately is a great asset of the tissue slice technique there is one serious disadvantage: there are indications that the rate of oxygen consumption of slices is rather lower than that of the intact urine-producing whole kidney. The basal oxygen consumption of the isolated perfused organ of the rat, when no substrate has been added, is almost twice as high as that of slices of the cortex and about five times as high as that of slices of the inner medulla (see Table 1). This is no doubt connected with the fact that the secretory work of slices is very low. The increments in respiration caused by the addition of substrates e. g. lactate, on the other hand, are about the same in the perfused organ and in slices.

Similar differences between the perfused organ and slices have been found with rat liver where the rates of oxygen consumption, gluconeogenesis and ketone body formation are considerably greater in the perfused organ than in slices (Table 2 and 3).

The inference is that metabolic rates observed in slices may be lower than in the *in vivo* rates. However, this does not necessarily apply to all metabolic processes. Thus the rates of gluconeogenesis, on a tissue weight basis, are slightly higher in rat kidney cortex slices than in the perfused organ. Since gluconeogenesis occurs in the cortex only but not

Table 2. *Comparison of rates of gluconeogenesis in perfused and sliced rat liver.*
For full details of procedures and statistical information see ROSS, HEMS & KREBS (12), and KREBS (13). The rats were starver for 48 hrs. The rates of gluconeogenesis are expressed as µmole/min./g. wet wt.

Substrate	Perfused organ	Slices
None	0.14	
L-Lactate	1.06	0.55
Pyruvate	1.02	0.40
Glycerol	0.48	0.62
L-Alanine	0.66	0.23
L-Serine	0.98	0.20
L-Proline	0.55	0.17
Dihydroxyacetone	2.07	0.38
Fructose	2.68	0.81

Table 3. *Comparison of rates of total ketone body production in rat liver.*
The rats were starved for 48 hrs. The initial substrate concentration was 2 mM. The medium contained 2 mM DL-carnitine and 2.3% serum albumin. The rates are expressed as µmole/g. wet wt./hr. [from KREBS (13)].

Substrate added	Perfused organ		Slices	
	Total	Increment due to substrate	Total	Increment due to substrate
None	30		25	
Butyrate	94	64	41	16
Octanonate	128	98	48	23
Oleate	98	68	30	5
Linoleate	117	87	29	4

in the medulla, such differences are expected provided that slicing does not decrease the glucogenic capacity.

In spite, then, of the shortcomings of the slice technique, we have to use slices for some investigations because no better quantitative method is available for the study of the metabolism of the separate kidney segments.

As a final general comment I must mention that I shall not discuss in any detail the gaseous metabolism of the kidney as this will be dealt with by other contributors.

Metabolism of the Inner Medulla

As far as is known the medulla depends essentially on carbohydrate as a source of energy (14, 15, 16). Compared with the cortex the energy requirements of the medulla appear to be low and a large proportion of the energy is obtained from the conversion of glucose to lactate rather than the oxidation of glucose. Aerobic lactate formation is exceptionally high in the medulla, equalled only by that of the red and white blood cells and possibly the retina. The renal medulla belongs to the small number of animal tissues – others are the blood cells and nervous tissue – which seem to be unable to use to a major extent fuels other than carbohydrate.

The dependence of the renal medulla on carbohydrate as a source of energy and on the high rate of lactic acid production was first established in slice experiments (14, 15, 16, 17, 18) but has been confirmed for the intact kidney, especially by RUIZ-GUINAZU et al. (17) who compared the glucose and lactate concentrations in the renal artery and the vasa recta and found a fall in the glucose concentration and a rise in the lactate concentration.

Slices represent essentially (as already mentioned) the non-secreting, i. e. resting or partially resting kidney. Whether carbohydrate is also the sole fuel of maximally working inner medulla should perhaps be regarded as an open question. It is known for the mammalian heart that the nature of the fuel can change in relation to the work done. The basal fuel of the heart is provided mainly by fatty acids but for maximum work carbohydrate appears to be necessary. This also applies to some skeletal muscles.

Metabolism of the Renal Cortex

The special metabolic functions of the kidney all seem to be located in the cortex – those which serve the organism as a whole rather than the production of urine. I propose to limit the discussion of special metabolic functions to two aspects, the fuel of respiration and gluconeogenesis.

Under normal condition renal cortex uses long chain fatty acids as the *main* fuel of respiration. The recent work by LEE, VANCE and CAHILL (20), GOLD and SPITZER (21) and NIETH and SCHOLLMEYER (22) confirms the long-standing observation that the respiratory quotient of kidney is low [DICKENS and SIMER (23)]. Experiments by WEIDEMANN (24) show that rat kidney cortex slices readily oxidise all even-membered fatty acids between chain lengths C_2 to C_{18}. Added butyrate at 10 mM can contribute about 70% and added oleate at 2 mM about 50% to the respiratory fuel. The remaining fuel appears to be mainly endogenous fat.

In addition to forming respiratory CO_2 fatty acids can also give rise to the formation of ketone bodies, the maximum rates being about 80 µmoles/g. dry wt./hr., when butyrate or octanoate are the substrates (Table 4). The rates of ketone body formation

Table 4. *Renal ketogenesis.*
The data on rat kidney cortex were obtained with slices of rat kidney cortex suspended in a bicarbonate-buffered saline medium saturated with 5% CO_2 in O_2. Optimal concentrations of substrate are given. The period of starvation was 48 hrs. Acetoacetate and β-hydroxybutyrate were measured enzymically. Unpublished observations by M. J. WEIDEMANN. The data on the perfused rat liver are taken from unpublished work by WALLACE, HEMS and KREBS (see 13).

Added substrate	Nutritional state	Rate of total ketone body formation (µmole/g. dry wt./hr.)	Rate of total ketone body formation in the perfused rat liver (µmole/g. dry wt./hr.)
None	well fed	3	
None	starved	4	144
Butyrate (10 mM)	well fed	81	
Butyrate (10 mM)	starved	81	340
Octanoate (0.5 mM)	starved	60	460
Octanoate (0.5 mM); DL-carnitine (1 mM)	starved	80	460
Oleate (2 mM); albumin (2%)	well fed	4	
Oleate (2 mM); albumin (2%); carnitine (1 mM)	well fed	8	
Oleate (2 mM); albumin (2%)	starved	12	350
Oleate (2 mM); albumin (2%); carnitine (1 mM)	starved	40	350

from long-chain fatty acids are lower and unlike that from butyrate are dependent, in slice experiments, on the addition of carnitine. Thus after 48 hrs. starvation 2 mM oleate formed 12 µmoles ketone bodies without added carnitine but 40 µmoles on addition of 1 mM DL-carnitine. The ketone body formation from long-chain fatty acids by renal cortex slices was not greatly increased by starvation but with oleate as a precursor the rate increased 5-fold after 48 hours starvation (Table 4). Maximal rates of renal ketogenesis, it should be emphasised, are much lower than those of hepatic ketogenesis. Maximal rates of ketogenesis from oleate in kidney cortex slices in these experiments were about 11% of the maximal rates found in the perfused starved rat liver. With butyrate as a substrate, the rates of ketogenesis of kidney cortex slices may reach 25% of maximal hepatic ketogenesis.

Ketone bodies are also readily oxidised by renal cortex (25). The rate of oxidation of ketone bodies depends on their concentration. There appears to be a concentration-dependent competition between acetoacetate and endogenous fuels, based presumably on competition between acetoacetate and fatty acids for the available coenzyme A. At 5 mM acetoacetate (a concentration of which can be reached in diabetic acidosis) acetoacetate can contribute up to 70% to the fuel of respiration of the well-fed kidney. In the kidneys of starved rats the rate of oxidation of acetoacetate is somewhat lower owing to the increased concentration of fatty acids which competitively depresses the oxidation of acetoacetate.

As far as cortical carbohydrate metabolism is concerned, the maximal rates of carbohydrate oxidation appear to be small in relation to the energy requirements (see 26, 27) which are exceptionally high in kidney cortex, exceeded only by those of the working heart, flight muscles and possibly the retina. The potential capacity of rat kidney cortex to degrade glucose to lactate is revealed by anaerobic incubation of slices (27) which can under some conditions be high enough to supply 270 μmoles lactate/g. dry wt./hr. (see Table 5), and if this lactate were also formed anaerobically and completely oxidised it could supply up to 40% of the fuel of cortical respiration. But the low values of the respiratory quotients suggest that this does in fact not occur. It is possible that the degradation of glucose which shows itself anaerobically as a formation of lactate is, under physiological conditions, part of the pathway bringing about the conversion of carbohydrate to fat. In the first stage of this conversion carbohydrate is broken down by glycolysis to pyruvate and acetyl-CoA.

There appears to be a good physiological reason why the renal cortex does not use carbohydrate as a major fuel of respiration; the cortex (as already mentioned) is the site of gluconeogenesis, and gluconeogenesis and carbohydrate degradation cannot occur in the same cell at the same time. Gluconeogenesis from lactate (and many other precursors) is a process which on balance essentially reverses glycolysis, and many of the inter-

Table 5. *Maximal rates of glycolysis and gluconeogenesis from lactate in rat kidney and rat liver.* The data are taken from 9, 13, 27, 28, 29, 30, 31 and 32. All values represent rates of lactate metabolism in terms of μmole/g. dry wt./hr. The ratio wet wt./dry wt. was taken to be 3.5 for rat liver. In terms of lactate removed the rates of gluconeogenesis from lactate are twice the values of glucose formed. Maximal rates of glycolysis were found to occur anaerobically or aerobically after addition of 1 mM HCN. Liver glycolysis is largely dependent on the presence of glycogen in the tissue or high (20 mM) glucose concentrations in the external medium, whilst kidney utilised added glucose at low concentrations. The Table illustrates the effects of starvation and compares slices with perfused organs.

Tissue	Maximal rates of glycolysis		Maximal rates of gluconeogenesis from lactate	
	Slices	Perfused organ (whole organ)	Slices	Perfused organ (whole organ)
Kidney, well fed	270 (cortex) 1250 (inner medulla)	560	194	
Kidney, starved 48 hrs.	290 (cortex)	450	360	300
Liver, well fed	540	600		190
Liver, starved 48 hrs.	70	50	230	970

mediate steps of gluconeogenesis (though not all) are identical with those of glycolysis – except that they occur in the opposite direction.

Only one other mammalian tissue, the liver, shares with the kidney cortex a capacity for both glycolysis and gluconeogenesis. In both tissues the capacity for glucose degradation and for gluconeogenesis depends on the nutritional state (Table 5). In the liver the maximal rates of glycolysis in the well-fed state fall to about one tenth on starvation. In renal cortex the differences are less marked but in this tissue rates of glycolysis are already low in the well-fed state in relation to the energy requirements (as already mentioned). On the other hand the capacity for gluconeogenesis from lactate rises on starvation. These changes are known to be due to adaptive variations of enzyme concentrations and/or enzyme activity (see 33).

Illustrative data concerning glucose formation from various precursors are shown in Tables 6 and 7. The highest renal rates of glucose formation are found when fructose, D-glyceraldehyde, dihydroxyacetone, pyruvate, glycerol and the intermediates of the tricarboxylic acid cycle are precursors. Almost every substance which is known to be glucogenic in the intact mammalian body can also form glucose in kidney cortex. These include the glucogenic amino acids (glutamate, aspartate, proline, ornithine, arginine), propionate, galactose, mannose, pentoses (xylose) and pentitols (xylitol, ribitol). In the case of glutamate, aspartate and the intermediates of the tricarboxylic acid cycle, the rates of gluconeogenesis observed in the perfused rat kidney are very much higher than those found in the perfused rat liver. The reason for this difference appears to be a slow penetration into the liver cell of doubly or trebly charged anionic substances (34).

Table 6. *Glucose formation from various precursors in rat kidney cortex slices* (1, 2)
Rates are expressed as μmole/g. dry wt./hr. Standard diet.

L-Lactate	103	Fumarate	208
D-Fructose	423	Oxoglutarate	220
D-Glyceraldehyde	322	Glutamate	157
Dihydroxyacetone	268	Aspartate	90
Pyruvate	250	Proline	62
Xylitol	106	Ornithine	36
D-Xylose	40	Arginine	23

Table 7. *Effect of diet on glucose formation from various substrates in rat kidney cortex slices* (1). Adult rats. The data represent μmole glucose/g. dry wt./hr.

Substrate added	Standard mixed diet	Low carbohydrate diet (casein-margarine)
None	11	25
L-Lactate	97	181
Pyruvate	250	404
Fumarate	273	355
Aspartate	33	73
Glutamate	137	269

Regulatory Mechanisms

Regulatory mechanisms exist which see to it that the simultaneous occurrence of glycolysis and gluconeogenesis in the same cell at the same time is prevented. One of the main control sites is known to be at the stage where fructose-6-phosphate (F-6-P) and fructose, 1-6-diphosphate (FDP) are interconverted. In glycolysis this step is catalysed by phosphofructokinase (PFK) and involves the participation of ATP:

$$\text{F-6-P} + \text{ATP} \rightarrow \text{FDP} + \text{ADP}$$

In gluconeogenesis the enzymic mechanism of the interconversion is different; it represents an hydrolysis of the 1-phosphate group and is catalysed by fructose diphosphatase (FDPase):

$$\text{FDP} \rightarrow \text{F-6-P} + \text{Phosphate}$$

Both enzymes have built-in regulatory properties which are essentially the same in kidney cortex and in liver. Among these regulatory properties the most important, though not the only one, is the sensitivity of the enzymes towards ATP and AMP. This property correlates the activity of the two enzymes to the energy status of the cell, i. e. to the relative concentrations of ATP and AMP. When the cell is adequately supplied with a source of energy, and when, therefore, the concentration of ATP is high and that of AMP low, glucose degradation ceases because PFK is inhibited by high concentrations of ATP. When the concentration of ATP falls and that of AMP rises, PFK becomes activated and glucose degradation is promoted, causing an increased rate of ATP synthesis. On the other hand FDPase is inhibited by AMP and therefore gluconeogenesis ceases when a shortage of AMP calls for the promotion of reactions which lead to a synthesis of ATP and a restriction of processes, like gluconeogenesis, which consume ATP.

Somewhat analogous control mechanisms exist at the stages where pyruvate and phosphopyruvate are interconverted. Again different enzymic mechanisms operate in glycolysis and gluconeogenesis. A high ATP concentration and a surplus of acetyl-CoA favour the gluconeogenic direction, whilst high ADP concentrations and low acetyl-CoA concentrations, i. e. the lack of a substrate for the tricarboxylic acid cycle, promote glucose degradation (see 33).

Concluding Remarks

It might be asked why a specialised biosynthetic process like gluconeogenesis is located in the kidney, an organ which has primarily evolved as a secretory system. Any answer would at this stage be a matter of speculation. Maybe gluconeogenesis in the cortex serves to supply glucose to the medulla where it is an essential fuel.

Since the arterio-venous differences in glucose concentrations under many conditions do not show a net production of glucose by the whole kidney the question has been raised to what extent the glucogenic capacity measured at somewhat high substrate concentrations operates *in situ*. The fact that the gluconeogenic capacity of the kidney readily adjusts itself to physiological needs for carbohydrate, as it does in starvation (Tables 5 and 7) and after continual strenuous exercise (35), indicates that renal gluconeogenesis is of physiological importance.

References

1. Krebs, H. A., D. A. H. Bennett, P. de Gasquet, T. Gascoyne and T. Yoshida: Biochem. J., **86**, 22 (1963).
2. Krebs, H. A. and P. Lund: Biochem. J., **98**, 210 (1966).
3. Cohen, P. P. and R. W. McGilroy: J. biol. Chem., **169**, 119 (1947).
4. Krebs, H. A.: Biochem. J., **29**, 1951 (1935).
5. Wu, C.: Compar. Biochem. Physiol., **8**, 335 (1963).
6. Borsook, H. and J. W. Dubnoff: J. biol. Chem., **141**, 717 (1941).
7. Koszalka, T. R. and A. N. Bauman: Nature, **212**, 691 (1966).
8. Gerber, G. B., T. R. Koszalka, G. Gerber and K. I. Altman: Nature, **196**, 286 (1962).
9. Nishiitsutsuji-Uwo, J. M., B. D. Ross and H. A. Krebs: Biochem. J., **103**, 852 (1967).
10. Krebs, H. A., R. Hems and T. Gascoyne: Acta biol. med. germ., **11**, 607 (1963).
11. Krebs, H. A., R. N. Speake and R. Hems: Biochem. J., **94**, 712 (1965).
12. Ross, B. D., R. Hems and H. A. Krebs: Biochem. J., **102**, 942 (1967).
13. Krebs, H. A.: In 3 Konf. Ges. Physiol. Chem., Stoffwechsel der isoliert perfundierten Leber, edited by Staib, W. and R. Scholz: Berlin, Springer Verlag, p. 129.
14. György, P., W. Keller and Th. Brehme: Biochem. Z., **200**, 356 (1928).
15. Kean, E. L.: Energy metabolism and ion transport in the renal medulla, Ph. D. Thesis, University of Pennsylvania, 1961.
16. Kean, E. L., P. H. Adams, R. W. Winters and R. E. Davies: Biochem. Biophys. Acta, **54**, 474 (1961).
17. Dickens, F. and H. Weil-Malherbe: Biochem. J., **30**, 659 (1936).
18. Grupp, G. and K. Hierholzer: Z. Biol., **109**, 997 (1957).
19. Ruiz-Guinazu, A., G. Pehling, G. Rumrich and K. J. Ullrich: Pflüg. Arch., **274**, 311 (1961).
20. Lee, T. B., V. K. Vance and G. F. Cahill: Amer. J. Physiol., **203**, 27 (1962).
21. Gold, M. and J. J. Spitzer: Amer. J. Physiol., **206**, 153 (1964).
22. Nieth, H. and P. Schollmeyer: Nature, **209**, 1244 (1966).
23. Dickens, F. and F. Simer: Biochem. J., **24**, 905 (1930).
24. Weidemann, M. J.: (Unpublished results.)
25. Krebs, H. A., R. Hems, M. J. Weidemann and R. N. Speake: Biochem. J., **101**, 242 (1966).
26. Underwood, A. H. and E. A. Newsholme: Biochem. J., **104**, 296 and 300 (1967).
27. Gaja, G., G. Ragnotti, F. Cajone and A. Bernelli-Zazzera: Biochem. J., **105**, 647 (1967).
28. Burk, D., M. Woods and J. Hunter: J. Nat. Inst. Cancer, **38**, 839 (1967).
29. Ross, B. D., R. Hems, R. A. Freedland and H. A. Krebs: Biochem. J., **105**, 869 (1967).
30. Ragnotti, G., F. Cajone and G. Gaja: Biochem. J., **105**, 47C (1967).
31. Bernelli-Zazzera, A., G. Gaja and G. Ragnotti: Biochem. J., **100**, 114 (1966).
32. Unpublished work from the Oxford laboratory by D. A. Hems, F. Gaja, F. Woods and R. Hems.
33. Newsholme, E. A. and W. Gevers: In Vitamins and Hormones, **25**, 1 (1967), New York, Academic Press Inc.
34. Krebs, H. A. and T. Gascoyne: T. Biochem. J., **108**, 513 (1968).
35. Krebs, H. A. and T. Yoshida: Biochem. Z., **338**, 241 (1963).

DEETJEN: Professor KREBS, I was surprised to learn from your table about the metabolic properties of rat kidneys that the kidneys are producing creatinine. Is this a specialty of rat kidneys which we know are also secreting creatinine ? Or do human or dog kidneys also have the ability to synthesize creatinine ?

KREBS: I only know of reports that *rat* kidney synthesizes creatine (see KOSZALKA and BAUMAN, Nature, **212,** 691, 1966). I have no information on other species. Creatine is formed from glycine which interacts with arginine to form glycocyamine. This in turn is methylated by methyl transfer from methionine. The creatine formed enters the circulation and is utilized by various tissues for the synthesis of phosphocreatine. I do not think that the synthesis of creatine is directly connected with the excretion of creatinine. There are well known species differences in the capacity of the kidney to synthesize glutamine. It is possible that they also exist in the case of creatine.

EPSTEIN: Professor KREBS, is there any evidence that the predominant utilization of fat as a fuel by the kidney is altered by diet, for example, will the kidney preferentially use carbohydrate for its energy needs if the perfused kidney is taken from an animal fed on a high carbohydrate diet ?

KREBS: The capacity of the rat kidney to utilize carbohydrate does not appreciably increase on a high carbohydrate diet.

KRAMER: Is there any uptake of glucose or increase of O_2 consumption detectable when glucose is added to the perfusate containing no other fuel ?

KREBS: We have not carried out this kind of experiment on the perfused kidney. The oxygen consumption of slices (which are more convenient material) does not increase on addition of glucose. Altogether, the information obtained from slices suggests that availability of glucose makes no difference to the fuel used by the cortex. The situation is, of course, different in the medulla.

KRAMER: Our experiments are in good agreement with yours. We have not found any increase in O_2 consumption following glucose infusion. One word to the "anaerobic" situation of the medulla. We have found that the O_2 tension of the medulla even at the tip is still 20 mm Hg. Would you think that an in vivo medulla would have a high glycolysis under the conditions of relatively high O_2 tension ?

DEETJEN: It should be emphasized that oxygen tension of the medulla is not really high. The critical oxygen tension of this tissue is about 12 mm Hg. The difference to 20 mm Hg is not large. Furthermore, there is some evidence that in the medulla oxygen is undergoing a countercurrent diffusion which makes it difficult for oxygen to reach the papilla. The countercurrent diffusion is most effective when medullary blood flow is low. This particularly happens during antidiuresis when, on the other hand, this region has its relatively highest demand of energy to transport sodium for concentrating purposes.

ULLRICH: Several years ago, we measured the glucose and lactate concentration in the vasa recta plasma at the tip of the renal papilla. Compared with the concentration in the aterial blood an increase in lactate concentration of 2.3 mmol/l and a decrease in glucose concentration of 3.1 mmol/l was found. From this, one could conclude that lactic acid is formed in the kidney medulla, when the conditions for the whole organ are aerobic. A quantitative account for glucose metabolized to lactic acid is not possible because the plasma concentration changes of both substances are multiplied by the countercurrent system.

LEAF: In frog skin and toad bladder, which also have active sodium transport systems, a considerable aerobic glycolysis can be demonstrated in vitro under oxygen tensions equal to atmospheric conditions. This suggests that the aerobic glycolysis is not dependent on whether oxygen is available or not.

EDELMAN: Professor KREBS, does renal cortex, either in a slice or in perfusion systems, show a Pasteur effect ?

KREBS: Yes, there is a Pasteur effect. In slices the aerobic glycolysis is always lower than the anaerobic glycolysis. In fact in the cortex there is virtually no lactic acid production under aerobic conditions. The reason for the aerobic lactic acid production in the medulla seems to be due to the low rate of respiration but not to an inefficiency of respiration.

Renal Metabolism of Amino Acids and Ammonia*)

R. F. PITTS

In a quantitative sense, the renal metabolism of amino acids is predominantly concerned with two processes: the production of ammonia in acidosis, and the synthesis and addition to renal venous blood of certain amino acids, most notably alanine and serine. No doubt amino acids are also utilized in smaller quantities as building blocks of enzymes and structural proteins degraded in normal wear and tear or added as tissue mass under conditions which lead to renal hypertrophy. They are probably also used in even smaller quantities in the synthesis of such hormones as erythropoietin and renin. I shall consider only the problem of gross utilization of amino acids as precursors of ammonia and of other amino acids.

VAN SLYKE *et al.* in 1943 (1) observed in the acidotic dog that the extraction of glutamine by the kidney was large and adequate to account for most of the ammonia excreted in the urine and added to renal venous blood. Extraction of glutamine was enhanced in metabolic acidosis and reduced in normal acid-base balance or metabolic alkalosis. The emphasis of VAN SLYKE was on the amide nitrogen of glutamine as the major precursor of ammonia. A minor fraction of the ammonia produced by the kidney was presumed to be derived from unspecified amino acids.

Measurements of arterio-venous differences of glutamine and a variety of circulating amino acids, using methods of column chromatography, by SHALHOUB *et al.* (2) in the dog, by OWEN and ROBINSON (3) in man and by LYON (4) in the rat have confirmed and considerably extended these observations of VAN SLYKE. The data shown in Fig. 1 are taken from the work of SHALHOUB. On the left are shown the arterial and renal venous plasma concentrations of some 23 amino acids, expressed as μmoles/ml. Data are the means of measurements on 20 dogs in acidosis. The upper black bar of each pair describes arterial concentration. The lower clear bar describes renal venous concentration. On the left are shown arterio-venous differences, similarly expressed as μmoles/ml.; black, if the amino acid is extracted by the kidney; clear, if the amino acid is synthesized in the kidney and added in net amounts to renal venous blood. There are three points I wish to call to your attention. First, in confirmation of VAN SLYKE, the renal extraction of glutamine greatly exceeds that of any other amino acid, although appreciable amounts of glycine are also extracted. Second, alanine and serine are synthesized in significant amounts by the kidney and added to renal venous blood. Third, only a small amount of glutamate is added to venous blood, much less than the equivalent of the glutamine

*) Aided by research and training grants from the National Heart Institute, National Institutes of Health and grants in aid from the Life Insurance Medical Research Fund.

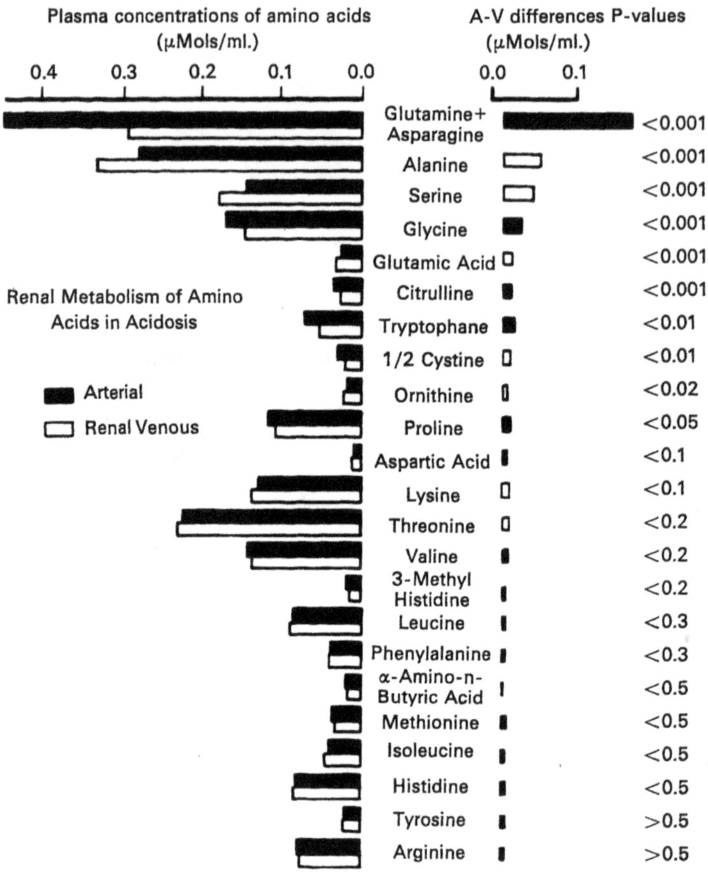

Fig. 1. Renal extraction of amino acids in the acidotic dog. Left, mean concentrations of free amino acids in simultaneously collected samples of arterial and renal venous plasma of 20 dogs. Center, arterio-venous differences in concentration. Right, P-values: probabilities that arterio-venous differences could have been fortuitous (2).

extracted. None is excreted in the urine. Therefore, both the amide and amino nitrogens of glutamine must be utilized by the kidney.

By combining measurements of blood flow, blood ammonia concentration, urinary excretion of ammonia and amino acid extraction, it is possible to strike a balance between rate of renal production of ammonia and rate of utilization of precursors of ammonia. Table 1 illustrates such measurements on 8 dogs in acidosis (5). The total amide and amino nitrogen extracted, largely glutamine and glycine, was 86.0 μmoles/min. The amino nitrogen synthesized in the kidney and added to renal venous blood, largely alanine and serine, was 31.1 μmoles/min. The net extraction amounted to 54.9 μmoles/min. The total ammonia produced by the kidney, namely the sum of that added to renal venous blood and that excreted in the urine, amounted to 57.5 μmoles/min. Accordingly, no less than 95% of the ammonia produced by the acidotic kidney of the dog can be

Table 1. Renal balance of amino, amide and ammonia nitrogen in the dog in chronic metabolic acidosis. Mean of nine experimental studies on eight dogs (5).

Data	μM Nitrogen/min
Total amide and amino nitrogen extracted from plasma	86.0
Amino nitrogen added to plasma	31.1
Net amide and amino nitrogen extracted from plasma	54.9
Ammonia nitrogen added to renal venous plasma	14.4
Ammonia nitrogen excreted in urine	43.1
Total ammonia nitrogen produced in kidney	57.5

Note:

$$\frac{\text{Net nitrogen extracted}}{\text{Ammonia produced}} = \frac{54.9}{57.5} \times 100 = 95 \text{ per cent.}$$

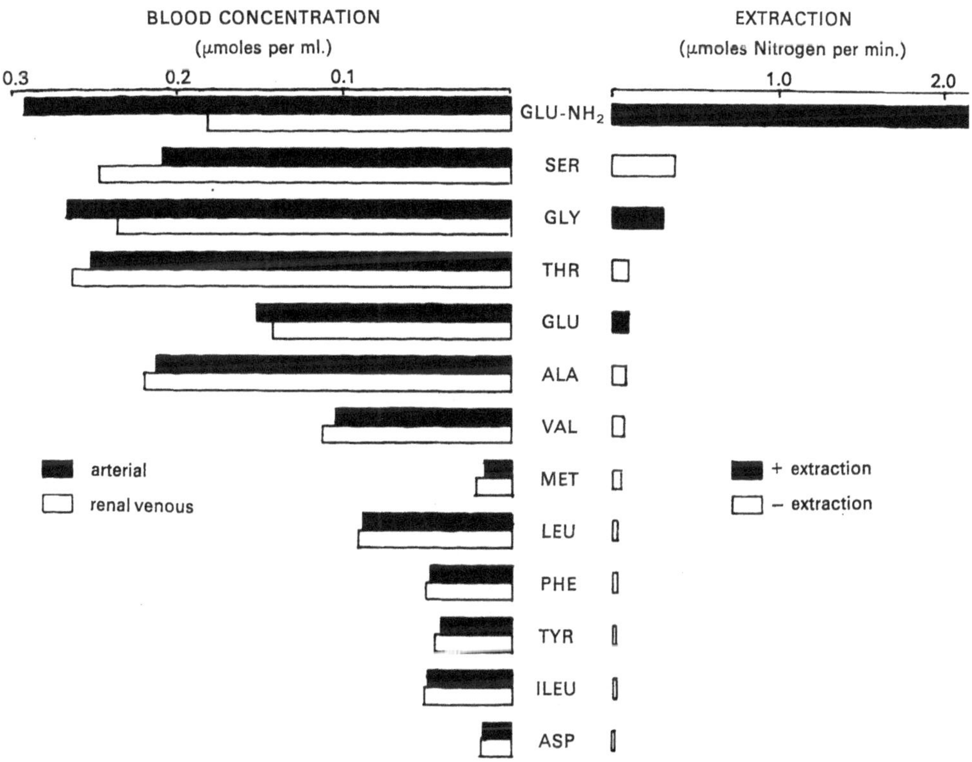

Fig. 2. Renal extraction of amino acids in the acidotic rat. Left, mean concentrations of free amino acids in simultaneously collected samples of arterial and renal venous blood of 4 rats. Right, renal extractions calculated from arterio-venous differences in concentration and blood flow (4).

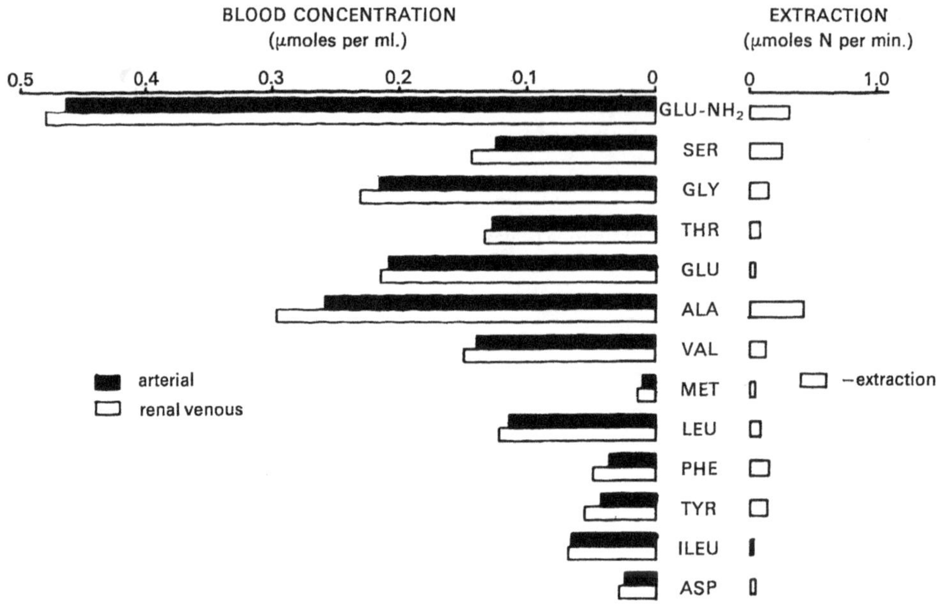

Fig. 3. Renal extraction of amino acids in the alkalotic rat. Left, mean concentrations of free amino acids in simultaneously collected samples of arterial and renal venous blood of 4 rats. Right, renal extractions calculated from arterio-venous differences in concentration and blood flow (4).

accounted for on the basis of the moment to moment extraction of the amide and amino nitrogen of circulating plasma amino acids.

In general, recent results of LYON (4) obtained on the acidotic rat are in agreement with those of SHALHOUB on the dog and those of OWEN and ROBINSON on man. Fig. 2 is similar to Fig. 1 of SHALHOUB, except that extraction is expressed in terms of μmoles/min. of nitrogen, rather than as A-V difference. However, the major amino acids extracted by the acidotic rat are glutamine and glycine and the major one synthesized is serine.

In contrast, the rat in metabolic alkalosis, Fig. 3, no longer extracts glutamine and glycine as does the rat in metabolic acidosis. Indeed, I call your attention to a small production and addition to renal venous blood of both glutamine and glycine. I shall return to the problem of the synthesis of glutamine later in this paper.

Renal balance studies such as those which I have illustrated on the dog can only give evidence of overall equivalence of production of ammonia and utilization of precursors. They cannot distinguish, in any precise way, the contribution of a specific amino acid to ammonia production or to the production of alanine and serine. To do so requires the performance of tracer experiments in which amino acids labelled with nitrogen-15 are used. Fig. 4 illustrates the method we use in such studies (6). The two ureters of a dog are catheterized to permit the collection of urine separately from the two kidneys. A solution of an amino acid, for example glutamine labeled with nitrogen-15 in high activity in the amide position, is infused into the left renal artery at a precisely controlled and known rate. The rate of administration of the isotope is low, i. e. a tracer rate, so that the concentration of glutamine in the blood perfusing the left kidney is increased only a few per cent. In this diagram, glutamine labeled with nitrogen-15 in the amide position is represented by a capital *G*. Normally circulating nitrogen-14 glutamine is represented by a small *g*. Similarly, nitrogen-15 ammonia derived from labeled glutamine is represented by a capital *A*; nitrogen-14 ammonia, by a small *a*.

Since the ammonia produced by the infused kidney is rich in isotope, the amide nitrogen of glutamine must in part be extracted and converted to ammonia in its initial passage through the kidney. In part, it passes into the renal vein, into the general circulation, and is then returned to both kidneys equally. If one subtracts atoms % excess N^{15} ammonia in the urine formed by the control kidney from that formed by the infused kidney, one corrects for recirculation. Dividing corrected atoms % excess N^{15} ammonia in the urine by atoms per cent excess N^{15} plasma glutamine and multiplying by 100, yields the per cent of the renal pool of ammonia derived from the amide nitrogen of glutamine. By renal pool is meant not only that excreted in the urine but also that added to renal venous blood.

Table 2 summarizes results obtained in 36 such experiments, in each one of which a single labeled precursor was infused (7, 8, 9, 10, 11). It is evident on an average that the amide nitrogen of glutamine accounts for 43.3% of the renal pool of ammonia, whereas the amino nitrogen of glutamine accounts for nearly half this amount. Together the two nitrogens of glutamine contribute two-thirds of the ammonia of the pool. Since preformed ammonia brought to the kidney in arterial blood mixes completely with the renal pool, the proportion of the total pool derived from this source is large, about 35% to be exact. Minor and decreasing percentages of the pool are derived from the amino nitrogens of plasma alanine, glycine and glutamate. We consider the mean derivation of

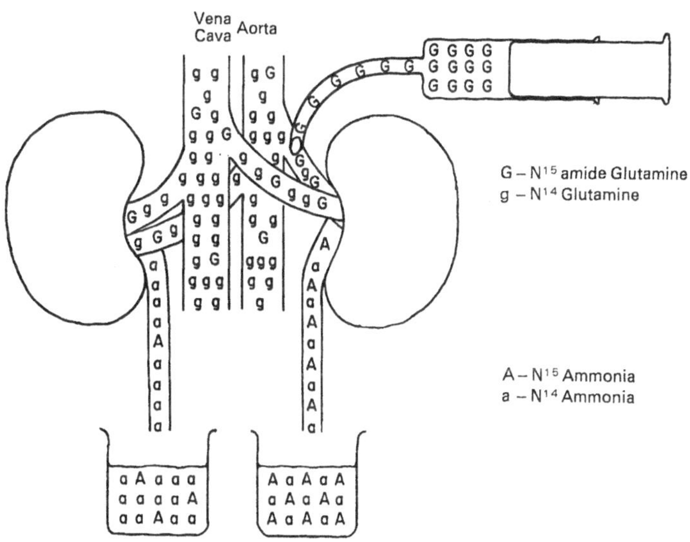

Fig. 4. Use of N^{15} amide-labeled glutamine in the study of the origin of urinary ammonia in the acidotic dog (6).

Table 2. Contribution of five amino acid precursor nitrogens to the ammonia produced in the kidney of the dog in chronic metabolic acidosis (10).

Number of Experiments	Ammonia Excreted and Added to Renal Venous Blood		
	Source	Mean Per Cent	Range Per Cent
9	Amide Nitrogen of Glutamine	43.3	35.3 – 51.4
6	Amino Nitrogen of Glutamine	18.3	10.1 – 25.5
8	Amino Nitrogen of Alanine	5.71	3.03 – 8.41
5	Amino Nitrogen of Glycine	3.76	2.92 – 5.55
2	Amino Nitrogen of Glutamate	1.88	1.43 – 2.34
6	Arterial Ammonia	35.0	23.0 – 48.0
		Sum 108.0	

the pool of 108% from these 6 sources to be within the limit of accuracy of the summed values in a series of 36 experiments. If one considers only the ammonia formed *de novo* within the kidney and thus excludes preformed arterial ammonia, then over 80% is derived from the two nitrogens of glutamine.

Let us turn for the moment from a consideration of the utilization of amide and amino nitrogens as precursors of ammonia to a consideration of the production and utilization of the amino acid alanine. These experiments are taken from the work of PITTS and STONE (9). From Table 2 and from the graph at the left of Fig. 5, it is evident, at normal plasma concentrations of alanine of 0.2 to 0.3 μmoles/ml, that some 3 to 8% of urinary

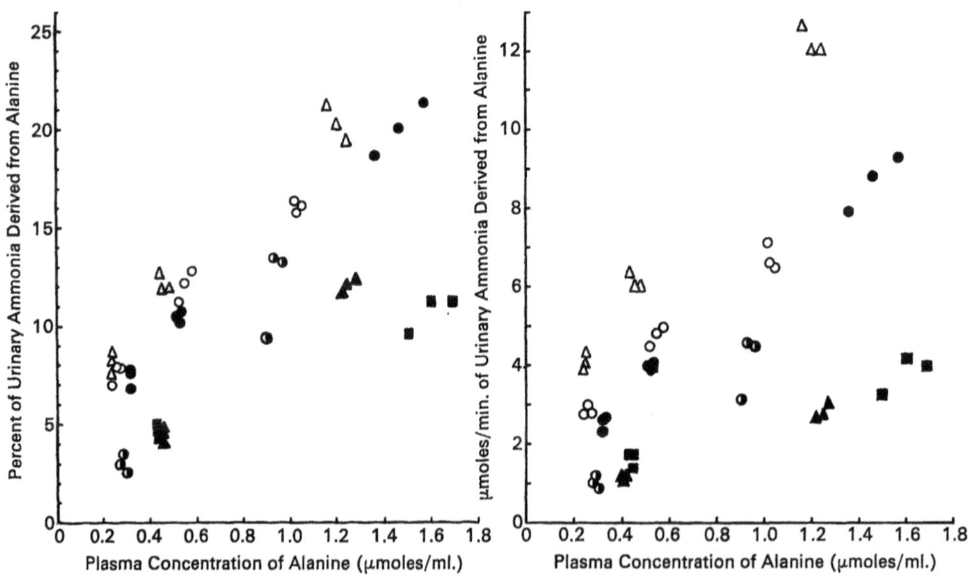

Fig. 5. Utilization of alanine as a precursor of ammonia in the acidotic dog. Left, per cent of urinary ammonia, right, μmoles/min of urinary ammonia, derived from plasma alanine during elevation of plasma concentration by intravenous infusion of alanine (9).

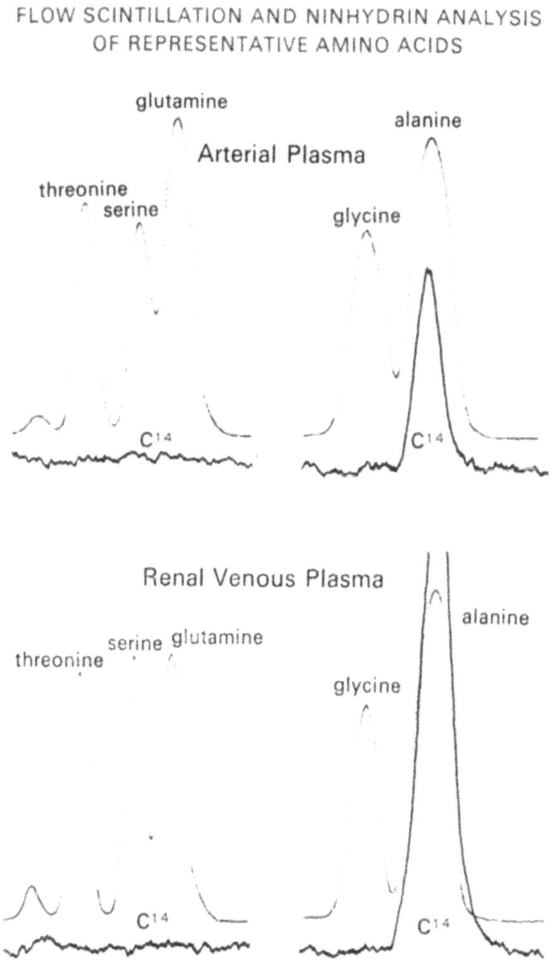

Fig. 6. Incorporation of 1-C^{14} pyruvate infused into one renal artery into the alanine synthetized by that kidney and added to renal venous blood. Upper traces of each pair, concentrations of representative amino acids in femoral arterial and renal venous plasma. Lower traces, C^{14} activities of these same amino acids in femoral arterial and renal venous plasma (9).

ammonia is derived from alanine. Fig. 5 demonstrates that as plasma concentration of alanine is raised over the range of 0.3 and 1.6 μmoles/ml by the intravenous infusion of alanine, the per cent of the ammonia derived from this source increases. The graph on the right of Fig. 5 illustrates this same fact in terms of μmoles/min of urinary ammonia derived from alanine. The four different symbols in these figures refer to four different experiments. Although it seems at first glance that the scatter is great, each separate experiment exhibits a reasonably linear relationship between plasma alanine concentration and either per cent of ammonia or μmoles/min of ammonia derived from alanine. Such a relationship is not peculiar to alanine. It is likewise true of all other amino acids which can serve as precursors of ammonia; the higher the plasma concentration of that amino acid, the more extensively it is used as a precursor of ammonia.

At the same time that alanine is utilized as a source of ammonia, it is also produced by the kidney and added to renal venous blood. The experiment described in Fig. 6

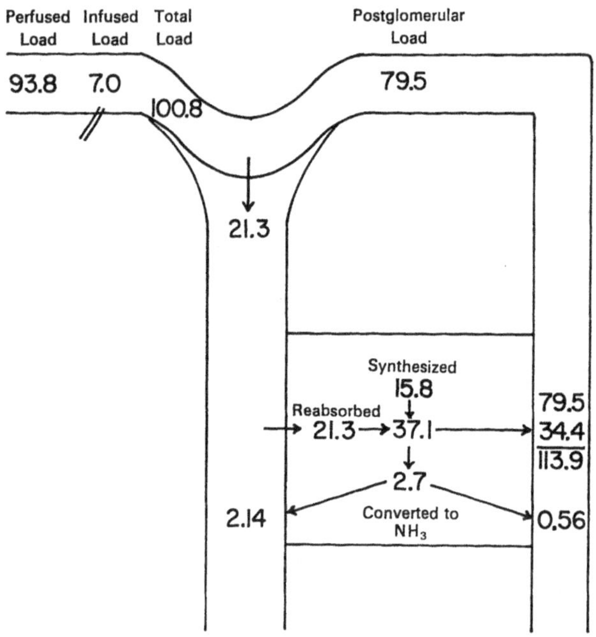

Fig. 7. Data obtained on the kidney of an acidotic dog which illustrate simultaneous production of alanine and utilization of alanine as a precursor of ammonia (11).

illustrates the incorporation of the C^{14} label of pyruvate, infused into one renal artery, into the alanine liberated into the renal vein of that same kidney. Because of recirculation of labeled alanine, some is present in arterial blood entering the kidney. However, as shown at the lower right, incorporation of the C^{14} label of pyruvate into alanine by the kidney is extensive. Furthermore the label is not incorporated into other amino acids, 4 of which are shown in the ninhydrin traces of this experiment.

Fig. 7 is a much simplified representation of a kidney, consisting of glomerulus, renal tubule, one tubular cell, and a single peritubular capillary. The data illustrate observations made on simultaneous production and utilization of alanine by the kidney of an acidotic dog in one of several experiments. Since the plasma concentration of alanine was normal, utilization of alanine as a source of ammonia was low. Synthesis of alanine and addition to renal venous blood was relatively high.

The product of arterial plasma alanine concentration and arterial plasma inflow, namely the normal perfused load of alanine entering the kidney, was 93.8 μmoles/min. Seven μmoles/min of N^{15}-labeled alanine were infused into the renal artery, giving a total alanine load of 100.8 μmoles per min. Leaving the kidney in the renal vein were 113.9 μmoles/min. Thus the net renal production of alanine amounted to 13.1 μmoles/min. The filtered load of alanine was 21.3 μmoles/min. Since no alanine was excreted, all 21.3 μmoles/min were reabsorbed. However 2.7 μmoles of cellular alanine were utilized for ammonia formation, demanding an overall synthesis of 15.8 μmoles/min. The cellular pool of alanine therefore turned over at a rate of 37.1 μmoles per min, i. e. 21.3 μmoles/min reabsorbed plus 15.8 μmoles/min synthesized. The specific activity of this cellular pool, calculated from the specific activity of the infused alanine and the rates of glomerular filtration and tubular reabsorption, was 3.60 atoms % N^{15} excess. The kidney was removed and free tissue alanine was separated on a preparative column. The measured specific activity of renal alanine was 3.79 atoms % N^{15} excess, a value 105% of that calculated.

This experiment demonstrates that the renal pool of alanine is small, that it turns over rapidly, and that it consists of reabsorbed and newly synthesized moieties from which is subtracted the fraction utilized for ammonia production. All of our findings are consonant with the view that production of alanine is by transamination of pyruvate by the amino nitrogen of glutamine, either directly or after conversion of glutamine to glutamate. Utilization of alanine in the renal production of ammonia is by transamination of α-ketoglutarate, followed by oxidative deamination of the resulting glutamate.

An appreciation of the quantitative significance of the amide nitrogen of glutamine as a major precursor of renal ammonia led KAMIN and HANDLER (12), RICHTERICH and GOLDSTEIN (13), and LOTSPEICH (14) some years ago to postulate that all ammonia secreted into the urine is directly derived from intracellular glutamine. This view is difficult to reconcile with recent evidence (10, 15, 16) that ammonia enters both urine and peritubular blood by passive diffusion of the uncharged free base, NH_3, and that diffusion equilibrium for the free base exists throughout the kidney.

Experiments of LYON and PITTS (17) on the dog provide direct evidence that the incorporation of amino and ammonia nitrogen into the amide group of cellular glutamine is not an obligatory step in the transport of ammonia into the urine. Mean values of two experiments in acidosis and two in alkalosis are summarized in Fig. 8. C^{14}-α-keto-

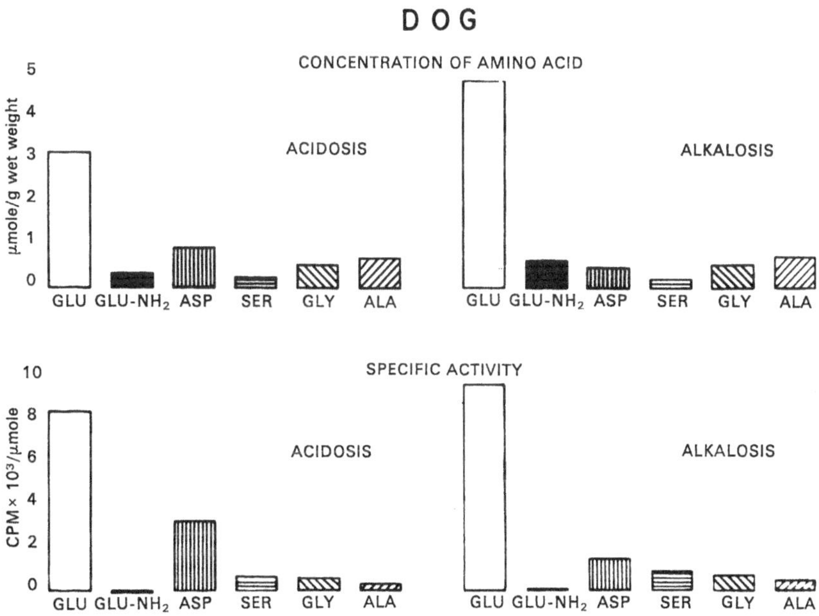

Fig. 8. Data which illustrate the failure of the kidney of either the acidotic or alkalotic dog to convert tissue glutamate into glutamine (17).

glutarate was infused into one renal artery of the dog for 40 min prior to removing the kidneys and measuring concentrations and C^{14} activities of free tissue amino acids. Amino acid concentrations are shown in the upper half of the figure; C^{14}-specific activities, corrected for recirculated label, are shown in the lower half. Glutamate, which is present in the acidotic kidney of the dog in a concentration of 3 μmoles/gram wet weight, is highly labeled, approximately 8000 cts/min/μmole. Glutamine present in the acidotic kidney in a concentration of 0.315 μmoles/gram wet weight is not labeled at all. In fact specific activity is slightly less than background. If incorporation of all nitrogen into the amide group of cellular glutamine were an obligatory step in secretory transport of ammonia, one would predict high labeling of glutamine in acidosis, for as much as 50% of urinary ammonia is derived from preformed ammonia, and from the amino nitrogens of glutamine and other amino acids. As shown on the right, the situation is similar in alkalosis except that the concentrations of free tissue glutamate and glutamine are higher than in acidosis. Specific activity of glutamate is also higher. However no significant amount of label was incorporated into cellular glutamine.

In sharp contrast, the kidney of the rat incorporates significant amounts of C^{14}, administered as α-ketoglutarate, into cellular glutamine in acidosis and even greater amounts in alkalosis (Fig. 9). No doubt the high labeling of glutamate in both the dog and rat is a consequence of the rapid attainment of equilibrium of the pyridoxamine phosphate form of transaminase enzymes with tracer amounts of α-ketoglutarate. In the rat the labeled glutamate is further amidated to glutamine by the glutamine synthetase system. In the dog, it is not. The fact that the kidney of the rat synthesizes glutamine does not necessarily indicate that cellular glutamine is an obligatory step in the secretion

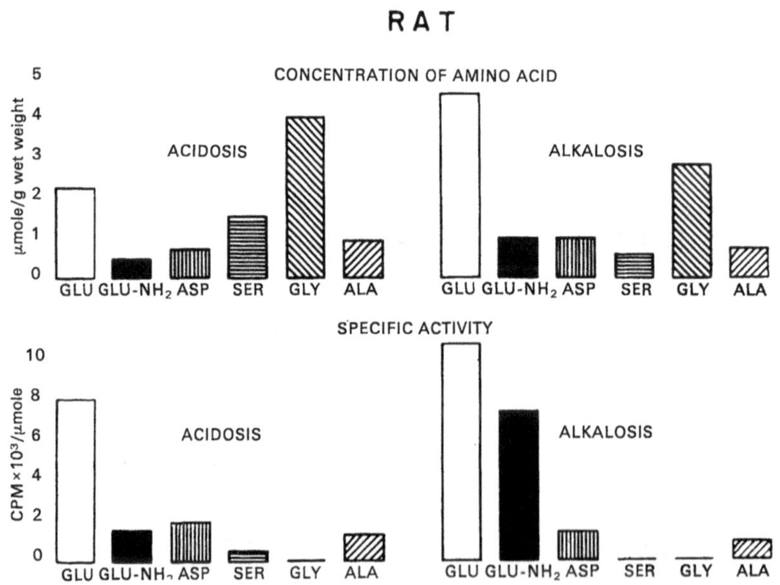

Fig. 9. Data which illustrate the ability of the kidney of both the acidotic and alkalotic rat to convert tissue glutamate into glutamine (17).

of ammonia into the urine. As I pointed out in connection with experiments on the dog, one would predict greater labeling of glutamine in acidosis than in alkalosis if this were true. Actually, in acidosis, the specific activity of glutamine is 20% of that of glutamate, whereas in alkalosis, it is 78%.

The cat kidney is similar to the dog kidney; neither synthesizes glutamine *in vivo*. On the other hand, the guinea pig kidney is similar to the rat kidney; both synthesize glutamine *in vivo*. These findings are reminiscent of those of KREBS published in 1935 (18). He observed that slices of kidneys of the dog and cat, incubated with ammonia and glutamate, synthesize no glutamine; whereas slices of kidneys of rabbits, guinea pigs and rats synthesize glutamine.

You recall from the studies of LYON, presented as Fig. 3, that the kidney of the rat in alkalosis does not extract glutamine from arterial blood; rather it synthesizes glutamine and adds it in moderate net amounts to renal venous blood. This poses the interesting questions: what is the rate of glutamine synthesis of the rat kidney *in vivo*, and how does it vary with acid-base balance?

These questions have been approached in the rat by DAMIAN (19), who employed a method of pulse labeling of glutamate by the rapid injection of C^{14}-α-ketoglutarate into one renal artery. This leads to instantaneous labeling of glutamate, the specific activity of which remains essentially constant for up to 30 to 45 seconds. By removing kidneys at 10, 15 and 30 seconds and dropping them into liquid nitrogen, one can follow the synthesis of glutamine from glutamate. From the slopes of these lines, shown in Fig. 10, one may calculate rates of synthesis. Each point on these lines is the mean of from 3 to 5 rats.

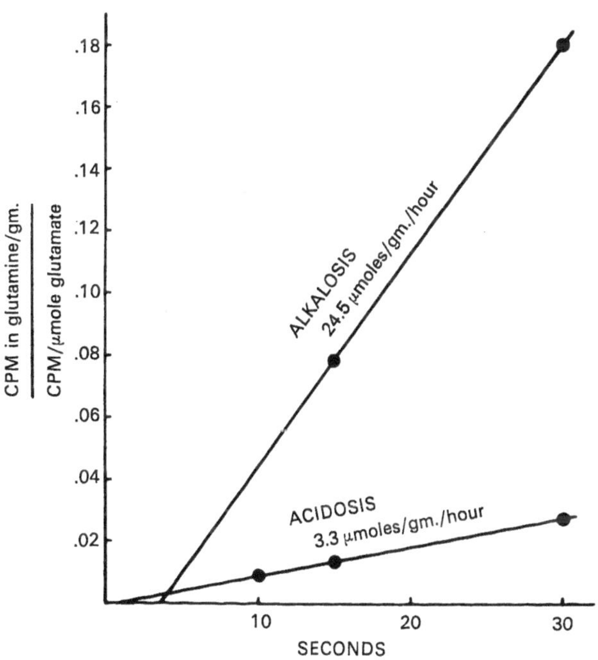

Fig. 10. The rate of synthesis of glutamine in vivo by the kidney of the rat in acidosis and in alkalosis (19).

The rate of synthesis of glutamine in metabolic acidosis is 3.3 μmoles/g. wet weight/hour. In metabolic alkalosis it increases 7 fold to 24.5 μmoles/g. wet weight/hour. Miss LUND, in Professor KREBS' laboratory, has observed that the glutamine synthetase activity of homogenates of rat kidneys under optimum conditions is about 50 μmoles/g. wet weight/hour (20), thus, about twice the *in vivo* rate in alkalosis. Furthermore synthetase activity is the same in the kidneys of rats in normal acid-base balance and in chronic metabolic acidosis. These findings suggest that the differing rates of glutamine synthesis which DAMIAN has observed *in vivo* in alkalosis and acidosis are a consequence of altered intracellular milieu, not of enzyme induction. Furthermore the rate of cellular synthesis of glutamine in alkalosis is from three to four times greater than the rate of addition of glutamine to renal venous blood in alkalosis. This suggests that intracellular cycling of glutamine synthesis and glutamine hydrolysis may play some role in control of production of renal ammonia in the rat. It definitely is not a mechanism of control in the dog and cat, in which forms synthesis does not occur.

The control of ammonia production has been explained by GOODMAN *et al.* (21), by GOLDSTEIN (22) and by ALLEYNE (23) in the following terms. Acidosis enhances the activity of the enzyme, phosphoenolpyruvate carboxykinase, which catalyzes the conversion of oxaloacetate to enolphosphopyruvate. This increase in enzyme activity reduces the cellular concentration of oxaloacetate and of intermediates of the TCA cycle back to α-ketoglutarate. As a consequence of reduction of the concentration of α-ketoglutarate, product inhibition of glutamic dehydrogenase is reduced and production of ammonia from glutamate increase. As a further consequence of reduction of cellular glutamate, the inhibition which it exerts on the hydrolysis of glutamine is reduced, and ammonia production from the amide nitrogen of glutamine increases. Whether the demonstrated decreases in concentration of α-ketoglutarate and glutamate which occur in acidosis adequately account for increased production of ammonia from glutamate and glutamine, remains to be demonstrated.

References

1. VAN SLYKE, D. D., R. A. PHILLIPS, P. B. HAMILTON, R. M. ARCHIBALD, P. H. FUTCHER and A. HILLER: Glutamine as source material of urinary ammonia. J. biol. Chem., **150,** 481 (1943).
2. SHALHOUB, R., W. WEBBER, S. GLABMAN, M. CANESSA-FISCHER, J. KLEIN, J. DE HAAS and R. F. PITTS: Extraction of amino acids from and their addition to renal blood plasma. Amer. J. Physiol., **204,** 181 (1963).
3. OWEN, E. E. and R. R. ROBINSON: Amino acid extraction and ammonia metabolism by the human kidney during the prolonged administration of ammonium chloride. J. clin. Invest. **42,** 263 (1963).
4. LYON, M.: (Unpublished observations.)
5. PITTS, R. F., J. DE HAAS and J. KLEIN: Relation of renal amino and amide nitrogen extraction to ammonia production. Amer. J. Physiol. **204,** 187 (1963).
6. PITTS, R. F.: The renal metabolism of ammonia. Physiologist. **9,** 97 (1966).
7. PITTS, R. F., L. A. PILKINGTON and J. C. M. DE HAAS: N^{15} tracer studies on the origin of urinary ammonia in the acidotic dog, with notes on the enzymatic synthesis of labeled glutamic acids and glutamines. J. clin. Invest. **44,** 731 (1965).
8. PITTS, R. F. and L. A. PILKINGTON: The relation between plasma concentrations of glutamine and glycine and utilization of their nitrogens as sources of urinary ammonia. J. clin. Invest. **45,** 86 (1966).

9. PITTS, R. F. and W. J. STONE: Renal metabolism of alanine. J. clin. Invest. **46,** 530 (1967).
10. STONE, W. J., S. BALAGURA and R. F. PITTS: Diffusion equilibrium for ammonia in the kidney of the acidotic dog. J. clin. Invest. **46,** 1603 (1967).
11. STONE, W. J. and R. F. PITTS: Pathways of ammonia metabolism in the intact functioning kidney of the dog. J. clin. Invest. **46,** 1141 (1967).
12. KAMIN, H. and P. HANDLER: The metabolism of parenterally administered amino acids: III. Ammonia formation. J. biol. Chem. **193,** 873 (1951).
13. RICHTERICH, R. W. and L. GOLDSTEIN: Distribution of glutamine metabolizing enzymes and production of urinary ammonia in the mammalian kidney. Amer. J. Physiol. **195,** 316 (1958).
14. LOTSPEICH, W. D.: Metabolic Aspects of Renal Function. C. C. Thomas, Springfield, Ill. 1959.
15. BALAGURA, S. and R. F. PITTS: Excretion of ammonia injected into renal artery. Amer. J. Physiol. **203,** 11 (1962).
16. DENIS, G., H. PREUSS and R. F. PITTS: The pNH_3 of renal tubular cells. J. clin. Invest. **43,** 571 (1964).
17. LYON, M. and R. F. PITTS: Species differences in renal glutamine synthesis in vivo. Amer. J. Physiol. **216,** 117 (1969).
18. KREBS, H. A.: Metabolism of amino acids. IV, The synthesis of glutamine from glutamic acid and ammonia, and the enzymatic hydrolysis of glutamine in animal tissues. Biochem. J. **29,** 1935 (1951).
19. DAMIAN, A.: (Personal communication.)
20. LUND, P.: (Personal communication.)
21. GOODMAN, A. D., R. E. FUISZ and G. E. CAHILL: Renal gluconeogenesis in acidosis, alkalosis, and potassium deficiency: Its possible role in the regulation of renal ammonia production. J. clin. Invest. **45,** 612 (1966).
22. GOLDSTEIN, L. and J. M. SCHOOLER: Regulation of ammonia production in the rat kidney. Adv. Enz. Reg. **5,** 71 (1966).
23. ALLEYNE, G. A.: Concentrations of metabolic intermediates in kidneys of rats with metabolic acidosis. Nature. **217,** 847 (1968).

KRAMER: May I ask Dr. OELERT to present his prepared discussion to Dr. PITTS' paper.

Transport of Ammonia in the Mammalian Cortical Nephron

H. OELERT, E. UHLICH, A. G. HILLS

DENIS, PREUSS and PITTS (1) have proven the equality of ammonia pressure between the cells of the cortical tubules and renal venous blood, and predicted that the tubular urine would also be equilibrated. In order to study the question directly, we have determined P_{NH_3} on simultaneously obtained samples of cortical tubular fluid and renal venous blood of the rat kidney. The tubular fluid represented both free flow and microperfusion samples. Microperfusion allows perfusion of isolated proximal and distal convolutions independently of glomerular filtrate. In order to prevent the disequilibrium pH described by RECTOR et al. (3) from developing in the distal free-flow samples, carbonic anhydrase was intravenously infused at a constant rate into the experimental animals. The fluid used for the perfusion experiments consisted of an ammonia-free phosphate buffer solution at pH 6.3 containing carbonic anhydrase and sodium bicarbonate. The free-base ammonia concentration of the samples was determined from their total ammonia and pH according to the Henderson-Hasselbalch equation and

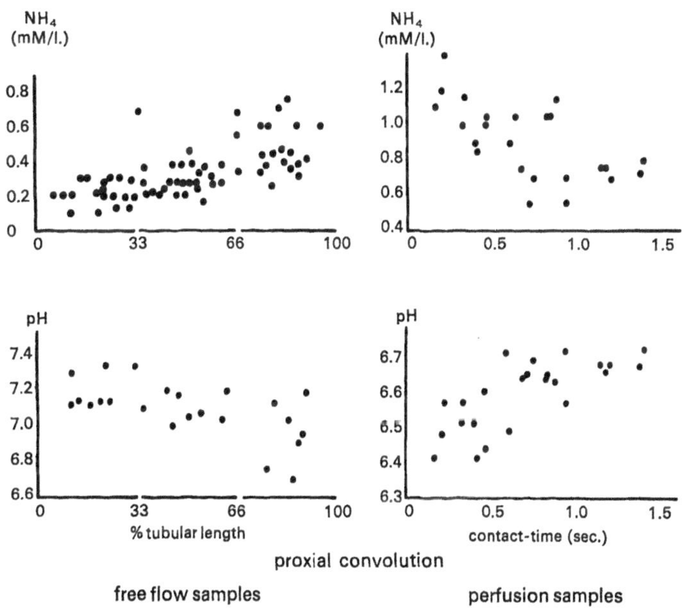

Fig. 1.

P_{NH_3} from the ammonia absorption co-efficient determined according to JACQUEZ et al. (2).

In both free-flow and perfusion samples (Fig. 1) pH values and total ammonia concentration are inversely related. The pH value of free-flow samples steadily declines along the proximal convolution while the concentration of total ammonia rises. By contrast, the pH value of the microperfusion samples rises as a function of the length of tubule perfused, while total ammonia concentration, which is immediately high at very short contact-times of the perfusate, declines. Equilibration is established between NH_3 and NH_4^+ in accordance with the law of mass action, so that the cations formed out of the undissociated molecule are distributed on the same side of the tubular membrane as the higher concentration of hydrogen ions.

The table summarizes the results. Although there is a large variation of pH values and total ammonia concentrations in the individual samples, mean values for P_{NH_3} in the proximal and distal convolution are equal in the free-flow as well as in the perfusion samples. Calculated P_{NH_3} of the renal venous blood of the same experimental animals disclosed no significant deviation of cortical P_{NH_3} from mean values for ammonia pressure of cortical tubular fluid. There appears to be no measurable difference of ammonia pressure, therefore, between luminal fluid and the remainder of the cortical tissue.

The P_{NH_3} of perfusion samples (Fig. 2) was independent both of the length of the tubule perfused and of the duration of perfusion. In both proximal and distal convolution, perfusion times of 0.15 seconds sufficed for equilibration of ammonia pressures between cortex and ammonia-free perfusion fluid. Since our methods do not allow accurate measurement of perfusion times less than 0.15 seconds, we cannot calculate the slope of the initial change of concentration of ammonia in the perfusion fluid, and consequently cannot give an accurate value for permeability of the tubular membrane to ammonia. There can be no question, however, that the transit time of both urine and blood through the renal cortex amply suffice for complete equilibration of ammonia pressure between compartments.

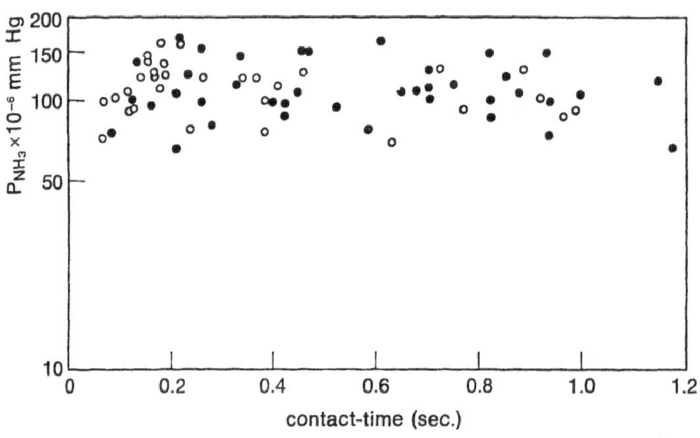

Fig. 2.

It has been clear from many earlier investigations that ammonia transport from capillary blood and tubular cells into the luminal fluid and also transport in the reverse direction must be very rapid and that it is strongly pH dependent (5). The theory of non-ionic diffusion gives an explanation for the pH dependence of transport through the tubular membrane of a number of weak organic acids and bases as well as ammonia. The theory states that the non-ionized congener diffuses through the cell-membrane more readily than the ionized portion because of its superior lipid solubility. The degree of permeability for several weak organic acids and bases has been correlated with the solubility of the undissociated molecule in organic solvents (4). Nevertheless, the high permeability for ammonia of the tubular cell probably does not depend upon particulary high solubility in the lipids of the cell membrane, because the undissociated ammonia molecule has been found to be practically insoluble, even in strongly alkaline solutions, in the organic solvents investigated: namely chloroform, toluol, and olive oil.

Organic solvents may differ markedly from the lipids of the cell membrane in their capacity to dissolve NH_3. But since all membranes which are highly permeable to water are also permeable to NH_3, transport of ammonia through the tubular cell probably reflects passage of molecular NH_3 through the aqueous portions of the membrane, and not through the lipid. Because of the small molecular size of NH_3 the available water-filled pores might suffice for the extremely rapid equilibration of ammonia across both the proximal and distal tubular membrane.

Free flow samples	proximal convolution:	$118 \pm 27 \cdot 10^{-6}$ mm Hg
	distal convolution:	$121 \pm 29 \cdot 10^{-6}$ mm Hg
Perfusion samples	proximal convolution:	$115 \pm 32 \cdot 10^{-6}$ mm Hg
	distal convolution:	$116 \pm 30 \cdot 10^{-6}$ mm Hg
Renal venous blood		$109 \pm 20 \cdot 10^{-6}$ mm Hg

References

1. Denis, G., H. Preuss and R. F. Pitts: The P_{NH_3} of renal tubular cells. J. Clin. Invest. **43**, 571 (1964).
2. Jacquez, J. A., J. W. Poppell and R. Jeltsch: Solubility of ammonia in human plasma. J. Appl. Physiol. **14**, 255 (1959).
3. Rector, F. C., jr., N. W. Carter and D. W. Seldin: The mechanism of bicarbonate reabsorption in the proximal and distal tubules of the kidney. J. Clin. Invest. **44**, 278 (1965).
4. Sonnenberg, H., H. Oelert and K. Baumann: Proximal tubular reabsorption of some organic acids in the rat kidney in vivo. Pflügers Arch. ges. Physiol. **286**, 171 (1965).
5. Sullivan, L. P. and M. McVaugh: Effect of rapid and transitory changes in blood and urin pH on NH_4 excretion. Am. J. Physiol. **204**, 1077 (1963).

Pitts: My only comment is that I have never measured lipid solubility of ammonia so I accept your statement regarding its partition between aqueous and lipid phases. However, I am very pleased that you have confirmed the essential observation that ammonia is very rapidly transported as a free base.

KRÜCK: Dr. PITTS, you stated that approximately 95% of the urinary ammonia derives from extraction of precursors from arterial blood. In patients with chronic renal insufficiency we have found a very close correlation between the reduction of urinary ammonia excretion and the reduction of renal plasma flow and glomerular filtration rate. Would you think that the diminished renal blood flow is the only reason for the reduced ammonia excretion or do we have to postulate some additional intrinsic defects of the tubular cells ?

PITTS: I really cannot answer your question directly, but the capacity of the diseased kidney in advanced renal insufficiency to form ammonia seems to be reduced to a greater extent than its capacity to acidify the urine. It seems, therefore, that it would be related to some intrinsic inability of the kidney to metabolize amino acids. It is possible that this inability to produce ammonia is a consequence of decreased delivery of amino acids to tubular cells because of reduced blood flow or filtration rate.

Remarks on Renal Gaseous Metabolism*)

K. KRAMER, E. BASSENGE, H. BRECHTELSBAUER

Summary: 1. Excess O_2 consumption of the kidney is mainly determined by the Na load and its reabsorption by tubular transport.

2. In dogs the ratio of $\frac{\text{Na transported}}{O_2 \text{ consumed}}$ amounts to 7. A similar value has been found in man.

3. Continuous recordings of CO_2 contents in arterial and renal venous blood using Technicon analyzers revealed large variations depending on breathing; hence, throwing doubt on the value of any random sampling.

4. Using integrated AVD_{CO_2} values and oximeter readings both derived from continuous recordings RQ values are obtained in the range of 0.63 to 0.83 indicating a much smaller scatter than any data previously published based on sampling at random.

5. The RQs found in the present experiments are in good agreement with the significant extraction of fatty acids found in kidneys.

In their studies on exteriorized kidneys in dogs VAN SLYKE et al. found that in a large range of blood flow variations O_2 consumption of the kidney relates linearly to flow (13). This has been explained in the last decade. In a normal kidney the resistance of preglomerular vessels determines not only blood flow but also glomerular filtration rate, and the latter determines the load of reabsorbable substances to the tubular system. Sodium salts represent about 95% of these substances and must be reabsorbed by active processes. The overall cost of this transport can be expressed in terms of O_2 consumption. It was found by DEETJEN and KRAMER (3, 4) that in a great variety of circumstances the renal O_2 consumption of dogs depends on Na load and its reabsorption (Fig. 1).

The ratio $\frac{\text{Na transported}}{O_2 \text{ consumed}}$ amounts to about 7 on the basis of milliequivalents. In these experiments net tubular sodium reabsorption was changed by a variety of experimental procedures, i. e. changing tubular sodium load by renal artery clamping, or changing tubular sodium reabsorption by osmotic diuresis or natriuretic drugs. Also a decreased tubular sodium load induced by dilating drugs which lower effective filtration pressure in the presence of high renal blood flow, is associated with a similar ratio of $\frac{\text{Na transported}}{O_2 \text{ consumed}}$. This ratio amounting to 7 has recently been confirmed on man with a mean ratio of 6.7 (12).

The only exception from this rule is found in osmotic diuresis with mannitol (5) and in Na_2SO_4-diuresis as discovered by BARCROFT and BRODIE (1) about 60 years ago. The

* This work was supported by a grant of the "Deutsche Forschungsgemeinschaft".

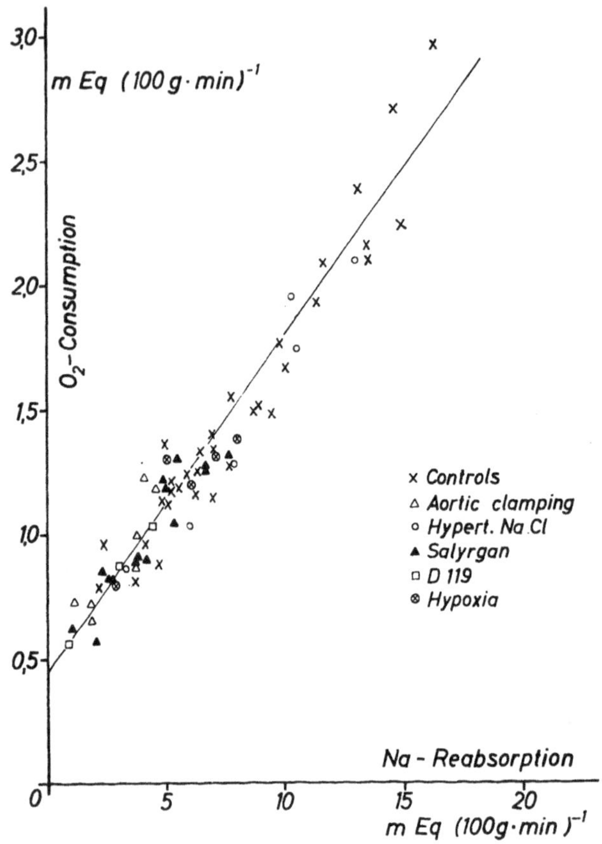

Fig. 1. Relationship between renal oxygen consumption and Na reabsorption under various conditions of renal functions and blood flow.

D 119 is a papaverine derivative. Modified from P. DEETJEN and K. KRAMER (4).

oxygen consumption per Na reabsorbed is increased (Fig. 2). This could possibly be explained by the fact that because of the smaller proximal tubular Na reabsorption a greater load is imposed on the ascending limb of HENLE and the distal tubule where the electro-chemical gradient is much larger than in the proximal tubule, causing higher costs for Na transport.

The classical concept of VOIT is that the respiratory quotient $\frac{CO_2}{O_2}$ relates to the foodstuffs consumed and broken down to CO_2 and H_2O. This concept can hardly be applied on the basis of values found in the kidney which show large deviations from the normal range (2, 12). The authors found a surprisingly great scatter of RQ values under different conditions of renal function. In their figures RQ values fluctuate between 0.4 and 2.7. In COHEN's experiments the mean values are above 1 (1.14–1.33). Although COHEN proposes possible explanations for these high RQs, which are based on excess CO_2 production under anaerobic conditions, some sources of experimental errors may not have been entirely excluded. For it is generally accepted that the errors which occur with two pairs of O_2 and CO_2 determinations in arterial and venous blood which are

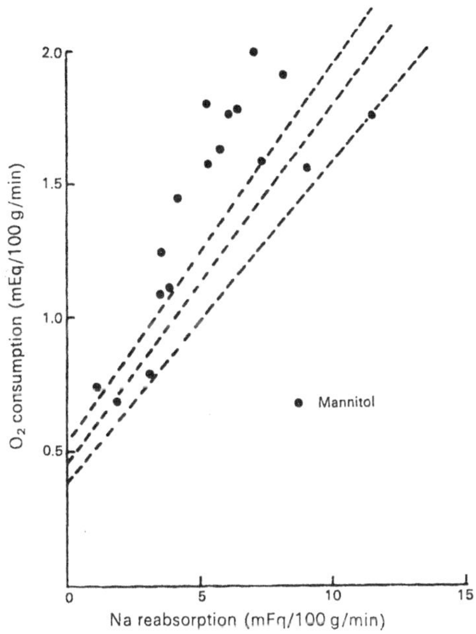

Fig. 2. Deviation of renal O_2 consumption per Na transported from normal range under mannitol diuresis. Data from K. KRAMER and P. DEETJEN (7).

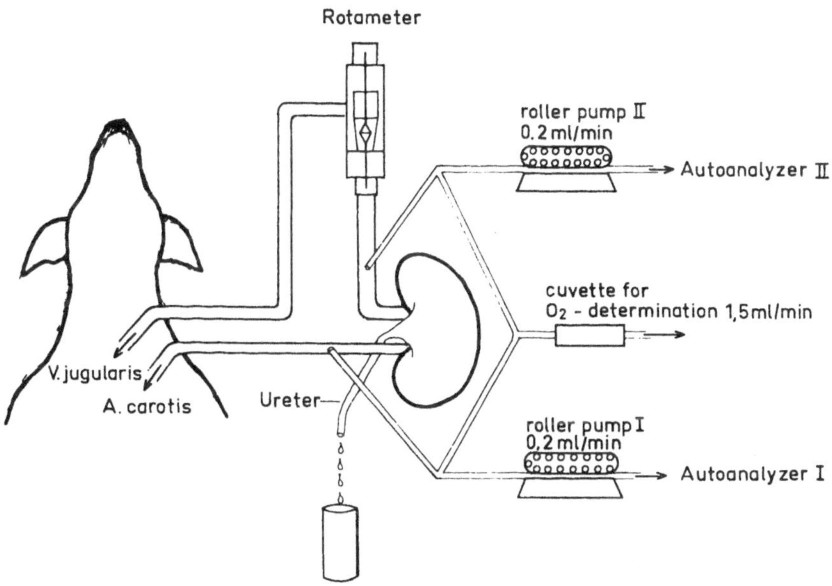

Fig. 3. Experimental set-up for O_2 and CO_2 determinations in a kidney transplanted to the neck of a donor dog.

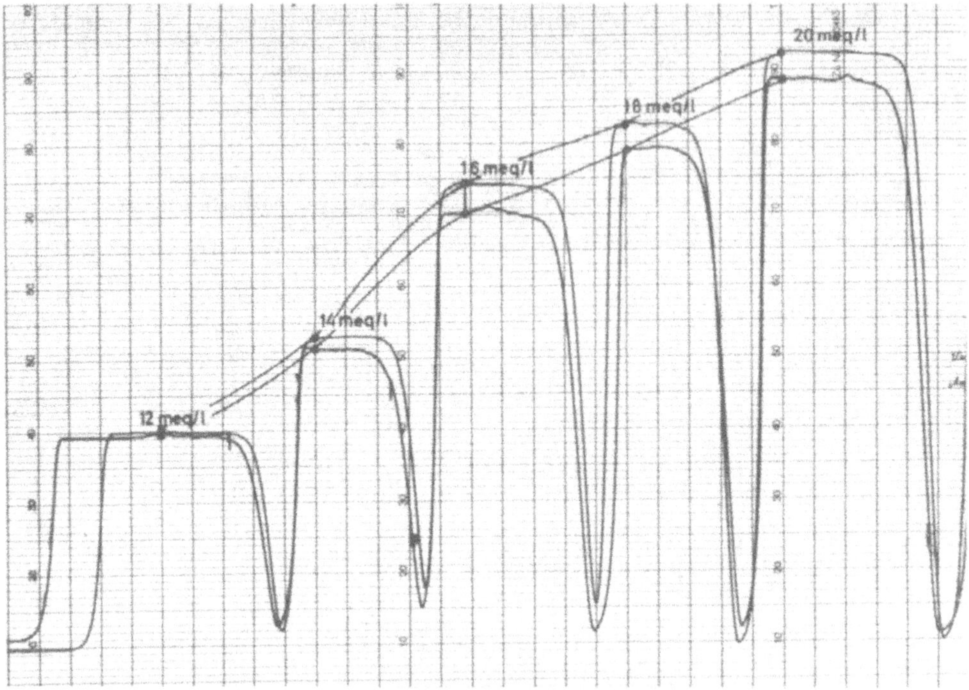

Fig. 4. Calibration curve of continuous CO_2 determination in Technicon analyzer obtained by recordings of 5 different standards from 12.0 to 20.0 m Eq/l.

necessary to obtain a single RQ value, are partly responsible for the large scatter of the results. Because of the low renal extraction the errors in each single determination may exceed $\pm 10\%$. This would result in RQ values maximally deviating from 1.0 to the extent of 0.66 to 1.50. Moreover, blood samples taken at random over short periods of time could provide reliable results only under strict steady state conditions. This, however, is barely the case in anaesthetized animals which show irregular breathing, rhythmic changes of blood flow and energy output. Therefore, we decided to try to obtain integrated values of RQ over *longer* periods of time. This was achieved by carrying out continuous measurements of O_2 and CO_2 contents in arterial and venous blood.

The experiments were carried out on 8 kidneys transplanted to the neck of donor dogs, anaesthetized with Nembutal. The technique of REINHARDT et al. (11) was adapted to our purpose. The measurements of O_2 and CO_2 contents were carried out on renal venous and brachial arterial blood which was drawn by pumps through an oximeter unit and Technicon CO_2 analyzers. The oximeter unit was used alternatively for venous and arterial blood (Fig. 3), a technique which had the advantage of only one calibration procedure (6). Using the oximeter O_2 saturation readings and the O_2 capacity derived from cyanhemoglobin determinations the oxygen content was calculated. Arterial and venous CO_2 contents were recorded simultaneously using two Technicon analyzers (Fig. 3). The principle of CO_2 determination was a photometric procedure in which the decoloration of phenolphthalein was measured; this was due to the acidification by CO_2 liberated from the blood by addition of sulphuric acid. Calibration curves were obtained by recordings of 5 different carbonate solutions with concentrations ranging from 10 to 20 mEq/l. A calibration curve is demonstrated in Fig. 4. Since the analyzing procedure incorporates constant volume flows, an exact control of the analyzer roller pump is essential for a correct CO_2 determination. It was found that the lift of the roller pump depended on the blood pressure at the input side. This means that the deflection of the CO_2 channel also depends on pressure. Therefore, the arterial CO_2 readings had to be corrected. Fig. 5 shows the dependency of CO_2 recordings on blood pressure ranging from 0 to 200 mg Hg. In this range the relationship is linear and amounts to deviations of 0.0057 mEq/mm Hg. Although the pressure effect causes only small deviations from actual values, its influence is not negligible because of the smallness of AVD_{CO_2}.

Results

In all experiments continuous recordings of arterial and venous CO_2 contents showed large variations depending on the respiratory rate of the animals. Therefore, blood samples taken at random over short periods (1 min or less) – a technique commonly applied – furnished a large scatter of AVD_{CO_2}. Fig. 6 shows that the values taken at random range from 1.5 to 3.6 Vol% CO_2, and this in spite of small respiratory variations.

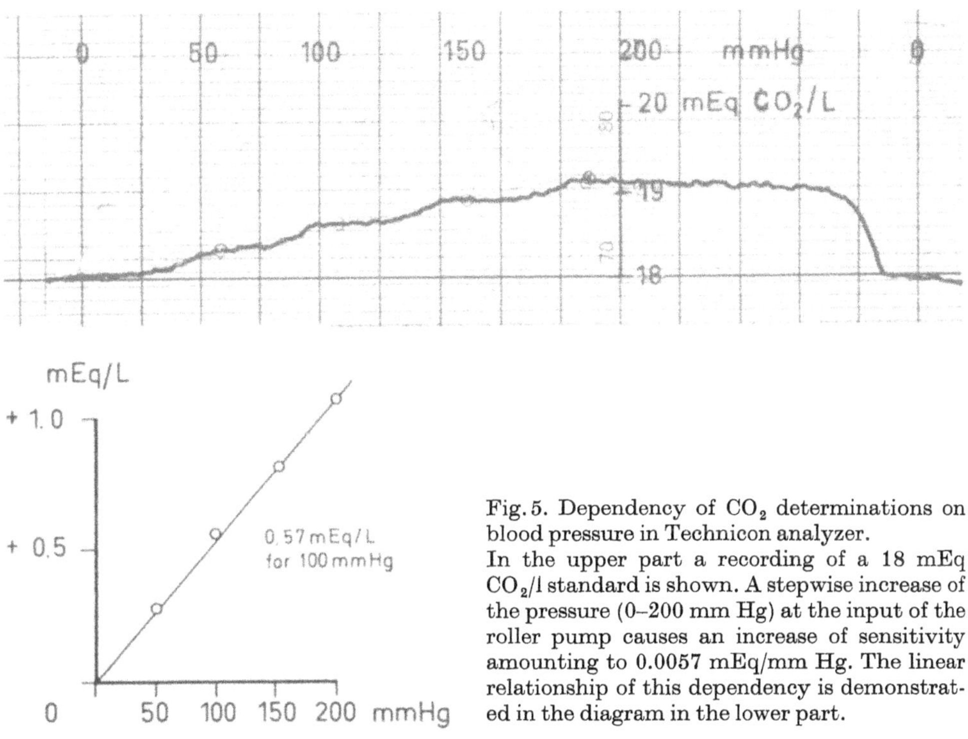

Fig. 5. Dependency of CO_2 determinations on blood pressure in Technicon analyzer. In the upper part a recording of a 18 mEq CO_2/l standard is shown. A stepwise increase of the pressure (0–200 mm Hg) at the input of the roller pump causes an increase of sensitivity amounting to 0.0057 mEq/mm Hg. The linear relationship of this dependency is demonstrated in the diagram in the lower part.

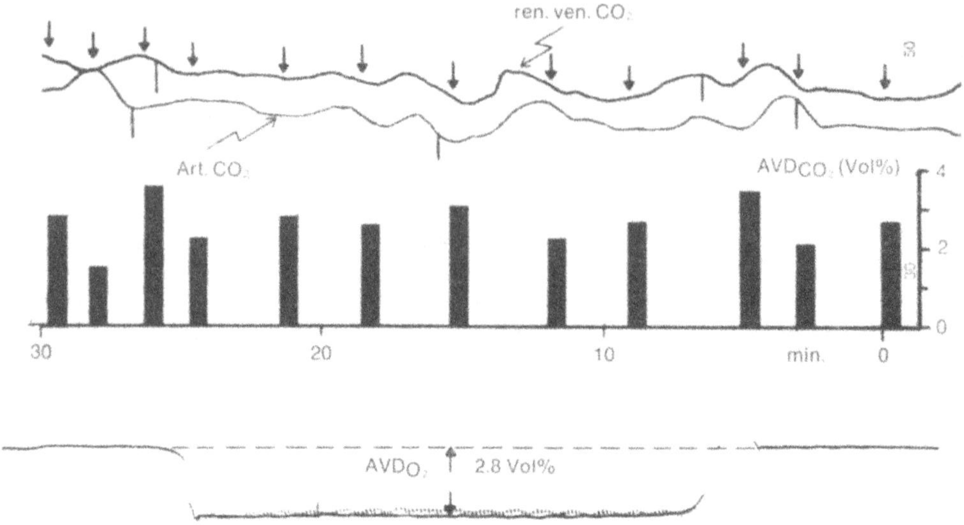

Fig. 6. Upper part: CO_2 recordings of arterial and renal venous blood. The $AVDco_2$ of random samples taken at the arrows range from 1.5–3.3 vol%. Simultaneously recorded O_2 contents (lower part) do not fluctuate and show a value of 2.8 vol%. The calculated RQ values range from 0.5–1.3. RQ values from left to right: 1.0, 0.54, 1.3, 0.8, 1.0, 0.93, 1.09, 0.8, 0.96, 1.23, 0.75, 0.96.

No detectable fluctuations of AVD_{O_2} occurred during this period. In the following period of the experiment (Fig. 7) a glucose infusion caused a decrease of respiratory rate from 36/min. to 18/min. which returned to normal within 50 min. This decrease was

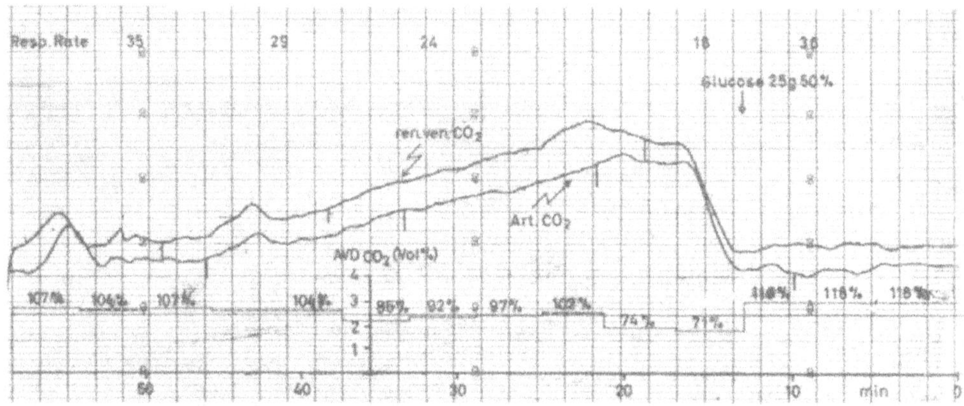

Fig. 7. Upper part: Continuous recordings of arterial and renal venous CO_2 contents over 60 min. Curves are recorded from right to left. Arrow at right marks a glucose infusion which results in a decrease of respiration rate from 36/min to 18/min.
Lower part: $AVDco_2$ in vol%. Line at 2.4 vol% shows mean value integrated over one hour = 100%. Figures show $AVDco_2$ of integrated 4 min periods in % of mean value.

accompanied by a large increase of arterial CO_2 content ranging from 29 to 33.6 vol% CO_2. Venous CO_2 variations followed with a delay of 15 to 120 seconds. The large CO_2 variations with respiration were expected in view of the steepness of the CO_2 blood dissociation curve. This consideration does not apply to the O_2 curve which is nearly horizontal in the same respiratory situation.

In order to investigate the influence of sampling time on the variation of AVD_{CO_2} 4 min. periods of the records were integrated. The results shown in the same figure (Fig. 7) demonstrated a reduction of the AVD_{CO_2} scatter as compared with the shorter sampling time (Fig. 6). However, the deviation of the above values from the mean integrated over a period of one hour is still considerable, ranging from 71 to 118% of the mean while AVD_{O_2} is almost constant. We may, therefore, conclude that the scatter of RQ readings of even 4 min periods depends mainly on CO_2 fluctuations. Renal metabolic changes due to the infusion of glucose are improbable since it is generally accepted that glucose is not used by the kidney as fuel in significant amounts. Glucose metabolism being essential for renal medullary tissue (9) can be neglected since the overall metabolism of the renal medulla in the intact kidney does not exceed 2% (8).

According to the fact that no experimental conditions with strict steady states do occur we have integrated the continuously recorded CO_2 values over periods of 28 minutes. The scatter of random samples was notably reduced. Simultaneous determinations of AVD_{O_2} allowed the calculation of RQs which are presented in Table 1. Such values taken from 6 experiments showed only variations between 0.63 and 0.83. The results obtained to date are in good agreement with findings which indicate that the kidney uses mainly fatty acids for its requirements (10).

Table 1. Comparison of RQ values integrated over 28 and 4 min periods.

RQ values integrated over 28 min periods:

Dog No.	1	2	3	4	5	6
	0.65 0.73 0.68	0.63 0.67 0.69 0.66	0.68 0.78 0.75 0.66 0.79	0.83	0.77 0.77 0.63	0.65 0.65
Mean	0.69	0.66	0.73	0.83	0.72	0.65

Range of RQ values integrated over 4 min periods:

Dog No.	1	2	3	4	5	6
	0.52–0.78	0.42–0.96	0.49–0.99	0.47–1.0	0.48–1.15	0.55–0.82

RQ values listed in this table are obtained from 28 and 4 min periods. Only periods are selected out of the continuous recordings of O_2 and CO_2 contents which show smallest fluctuations. Note the greater scatter of 4 min values as compared to the 28 min values. The mean values of the latter signify a preferential fatty acid combustion which could be due to the high fatty acid levels in arterial blood (1.68 m Eq/l).

References

1. BARCROFT, J. and T. G. BRODIE: J. Physiol. **33,** 52 (1905), **32,** 18 (1905).
2. COHEN, J. J.: Amer. J. Physiol. **199,** 560 (1960).
3. DEETJEN, P.: Habilitationsschrift Göttingen 1963.
4. DEETJEN, P. und K. KRAMER: Pflügers Arch. ges. Physiol. **273,** 636 (1961).
5. KIIL, F., K. AUKLAND and H. REFSUM: Amer. J. Physiol. **201,** 511 (1961).
6. KRAMER, K. und P. DEETJEN: Pflügers Arch. ges. Physiol. **271,** 782 (1960).
7. KRAMER, K. and P. DEETJEN: Pergamon Press, London 1963.
8. KRAMER, K., K. THURAU und P. DEETJEN: Pflügers Arch. ges. Physiol. **270,** 252 (1960).
9. KREBS, H. A.: This symposium.
10. NIETH, H. and P. SCHOLLMEYER: Nature **209,** 1244 (1966).
11. REINHARDT, H. W., H. J. KLOSE, K. ELLINGHAUS, H. BRECHTELSBAUER und D.W. BEHRENBECK: Pflügers Arch. ges. Physiol. **297,** 71 (1967).
12. SCHOLLMEYER, P.: Habilitationsschrift Tübingen 1966.
13. VAN SLYKE, D. D., C. P. RHOADS, A. HILLER and A. S. ALVING: Amer. J. Physiol. **109,** 336 (1934).

REUBI: I would like to comment briefly on oxygen consumption in the human kidney. It is extremely difficult in the human to decrease significantly the tubular reabsorption of sodium without modifying the glomerular filtration rate and the renal blood flow. Thus, if you correlate the oxygen consumption with one of these parameters, you usually get good correlation with either one of the three. Therefore, we should try to selectively block the sodium reabsorption. The trouble is, if you give a diuretic, in normal subjects you reduce the sodium reabsorption only by 5–10%. Several years ago we tried hydrochlorothiazide in patients with reduced renal function. In these patients tubular rejection fraction is always higher and the difference may become significant. Unfortunately, hydrochlorothiazide also diminishes renal blood flow and glomerular filtration rate. More recently, we used furosemide because furosemide is a very potent diuretic and at least during the first 10 or 20 minutes it increases renal blood flow and glomerular filtration rate. We actually found in our patients an increase in renal blood flow, an increase in glomerular filtration rate, a decrease in oxygen consumption and a decrease in sodium reabsorption. These data seem to support Dr. KRAMER's hypothesis.

GROSS: Dr. KRAMER, did you see a difference in a sodium losing and a sodium retaining kidney, regarding oxygen consumption?

I did not follow exactly the experiments you demonstrated on the first slide where you showed the dependence of sodium reabsorption on oxygen consumption. But I wonder whether in a negative sodium balance e. g. in adrenalectomized animals or in a positive sodium balance, e. g. after an overdosage of desoxycorticosterone or fluorocortisol and salt, a difference in oxygen consumption between the sodium losing and the sodium retaining kidney can be demonstrated.

KRAMER: This is a fine suggestion. Unfortunately, we have not done these experiments. So I cannot answer it. But these experiments should be done just to complete the oxygen story.

Relationship Between Cell Structures of Renal Tubules and Transport Mechanisms*) **)

W. THOENES, K. H. LANGER

The use of the electron microscope in morphological research has led to substantial information concerning the fine structure of cells and hence, that of the nephron itself. New techniques have greatly facilitated this research during the last few years. I would like to emphasize the following new methods:

1. Intravital fixation in order to avoid supravital artifacts, previously a source of misinterpretation,
2. Cytochemical and, especially, enzyme-cytochemical methods and
3. Tubular micropuncture.

These methodological improvements permit us to deal with and discuss a few new aspects of the cytomorphology of the mammalian nephron. I would like to divide my talk into two parts. Firstly, I shall discuss the differentiation of the cell structures along the nephron and in the second part I shall report a few of our recent morphological findings concerning certain transport mechanisms in the convoluted tubules.

I. Cell differentiations along the nephron[1])

With the aid of the above mentioned intravital fixation it is possible to maintain the shape of the tubules and thus also the shape of the associated epithelial cells and the arrangement of their subunits. Even though it may not be possible to preserve them in a "true to life" condition, it is, nevertheless, possible to keep them in a condition which certainly approximates the in vivo condition. Certain structural principles have, therefore, been demonstrated more clearly than ever before and we are thus enabled at the present time to carry out a comparative analysis of the cell types involved in the structure of the nephron with greater significance than had previously been possible.

A. General remarks

In the center of such an evaluation I shall place the external structure of the cell and in connection with that the interdigitation of the tubular epithelia (32). The latter follows

*) Dedicated to Professor Dr. HELMUT RUSKA, Düsseldorf, on the occasion of his 60th birthday.

**) The work was supported by the Deutsche Forschungsgemeinschaft.

1) According to the classical definition the "nephron" terminates at the beginning of the collecting system. In this report the term is more loosely defined based on cytological and functional aspects and includes the collecting system.

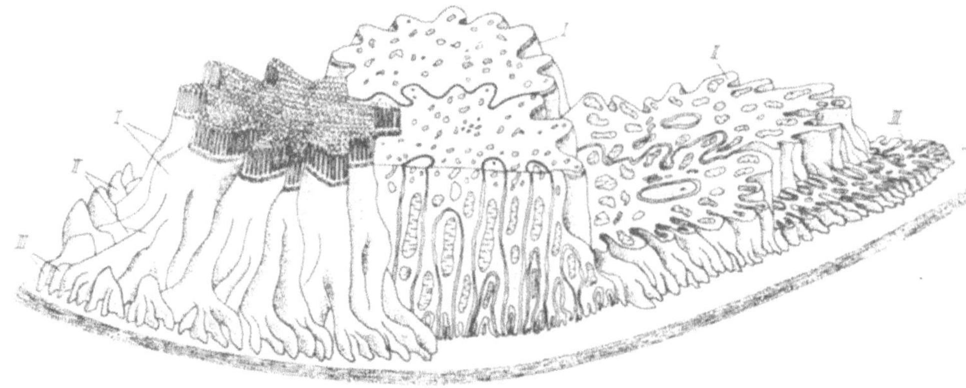

Fig. 1. Schematic three-dimensional reproduction of the epithelium in the proximal convoluted tubule (adapted from Yoshimura and Nakamura, 59) to explain the "principle of multiple interdigitation": Processes of the Ist, IInd and IIIrd order with their respective interdigitation in the apical, intermediate and basal cell-regions can be differentiated. The processes can be clearly recognized in the vertical section (center of the picture, front) and in the various horizontal planes of sections, compare to Fig. 2 and 3.

a principle which has previously been mentioned when the structure of Henle's thin loop was analyzed (47, 48). On the basis of more recent findings this principle will be extended and defined more precisely. We shall call it the "*principle of multiple interdigitation*". Our line of thought which is based on cellular shape will furthermore provide us with an opportunity to point out intracellular characteristics which are significant for the morphological characterization of individual segments of the nephron.

The "principle of multiple interdigitation" of the epithelia of the renal tubules is illustrated in a three dimensional schematic diagram of the tubular epithelia in the first segment of the proximal tubule (Fig. 1, adapted from Yoshimura and Nakamura, 59): The complete epithelial cell to the left clearly shows a systematic subdivision of the cell body progressing from the apex in a basal direction. In this context it is possible to differentiate processes of the Ist, IInd and IIIrd order. Horizontal sections through the apical, intermediate and basal cell-region reveal that the other epithelia are of the same shape and that the processes of adjacent cells are fairly systematically

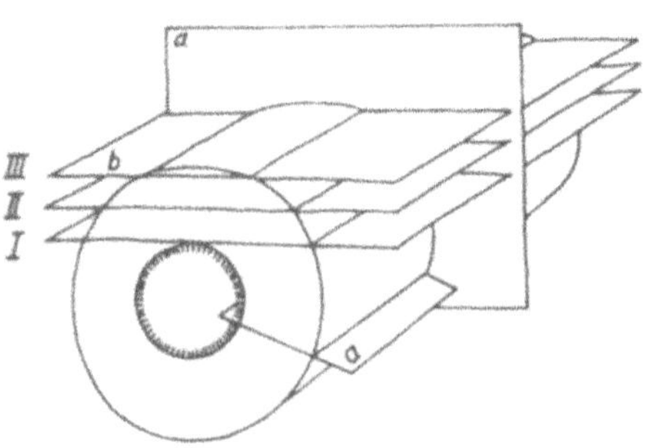

Fig. 2 Illustration of the electron microscopic appearance of sections through the proximal convoluted tubule as presented in Fig. 3: a) vertical or radial to the axis of the tubule; b) parallel to the axis of the tubule: at the level of the terminal bars near the lumen (I), at the intermediate region (II), near the base (III) of the tubular epithelial wall.

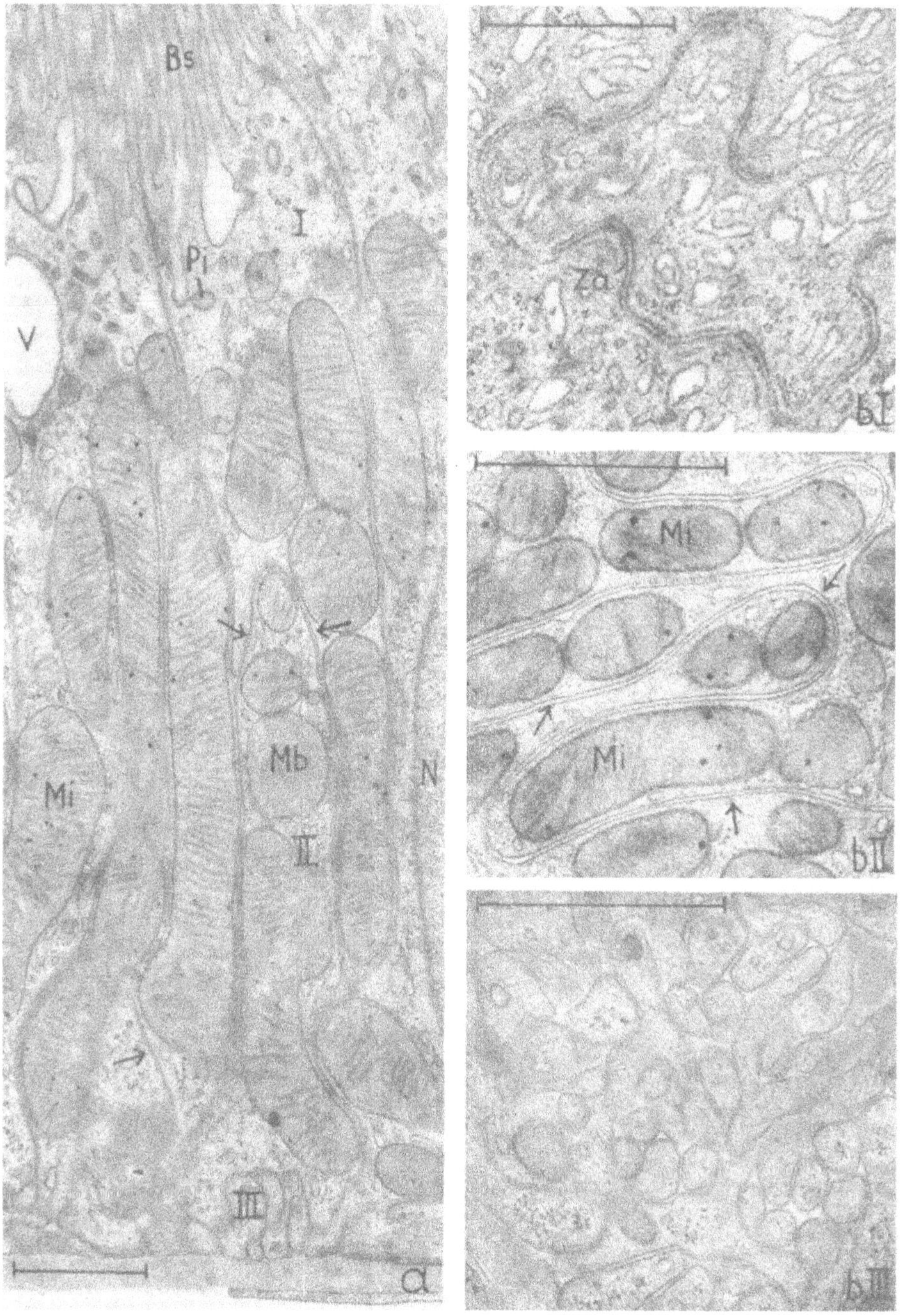

Fig. 3. Sections of the proximal convoluted tubule of the rat kidney with threefold interdigitation of the epithelium: a) vertical or radial section (18,000:1), b) longitudinal sections; I: at the level of the terminal bars (zonula adhaerens, *Za*) near the lumen (26,000:I), II: at the intermediate cell-region (33,000:1), III: near the base of the tubule (33,000:1). For explanation, see text. *BB* brush border, *Pi* pinocytosis vesicles, *V* apical vacuole, *Mi* mitochondria, *Mb* microbodies, *N* cell nucleus → Intercellular spaces between processes of the IInd order.

interdigitated. One may therefore refer to an interdigitation of the Ist, IInd and IIIrd order. The appearance in an electron micrograph of the multiple interdigitation varies, depending on the plane of section (see Fig. 2: perpendicular and radial, respectively *(a)*, parallel *(b I, II, III)* to the axis of the tubule). In Fig. 3 the interdigitation of the Ist order manifests itself in vertical or in radial sections *(a)* by the short distance of the terminal bars, in horizontal sections *(b I)* by the meandering course of the contact line along which the adjacent cells are firmly attached to one another. Below the terminal bars the subapical cell territories are separated from one another by the intercellular space. For the most part they contain the elements of micropinocytosis, including the subapical vacuoles and a few mitochondria and ribosomes. In vertical sections through intermediate cell regions narrow cytoplasmic compartments correspond to the interdigitation of the IInd order. In the vertical section (Fig. 3: *a*) the compartments are separated by a straight intercellular space, in the longitudinal sections *(b II)* by meandering ones. In addition to the profiles of the ER, free ribosomes and lytic vacuoles the compartments contain the bulk of the mitochondria. Finally, the interdigitation of the IIIrd order is caused by very small cell processes which only contain cytoplasmic matrix, a few microvesicles and ribosomes. The morphological substrate of this fine basal interdigitation is also presented in Fig. 3 (*a* shows the vertical section, *b III* the horizontal

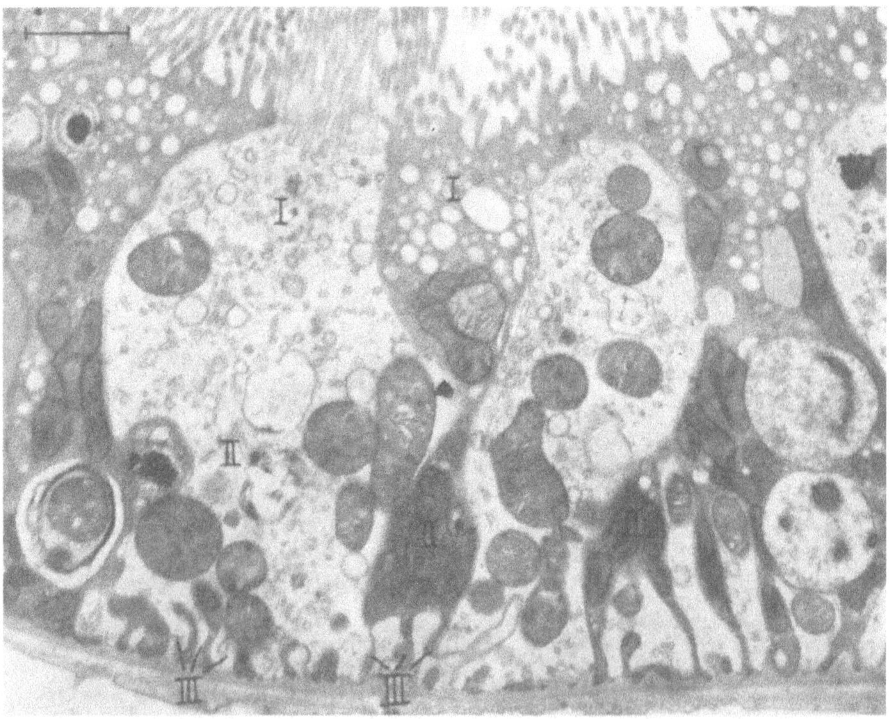

Fig. 4. Threefold interdigitation of the proximal epithelium of the renal tubule, demonstrated by hydrops of a cell (produced by the action of KCN, 53): The alternatingly interdigitated cellular processes of the Ist, IInd and IIIrd order can be clearly recognized. 14,000 : 1.

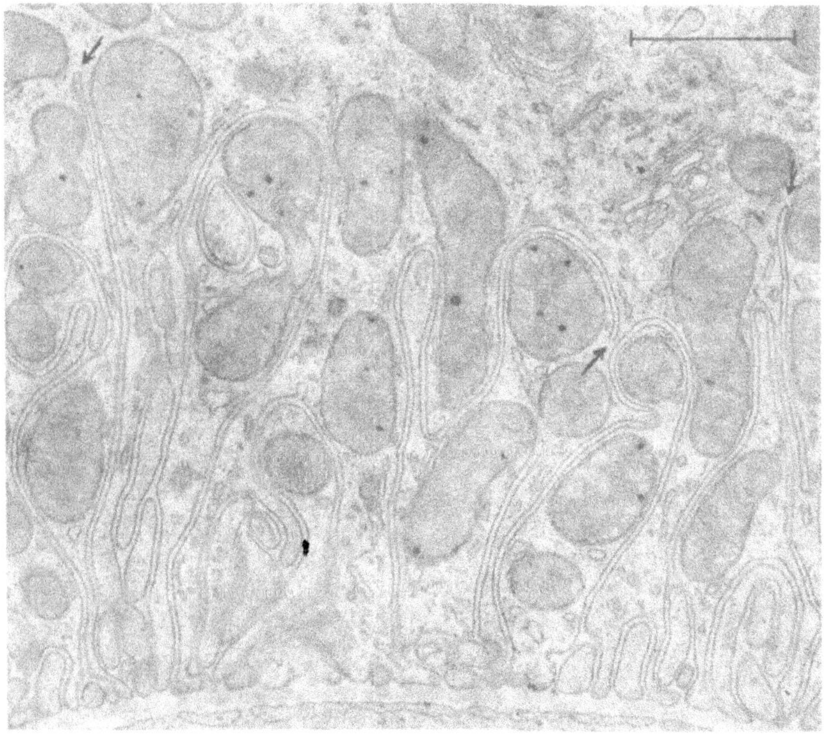

Fig. 5. Blind labyrinth spaces (→) in the terminal section of the distal convoluted tubule. 24,300 : 1.

section). The fact that the processes do indeed originate from different cells can be demonstrated if, for some reason, one of the interdigitated epithelial cells has become hydropic (Fig. 4), thus permitting exact identification of their processes. In this case the effect was caused by the action of potassium cyanide (54). In the terminal segment of the distal convoluted tubule which otherwise shows the same interdigitation principle, additional blind labyrinthic clefts occur with a certain regularity i. e., membrane-folds without demonstrable interdigitation (Fig. 5).

For most segments of the renal tubules the interdigitation is connected with the existence of the *labyrinth system* in the epithelial wall. The above described threefold interdigitation which exists in the proximal convoluted tubule and in the distal convoluted tubule, is associated with a subdivision of the labyrinth system which becomes more pronounced towards the basis of the cell. Therefore it is particularly obvious at the base of the tubule ("basal labyrinth" 35). One has to keep in mind, however, that the labyrinth is not limited to the basal region. Basically we are dealing with a complicated, predominantly intercellular system of clefts which extends as a uniform diffusion space from the terminal bars to the tubular basal membrane. This fact can be experimentally confirmed by injection of ferritin under high pressure into the renal vascular system (49). The ferritin penetrates from the capillary through the basal membrane into the entire

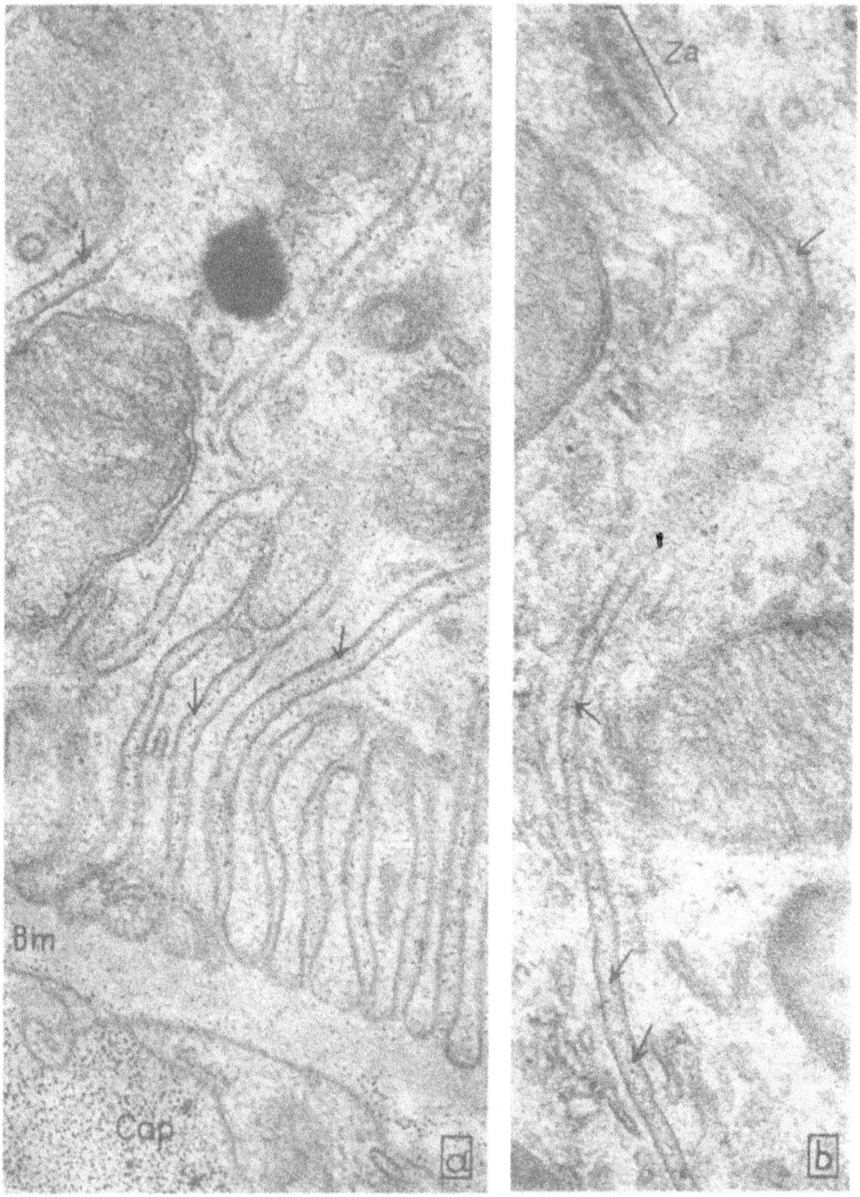

Fig. 6. a–b. Retrograde inflow of ferritin from the peritubular capillary *(Cap)* through the tubular basal membrane *(Bm)* into the labyrinth of the distal convoluted tubule (→) as far as close to the zonula adhaerens *(Za)* of the junctional complex, a) 76,800 : 1, b) 78,800 : 1.

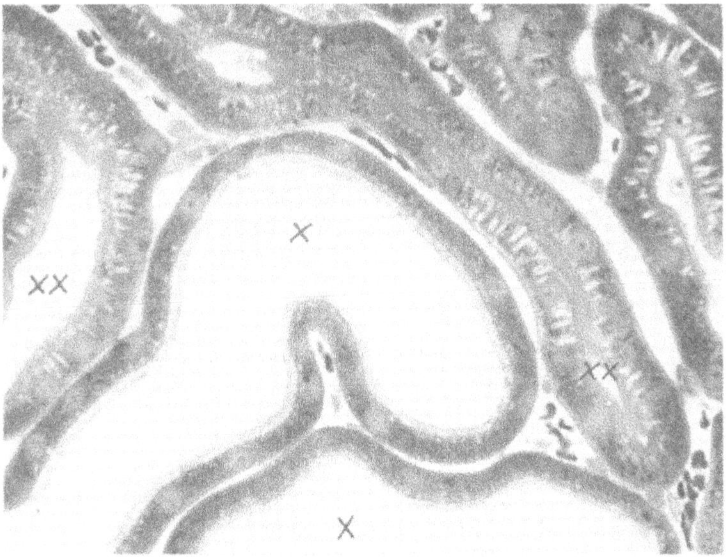

Fig. 7. Loops of proximal tubule (x) which were intravitally fixed by free flow-microperfusion with 1% OsO_4, show a homogenous epithelial wall; in contrast to this, the adjacent tubular loops which were exposed to ischemia two minutes after the start of perfusion (xx) show numerous clefts (expanded labyrinth). Light-microscope, Giemsa, 485:1.

labyrinth system towards the zonula adhaerens of the terminal junctional complex (Fig. 6, see also 49).

Two additional findings must be mentioned to further characterize the morphology of the labyrinth system: The labyrinth spaces of the tubules of normal antidiuretic rat kidneys intravitally fixed with osmium tetroxide are always quite narrow and show a fairly constant width. In sections, the mean width in the proximal convoluted tubule was approximately 20 nm, in the distal convoluted tubule about 30 nm (49). A dilated labyrinth system in normal antidiuretic kidneys must always create the suspicion of inadequate fixation (compare 17) or suggests that the respective tubules were exposed to ischemia prior to fixation.

This can be clearly shown by a microperfusion experiment (method see 50): Puncture of a segment of the proximal convoluted tubule; perfusion with 1% isotonic OsO_4-solution for 2 minutes; clamping of the renal artery and continuation of the OsO_4-perfusion of the same tubule for another 3 minutes. The perfused tubule shows a narrow labyrinth. Contrarily, the adjacent tubule which obviously belongs to another nephron, not yet fixed at the time of ischemia, shows a wide labyrinth (Fig. 7). If, on the other hand, intravital fixation by microperfusion is carried out for a prolonged period of time – without ischemia – the adjacent tubules also show a narrow labyrinth.

Furthermore, microdensitometric tests have shown that the labyrinth spaces contain a loose substance with a density corresponding approximately to that of the cytoplasmic matrix of intravitally fixed tubular epithelia (49). We are probably dealing here with mucopolysaccharides (29) which are also present in the so-called glycocalyx (2).

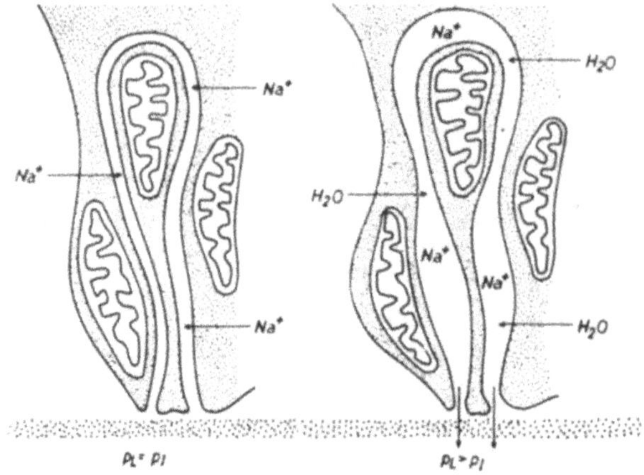

Fig. 8. On the "pressure transformer" function of the basal labyrinth according to RUSKA (37): An increase of the osmotic pressure by ion-transport into the labyrinth (left) is followed by the inflow of water (right). The direction of the fluid-movement between the labyrinth and the interstitium depends on the respective hydrostatic pressure, PL and PI.

The significance of these findings for the *function of the labyrinth* cannot be estimated as yet. The idea that the labyrinth of the renal tubule functions as a pressure transformer ("Druckwandler-Funktion") (Fig. 8) was first introduced by RUSKA et al. (35, 36, 37) in order to explain the fluid transport from the labyrinth to the capillary ("Endstreckentransport", 45) during the reabsorption process. The compartment model later developed for the epithelium of the intestine by CURRAN and MCINTOSH (4) was based on the same concept. It had previously been pointed out that the epithelia of the small intestine and that of the renal tubule are in some respects comparable to one another (47). In the epithelium of the small intestine (compare 34) and in the related epithelium of the gallbladder (8) widening of the intercellular spaces occurs during intensive reabsorption. Till now, no similar results have been available for the renal cortical tubules. It remains questionable, however, whether or not the pressure transformer mechanism necessarily leads to a widening of the intercellular spaces in all types of absorbing epithelia, including the renal tubule. We are planning specific experiments to further clarify this point. The work by CURRAN and MCINTOSH (4) which was able to confirm the pressure transformer mechanism for a model system is in any case quite significant for the conditions prevailing in the renal tubule (see 57).

Since the compartment model has increasingly become a current concept in renal physiology, it is particularly interesting to analyze more closely the type and extent of the epithelial labyrinth along the nephron.

B. Cytological characteristics of the individual tubular segments

Fig. 9 is a schematic reproduction of the main characteristics of the individual tubular segments and subsegments. In addition to other criteria (e. g. number of mitochondria, presence of brush border or of short microvilli, number of ribosomes, vacuoles, etc.), the mode of interdigitation and of the labyrinth respectively is obviously a decisive but quite variable characteristic of the individual segments of the tubule (see also Table 1). In addition we would like to emphasize the following more recent results of the cytomorphology of the nephron with reference to previous reviews (31, 32, 39, 45, 47, 48 and others).

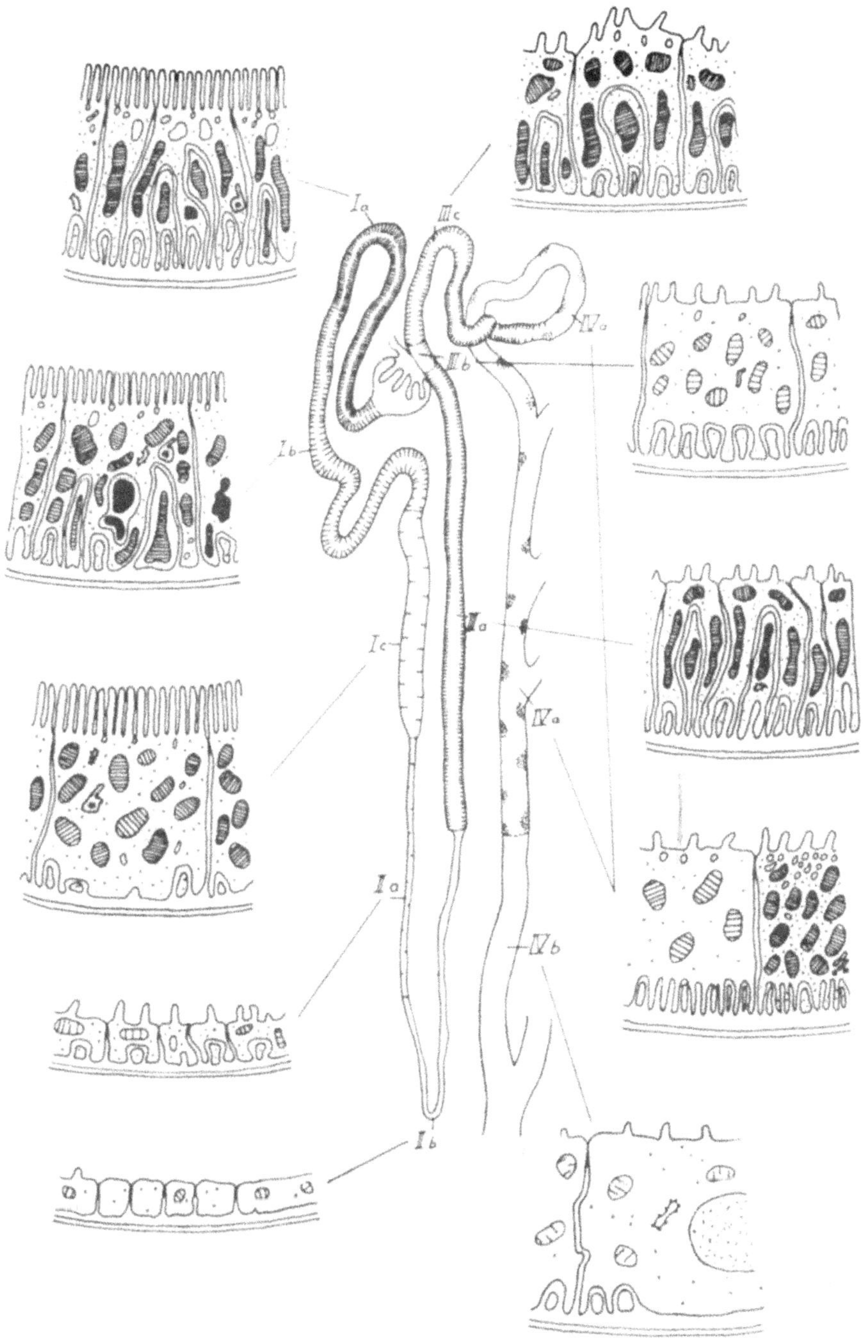

Fig. 9. Differentiations of the renal tubular epithelium along the nephron, with particular consideration of the labyrinth system (compare Table 1).

Table 1. Scheme of interdigitation and labyrinth formation according to the "principle of multiple interdigitation" along the nephron (I^{st}, IInd and IIIrd order: + = fully developed, (+) = less fully developed, – absent, compare this to Fig. 9).

Tubule Segment		Interdigitation		
No. in Fig. 9	Designation	I	II	III
I	*Proximal tubule* (Hauptstück)			
a	Segment I (Pars convoluta)	+	+	+
b	Segment II (P. conv.-recta)	(+)	(+)	(+)
c	Segment III (Pars recta)	–	–	(+)
II	*Thin segment of Henle's loop* (Überleitungsstück)			
a	Pars descendens	+	–	+
b	Pars ascendens	+	–	–
III	*Distal tubule* (Mittelstück)			
a	Pars recta	+	+	+
b	Macula densa	–	–	+
c	Pars convoluta	(+)	+	+

1. Proximal tubule (Hauptstück)

With reference to light microscopical findings of SJÖSTRAND (40), electron microscopic data and combined phase-contrast, fluorescent and electron microscopic investigations MAUNSBACH (16) differentiated three segments in the proximal tubule (Figs. 9, 10). The first segment covers the first third or one half of the pars convoluta and the beginning of the pars recta, the second segment the remaining part of the pars convoluta and the beginning of the pars recta. The third segment comprises the major part of the pars recta which extends to the external part of the outer medullary zone.

The emphasis on the second segment is new. It is characterized by the frequent occurence of large autofluorescent, periodate-reactive "granules". In the electron micrograph the latter appear as dense homogenous lumps confined to vacuoles which are surrounded by membranes (Fig. 10b). The reaction product of acid phosphatase which can be demonstrated cytochemically (PFEIFER, 27) confirms the lysosomal nature of these granules or vacuoles. The distinct separation of the second segment from the proximal and distal part of the proximal tubule thus is primarily based on the special type, number and size of the lysosomes which indicate a considerable activity of intracellular digestive processes.

The *microbodies* (31) are of particular significance. They are found exclusively in the proximal tubule but here they are present in all three segments. They differ from the microbodies of the hepatic parenchymal cells by the absence of the crystalline (urikase-containing) "nucleoid" and by the formation of peculiar "rods" (7, 12, 15c), whose ultrastructure has recently been elucidated (12).

Apart from the "peroxisomal" nature of the microbodies (DE DUVE, 5) it is worth mentioning that the renal microbodies do not only contain amino acid oxydase for the d-types (liver), but also for the natural l-types of the amino acids. Furthermore, the relationship of the microbodies to gluconeogenesis must be pointed out (5a). Its import-

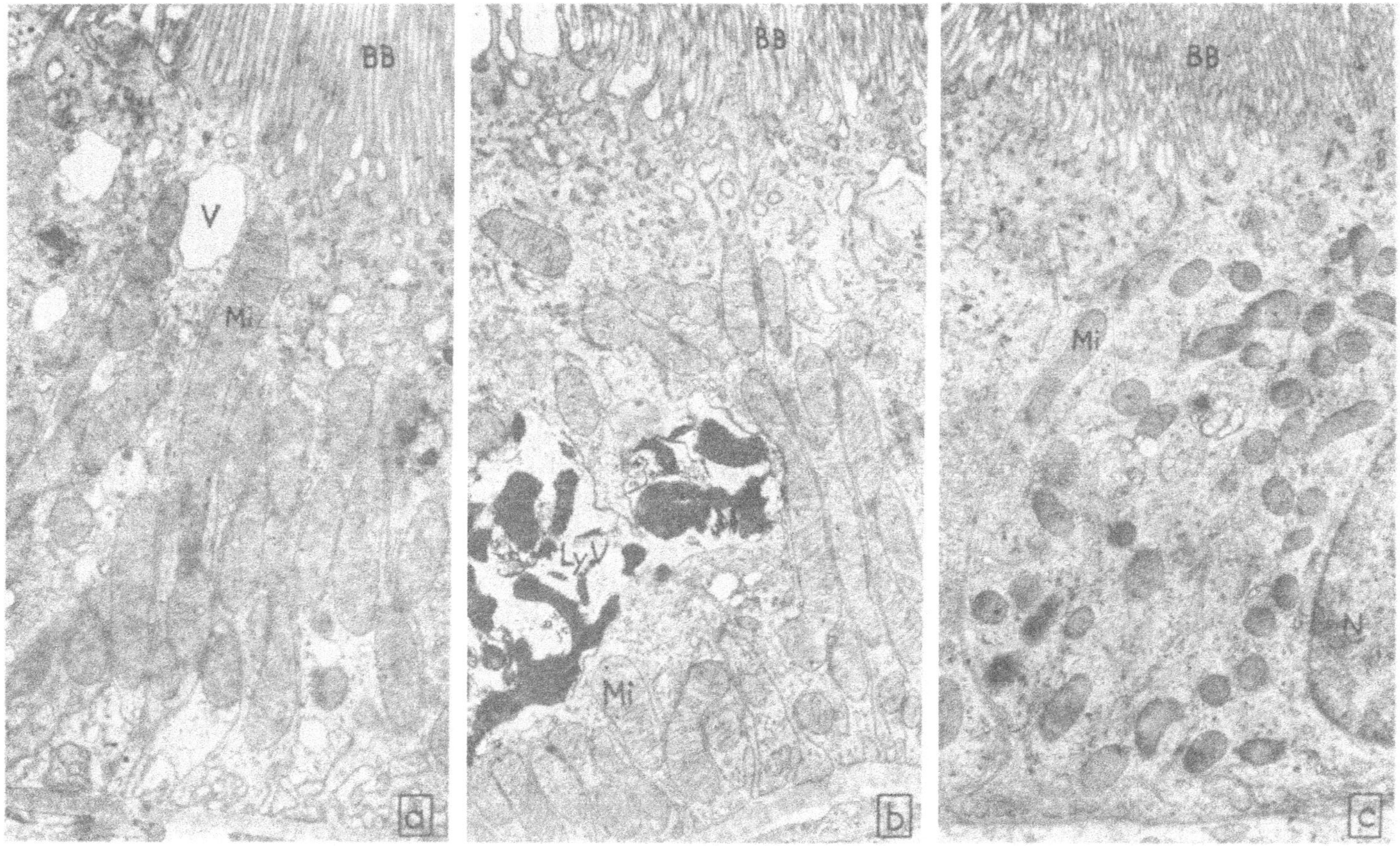

Fig. 10. a–c. Three segments of the proximal tubule (compare to I a, b, c in Fig. 7 and Table 1). *BB* brush border, *V* apical vacuole, *LyV* lytic vacuole with compact material, *Mi* mitochondria. *N* cell nucleus 10,000 : 1.

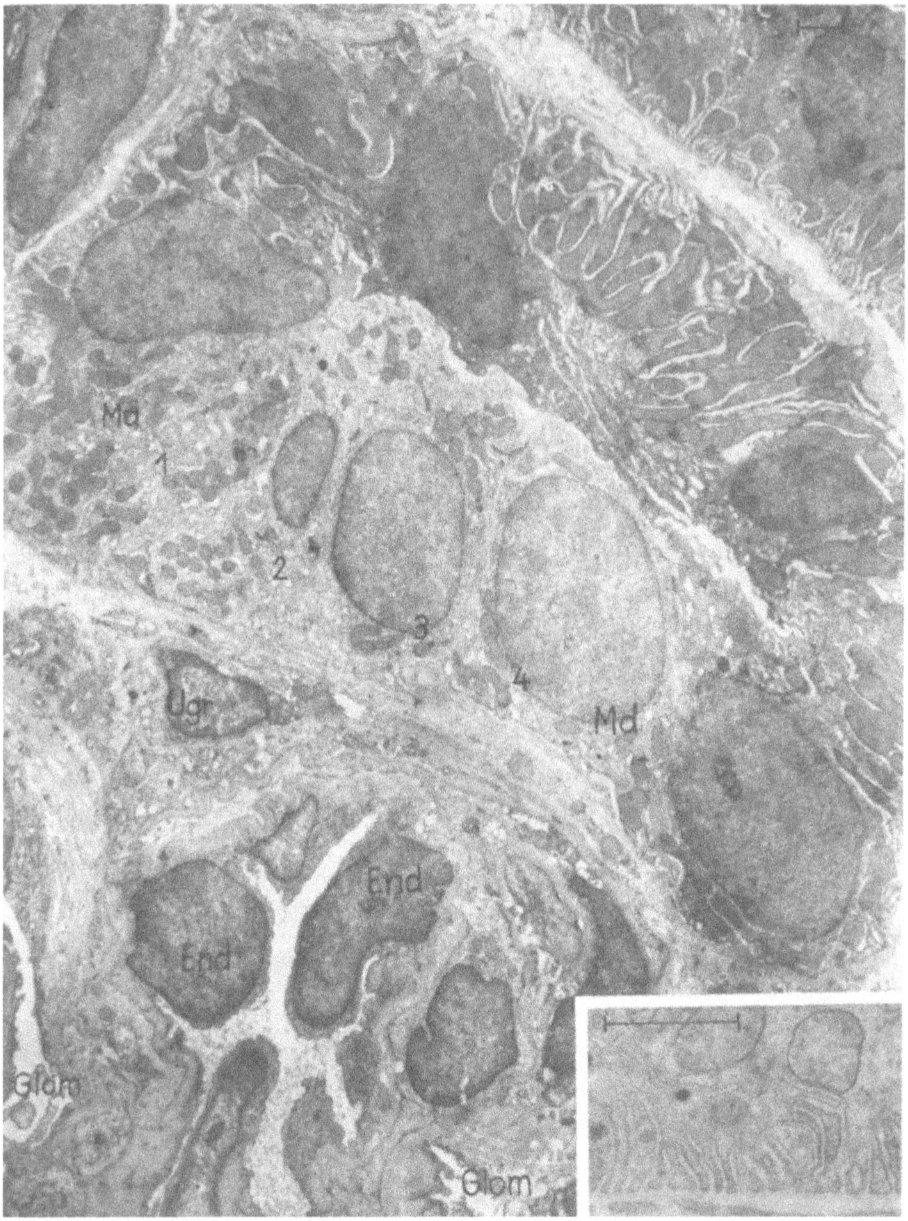

Fig. 11. Transverse section of the macula densa segment of the distal tubule. Below, the vascular pole of the glomerulus (Glom) with the hilus vessel (*End* endothelium) and non-granulated juxtaglomerular cells (Ugr.). Above, the macula densa (Md) consisting of epithelia (1–4) which contain relatively few mitochondria with a small, exclusively basal labyrinth (insert right below). Compare the large number of mitochondria and the deep-reaching threefold interdigitation of the epithelium on the side of the same tubular segment which faces away from the glomerulus. 5,500:1 (insert 18,000:1).

ance for the metabolism of the renal cortex has been emphasized by KREBS at this meeting (11).

2. The thin segment of Henle's loop (Überleitungsstück)

As is obvious from Table 1 and Fig. 9 (compare Fig. 11a, b in 47), the descending and ascending part show a different mode of interdigitation. In the initial part of the descending limb a double (I^{st} and IIIrd order) interdigitation (see 47) is found, whereas the entire ascending limb shows simple interdigitation only (I^{st} order). This finding, first described by LAPP and NOLTE (13), has been confirmed by several investigators (26, 47). In the transition zone from or to the pars recta of the proximal or distal tubule the results are less clear cut (compare 47 and 26). Additional differences between the two limbs of the thin loop concern the microvilli, mitochondria and ribosomes which are more numerous in the more strongly interdigitated cells of the descending limb than in the less differentiated cells of the ascending limb. One may therefore say that along the thin loop a loss of differentiation of the epithelium occurs, faint as it may be. It obviously starts already in the descending limb and in any case does not coincide with the tip of the loop.

3. Distal tubule (Mittelstück) – **collecting tubule** (Sammelrohr)

The epithelium of the pars recta (= thick ascending part of the loop of Henle) and of the pars convoluta (Schaltstück) of the distal tubule shows threefold interdigitations similar to the proximal convoluted tubule. In both segments the interdigitation of the IInd and IIIrd order is quite intensive, whereas the interdigitation of the I^{st} order, characterized by the mean distance of the terminal bars, is less pronounced in the convoluted tubule than in the pars recta [see schematic Fig. 9 in this paper as well as electronmicroscopic Fig. 6 in (47)].

In contrast to this the *macula densa*, whose epithelium shows relatively few mitochondria and exclusively basal short infoldings of the membrane (corresponding to the processes of the IIIrd order), stands out clearly (Fig. 11, see 3, 14, 46). This structural difference indicates that the capacity for solute transport which must be carried out by the cells of the macula – serving the juxtaglomerular transmission of information – is less than that of the preceding and following segments of the distal tubule. To interpret the relationship between structure and function of the epithelia of the macula we had, therefore, suggested that the information might only concern certain solutes, e. g. sodium ions (46). Thus we find complete agreement between the morphology and the functional behavior as observed by THURAU and SCHNERMANN (56) with the aid of micropuncture.

The relationship between the distal convoluted tubule and the collecting tubule must be discussed in somewhat more detail. We investigated this problem together with STEIDL starting with the question: What are the so-called "early-distal" and "late-distal" tubules, which can be differentiated on the renal surface by intravital microscopy after lissamine-green passage according to STEINHAUSEN (41). Let me immediately present the main results (identification of the two segments of the tubule in the histological section was carried out by intraluminal oil-injection): The so-called "early-distal tubule" corresponds to the distal convolute per se ("Schaltstück" in the nomenclature of v. MÖLLENDORFF, 22) showing the above mentioned epithelia with numerous mito-

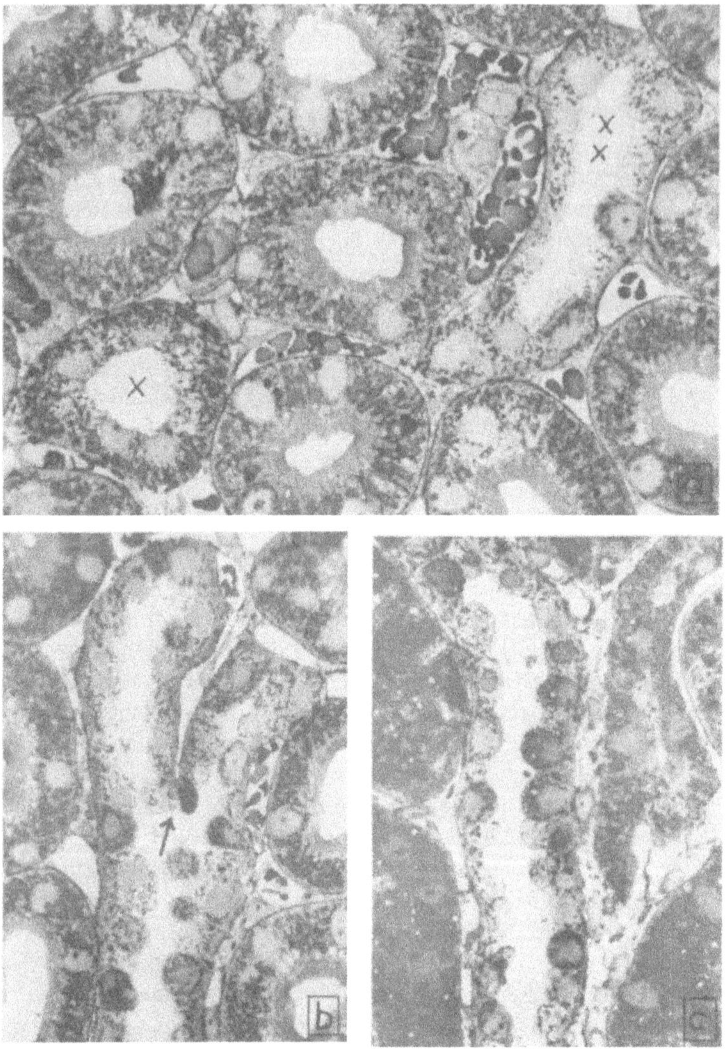

Fig. 12. The relationship between the distal convoluted tubule and the cortical collecting tubule (rat kidney). a) Section from the subcapsular area of the renal cortex. Below left (x): distal convoluted tubule (tubulus contortus II, Schaltstück, so-called "early-distal" tubule, compare this to Fig. 13a). Above right (xx): pars contorta of the cortical collecting tubule with a few dark intercalated cells (so-called "late-distal" tubule, compare this to Fig. 13b). b) The cortical collecting tubule at the point of entry into the "Markstrahl" also showing the point of confluence (→). c) Collecting tubule in the area of the outer medullary zone. – Notice the increase of the number of intercalated cells from a – c. Light-microscope, silver methenamine. a: 660:1, b and c 510:1.

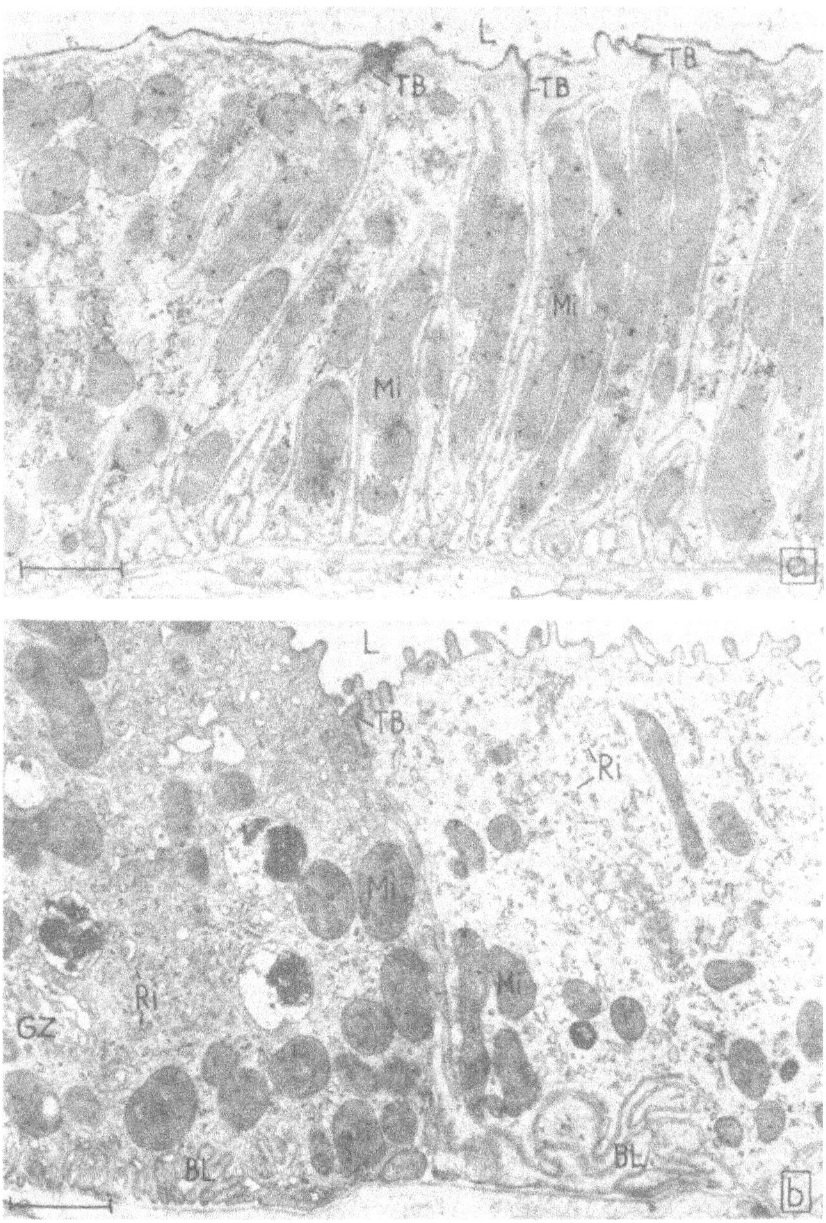

Fig. 13. a) Distal convoluted tubule (Schaltstück) with threefold interdigitated epithelium containing many mitochondria ("early-distal" tubule). b) Pars contorta of the cortical collecting tubule ("late-distal" tubule) with light (right) and dark epithelia (left, intercalated cell). The labyrinth is only found at the base (BL), mainly without interdigitation. – *L* lumen of the tubule, *TB* terminal bars, *Mi* mitochondria, *Ri* free ribosomes, *GZ* Golgizone. a and b 15,000 : 1.

chondria and a threefold interdigitation (Figs. 12a, 13a). In contrast to this, the so-called "late-distal tubule" consists of relatively light epithelia which contain few mitochondria. Darker cells are interspersed between the light cells (the ratio of light to dark epithelial cells is approximately 3:1) (Fig. 12b). The dark "intercalated cells" (Schaltzellen, ref. 22, 32, 45) contain a relatively great number of cristae-rich mitochondria per unit volume of the cytoplasm and, in addition, they contain numerous vesicular or tubular endoplasmatic profiles, Golgi-zones and free ribosomes (Fig. 13b). Both the light and the dark epithelia show a labyrinth which is exclusively confined to the cell base. In this labyrinth – in contrast to the renal tubules which have hitherto been discussed – the interdigitation obviously only plays a minor role and thus is for the main part only due to simple infoldings of the basal cell membrane. In vertical and horizontal sections numerous blind clefts are found and, in addition, repeated rows of vesicles. The latter may be taken as an indication of the continuous breakdown and reconstruction of these clefts. If the so-called "late-distal" tubule is followed in a distal direction a basically identical picture is found at the first points where conflux takes place (compare Fig. 12b to 12a). The situation is similar along the subsequent descending course up to the transition between the outer and inner medullary zone only changing in degree (Fig. 12c) insofar as the difference between light and dark epithelia becomes more pronounced and the numerical ratio of light to dark cells decreases to 2:1. On the basis of these findings one may conclude that the so-called "late-distal" tubule does not really deserve this name but already marks the beginning of the collecting tubule and is better designated as "*pars convoluta of the cortical collecting tubule*". It must thus be pointed out that the collecting tubule starts some distance before reaching the "Markstrahl".

Furthermore, it must be emphasized that the cell structure in the transition area between the distal convoluted tubule ("early-distal" tubule) and the initial convoluted collecting tubule ("late-distal" tubule) does not change abruptly but gradually (cytomorphological proof of this finding will be presented elsewhere).

The fact that the *medullary part of the collecting tubule*, i. e. the part located in the inner medullary zone, consists exclusively of light epithelia with few mitochondria is shown under IV b in Fig. 9 [compare 16b in (47)]. In this location we also find a labyrinth which is exclusively located basally, but which is much less well developed than in the cortical collecting tubule.

I would now like to conclude my cytomorphological survey of the renal tubules of the mammalian kidney. It has been mentioned that the renal tubules of the "nephron" in the classical definition (including the distal convoluted tubule) gradually blend into the collecting tubule, even though embryologically they originate from different blastemata. In contrast to this gradual transformation the character of the epithelium changes fairly rapidly in other locations (e. g., at the transitions: proximal tubule – thin loop of Henle – distal tubule or even within the macula densa-segment of the distal tubule). v. Möllendorff (22) already pointed out that this reflects the prevalence of the function over the histogenesis or cytogenesis. At the same time it becomes obvious in this context how far these cell structures must indeed be regarded as functional structures.

II. Contributions of functional morphology to transport problems in the convoluted tubules (with special reference to reabsorption)

Two basic mechanisms have to be considered for the crossing of the cell membrane barrier during reabsorption: 1. *membrane permeation*, i. e., the passage through the closed membrane without morphologically demonstrable changes, and 2. *membrane flow*, i. e., a morphologically demonstrable, directional flow process of the membrane as, e. g., vesiculation during micropinocytosis. Whether one or the other mechanism is preferentially or exclusively used will probably depend on the size of the molecule. From this point of view we have tested both the absorption spectrum of sodium- and chloride-ions and that of proteins. For the selective administration of reaction mixtures and test substances, respectively, into the lumen of the tubule we used tubular micropuncture under in vivo conditions with simultaneous or subsequent intravital fixation. Technical details and some of the results have already been reported (51, 52, 53, 55, 58).

A. Sodium$^+$ and chloride$^-$

Komnick (9) has given cytochemical methods for the contrasting of sodium and chloride. These methods are based on the precipitation of Na^+ as sodium hexahydroxo-antimonate and of Cl^- as silver chloride.

Previously, ion-contrasting had only been carried out supravitally on excised tissue specimens by immersion in the reaction mixture. In such tests carried out by Komnick and Komnick (10) on the salt-secreting gland of the gull and by Nolte (24) on the rat kidney the sodium antimonate precipitates were only found *intra*cellularly and the silver chloride precipitates only *inter*cellularly. On this basis the authors have concluded that a separate transport mechanism exists for each of these two ions.

Our own in vivo micropuncture experiments have led to the following results: Except for a partial finding which will be discussed later (Fig. 15b) the *sodium* ion contrasting turned out to be fairly variable despite manifold variations of the method (increasing the antimonate concentration in the perfusion solution to 4%, the perfusion times from 3 to 15 minutes, and utilization of the split oil-drop method). In part, the precipitates were only found intracellularly and in part they were also found in the labyrinth. A definite principle could not be recognized. This unsatisfactory result does not detract from the contrast method as such, but it shows the special conditions with which one is confronted in the in vivo use of certain cytochemical methods. This poses new basic questions which cannot be discussed in detail at this point. At present, we therefore cannot provide any new data concerning the localization of sodium.

In contrast, we did obtain uniform findings with the *chloride* ion contrasting (52): Immediately after intratubular injection of the silver lactate mixture the characteristic white precipitate of silver chloride forms in the lumen and quickly spreads to the wall of the epithelium (Fig. 14a). Even under the light-microscope the straight diffusion front of the reagent in the epithelial wall may be clearly visible (Fig. 14b). Under the electron-microscope heavy precipitates are found in the region of the labyrinthian clefts. The entire area of the terminal bars near the lumen is also clearly marked (Fig. 14c, d). In contrast to the findings obtained with the supravital immersion method, small amounts of silver precipitates can be demonstrated in the intravitally perfused renal tubules and

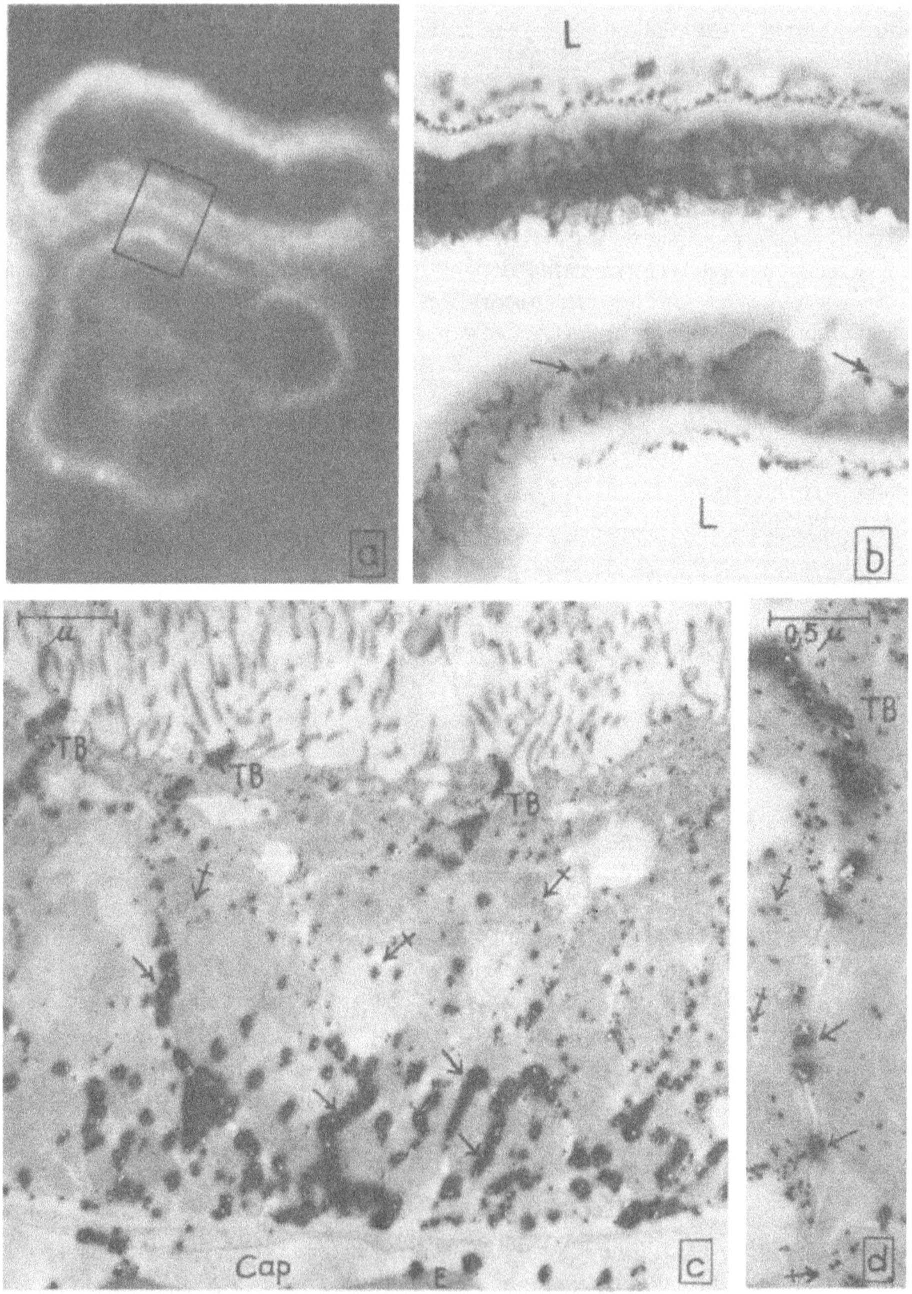

Fig. 14. Chloride-ion contrasting at the proximal convoluted tubule of the rat kidney (precipitation of the Cl^- as silver chloride by 0.25% silver lactate, 9) in vivo with the aid of tubular microperfusion. a) In the epithelial wall of the perfused proximal tubular loops white precipitation can still be recognized after embedding in the plastic. b) Two tubular loops after chloride-ion contrasting (corresponding to the section in a). The straight diffusion front of

can also be regularly demonstrated intracellularly in all regions of the cytoplasm (Fig. 14c, d) and in the cell nucleus. All findings are equally valid for the distal tubule.

Concerning the question whether the findings obtained with supravital immersion technique and with the intravital microperfusion technique differ truely or only artifactually, I would like to mention two points: 1. The precipitation density after chloride-ion contrasting in excised tissue specimens is generally, and thus also in the intercellular spaces, considerably smaller than it is after tubular microperfusion. The latter, therefore, leads to a considerably stronger reaction. To explain the difference it is important to know that during the contrasting of an excised specimen a heavy precipitate of silver chloride forms on the surface of the tissue block. The precipitation is maintained by the escape of chloride from the interior of the tissue and, in addition, retards penetration of the reagent into the inner layers of the block (1, 1a). During tubular micropuncture, on the other hand, the reagent is brought directly into contact with the epithelium of the tubule. In this manner it appears to be possible to precipitate not only the numerous extracellular but also the relatively few intracellular chloride-ions and to demonstrate them cytochemically. 2. Furthermore, it remains open for discussion whether or not the above mentioned intercellular substance (29, 49) contributes in any way (be it by "stationary" chloride binding or by the affinity of the silver components) to the preferred marking of the intercellular spaces.

We would like to make the following statements concerning the interpretation of our findings: If we assume that the chloride specificity of the reaction does exist, the result of contrasting obtained by micropuncture would mean that a relatively high chloride-ion concentration in the intercellular space is faced by a lower chloride-ion concentration inside the cell. We are thus once more faced with the problem of the transport mechanism for chloride; Komnick's (10) and also Nolte's (24) conclusion that chloride passes the epithelial wall only intercellularly is based on the selective location of the silver precipitates in the intercellular clefts after incubation of tissue specimens. Assuming that our finding is correct, i. e. that chloride does occur *intra*cellularly in significant amounts, it appears to me that the problem of the pathway for chloride is once again completely open. Taking these findings into consideration it will no longer be possible to simply deny the *trans*cellular chloride flow. We would like to limit ourselves to this statement, since anything in excess of it would mean an overinterpretation of the cytochemical results.

B. Protein

Basic studies by Miller et al. (18, 19, 20, 21), Ericsson (6), Maunsbach (15a–c) and others are available on the mechanism of cellular protein absorption in the proximal tubule as an example of a transport process by membrane flow. Nevertheless, a few

---

Fig. 14. cont'd.

the reagent in the lower loop is marked by arrows (→) L = lumen of the tubule. Light microscope, Giemsa, 1760:1. c) and d): The electron microscopic picture shows that the precipitates are deposited very densely at the terminal bars (TB) and over the intercellular labyrinth spaces (→), less densely but regularly over the cytoplasm (→). *Cap* Lumen of the capillary, *E* erythrocytes. c) 13,500:1, d) 26,000:1.

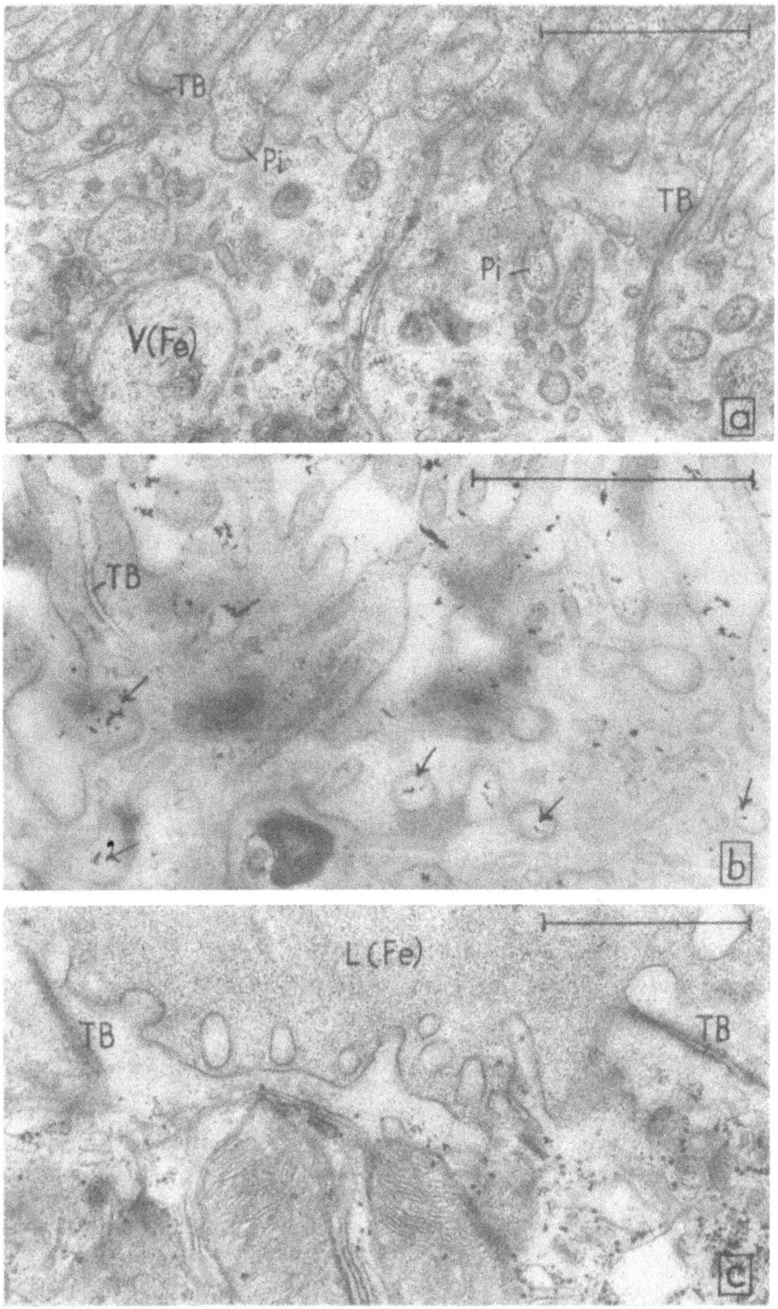

Fig. 15. a) I. phase of protein absorption in the proximal tubule: absorption of ferritin by micropinocytosis *Pi* (5 minutes after intratubular injection). Ferritin can already be demonstrated in the apical absorption vacuoles (VFe). 28,000 : 1. b) Sodium hexahydroxo-antimonate

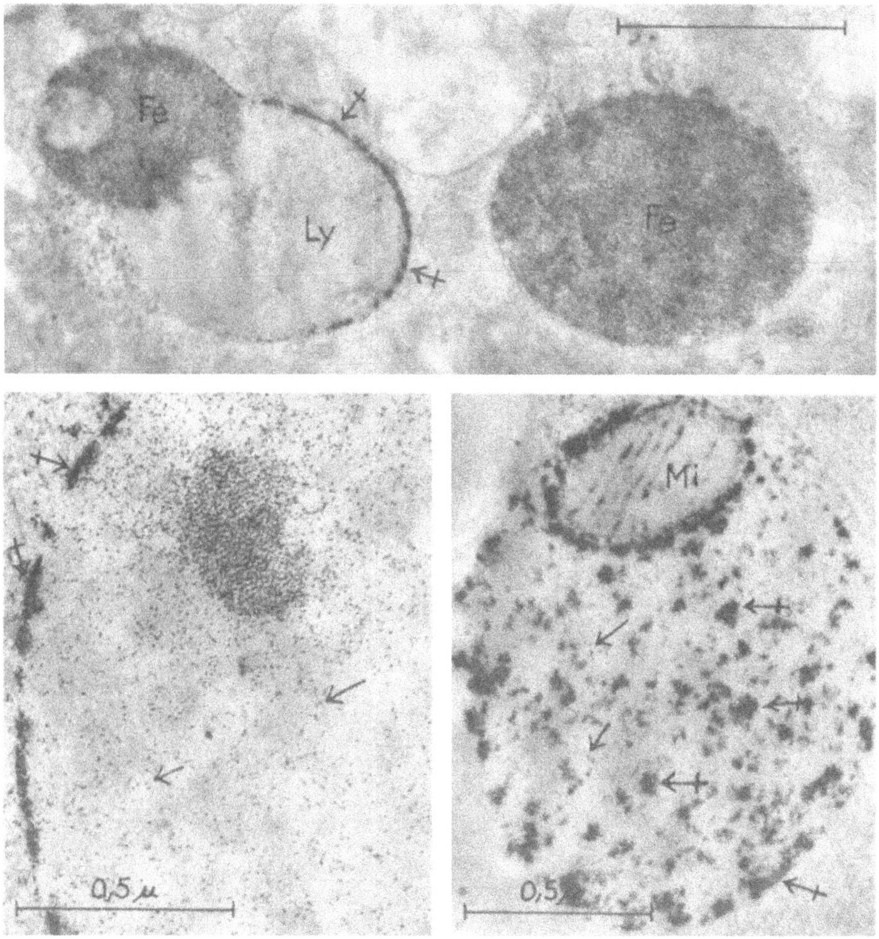

Fig. 16. II. phase of protein absorption in the epithelium of the proximal lubule (intratubular ferritin-injection, cytochemical demonstration of acid phosphatase): a) To the right, "primary" ferritin-absorption droplet (Fe), to the left, fusion of a primary ferritin droplet with a pre-existing lysosome *LY* (170 minutes after the start of absorption) 31,200:1. b) Pre-existing lysosome with incorporated ferritin droplets and ferritin molecules which are loosely distributed within the lysosomal matrix. (140 minutes after the start of absorption) 60,000:1. c) Pre-existing lysosome with a few loosely distributed ferritin molecules and an enclosed mitochondrion *Mi* (170 minutes after the start of absorption) 51,000:1. → Ferritin, ⇸ Reaction product of acid phosphatase. From studies by Thoenes, Langer, and Pfeifer (53).

Fig. 15. cont'd.

precipitates (→) in numerous micropinocytotic vesicles (after intravital tubular microperfusion for 5 minutes with 2% K [Sb $(OH)_6$] 37,500:1. c) No absorption of ferritin located in the lumen [L (Fe)] in the distal convoluted tubule (20 minutes after intratubular injection) 28,000:1. TB = terminal bars.

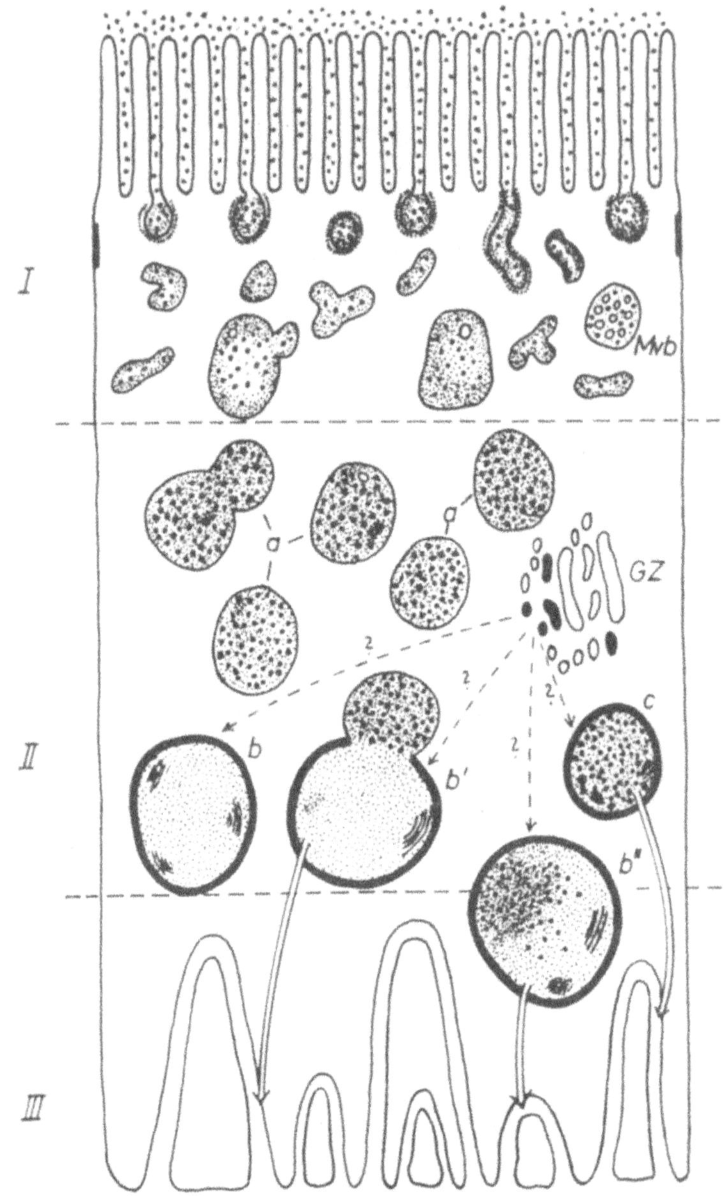

Fig. 17. Schematic diagram of cellular protein absorption in the proximal tubule. Presented on the basis of observations on ferritin-absorbing tubular epithelia of the rat kidney (53), up to 3 hours after the start of absorption (simple vacuoles are characterized by thin membranes and lysosomal vacuoles are characterized by thick membranes). *I. phase:* Micropinocytosis at the base of the brush border up to apical absorption vacuoles. *Mvb* = multivesicular body with stored ferritin. *II. phase:* a) Ferritin-filled vacuoles which have migrated in basal direction = "primary" protein absorption-droplets, b) pre-existing lysosome, b') fusion between a "primary" absorption droplet and a pre-existing lysosome; b") pre-existing lysosome with an in-

important details have remained open or are debated. Among others they concern the course of events, the relation to other cell structures and the mechanism of lysosomal digestion. We have studied these problems with the aid of the split oil droplet method (51, 53, 55). At the same time we investigated whether or not the epithelia are preserved in the tubular segments blocked by oil (58). A 10% commercial ferritin solution was used as marker protein (see also 15b). The time of absorption was varied from 2 minutes to 3 hours. Strictly morphological studies (51, 55) were combined in a second test series (together with PFEIFER, 53) with the enzyme-cytochemical demonstration of acid phosphatase as the main lysosomal enzyme, according to the method of MILLER and PALADE (21). Here we shall only emphasize the most significant results.

On the basis of the course of events and the morphologically demonstrable processes in the "vacuolar apparatus" (38) we can differentiate three phases of the cellular absorption process in the proximal tubule (Fig. 17):

The *I^st^ phase* includes the formation of membranous invaginations at the base of the brush border as well as their separation from the cell membrane and their advancement until large apical absorption vacuoles are formed (Fig. 15a, b); (18; 55a, b). These represent the end of the first phase. The transport from the lumen to the large apical vacuoles takes place very rapidly – within 2 to 5 minutes. At the moment the membrane invaginates, a characteristic "coat" is formed on the side of the cytoplasm (23, 33); this coat soon disappears. On the side of the lumen a loose, homogenous material appears into which the absorbed protein molecules become embedded. Here we are most likely dealing with mucopolysaccharides (compare 29) which are released in amounts larger than corresponding to the physiological glycocalyx, into the developing membrane invagination. Obviously their amount further increases during the following events (compare 38).

We would like to emphasize that the glycocalyx does not principally promote protein absorption. This is obvious from the fact that in the distal tubules – in contrast to the proximal ones – the luminal cell membrane shows a strong iron-colloid positive glycocalyx (28). Probably the glycocalyxes of various cell-types are chemically and thus also functionally different.

Concerning the problem whether or not low-molecular resorbates are also taken up during micropinocytosis we would like to refer to the sodium-contrast finding presented in Fig. 15b. The presence of antimonate precipitates in the pinocytosis vesicles was fairly reproducible in perfusion experiments. This must be regarded as an indication that salt and water are taken up simultaneously with the macromolecular substances. Their amount is insignificant, however, as far as the total absorption volume is concerned.

With regard to protein absorption it is worth mentioning that in the distal tubule the luminal cell membrane is quite indifferent towards the same protein, i. e., it practically

---

Fig. 17. cont'd.

corporated protein absorption-droplet. c) dense protein droplet (comparable to a) with demonstration of acid phosphatase, probably a protein absorption-drop directly transformed into a lysosome. GZ = Golgi-zone with a few acid phosphatase positive cisternae (painted black). *III. phase:* Release through the basal membrane of low-molecular fragments of the absorbed protein which were formed inside the lysosomes shown by double arrows.

fails to react with micropinocytosis (Fig. 15c) (compare 18). This observation further points at the functional difference of the luminal cell membranes in the proximal and distal tubule (compare 28).

In the *IInd phase* the ferritin-filled vacuoles or droplets now migrate considerably slower in a basal direction. The droplets reach the basal cell region after 90 to 120 minutes, at the earliest. Investigations by Miller and Palade (19, 20, 21) had very elegantly proven that the protein absorption droplets assume lysosomal status after a certain latent period of 1–2 hours. It was merely the mechanism of this process that had still been debated. Whereas Straus (42–44) and Ericsson (6) assume that the droplets are introduced into pre-existing lysosomes, Miller and Palade (21) favour a direct transformation of the primary protein absorption droplets into lysosomes. Our experiments have shown – contrary to our expectations – that regularly the "primary" ferritin-droplets indeed do merge secondarily with the lysosomes present in the cell, i. e., with the "pre-existing" lysosomes. In contrast to this, findings which could be interpreted in the sense of a direct transformation of ferritin-droplets into lysosomes were relatively rare. Fig. 16 shows ferritin-droplets before, during and after incorporation into pre-existing lysosomes (more than 2 hours after the start of absorption) and, in addition to this, it shows that the ferritin molecules after incorporation are slowly distributed in the lysosomal matrix. On the basis of the frequency with which these phenomena can be observed, we would like to conclude that the epithelia of the convoluted proximal tubule always have lytic vacuoles available in which absorbed material as well as segregated cytoplasmic material (Fig. 16c) is digested. However, a direct transformation of the protein absorption droplets into lysosomes is also possible (Fig. 17 c). Perhaps this mechanism is more predominant if the cell is charged with absorbed protein. Further investigations in this direction are necessary.

With regard to the problem where the lysosomal enzymes are formed and how they reach the lysosomes, our studies have as yet not yielded a definite answer. Consistent with previous studies (21, 25) we were frequently able to demonstrate the reaction product of acid phosphatase in the cisternae and vesicles of the Golgi-apparatus (Fig. 17, GZ). Never, however, we were able to demonstrate the migration of an acid phosphatase-positive Golgi vesicle to a pre-existing lysosome or to a (primary) ferritin-droplet. For this reason we put in Fig. 17 the question marks next to the broken arrows between the Golgizone and the lysosomes (ref. 25).

The *IIIrd phase* includes the release of the low-molecular fragments of the absorbed material which were formed in the lysosomes into the extracellular space (double-arrows in Fig. 17). On account of the small size of the molecules this process has as yet not been visualized morphologically – which is not surprising. Contrary to the findings of Reger (30), we did not observe migration of single ferritin molecules through the basal cell membrane. Despite the lack of morphological proof, the basal release of low-molecular substances formed inside the lysosomes must be regarded as certain, since the exit of entire vacuoles or smaller parts of vacuoles has never been observed in the epithelium of the renal tubules while the absorbed protein disappears from the cell. This has also been known for a long time from the corresponding pathological conditions in humans (protein nephrosis, hemoglobinuria).

The presented morphological investigations attempt to relate cell structures to the functional processes of these structures. To conclude, we would like to emphasize that the last transport mechanism discussed – protein absorption of the renal tubule – is closely related to a human disease, i. e. nephrosis. This documents a continuous transition to problems of cytopathology.

References

1. AMON, H.: Kritische Untersuchungen zum Chlorid-Nachweis im Gewebe. Verh. Dtsch. Ges. Elektronenmikroskopie Marburg 1967. Mikroskopie **23**, 126 (1968).

1a. AMON, H.: Methodische Untersuchungen zum histochemischen Nachweis von Elektrolyten. I. Die lichtmikroskopische Darstellung von Cl^-. Histochemie **14**, 168–188 (1968).

2. BENNETT, H. S.: Morphological aspects of extracellular polysaccharides. J. Histochem. Cytochem. **11**, 15–23 (1963).

3. BUCHER, O. und E. REALE: Zur elektronenmikroskopischen Untersuchung der juxtaglomerulären Spezialeinrichtung der Niere. II. Über die Macula densa des Mittelstückes. Zschr. mikr.-anat. Forsch. **67**, 514-528 (1961).

4. CURRAN, P. F. and J. R. MCINTOSH: A model system for biological water transport. Nature (London) **193**, 347–348 (1962).

5. DE DUVE, C.: Functions of microbodies (Peroxisomes). J. Cell Biol. **27**, 25A–26A (1965).

5a. DE DUVE, C. and P. BAUDHUIN: Peroxisomes (Microbodies and related particles). Physiol. Rev. **46**, 323–357 (1966).

6. ERICSSON, J. L. E.: Absorption and decomposition of homologous hemoglobin in renal proximal tubular cells. An experimental light and electron microscopic study. Acta path. microbiol. scand. Suppl. **168**, 1–121 (1964).

7. ERICSSON, J. E. and B. F. TRUMP: Electron microscopic studies of the epithelium of the proximal tubule of the rat kidney. III. Lab. Invest. **15**, 1610–1633 (1966).

8. KAYE, G. I., H. O. WHEELER, R. T. WHITLOCK and N. LANE: Fluid Transport in the rabbit gallbladder. A combined physiological and electron microscopic study. J. Cell Biol. **30**, 237–268 (1966).

9. KOMNICK, H.: Elektronenmikroskopische Lokalisation von Na^+ und Cl^- in Zellen und Geweben. Protoplasma **55**, 414–418 (1962).

10. KOMNICK, H. und U. KOMNICK: Elektronenmikroskopische Untersuchungen zur funktionellen Morphologie des Ionentransportes in der Salzdrüse von Larus argentatus V. Teil: Experimenteller Nachweis der Transportwege. Z. Zellforsch. **60**, 163–203 (1963).

11. KREBS, U. A.: Carbohydrate and fatty acid metabolism. In: Renaler Transport und Diuretica. Int. Symposion Feldafing 1968. Heidelberg/Wien/New York, Springer 1969.

12. LANGER, K. H.: Feinstrukturen der Mikrokörper (Microbodies) des proximalen Nierentubulus. Z. Zellforsch. **90**, 432–446 (1968).

13. LAPP, H. und A. NOLTE: Vergleichende elektronenmikroskopische Untersuchungen am Mark der Rattenniere bei Harnkonzentrierung und Harnverdünnung. Frankf. Z. Path. **71**, 617–633 (1962).

14. LATTA, H. and A. B. MAUNSBACH: The juxtaglomerular apparatus as studied electron microscopically. J. Ultrastruct. Res. **6**, 547–561 (1962).

15a. MAUNSBACH, A. B.: Absorption of I^{125}-labeled homologous albumin by rat kidney proximal tubule cells. J. Ultrastruct. Res. **15**, 197–241 (1966).

15b. MAUNSBACH, A. B.: Absorption of ferritin by rat kidney proximal tubule cells. Electron microscopic observations of the initiale uptake phase in cells of microperfused single tubules. J. Ultrastruct. Res. **16**, 1–12 (1966).

15c. MAUNSBACH, A. B.: Observations on the ultrastructure and acid phosphatase activity of the cytoplasmic bodies in rat kidney proximal tubule cells. J. Ultrastruct. Res. **16**, 197–238 (1966).

16. Maunsbach, A. B.: Observations on the segmentation of the proximal tubule in the rat kidney. Comparison of results from phase contrast, fluorescence and electron microscopy. J. Ultrastruct. Res. **16**, 239–258 (1966).
17. Maunsbach, A. B., S. C. Madden and H. Latta: Variations in fine structure of renal tubular epithelium under different conditions of fixation. J. Ultrastruct. Res. **6**, 511–530 (1962).
18. Miller, F.: Hemoglobin absorption by the cells of the proximal convoluted tubule in mouse kidney. J. biophys. biochem. Cytol. **8**, 689–718 (1960).
19. Miller, F.: Acid phosphatase localization in renal protein absorption droplets. In: Electron Microscopy. V. Int. Kongr. Electron Microscopy, Philadelphia Q–2. New York – London: Academic Press 1962.
20. Miller, F. und G. E. Palade: Elektronenmikroskopische und histochemische Untersuchungen an den Lysosomen der Niere. Verh. Dtsch. Ges. Path. **47**, 346–350. Stuttgart: Fischer 1963.
21. Miller, F. and G. E. Palade: Lytic activities in renal protein absorption droplets. An electron microscopical cytochemical study. J. Cell Biol. **23**, 519–552 (1964).
22. Möllendorff, W. von: Der Exkretionsapparat. In: Handb. mikr. Anat. d. Menschen Bd. VII, 1., S. 1–328. Berlin: Springer (1930).
23. Nickel, E., A. Vogel und P. G. Waser: Coated vesicles in der Umgebung der neuromuskulären Synapsen. Z. Zellforsch. **78**, 261–266 (1967).
24. Nolte, A.: Elektronenmikroskopischer Nachweis und die Lokalisation von Natrium- und Chlorionen im proximalen Tubulusepithel der Rattenniere. In: Normale und pathologische Funktionen des Nierentubulus. III. Symp. Ges. Nephrologie, S. 299–307. Bern: Huber 1965.
25. Novikoff, A. B., E. Essner and N. Quintana: Golgi apparatus and lysosomes. Fed. Proc. **23**, 1010–1022 (1964).
26. Osvaldo, L. and H. Latta: The thin limbs of the loop of Henle. J. Ultrastruct. Res. **15**, 144–168 (1966).
27. Pfeifer, U.: Pers. Mitteilung.
28. Pfeifer, U. und W. Thoenes: "Coat"-Differenzen an der luminalen Zellmembran im proximalen und distalen Tubuluskonvolut der Rattenniere. J. Microscopie **7**, 575–580 (1968).
29. Rambourg, A. and C. P. Leblond: Electron microscope observations on the carbohydrate-rich cell coat present at the surface of cells in the rat. J. Cell Biol. **32**, 27–53 (1967).
30. Reger, J. F., M. P. Hutt and H. B. Neustein: The fine structure of human hemoglobinuric kidney cells with particular reference to hyalin droplets and iron micelle localization. J. Ultrastruct. Res. **5**, 28–43 (1961).
31. Rhodin, J.: Correlation of ultrastructural organization and function in normal and experimentally changed proximal convoluted tubule cells of the mouse kidney. Stockholm: Aktiebolaget Godvil, 1954.
32. Rhodin, J.: Anatomy of kidney tubules. Int. Rev. Cytol, **7**, 485–534 (1958).
33. Roth, T. F. and K. R. Porter: Specialized sites of the cell surface for protein uptake. In: Electron Microscopy, Vol. II, LL-3. New York and London: Academic Press 1962.
34. Ruska, C.: Die Zellstrukturen des Dünndarmepithels in ihrer Abhängigkeit von der physikalisch-chemischen Beschaffenheit des Darminhalts. I. Wasser u. Natriumchlorid. Z. Zellforsch. **52**, 748–777 (1960).
35. Ruska, H., D. H. Moore and J. Weinstock: The base of the proximal convoluted tubule cells of rat kidney. J. biophys. biochem. Cytol, **3**, 249–254 (1957).
36. Ruska, H.: Der Einfluß der Elektronenmikroskopie auf die biologische Forschung. Marburger Sitz. Berichte Ges. Beförderg. Naturwissenschaften **82**, 3–40 (1959).
37. Ruska, H.: Über funktionelle Konsequenzen der Vielphasigkeit der Zelle. IV. Int. Kongr. Neuropathologie München 1961. Proc. Vol. II, 42–49 Stuttgart: Thieme 1962.
38. Schmidt, W.: Licht- und elektronenmikroskopische Untersuchungen über die intrazelluläre Verarbeitung von Vitalfarbstoffen. Z. Zellforsch. **58**, 573–637 (1962).
39. Sitte, H.: Beziehungen zwischen Zellstruktur und Stofftransport in der Niere. In: Funk-

tionelle u. morphologische Organisation der Zelle. Sekretion u. Exkretion. S. 343–370. Berlin-Heidelberg-New York: Springer (1965).

40. SJÖSTRAND, F. S.: Über die Eigenfluoreszenz tierischer Gewebe mit besonderer Berücksichtigung der Säugerniere. Acta anat. I (Suppl. 1) 1–163 (1944).

41. STEINHAUSEN, M.: Eine Methode zur Differenzierung proximaler und distaler Tubuli der Nierenrinde von Ratten in vivo und ihre Anwendung zur Bestimmung tubulärer Strömungsgeschwindigkeiten. Pflügers Arch. ges. Physiol. **277,** 23–35 (1963).

42. STRAUS, W.: Comparative observations on lysosomes and phagosomes in kidney and liver of rats after administration of horse-radish peroxidase. In: Ciba Found. Symp. on Lysosomes S. 151–175. London-New York: Churchill Ltd. (1963).

43. STRAUS, W.: Cytochemical observations on the relationship between lysosomes and phagosomes in kidney and liver by combined staining for acid phosphatase and intravenously injected horseradish peroxidase. J. Cell Biol. **20,** 497–507 (1964).

44. STRAUS, W.: Occurrence of Phagosomes and Phagolysosomes in different segments of the nephron in relation to the reabsorption, transport digestion, and extrusion of intravenously injected horseradish peroxidase. J. Cell Biol. **21,** 295–308 (1964).

45. THOENES, W.: Die Mikromorphologie des Nephron in ihrer Beziehung zur Funktion. Teil I: Funktionseinheit: Glomerulum, proximales u. distales Konv. Klin. Wschr. **39,** 504–518 (1961).

46. THOENES, W.: Zur Feinstruktur der Macula densa im Nephron der Maus. Z. Zellforsch. **55,** 486–499 (1961).

47. THOENES, W.: Transportwege in den Harnkanälchen der Säugerniere. In: Funktionelle und morphologische Organisation der Zelle. Sekretion und Exkretion. S. 315–340. Berlin-Heidelberg-New York: Springer 1965.

48. THOENES, W.: Feinstrukturen des normalen und des funktionsgestörten Nephron. Verh. Dtsch. Ges. Path. **49,** 14–45. Stuttgart: Fischer 1965.

49. THOENES, W.: Neue Befunde zur Beschaffenheit des basalen Labyrinthes im Nierentubulus. Z. Zellforsch. **86,** 351–363 (1968).

50. THOENES, W., K. HIERHOLZER und M. WIEDERHOLT: Gezielte Fixierung von Nierentubuli in vivo durch Mikroperfusion zur licht- und elektronenmikroskopischen Untersuchung. Klin. Wschr. **43,** 794–795 (1965).

51. THOENES, W. und K. H. LANGER: Eiweißresorptionsstudien am Nierentubulus (mit Hilfe intratubulärer Mikroinjektion. Verh. Dtsch. Ges. Elektronenmikroskopie Marburg 1967. Mikroskopie (Wien) **23,** 121–122 (1968).

52. THOENES, W. und K. H. LANGER: The localization of chloride ions in the proximal tubule, studied by a micropuncture method. In: Progress in Nephrology. V. Symp. Ges. Nephrologie Lausanne 1967. Berlin-Heidelberg-New York: Springer (1969).

53. THOENES, W., K. H. LANGER und U. PFEIFER: Eiweißresorption, Cytoplasmaeinschmelzung und lytische Aktivitäten im Nierentubulus. Untersuchungen am Ferritin-resorbierenden Einzeltubulus der Rattenniere. Verh. Dtsch. Ges. Path. **52,** 294–299. Stuttgart: Fischer (1968).

54. THOENES, W., K. H. LANGER und A. WARNING: Funktionsmorphologische Studien zur energetischen Insuffizienz des Nierentubulus. Klin. Wschr. **46,** 696–708 (1968).

55a. THOENES, W., K. H. LANGER und M. WIEDERHOLT: Resorption von Ferritin im proximalen Konvolut der Rattenniere (nach intratubulärer Applikation durch Mikropunktion). Klin. Wschr. **44,** 1379–1381 (1966).

55b. THOENES, W. und K. H. LANGER: Die Endocytose-Phase der Eiweißresorption im proximalen Nierentubulus. Untersuchungen am Ferritin-resorbierenden Einzeltubulus der Rattenniere. Virchows Arch. Abt. B. Zellpath. (im Druck).

56. THURAU, K. und J. SCHNERMANN: Die Natriumkonzentration an den Macula densa-Zellen als regulierender Faktor für das Glomerulumfiltrat (Mikropunktionsversuche). Klin. Wschr. **43,** 410–413 (1965).

57. ULLRICH, K. J.: Permeabilität der kortikalen Nephronabschnitte in Beziehung zu Transportvorgängen und Struktur. In: Funktionelle und morphologische Organisation der Zelle. Sekretion und Exkretion S. 392–401. Berlin-Heidelberg-New York: Springer 1965.

58. WIEDERHOLT, M., K. H. LANGER, W. THOENES und K. HIERHOLZER: Funktionelle und morphologische Untersuchungen am proximalen und distalen Konvolut der Rattenniere zur Methode der gespaltenen Ölsäule (split oil droplet method). Pflügers Arch. ges. Physiol. **302**, 166–191 (1968).
59. YOSHIMURA, F. and M. NAKAMURA: Light and electron microscopy on the proximal convoluted tubules during the postnatal development. Fol. Anat. Jap. **41**, 121–157 (1965).

THURAU: Ich möchte Herrn THOENES fragen, ob an der Zonula occludens die beteiligten Zellgrenzen fest aneinander liegen oder ob die beiden Membranen durch einen interzellulären Spalt getrennt sind. Diese Frage ist für die Transportwege bei den passiven transtubulären Flüssen von großer Bedeutung.

THOENES: Die elektronenmikroskopischen Aufnahmen geben keine Hinweise darauf, daß im Bereich der Zonula occludens noch ein Interzellularraum herkömmlichen Sinnes existiert. Man muß annehmen, daß sich in diesem Bereich die äußeren Eiweißlagen der beiden Zellmembranen direkt berühren.

HIERHOLZER: Es gibt funktionelle Unterschiede zwischen der ersten und zweiten Hälfte des distalen Konvolutes. Nach MALNIC et al. (1964) ist es z. B. die zweite Hälfte dieses Nephronabschnittes, in der die Netto-Sekretion von K^+ erfolgt. Hier ist auch die K^+-Gleichgewichtskonzentration höher als im Anfangsteil des distalen Konvolutes. Daß die K^+-Sekretion unter entsprechenden Bedingungen (Zufuhr von K^+-Salzen, Hemmung der Carboanhydratase) auch im Sammelrohrsystem weiterläuft, wurde bereits früher von uns nachgewiesen (HIERHOLZER, 1961).

BOHLE: Ich habe mehrere Fragen an Herrn THOENES:
1. Sind die Tubulusepithelien im apicalen Bereich durch Desmosomen "vernietet", oder handelt es sich bei den Desmosomen um Strukturen, die in allen Schnittebenen kontinuierlich verfolgt werden können?
2. Ist die Macula densa eine »dynamische« Struktur? Gibt es Anhaltspunkte die dafür sprechen, daß sich unter bestimmten Bedingungen Mittelstückepithelien in Maculazellen umwandeln?
3. Haben Sie im Bereich der Sammelrohre 25% Schaltzellen gezählt oder geschätzt? Ich frage deshalb, weil einer meiner Mitarbeiter (Dr. WOERNLE) bei normal ernährten und kaliummangel-ernährten Ratten im Innenstreifen der Außenzone der Nierenrinde das Verhältnis von normalen Sammelrohrepithelien zu Schaltzellen bestimmt (gezählt) und dabei gefunden hat, daß in dieser Zone 32% der Sammelrohrepithelien wie Schaltzellen aussehen (da-Fano-Versilberung).

THOENES: Zur ersten Frage: Man kann sicher sagen, daß die Schlußleisten in Lumennähe kontinuierlich sind. »Nietstellen«, die FARQUHAR als »Maculae« adhaerentes bzw. occludentes bezeichnet, sind den tieferen, also lumenfernen Zellabschnitten vorbehalten.

Zur zweiten Frage nach der Macula-densa-Struktur: An der Kontaktstelle zum Glomerulum habe ich bisher nur die hier gezeigte Zellstruktur mit wenig Mitochondrien und niedrigem Labyrinth gesehen. In diesem Bereich erscheint die Struktur recht konstant. Epithelien mit Macula-Struktur können allerdings auch auf der gegenüberliegenden, also der Glomerulum-abgewandten Seite dieses Tubulussegmentes vorkommen (Lit. 46). Dieser Befund könnte dafür sprechen, daß die üblichen distalen Tubulusepithelien gegebenenfalls in solche vom Macula-Typ umgewandelt werden können.

Und schließlich zu den Schaltzellen: Die Zahlenangaben beruhen auf zonalen Auszählungen im Verlauf des corticalen Sammelrohres. Das Verhältnis 1:3 hat sich im initialen Abschnitt des corticalen Sammelrohres ergeben, während wir im Bereich der äußeren Markzone ebenfalls ein Verhältnis von 1:2 gefunden haben. Die Schaltzellen nehmen also von proximal nach distal zu. Es besteht somit eine gute Übereinstimmung mit den von Ihnen genannten Befunden.

MERTZ: Lassen sich aus Ihren Befunden Hinweise auf die Kapazität und die Kinetik der Reabsorption von Eiweiß ableiten? Diese Frage hat u. U. Beziehung zum nephrotischen Syndrom.

THOENES: Wir haben die Eiweißresorption nur an kurzen Strecken des proximalen Konvolutes untersucht. Unter den gegebenen konstanten experimentellen Bedingungen – Ferritinangebot über eine Zeit bis zu 3 Stunden – zeigte der zelluläre Resorptionsprozeß eine Kinetik, welche in den geschilderten zwei bzw. drei Phasen zum Ausdruck kommt. Über die Kapazität des Tubulusepithels für resorbiertes Eiweiß geben die Untersuchungen keinen Aufschluß. Zweifellos stehen die Befunde in enger Beziehung zu dem Phänomen der hyalin-tropfigen Eiweißspeicherung beim nephrotischen Syndrom, worauf wir an anderer Stelle näher eingegangen sind (Lit. 53).

BURG: I would like to comment on some related work in our laboratory. We have been interested in the question of distension of the interspaces of the proximal tubule during water transport and in differences between the convoluted and straight portions of the proximal tubule. Drs. GRANTHAM, TUNE, TORMEY and ORLOFF of the National Institutes of Health collaborated in these studies.

We had previously found that the interspaces between cells of collecting tubules become distended during osmotic movement of water *in vitro* and that the distension can be readily observed both by light microscopy during the experimental measurements of water absorption and by electron microscopy.

We wanted to see if the basilar interspaces in isolated perfused proximal convoluted tubule are distended during coupled salt and water transport in a manner similar to the gall bladder. In contrast to the gall bladder, however, we found no distension either by light microscopy during measurement of normal water absorption or by electron microscopy of tubules fixed in the functioning state. This is in agreement with the findings just reported by Dr. THOENES, who found that the spaces were not distended in normal rat kidneys.

A second point concerns the morphological differences between the proximal convoluted and straight tubules. We have compared the function of these two segments experimentally and find differences in PAH transport and fluid absorption corresponding to the morphological differences shown by Dr. THOENES. I will not go into the details now since they will be included later in my formal presentation.

The Role of Sodium and Potassium ATPase in Renal Sodium Reabsorption

F. EPSTEIN

Active transport of sodium and potassium across cell membranes utilizes energy stored in the cell in the form of adenosine triphosphate. An enzymatic property of cell membranes which accelerates the breakdown of ATP in the presence of sodium and potassium has been described in many tissues and is present in the membranes of every animal cell in which it has been looked for (1). As you all know, considerable evidence has accumulated to support the concept that this sodium and potassium stimulated adenosine triphosphate is directly involved with or is part of an active cation transport system (2). This enzyme or group of enzymes catalyzes the hydrolysis of the terminal high energy bond of ATP in the presence of both sodium and potassium but not in the absence of either. The suggestion that it is linked to active transport is supported by the fact that the enzyme is located predominantly in those cellular fractions which contain the cell membranes and is selectively inhibited by digitalis glycosides which also inhibit active electrolyte transport. Most of the evidence linking sodium-potassium-ATPase to the transport of ions is derived from studies of coupled transfers of sodium and potassium in red blood cells or in red blood cell ghosts. In these cells sodium and potassium are transferred in opposite directions across the membrane. A role for sodium potassium ATPase in the bulk transfer of sodium across epithelial cell barriers, on the other hand, has not been established and has been little explored. The kidney would seem an ideal organ to test the hypothesis that sodium-potassium-ATPase is involved in the active transport of sodium since the enzymatic activity of kidney cell membranes is quite high (3) and the chief work of the kidney is the active reabsorption of sodium contained in the glomerular filtrate. The experiments which I should like to tell you about were therefore designed to investigate the possible connection between sodium-potassium-ATPase in active transport of sodium by the kidney and also by other organs (4).

I want first to say a word about the actual chemical assay. The activity of sodium-potassium-ATPase is determined by homogenizing the tissue with deoxycholate and EDTA, and incubating part of the broken cell suspension together with equimolar concentrations of magnesium and ATP in a shaking water bath at 37 degrees. The breakdown of ATP is measured by the liberation of inorganic phosphate into the medium. Sodium is present in a concentration of 100–120 millimoles per liter and potassium at 20 millimoles per liter. The activity of sodium-potassium-ATPase is determined as the difference between the inorganic phosphate liberated when both sodium and potassium are present and the amount liberated when ouabain is added, or when either sodium or potassium or both are omitted from the medium. The amount of ATP broken down when potassium is absent or when ouabain is added is referred to as residual ATPase or magnesium ATPase.

Fig. 1 shows the distribution of sodium-potassium-ATPase and residual or magnesium dependent ATPase in the different fractions of a homogenate of rat kidney. Approximately half of the sodium-potassium-ATPase activity found in the whole homogenate is present in the heavy and light microsomal fraction. The proportion of total ATPase activated by sodium and potassium was highest in the so-called light microsomes which sedimented between 39,000 and 100,000 g. and this fraction was therefore selected for subsequent assay of the enzyme.

A general method which has proved useful in elucidating the physiological role of enzymes is to correlate changes in enzymatic activity with changes in function. This has been particularly helpful in studies of the enzymes of intermediary metabolism. If traffic over a pathway catalyzed by an enzyme is augmented, the amount of enzyme within the cell and its specific activity per milligram of protein often but not always tends to increase. With a decrease in flow through the enzymatic pathway activity is frequently suppressed. Enzymes which are normally rate limiting are the most responsive to such maneuvers but enzymes which are not normally rate limiting may also change. It is clear that failure to adapt when function changes does not exclude a functional role for the enzyme system in question. The problem therefore was how to increase the reabsorptive load of sodium by the kidney by a substantial amount. Merely putting an animal on a salt free diet so that sodium disappears from the urine, or injecting aldosterone or desoxycorticosterone, changes total reabsorption of sodium very slightly. This is because the amount of sodium excreted in the urine is only a small fraction of that

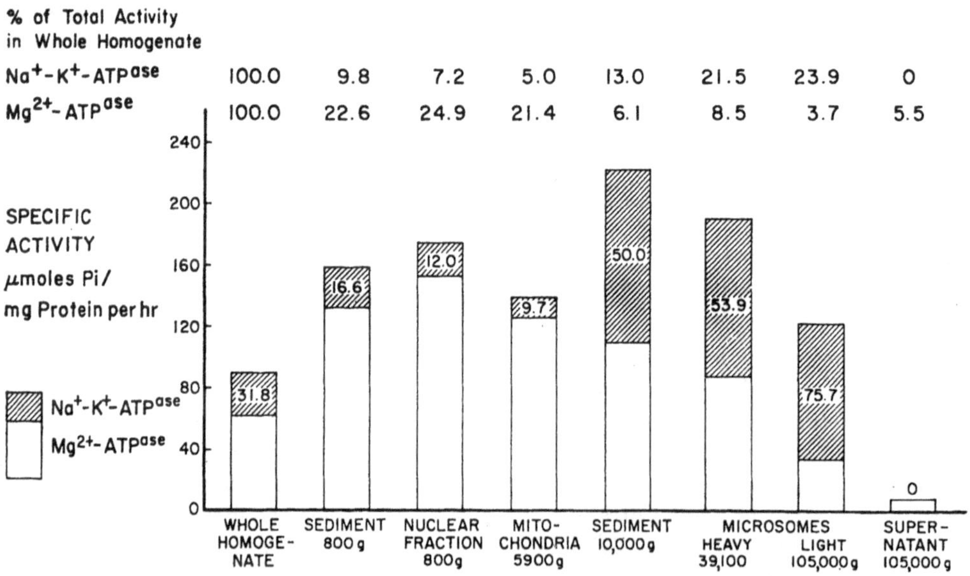

Fig. 1. Distribution of Na-K-ATPase and Mg-dependent ATPase in different fractions of a homogenate of rat kidney. Figures in the cross-hatched bars represent per cent of total activity which is stimulated by Na and K in each fraction.

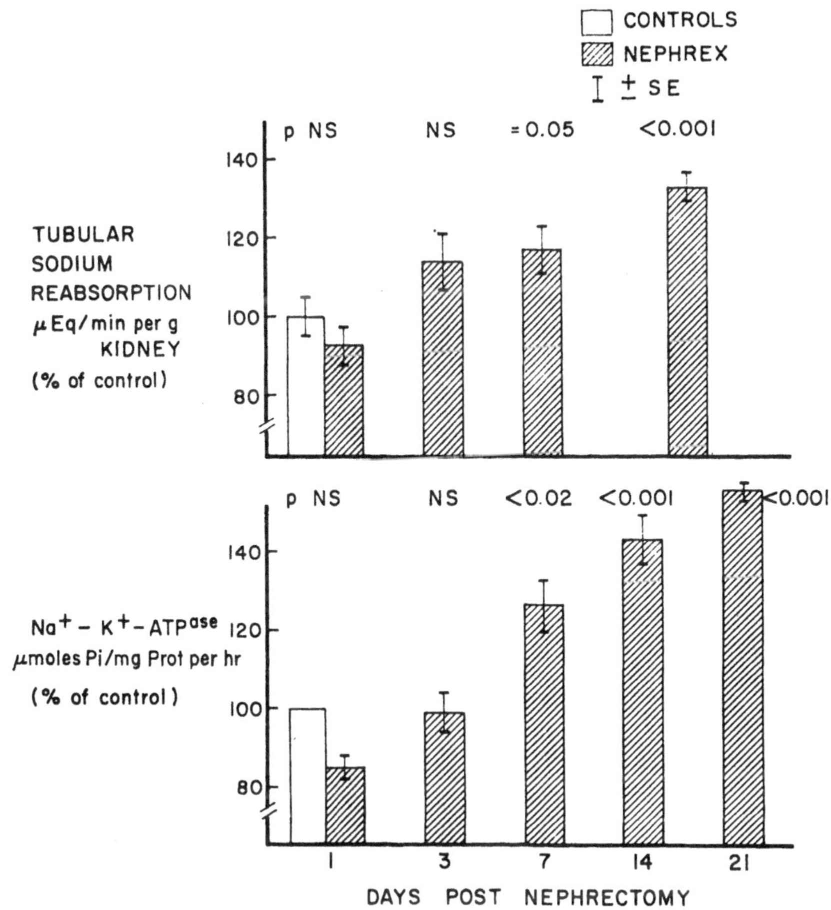

Fig. 2. The specific activity of Na-K-ATPase is compared with tubular reabsorption of sodium per gram of kidney (wet weight) at intervals after nephrectomy. Since there was no significant difference between the tubular reabsorption of sodium at 2 and 3 weeks after nephrectomy, a single average value for these periods is given.

filtered and reabsorbed. In order to change sodium reabsorption by the kidney drastically, it is necessary to change filtration rate. One way to do this is by partial nephrectomy. When one kidney is removed in the rat the opposite kidney hypertrophies and there is an increase in glomerular filtration rate. The increase in filtration rate, however, soon surpasses the increase in size so that after a few days the amount of sodium filtered per gram of kidney and the amount of sodium reabsorbed per gram of kidney is greatly increased. Fig. 2 illustrates this change in reabsorptive work and correlates it with the change in sodium-potassium-ATPase found in kidney microsomes of the remaining kidney in the course of compensatory renal hypertrophy. By three weeks after nephrectomy sodium reabsorption per gram of kidney had increased by 30 per cent. This was correlated with an increase in sodium-potassium-ATPase per milligram of microsomal protein that amounted to 40 or 50% above baseline levels. I should emphasize that the increase in sodium-potassium-ATPase per kidney was necessarily much larger than that depicted here because the kidney increased in size.

The increase in sodium-potassium-ATPase in rat kidney microsomes which occurred after nephrectomy has additional significance because it is not accompanied by changes in some other enzymes (Fig. 3). Glutaminase and succinic dehydrogenase, both mitochondrial enzymes, did not change. Two other microsomal phosphatases, glucose-6-phosphatase, and the residual or magnesium ATPase, also were unchanged after nephrectomy. The increase in sodium-potassium-ATPase that occurred with increased reabsorptive work therefore appeared to be relatively specific.

Another way to increase glomerular filtration and hence tubular reabsorption per gram of kidney tissue is by feeding rats a high protein diet. In rats fed a 50% protein diet for seven days there was also an increase in microsomal sodium-potassium-ATPase without any change in the other enzymes (Fig. 4).

The same change can be produced by giving rats methylprednisolone for 3 to 7 days as demonstrated in Fig. 5. This maneuver also increases glomerular filtration rate and sodium reabsorption and also produces an increase in sodium-potassium-ATPase. In this case glucose-6-phosphatase also increased. This was expected because of the greatly increased gluconeogenesis in the kidneys of animals treated with glucocorticoids.

After adrenalectomy, on the other hand, glomerular filtration and sodium reabsorption

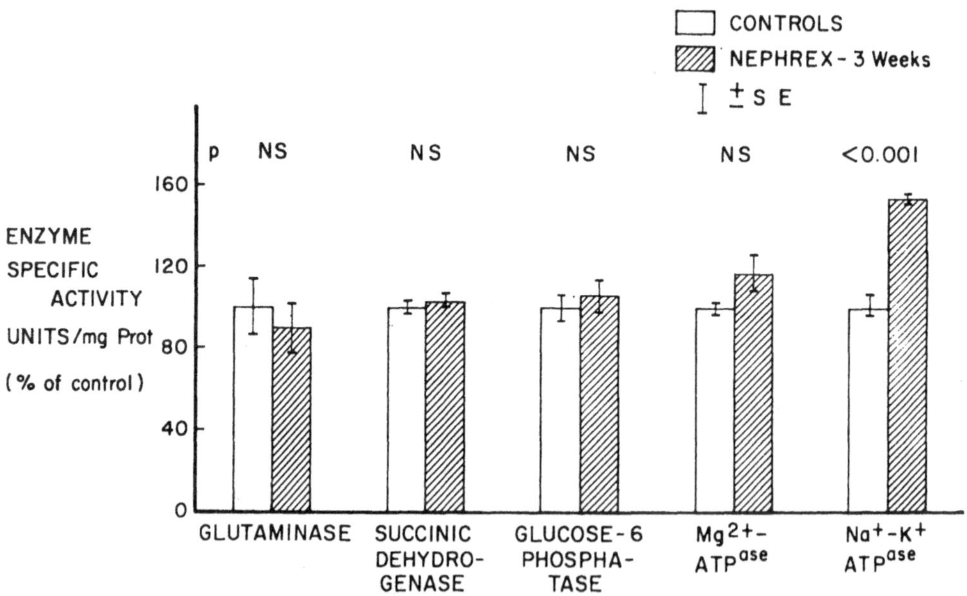

Fig. 3. Specific activity of renal enzymes in control rats 3 weeks after uninephrectomy. Glucose-6-phosphatase, Mg^{2+} ATPase, and Na-K-ATPase were assayed in the "light microsomal" fraction. Glutaminase and succinic dehydrogenase were assayed in the whole homogenate. Na-K-ATPase per milligram of microsomal protein increased in the remaining kidney after unilateral nephrectomy. There was no change in other enzymes.

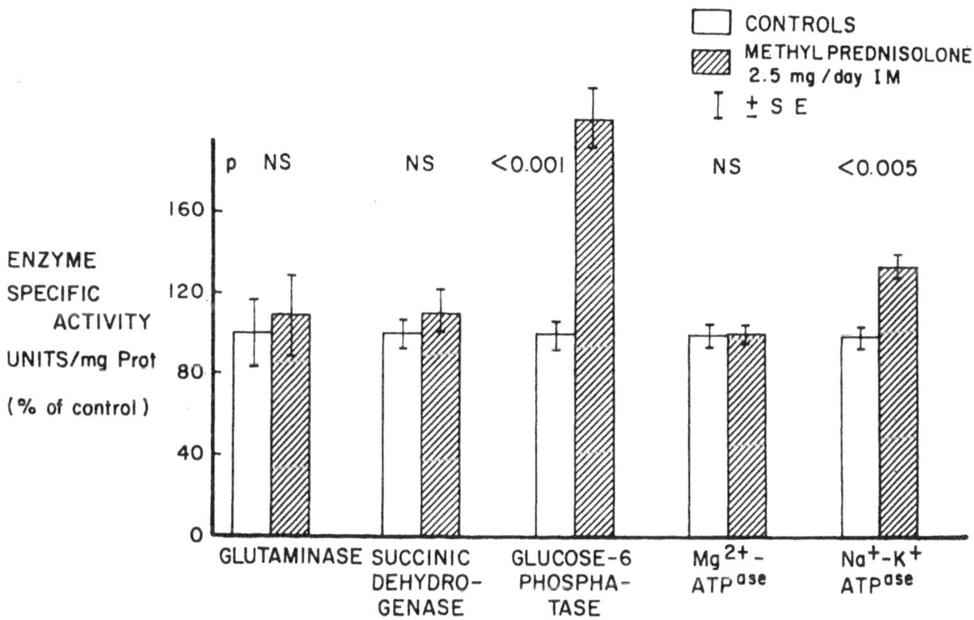

Fig. 4. Changes in specific activity of renal enzymes produced by methylprednisolone. Na-K-ATPase and glucose-6-phosphatase were increased by this large dose of glucocorticoid.

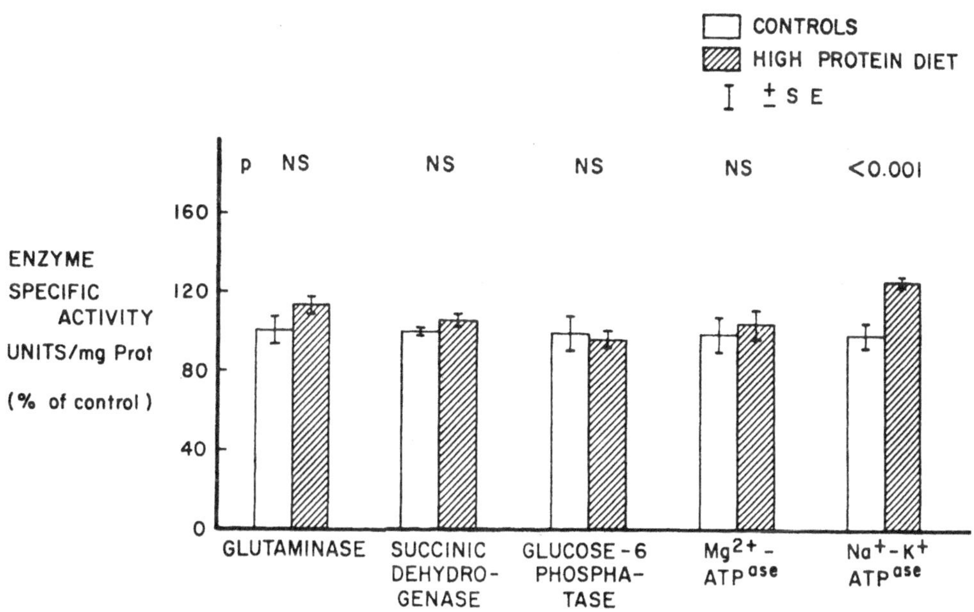

Fig. 5. Specific activity of renal enzymes in rats on a control diet (20% protein) and in rats fed a 50% protein diet for 7 days. High-protein feeding increased the specific activity of Na-K-ATPase in kidney microsomes.

both fall markedly (Fig. 6). Under these circumstances there is a decrease in sodium-potassium-ATPase in the kidney without a change in magnesium ATPase.

Might these changes in enzyme activities simply be reflections of renal hypertrophy? In order to test this, we made rats potassium deficient. Potassium-depleted rats have large kidneys with considerable increases in the specific activity of glutaminase in the whole homogenate. There is, however, no increase in glomerular filtration rate so that total sodium reabsorption is not changed. There is also no change in the specific activity of sodium-potassium-ATPase in the kidney microsomes. Similarly, rats made acidotic by feeding them ammonium chloride developed a considerable increase in glutaminase activity without evoking a change in sodium-potassium-ATPase.

The impression one gains from all these experiments is that in the rat sodium-potassium-ATPase changes in an adaptive way when renal reabsorption of sodium is chronically increased or diminished. The data therefore support the hypothesis that this enzyme system is closely involved in the process by which sodium is actively transported across the renal tubule.

Sodium-potassium-ATPase was detected in the highest concentrations in microsomes prepared from fragmented cells and it is here that changes in enzymatic activity are most marked when they are found at all. This poses a problem. The localization of enzyme activity in these small cell fragments is not easily correlated *a priori* with cation transport. There is no direct evidence that the endoplastic reticulum participates in the active movement of cations in the same way that the plasma membrane of the cell does. It seems entirely likely, however, that much of the sodium-potassium-ATPase containing

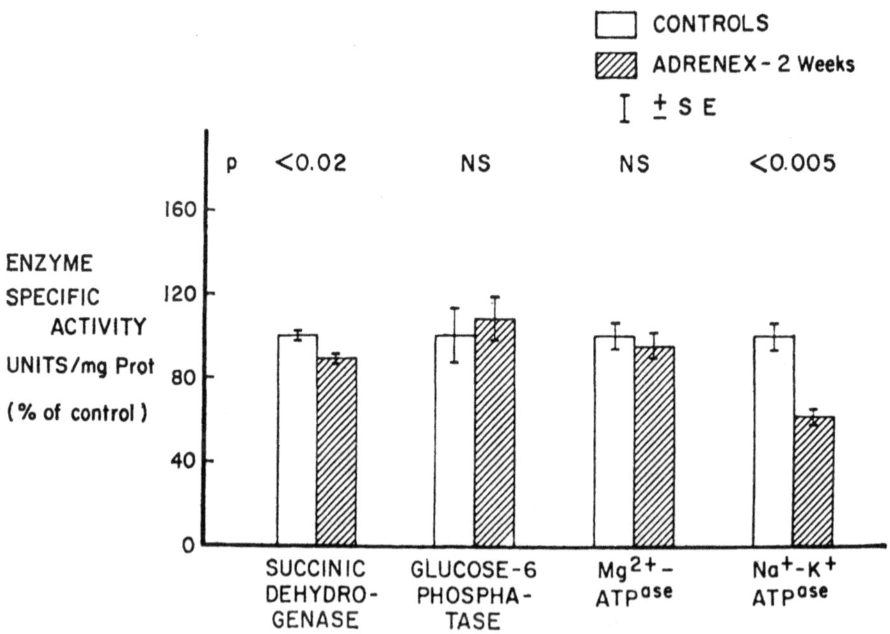

Fig. 6. Specific activity of renal enzymes after adrenalectomy. Na-K-ATPase and succinic dehydrogenase were decreased by adrenalectomy.

material in the microsomal fraction is derived from fragment of plasma membrane broken up in the homogenizing process. The microsomes prepared in the present experiments probably represent a mixture of cell membrane fragments some of which contain enzyme and some of which do not. It is therefore not possible to be entirely certain whether changes noted in the specific activity of enzyme in the microsomes reflect the specific activity of purified plasma membranes or a change in the proportion of enzyme containing membrane to non-enzyme containing material.

In order to try to approach this question Dr. ANDRZEJ MANITIUS has prepared purified plasma membrane from rat kidneys according to a modification of the technique of NEVILLE (5, 8). This involves the homogenization of tissue in distilled water and repeated washing and centrifugation of heavy membrane material with final purification on a sucrose gradient. We took a group of rats and treated them with methylprednisolone for 5 days and at the end of this time the sodium-potassium-ATPase specific activity had risen by about 50% in the whole homogenate. Despite this the specific activity of enzyme in the plasma membranes themselves was unchanged. It would appear from this experiment that the action of methylprednisolone is to increase the amount of plasma membrane per cell rather than increasing the amount of enzyme per unit of plasma membrane. This might happen, for example, if one of the changes induced by the steroid was to increase the basal infoldings of cell membrane on the antiluminal border of the tubular cell where sodium is presumably actively pumped.

The problem is not resolved by these experiments, however. The activity of Na-K-ATPase is greatly enhanced by exposing the homogenate to deoxycholate. (This is true of many enzymes bound to cell membranes) Changes induced by adrenalectomy and nephrectomy are most marked only when deoxycholate is used in the preparation. In order to prepare purified preparations of plasma membranes, on the other hand, it is necessary to homogenize tissue without deoxycholate. The technical problem of preparing adequate samples of pure plasma membranes needs some work before the real nature of the adaptive change in sodium-potassium-ATPase is resolved.

The changes which is possible to produce in transport work in the mammalian kidney are limited in magnitude. In the experiments we have just shown they amounted to perhaps 30 or 40%. Much larger changes in sodium transport can be produced in other organs when one goes outside the mammalian order. For example, the salt gland of the duck can be induced to transport enormous quantities of sodium by placing the duck on a salty diet. Under these circumstances there is a two-fold increase in sodium-potassium-ATPase activity in microsomes prepared from the gland.

The kidneys of teleost fish are another example of an organ in which large changes in sodium reabsorption can be produced. Fresh water fish must filter large quantities of fluid through their glomeruli and reabsorb almost all the sodium in order to excrete a copious dilute urine. When they are transferred to salt water glomerular circulation almost ceases, hence the reabsorptive load is very small. As you might expect, the kidneys of fish kept in fresh water have a relatively high sodium-potassium-ATPase content. When the same fish are transferred to salt water there is a decrease in the sodium-potassium-ATPase but not in the residual or magnesium ATPase.

Opposite changes take place in the gills (6). Salt water fish must continually drink sea water in order to keep from being desiccated. The burden of salt excretion falls on the gills so that the flux of sodium through the gills of salt water fish is many times higher than that through the gills of fish living in fresh water. In fish adapted for five months to fresh water the sodium-potassium-ATPase content of gill tissue is significantly lower than that from the gills of salt water adapted fish.

What do these experiments mean? I think they suggest strongly that the enzymatic activity we are measuring is closely connected with the active bulk transport of sodium across these epithelial membranes. It is quite true that in the kidney, the salt gland and the gill, there is not a reciprocal transfer of potassium across the sheet of epithelial cells in the opposite direction. But this is not a critical objection to the participation of a membrane pump analogous to that of the red cell. The sodium pump is thought to be located on the basal surface of the renal tubular cell. As sodium is pumped out potassium might be reciprocally transferred into the cell only to leak out again through the basal membrane which is known to be many times more permeable to potassium than the luminal surface of the tubular cell. That sodium reabsorption from tubular urine is to some degree dependent on the presence of potassium is suggested by the fact that perfusion of amphibian kidneys with potassium free solutions greatly reduces sodium absorption and increases the excretion of sodium in the urine (7). As Dr. LEAF has pointed out, active transport from mucosa to serosa by the toad bladder ceases when potassium is omitted from the solution bathing the serosal surface (9).

The mechanism by which enzyme activity is induced or suppressed remains unclear at present. We do not know as yet whether it is blocked by drugs which poison the manufacture of protein or of ribonucleic acid. It does seem increasingly likely that the induction of sodium-potassium-ATPase activity when sodium transport is greatly increased is a general biological phenomenon. If this proves to be correct it may help to establish an important link between the biochemical properties of cell fragments and the active movement of ions across epithelial membranes.

References

1. BONTING, S. L., L. L. CARAVAGGIO and N. M. HAWKINS: Studies on sodium-potassium-activated adenosinetriphosphatase. IV. Correlation with cation transport sensitive to cardiac glycosides. Arch. Biochem. Biophys. **98,** 413 (1962).
2. SKOU, J. C.: Enzymatic basis for active transport of Na^+ and K^+ across cell membrane. Physiol. Rev. **45,** 596 (1965).
3. LANDON, E. J. and J. L. NORRIS: Sodium- and potassium dependent adenosine triphosphatase activity in a rat kidney endoplasmic reticulum fraction. Biochem. Biophys. Acta. **71,** 266 (1963).
4. KATZ, A. I. and F. H. EPSTEIN: The role of sodium-potassium activated adenosine triphosphatase in the reabsorption of sodium by the kidney. J. Clin. Invest. **46,** 1999 (1967).
5. NEVILLE, D. J. Jr.: Biophys. Biochem. Cytol. **8,** 414 (1960).
6. EPSTEIN, F. H., A. I. KATZ and G. E. PICKFORD: Sodium and potassium activated adenosine triphosphatase of gills: Role in adaptation of teleost fish to salt water. Science, **156,** 1245 (1967).
7. VOGEL, G. and U. TERVOOREN: Die Bedeutung von Kalium für die renal-tubulären Transporte von Natrium und Calcium und für die Wirkung kardiotoner Steroide. Arch. ges. Physiol. **284,** 103 (1965).

8. MANITIUS, A., K. BEUSCH and F. H. EPSTEIN: Na-K-activated adenosine triphosphatase in kidney cell membranes of normal and methylprednisotone-treated rats. Biochem. Biophys. Acta, **150**. 563 (1968).
9. HAYS, R. M. and A. LEAF: The problem of clinical vasopressin resistance: in vitro studies. Annals Int. Med. **54**, 700 (1961).

HIERHOLZER: Dr. Ebel and Dr. DE SANTO in our group have also measured the activity of MgNa-K-ATPase in the kidneys of control rats and adrenalectomized rats. They have made the attempt to isolate not only the microsomal fraction but also a plasma cell membrane enriched fraction. In these experiments a decrease of the enzyme activity in adrenalectomized animals was *not* observed in the plasma membrane fraction, in contrast to the results obtained with the microsomal fraction. Perhaps Dr. Ebel would like to comment on this in more detail.

EBEL: From rat kidney homogenates a 700–1 200 g fraction was isolated, which was enriched with plasma cell membranes (PMF). The contamination with other subcellular fractions was evaluated by means of marker enzymes. The PMF contained only 10% microsomes. After treatment with Na-JaMgNa-K-ATPase could be demonstrated in the PMF. 80–90% of this activity was Na-K-ATPase. The properties of this enzyme resembled that of the microsomal ATPase: it was activated by Na, K in the presence of Mg and inhibited by ouabain. The enzyme exhibited a high substrate specifity; its pH optimum was in the range of 7,5.
After adrenalectomy no significant difference from controls was observed in specific ATPase activities both from the PMF and the microsomal fraction, if the animals were kept on isotonic saline. In adrenalectomized rats, maintained on tap water, the specific enzyme activities increased in the PMF but were reduced in microsomes. By kinetic studies an increase of V_{max} for MgATP, Na und K was demonstrated while K_m and the Hill-Coefficient "n" were found to be unchanged. Preliminary results obtained in experiments on six rats seem to indicate that the ATPase-activity is reduced by 7,5 μg/100 g $\times$ 24 h of d-aldosterone.
These results demonstrate a lack of direct correlation between the steroid dependent fraction of Na transport and Na-K-ATPase-activities in kidneys from adrenalectomized rats, in which local Na transport activity is inhibited in both the proximal and distal convolution, as shown previously (HIERHOLZER et al. 1966).

EPSTEIN: It may well be that what we call microsomes derive from something entirely different, from what we now call plasma membranes. I would like to ask whether you treated your microsomal fraction with sodium iodide in the same way that you did the plasma membrane fraction.

EBEL: As Chignell and Titus (1966) we have treated the microsomal fraction with desoxycholate. Plasma membranes have been treated either with desoxycholate or with sodium iodide. In both cases we observed the same qualitative changes in the plasma membrane enriched fraction.

EPSTEIN: Well, the problem of these discrepant results may well lie in the technique of preparing the membranes; that is, the variable unfolding and denaturation of membrane lipoproteins that occurs when they are treated in the unphysiological ways that are necessary to get measurable enzyme activities. It would certainly be nice if we could gently bathe them and could get out something that would act in the test tube as it did in the cell. But I suspect that the answer is connected with the variable denaturation that occurs no matter how these things are prepared.

EDELMAN: I would like to comment on the question of identification of plasma cell membranes in cell fractions. A colleague of mine, Dr. M. MAMELAK recently carried out a combined plasma membrane labelling and enzyme analysis on cell fractions of the epithelium of urinary bladder of the toad. The mucosal surface membranes were labelled with ^{3}H-polylysine (Mol. wgt. ~ 100,000) and isolations done by a method similar to that of EMMELÔT and Bos. Dr. MAMELAK found that the fraction that contained what appeared to be clean, cell envelopes had little Na^+-K^+ATP-ase-activity and only a small fraction of the ^{3}H-polylysine. The nuclear rich fraction, in contrast, was rich in both cation sensitive ATP-ase-activity and in radioactivity. Radioautographs done on these preparations by R. BOGOROCH showed that most of the radioactivity was associated with small membrane fragments and not with nuclei. These results suggest that microscopic criteria are inadequate in discrimination of plasma membranes from other membrane organelles and that varying results may be obtained from the application of a given fractionation procedure to diverse tissues. May I ask you two questions at this point: 1. Does the change in sodium transport activity precede that in enzyme activity? If so, the change in enzyme activity might only be a secondary effect of a general process rather than the determinant of the change in transport rates. 2. Are there parallel changes in ouabain-sensitive ATPase-activity and in ouabain-sensitive sodium transport?

EPSTEIN: It is clear that in the rat kidney the first thing that happens is the change in sodium transport. The changes in the specific activity of sodium potassium ATPase take place in the kidney only after a period of several days whereas it is quite clear that merely increasing filtration rate is associated with an immediate increase in the reabsorption of sodium by the renal tubules. This is consistent with the general rule that acute changes in the rate of enzymatic reactions are generally mediated by changes in substrate concentration, while over a longer period of time there is adaptation in the sense of enzyme induction or repression. In the kidney I think it is quite clear that first the traffic over the pathway increases and then it looks as if the amounts of enzymes increase.

The question whether ouabain-inhibitable sodium transport would change in the kidney is an excellent one. This is, of course, the way in which the problem has been attacked in the red cell. The difficulty about using ouabain as a tool in the intact kidney in the same way that it has been used in the red cell lies in the fact that if you get enough ouabain into the kidney to inhibit transport, the heart will stop.

BOHLE: Herr Dr. EPSTEIN, ich möchte Sie fragen, ob Sie Ihre Fermentbestimmungen (ATPase) auch an aglomerulären Teleostiern vornehmen konnten?

EPSTEIN: We are starting to measure the ATPase of the kidneys of aglomerular fish, but I do not have these results yet. The aglomerular kidney should not be devoid of enzymes concerned with transport since it carries on a great deal of secretory activity.

The Coupling of Solute and Water Transport in Epithelia

J. M. DIAMOND

The problem to be considered in this discussion is the question of how epithelial membranes such as those of the kidney proximal tubule, the intestine, the liver, and the gall bladder can form secretions and absorbates that have the same osmotic pressure as plasma. Traditionally this problem has been approached from two quite different points of view. On the one hand, physiologists have carried out experiments in which they regarded the epithelium as a black box and tried to deduce what solutes were being actively transported, to what extent water transport was coupled to solute transport, and what the coupling mechanism might be. On the other hand, anatomists have been impressed by the intricate and striking subcellular structures that one finds in fluid-transporting epithelia, such as basal labyrinths, tortuous intercellular spaces, brush borders, and systems of intracellular canals, and have speculated what role these structures might play in fluid transport. Within the past several years it has become increasingly clear that although each approach can make partial contributions, neither approach alone would be able to solve the problem, and that further progress could only come from an integrated physiological and anatomical effort. I shall present first some black-box physiological experiments to introduce the problem; then the combined physiological and anatomical experiments that Dr. JOHN TORMEY and I have been carrying out; and finally a model of fluid transport in epithelia that may help reconcile the physiological and anatomical observations.

The basic facts concerning isotonic fluid transport by epithelia are as follows. A major function of epithelia is the secretion or absorption of specific fluids that frequently differ greatly in composition from plasma. In many cases these fluids have the same osmotic pressure as plasma, that is to say, they are isotonic, and for more than a century physiologists have been fascinated by this problem of how an epithelium can manufacture a transported fluid in the absence of any external osmotic driving forces. Examples of this process are that the stomach secretes gastric juice, the proximal tubule of the kidney reabsorbs the glomerular filtrate, the gall bladder selectively reabsorbs bile, and the intestine reabsorbs the digesta. In the last century physiologists came to recognize that isotonic fluid transport by epithelia involves the consumption of metabolic energy by the epithelium: it is an active process. In the last 25 years it has been shown that this metabolic energy is channeled into active solute transport and that each epithelium specifically actively secretes or absorbs some solute (for instance, the stomach secretes hydrochloric acid, while the proximal tubule and the intestine actively absorb salts and sugars and amino acids). Within the past 10 years it has become clear that water transport is a passive and secondary consequence of active solute transport. This means that we have to rephrase the problem of isotonic water transport in the following terms:

What is the coupling mechanism by which the active transport of one solute molecule (whether that solute is a salt, an acid, or a non-electrolyte) leads to the transport of several hundred water molecules, the ratio in a solution isotonic to mammalian plasma?

The organ I have been using to approach this problem of the coupling mechanism is the gall bladder. Some words of explanation are appropriate why discussion of the gall bladder is even relevant at a symposium devoted to the kidney. The physiological function of the gall bladder is very similar to that of the proximal tubule and many other epithelia, namely, the isotonic absorption of salt and water (DIAMOND, 1962a; DIETSCHY, 1964; WHEELER, 1963). The ultrastructural anatomy of the gall bladder is basically similar to that of the proximal tubule and other epithelia. Numerous detailed parallels between the gall bladder, proximal tubule, and other epithelia indicate that the coupling mechanism between water and solute transport is probably the same in all these epithelia. The advantage of the gall bladder for studying this coupling mechanism is its physiological and anatomical simplicity. The gall bladder consists of a single large sack, in contrast to the mass of microscopic tubules in the kidney, and it has just a single active transport mechanism (for sodium chloride), in contrast to the large number of transport mechanisms in the kidney. The function of the gall bladder is selectively to reabsorb bile secreted by the liver, a function which it accomplishes by actively reabsorbing sodium chloride by means of an electrically neutral sodium chloride pump (DIAMOND, 1962b). What we are concerned with in this discussion is how water transport results from sodium chloride transport.

The experimental preparation is illustrated in Fig. 1. A gall bladder is removed from a fish or rabbit, the cystic duct is cannulated with a piece of polyethylene tubing, the gall bladder is filled with a physiological Ringer's solution and immersed in a bath of the same Ringer's solution, and the cannula is then plugged. The cannula and the gall bladder wall are very light, so that if one hangs the whole organ on a balance and weighs it, most of the weight is the fluid inside the gall bladder. As the gall bladder transports fluid from its inside to its outside, it loses weight. Thus, measurements of the weight of the gall bladder at intervals of 5 or 10 minutes provide an accurate and simple method

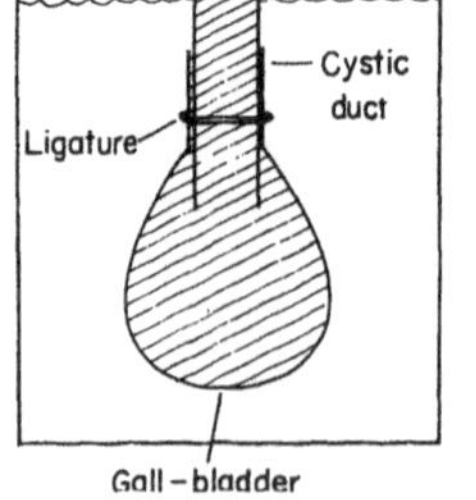

Fig. 1. An *in vitro* gall-bladder preparation in which fluid transport is followed by weighing. A cannula, with lateral flute holes to facilitate complete aspiration of luminal fluid, is ligated into the neck or cystic duct of a gall bladder. The organ is filled with Ringer's solution, and the cannula is closed by means of a glass plug to which a hook is attached. Absorption of fluid from the lumen results in a loss of weight of the whole preparation, monitored by weighing it at 5-min intervals, as illustrated in Fig. 2.

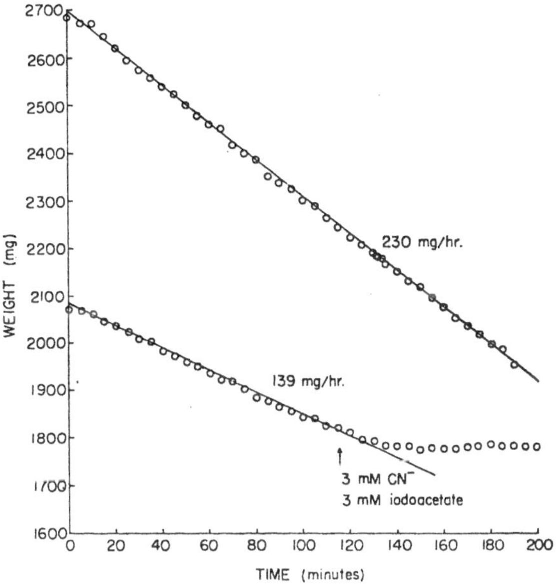

Fig. 2. Effect of cyanide plus iodoacetate on fluid absorption by two guinea-pig gall bladders *in vitro* as measured by weighing method (Fig. 1). Upper curve represents the weight at 5-min intervals of a preparation initially weighing 2 687 mg, of which 2 326 mg was the luminal fluid and 361 mg the cannula, plug, and gall-bladder wall. The linear loss of 230 mg per hour means that each hour 230 μl of luminal fluid is being transported across the gall-bladder wall into the external bathing solution. The gall-bladder preparation of the lower curve initially weighed 2 072 mg, of which 1 748 mg was luminal fluid and 324 mg was the cannula, plug, and gall-bladder wall. The preparation lost weight (reabsorbed luminal fluid) steadily for 2 hours at 139 mg per hour, but weight loss ceased after addition of 3 mM CN^- and 3 mM iodoacetate to the external bathing solution (after Diamond, 1964a).

of measuring water transport. Fig. 2 shows the results of a weighing experiment in which a guinea-pig gall bladder was filled with physiological Ringer's solution and immersed in a beaker of the same solution. Initially, the gall bladder weighed 2687 mg, of which about 2300 mg was the fluid inside the sack. When weighed at 5-minute intervals, the organ steadily lost weight at 230 mg per hour, meaning that it was transferring fluid from the inside to the outside of the sack at 230 μl per hour or reabsorbing about 10% of its volume per hour. The lower curve depicts weighing of another gall bladder which initially weighed 2072 mg; it lost weight at 139 mg per hour, meaning that fluid was absorbed at 139 μl per hour. At the end of two hours cyanide and iodoacetate were added to stop the metabolism of this second gall bladder, and its weight levelled off to a constant value, indicating that the process responsible for weight loss or fluid transport was powered by metabolism of the gall bladder, as one would expect for an active process. Analysis of the fluid left behind in the gall bladder at the end of a weighing experiment showed that NaCl as well as water was absorbed, in isotonic proportions.

This simple preparation was used to test theories of the coupling mechanism between water transport and solute transport. It became apparent that the coupling mechanism did not involve hydrostatic pressure, because the gall bladder could pump water against a hydrostatic pressure head. It did not involve electro-osmosis, because electro-osmotic forces were much too small and in the wrong direction. It did not involve pinocytosis, because if the gall bladder was filled not just with sodium chloride but with one or several of 22 other solutes, the 22 other solutes remained behind and only sodium chloride was reabsorbed (DIAMOND, 1962c and 1964a). A further possibility was that water transport depended upon external osmotic forces. Since we know that the renal proximal tubule and the gall bladder are actively reabsorbing sodium chloride, one might imagine that this reabsorption of sodium chloride lowered the osmotic pressure in the lumen of the proximal tubule or of the gall bladder, raised the osmotic pressure in the blood passing the proximal tubule or the gall bladder, and that water flowed out down this resulting external osmotic gradient. Fig. 3 shows, however, that external osmotic forces cannot be the mechanism of solute-linked water transport. This figure is based on an experiment with a fish gall bladder which was initially filled with a Ringer's solution and suspended in the same Ringer's solution. There was therefore no osmotic gradient across the organ, yet it lost weight (i. e., absorbed fluid) at 40 mg per hour. The lumen was then refilled with a solution made hypertonic by the addition of 20 m-moles of the impermeant non-electrolyte sucrose, so that the lumen was now hypertonic by half an atmosphere. If external osmotic forces had been the explanation of water transport, fluid should have flowed into the lumen, and the

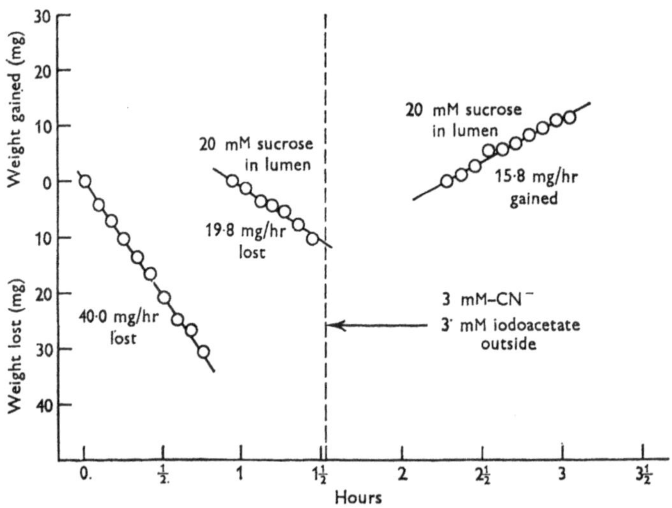

Fig. 3. Effect of osmotic gradients on water transport by a fish gall bladder. Ordinate, change in weight of the gall bladder preparation after the first weighing in each series. Weight loss means fluid movement out of the lumen, as in the first and second curves; weight gain means fluid movement into the lumen, as in the third curve. In the first curve identical Ringer's solutions were in the lumen and on the outside. In the second and third curves the luminal bathing solution contained 20 mM sucrose in addition to the usual components of Ringer's solution and was thus hypertonic. After t = 1.5 hours the metabolism of the gall bladder was stopped by addition of cyanide and iodoacetate as a neutral isotonic solution to the outer bathing fluid, to yield final concentrations of 3 mM. The third curve was thus obtained from a poisoned gall bladder (after DIAMOND, 1962c).

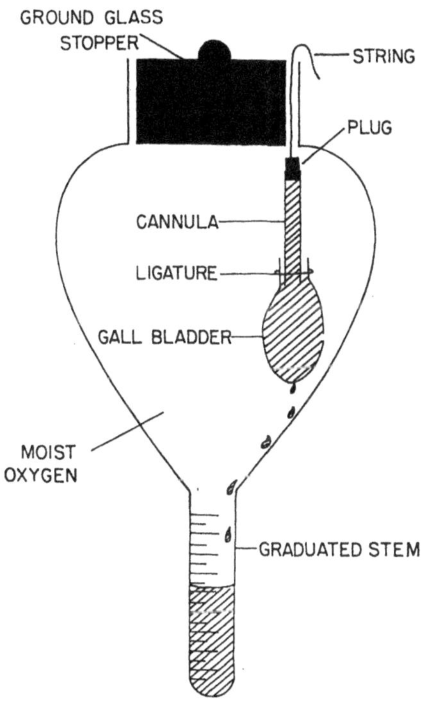

Fig. 4. "Unilateral" gall-bladder preparation. A cannulated gall bladder is suspended in a Goetz tube filled with moist oxygen, so that there is no outer bathing solution. Droplets of the pure absorbate transported out of the lumen appear on the outer surface of the gall bladder and drip off into the graduated stem. The absorbate composition may thus be determined by direct chemical analysis rather than by indirect calculations (after DIAMOND, 1964b).

organ should have gained weight. Nevertheless, the gall bladder continued to lose weight (absorb fluid), transferring fluid against the external osmotic gradient at 19.8 mg per hour. Finally, active sodium chloride transport was stopped with metabolic poisons (cyanide and iodoacetate); the same osmotic gradient – lumen hypertonic by half an atmosphere – was applied; and the organ was now found to gain weight, i. e., water flowed into the hypertonic solution, as one would expect for any non-living system. Thus, the gall bladder behaves as a simple osmometer under passive conditions, but active solute transport can carry water against an external osmotic gradient. Therefore, external osmotic forces are not the coupling mechanism. The same finding has been made in the renal proximal tubule, in the intestine, and in every other epithelium tested: external osmotic forces are not the mechanism of water transport because water can be transported against external osmotic gradients.

It is still possible, though, that osmotic forces are the explanation for water transport, but that the osmotic forces are local ones developed within the epithelium (DIAMOND, 1964b). One might imagine, for example, that sodium chloride is actively transported across the gall bladder and dumped into some small spaces near the epithelial cells, such as basal infoldings or lateral intercellular spaces. These small spaces would therefore become locally hypertonic, and fluid would cross the epithelium as a result of this local osmotic gradient. Fluid transport could then go on against external osmotic gradients until the external gradient was equal and opposite to the local osmotic gradient maintained within the epithelium by active solute transport.

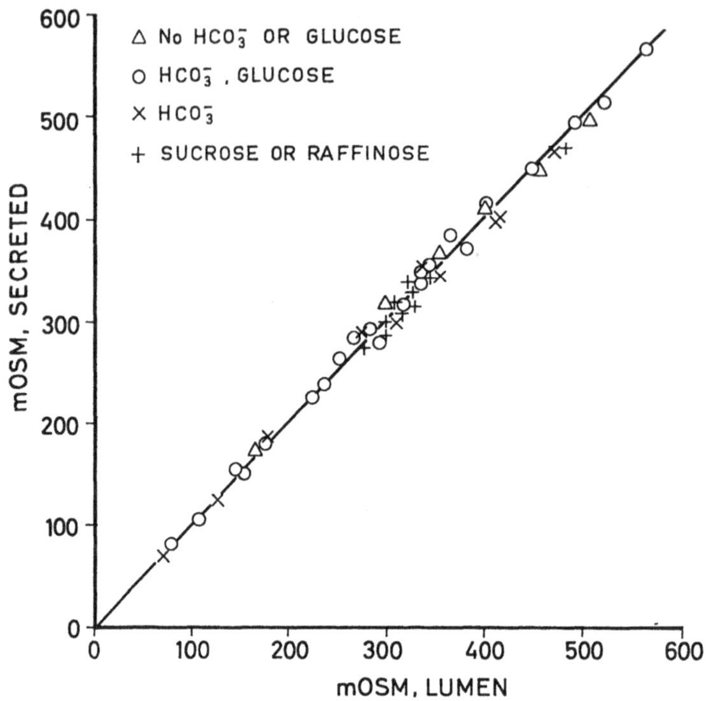

Fig. 5. Osmolarity of the fluid secreted by a rabbit gall bladder without an outer bathing solution (Fig. 4) as a function of the osmolarity of the luminal bathing solution. The straight line is the line of 45-degree slope. The luminal bathing solution was either mainly NaCl without HCO_3^- or glucose (△), NaCl with HCO_3^- and glucose (○), NaCl with HCO_3^- but no glucose (×), or NaCl plus HCO_3^- and glucose and either sucrose or raffinose (+) (after DIAMOND, 1964b).

The following experiment was devised to test whether local osmosis was the mechanism of water transport. We know that when the gall bladder is bathed in a Ringer's solution with an osmolarity of 300 m-osmol, the same osmolarity as plasma, then the absorbate is also 300 m-osmol. What would happen if the bathing solution were now 600 m-osmol, or 50 m-osmol? If local osmosis were the mechanism of water transport, water would equilibrate locally with the actively transported sodium chloride until the osmolarity of the bathing solution was attained. Thus, if the bathing solution were 600 m-osmol, the absorbate should also be 600 m-osmol. Similarly, if the bathing solution were 50 m-osmol, we should now find that the absorbate was also 50 m-osmol.

The experimental preparation devised to perform this test of local osmosis is illustrated in Fig. 4. A gall bladder is suspended in a tube filled with moist air or oxygen, not with fluid. The organ continues to transport fluid from its inside to its outside, and this fluid forms droplets which fall off the organ into the bottom of the tube. This is now the pure transported fluid elaborated by the gall bladder, and its composition can be determined directly by putting it into an osmometer or flame photometer. The experiment, then, was to vary the osmolarity of the luminal bathing solution and to observe the osmolarity of the pure transported fluid. This experiment was carried out in two ways, either by varying the sodium chloride concentration of the luminal bathing solution or by adding impermeant non-electrolytes such as sucrose or raffinose. As seen in Fig. 5, the results were the same in either case: when the bathing solution osmolarity was varied from 60 to 600 m-osmol, the osmolarity of the transported fluid varied in parallel and was identical to that of the bathing solution within the experimental error of about 1%. This result cannot be attributed to secondary equilibration within the connective tissue of an anisotonic primary transported fluid, since the measured water permeability of the gall-bladder is much too low. Thus, the primary transported fluid is always isotonic to the bathing solution whatever the bathing solution's osmolarity. The actively transported sodium chloride evidently undergoes complete osmotic equilibration with water locally within the tissue, and we can therefore say that local osmotic equilibration within the epithelium is the water-to-solute coupling mechanism in the gall bladder. The same experiment has now been carried out on the pancreas (CASE, HARPER and SCRATCHER, 1968), on the intestine (LEE, 1968), and on the Malpighian tubule of insects (BERRIDGE, 1968), with the same results. It seems likely that local osmosis is the coupling mechanism in most or all epithelia which carry out isotonic fluid transport.

In some ways, though, this conclusion raises as many problems as it solves. If the mechanism of fluid transport is local osmosis, where are the locally hypertonic regions responsible for water transport? Alternatively, one can ask: Why doesn't the actively transported sodium chloride simply diffuse out of the epithelium into the blood-stream before it can pull water across osmotically in isotonic proportions? These kinds of considerations suggested that it would be necessary to take into account the ultrastructure of the epithelium to arrive at a satisfactory solution.

At this point I had the good fortune to meet Dr. JOHN TORMEY, an electron microscopist interested in the same problem from an anatomical point of view, and we set out to do correlated physiological and anatomical experiments. Fig. 6 shows one of Dr. TORMEY's electron micrographs of rabbit gall bladder. The epithelium consists of a single layer of cells about 30 μ high. These cells have microvilli at their luminal surface, similar to those in the brush border of the proximal tubule and intestine. The cells also contain many mitochondria, whose concentration is higher at the luminal than at the basal end of the cell, a point to which I shall return (p. 93). But perhaps the most striking features of this electron micrograph are the empty spaces, the lateral intercellular spaces, separating adjacent epithelial cells from each other. These lateral intercellular spaces are closed at the luminal end by a tight junction but are open at the basal end, so that they are long and narrow dead-end channels – auf deutsch: lange und enge Sackgassen.

Our experiments consisted of studying the ultrastructure of the gall bladder under different physiological conditions (TORMEY and DIAMOND, 1967; KAYE, WHEELER, WHITLOCK and LANE, 1966). We always employed the same fixation procedure, but prior to fixation we varied the rate of transport in ten different ways – e. g., by varying temperature, by adding the transport inhibitor ouabain, by adding metabolic inhibitors, by replacing sodium with other cations, or by replacing chloride with other anions. We then looked for changes in structure correlated with changes in transport. The result was that the most striking changes in structure concerned the lateral intercellular spaces.

In transporting preparations the lateral intercellular spaces were distended (cf. Fig. 6). In preparations in which transport had been inhibited by whatever means, the lateral intercellular spaces were found to be collapsed so that the cytoplasmic projections from

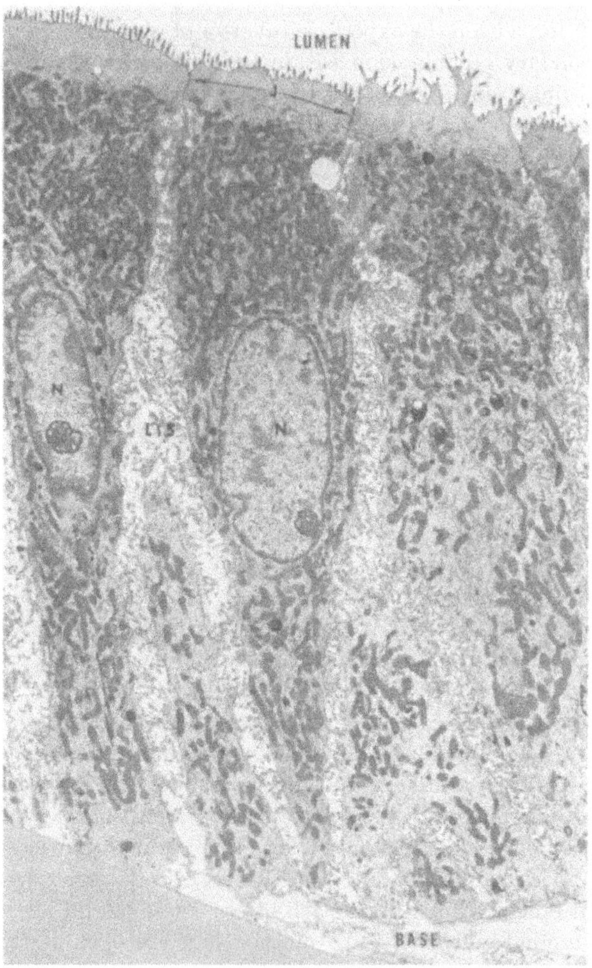

Fig. 6. Electron micrograph (2800 ×) of rabbit gall bladder epithelium, kindly provided by Dr. John M. Tormey. The lumen of the gall bladder is at the top of the picture, and the connective tissue layer begins to appear at the bottom, so that the direction of fluid transport is from top to bottom. At the luminal border (top) is an array of microvilli, followed by a short mitochondria-free zone and then by a mitochondria-rich region. The nucleus (labeled N) is visible in the middle of the left cell and the central cell. Adjacent cells are separated by clear, narrow channels, the lateral intercellular spaces (labeled LIS), into which numerous villus-like, fine, cytoplasmic projections extend from the adjacent cells. The spaces communicate with the connective-tissue layer (below), but are sealed off from the lumen (top) by tight junctions (labeled J). This gall bladder was transporting fluid; the width of the lateral intercellular spaces is slightly less than average for transporting gall bladders.

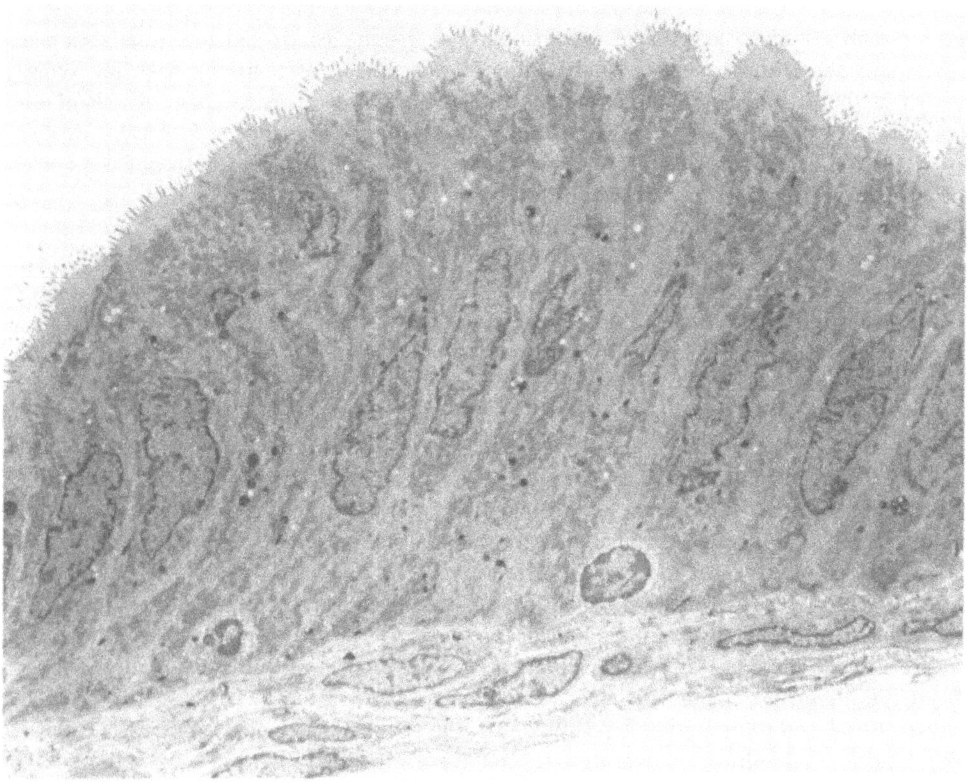

Fig. 7. Electron micrograph (2400 ×) of epithelium from rabbit gall bladder in which fluid transport had been brought to a halt by replacement of NaCl with sucrose in the luminal bathing solution; kindly provided by Dr. John M. Tormey. As compared with Fig. 6, the lateral intercellular spaces are closed so that they are hardly even visible at the magnification of this micrograph.

adjacent cells interdigitated. Fig. 7 is an electron micrograph of such a non-transporting gall bladder. It happens that the reason this particular gall bladder was not transporting was that all sodium chloride in the lumen had been replaced by sucrose. However, essentially the same picture was obtained from gall bladders whose transport had been inhibited by other means. Note that the lateral intercellular spaces are not even visible at the magnification of the electron micrograph of Fig. 7.

Prima facie, these results suggest that the route of fluid transport across the gall bladder involves the lateral intercellular spaces. But before we can jump to this conclusion, there are three questions we have to ask first. Is this conclusion simply a matter of desire influencing belief? The variability in some electron micrographs is sufficiently large that adoption of a random sampling procedure appeared desirable to substantiate one's first impression. The procedure we used was to measure off distances of 75 μ along the epithelium; at these 75-μ intervals we measured the width of the nearest intercellular space half way between lumen and base; and we did this for several dozen cells under each set of experimental conditions. The results confirmed our qualitative impressions: the transporting epithelia had lateral intercellular spaces with an average width of 0.9 μ, while non-transporting preparations had average space width of only 0.1 to 0.01 μ. One must ask next: are these results simply a fixation artifact? We obtained essentially the same results with osmium, with glutaraldehyde, and with unfixed frozen-dried preparations. More important, in any given experimental series the fixation conditions were always the same, and what was varied was only the physiological conditions and the transport rate. Finally, could these changes in the lateral spaces simply reflect changes in cell volume? For example, one might imagine that when transport is inhibited, the cells swell, pressing the spaces shut. In that case the state of the spaces would give no information about the route of fluid transport. We estimated cell volume by measuring the length and the width of the cells under various physiological conditions, and we found that, depending upon the means used to inhibit fluid transport, the cells either swelled, shrank, or remained unchanged in volume when transport was shut off. Therefore, there were no consistent changes in volume that could secondarily produce these changes in the lateral spaces. One may therefore return to the simplest interpretation, that the lateral intercellular spaces open during transport because these spaces represent the route of fluid transport.

Fig. 8 illustrates the route of fluid transport across the gall bladder deduced from these experiments. Evidently sodium chloride is continually being dumped into the lateral intercellular spaces, making them hypertonic. Water and sodium chloride enter the cells from the lumen (as suggested by other evidence: DIAMOND, 1962a; TORMEY and DIAMOND, 1967), sodium chloride is pumped into the spaces, water passes from the cells into the lateral intercellular spaces due to the resulting local osmotic gradient, and the sodium chloride and water then pass out the ends of the spaces towards the blood stream. This diagram of the route immediately answers one of the problems concerning local osmosis: the reason why sodium chloride does not simply diffuse away into the blood stream is this long diffusion pathway to the outside that holds back the salt until water can follow osmotically.

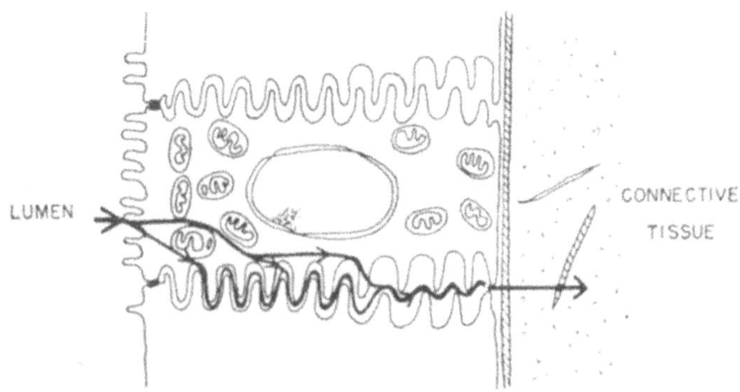

Fig. 8. Route of fluid transport across rabbit gall bladder, as deduced from combined physiological and anatomical experiments. Salt is pumped from the cells into the lateral intercellular spaces and makes them hypertonic. Water enters osmotically along the length of the spaces, distending them, and an isotonic NaCl solution emerges from the ends of the spaces facing the connective tissue (after DIAMOND and TORMEY, 1966).

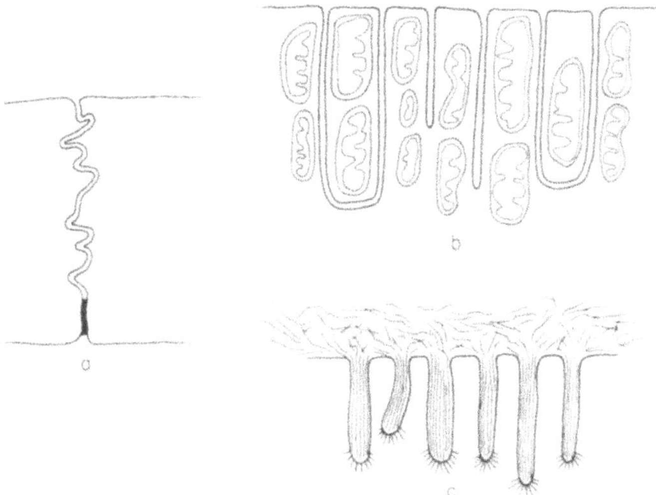

Fig. 9. Diagrammatic representation of some epithelial structures which may function as standing-gradient flow systems. (a) Lateral intercellular space (gall bladder, small intestine, large intestine, rat proximal tubule, lizard salt gland); (b) basal infoldings (ciliary body, avian salt gland, salivary gland striated duct, choroid plexus, proximal and distal tubule); (c) brush-border microvillus (gall bladder, intestine, proximal tubule, salivary gland duct). Other possible examples are intracellular canaliculi in gastric parietal cells and bile canaliculi in the liver.

In trying to work out the details of what goes on in the lateral intercellular spaces, Dr. TORMEY and I were impressed by the fact that structures of similar geometry are found in other fluid-transporting epithelia, as illustrated in Fig. 9. The essential feature of the lateral intercellular spaces is that they represent a long and narrow dead-end channel, closed in the direction from which fluid is being absorbed, but open in the direction towards which fluid is being transported. In other epithelia one finds structures with different names but with this same basic geometry of a long and narrow dead-end channel: for instance, the basal infoldings of the proximal tubule and other epithelia, the microvilli of the gall bladder, proximal tubule, and intestine, and the intracellular canaliculi of the stomach. The notion that this geometry might be important is reinforced by the complementary distribution of these structures in different organs. For example, in the salt gland of birds and the distal tubule of crocodiles the most prominent features are basal infoldings, while basal infoldings are little developed but lateral spaces prominent in the salt gland of reptiles and the distal tubule of lizards. In addition, in a number of other epithelia, such as frog skin and intestine, there are indications that these long and narrow channels distend during fluid transport as in the gall bladder, suggesting that they are the route of fluid transport. These considerations imply, then, that all these long and narrow dead-end channels may possess a common geometrical significance related to fluid transport.

Fig. 10 illustrates what this geometrical significance is likely to be (DIAMOND and TORMEY, 1966). If one has a long and narrow dead-end channel and solute is being dumped into the channel, making it hypertonic (upper half of Fig. 10), solute will diffuse down its concentration gradient towards the open end of the channel; water will flow from the outside of the channel across the channel wall into the channel lumen as a result of the osmotic gradient; and the water inflow will progressively dilute the solute

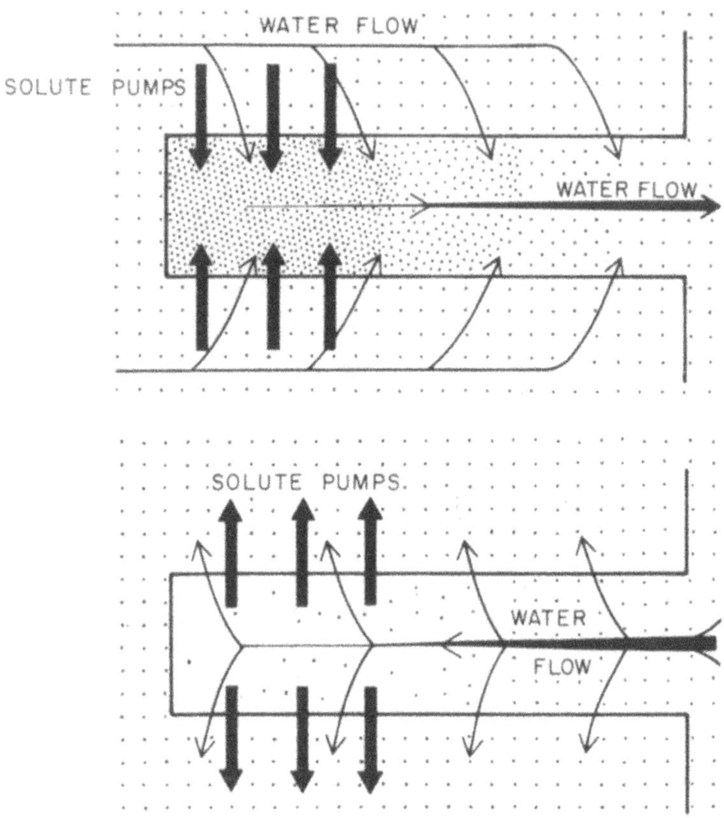

Fig. 10. Standing-gradient osmotic flow: a model for fluid transport across epithelia. Above, "forwards" operation: solute is actively transported into the channel across its walls, making the channel fluid hypertonic. As solute diffuses down its concentration gradient towards the open mouth, more and more water enters the channel across its walls due to the osmotic gradient. In the steady state a standing osmotic gradient will be maintained in the channel by solute transport, with the osmolarity decreasing progressively from the closed end to the open end; and a fluid of fixed osmolarity (isotonic or hypertonic, depending upon the values of such parameters as radius, length, and water permeability) will constantly emerge from the mouth. Below, "backwards" operation: solute is actively transported out of the channel across its walls, making the channel fluid hypotonic. As solute diffuses down its concentration gradient towards the closed end, more and more water leaves the channel across its walls owing to the osmotic gradient. In the steady state a standing osmotic gradient will be maintained in the channel by active solute transport, with the osmolarity decreasing progressively from the open end to the closed end; and a fluid of fixed osmolarity (isotonic or hypertonic, depending upon the parameters of the system) will constantly enter the channel mouth and be secreted across its walls. Solute pumps are depicted only at the bottom of the channel for illustrative purposes but may have different distributions along the channel. The density of dots indicates the solute concentration.

so that the osmolarity of the channel decreases continuously from the closed end to the open end. In the steady state this standing osmotic gradient will be maintained by active solute transport, and a fluid of fixed osmolarity, whose value depends on such factors as the permeability and length of the channel, will continually emerge from the open end. The lower half of Fig. 10 shows that if solute is continually transported out of the channel rather than dumped into it, the system works in reverse: the channel goes hypotonic, and water continually flows in the open end and moves by osmosis out of the channel across its walls. This is presumably the case in such epithelia as the choroid plexus and avian salt gland, where the channels are oriented "backwards", i. e., where the direction of fluid transport is from open end to closed end. I should emphasize that the geometry of epithelial channels makes the existence of standing osmotic gradients inevitable, provided that the channel contents are effectively unstirred.

In order to decide whether this reconstruction of events in the lateral spaces offered a quantitatively satisfactory explanation for fluid transport in epithelia, Dr. WILLIAM BOSSERT and I carried out an analysis of water-to-solute coupling in structures of this geometry (DIAMOND and BOSSERT, 1967, 1968). Using numerical values for the lengths and widths of spaces that one actually measures in electron micrographs, and using measured values for water permeability and transport rates, we analyzed coupling in a simple standing-gradient flow system consisting of a right circular cylinder closed at one end. The two differential equations describing flows and concentrations in such a system may be shown to be:

$$\frac{2\,N(x)}{r} + D\frac{d^2C}{dx^2} - C(x)\frac{dv}{dx} - v(x)\frac{dC}{dx} = 0$$

$$\frac{dv}{dx} = \frac{2\,P}{r}\,[C(x) - C_0]$$

where x = distance from the closed end, measured along the axis of the channel
L = length of the channel, so that the closed end is at $x = 0$ and the open end is at $x = L$
r = channel radius
P = water permeability or hydraulic conductivity of channel walls
D = diffusion coefficient of actively transported solute
N (x) = rate of active solute transport across the channel walls at any distance x along the channel axis
v (x) = linear velocity of water flow along the channel
C (x) = standing concentration of solute in channel at distance x
C_0 = bathing solution concentration

We want to solve this equation for the following expression, which is the osmolarity of fluid continually emerging in the steady state from the open end of the channel:

$$\frac{2\pi r \int_{x=0}^{x=L} N(x)\,dx}{\pi r^2\, v(L)}$$

Dr. BOSSERT and I carried out these calculations by computer and inserted into these equations describing a simplified standing-gradient flow system measured values of lengths and radii of lateral spaces, basal infoldings, and microvilli from electron micrographs and measured water permeabilities and transport rates in epithelia. The results are of physiological and anatomical interest and are summarized in the last six figures.

Fig. 11 illustrates the calculated standing osmotic gradients in a dead-end long and narrow channel for four particular combinations of values of the transport rate, perme-

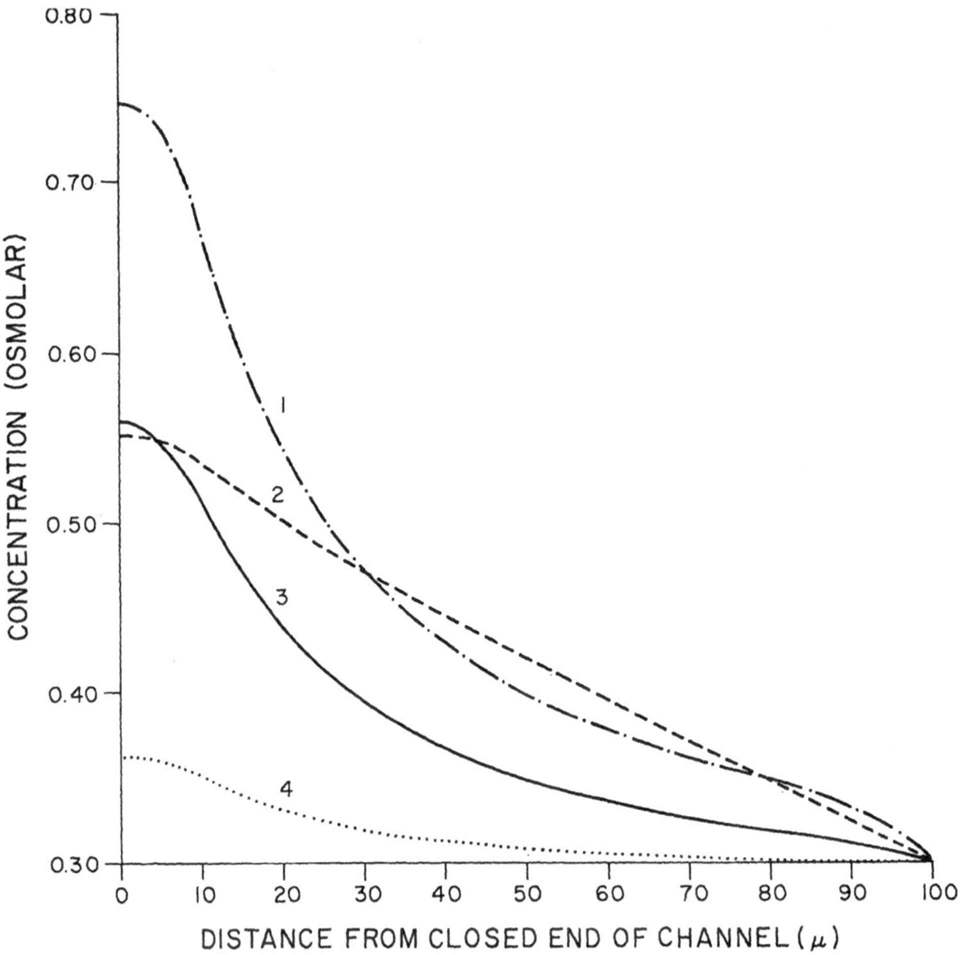

Fig. 11. Examples of concentration profiles in a standing-gradient flow system. The solute concentration in the channel in the steady state (ordinate) is plotted against x, the linear distance from the closed end of the channel (abscissa). L was held fixed at 100 μ, r at 0.05 μ, C_0 at 0.3 Osm, and D at 10^{-5} cm² per sec. N was held at 10^{-5} (curve 1), 5×10^{-6} (curve 3), or 10^{-6} (curves 2 and 4) milliosmols per cm², sec for $0 < x < 10$ μ, and at zero for $x > 10$ μ. P was held at 2×10^{-5} (curves 1, 3 and 4) or 1×10^{-6} (curve 2) cm per sec, Osm. The corresponding calculated concentrations of the emergent fluid were 0.342 (curve 1), 0.803 (curve 2), 0.318 (curve 3), and 0.304 (curve 4) Osm. (From DIAMOND and BOSSERT, 1967.)

ability, length, and radius. The bathing solution has an osmolarity of 0.3 osmol in these calculations. It is apparent that the solute concentration is highest at the closed end of the channel and decreases continually from the closed to the open end. The exact form of these standing concentration gradients depends upon the parameters of the system.

Fig. 12 shows the relation between the transported osmolarity and the length of the channel. For very long channels the transported fluid is 0.3 osmol, i. e. is isotonic to the bathing solution. The shorter the channel, the more hypertonic the transported fluid becomes. This conclusion is readily understood: the shorter the channel, the more likely solute is to diffuse away to the outside, and the shorter the length over which the osmotic

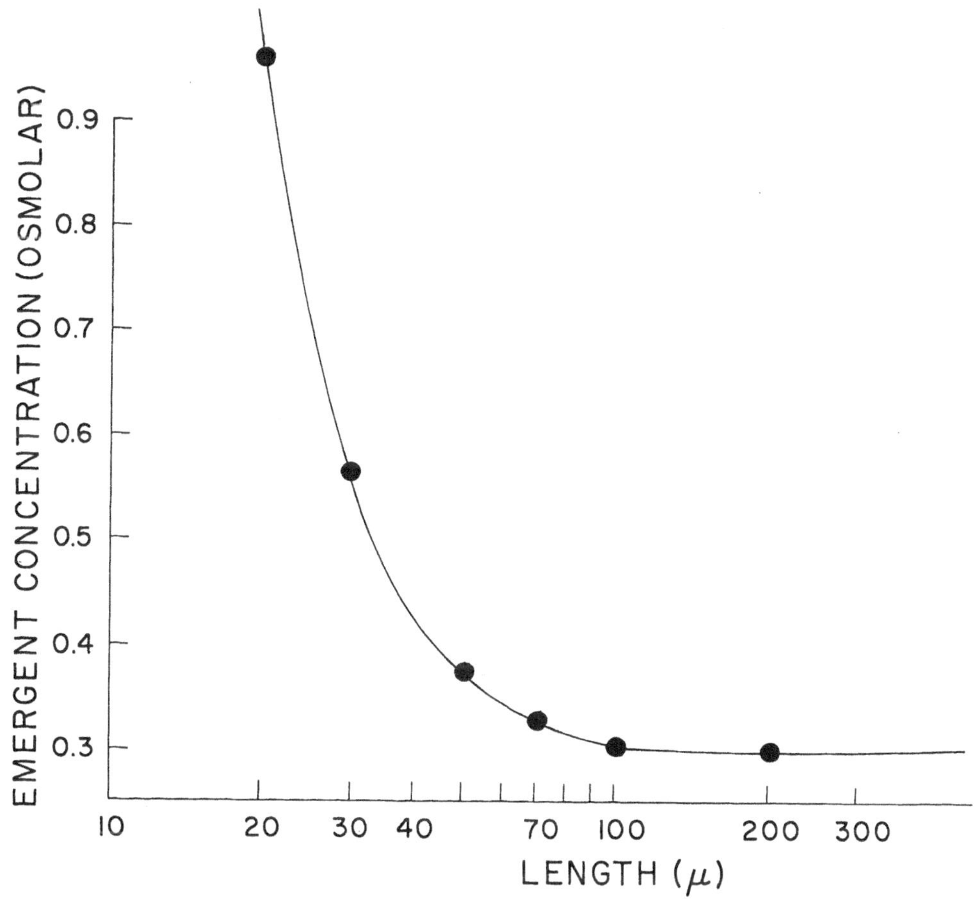

Fig. 12. The effect of varying channel length upon the osmolarity of fluid produced by a standing-gradient flow system. The parameters of the system other than length were held fixed at the following values: $P = 2 \times 10^{-5}$ cm per sec, Osm; $r = 0.05\ \mu$; $D = 10^{-5}$ cm^2 per sec; $C_0 = 0.3$ Osm; $N = 10^{-6}$ milliosmols per cm^2, sec from $x = 0$ to $x = 10\ \mu$, $N = 0$ for $x > 10\ \mu$. The abscissa is channel length plotted on a logarithmic scale. Note that the longer the channel, the more nearly isotonic (0.3 Osm) is the emergent fluid. (After DIAMOND and BOSSERT, 1967.)

gradients can pull water in, hence the more hypertonic the transported fluid. Fig. 13 shows the relation between transported osmolarity and channel radius. The calculation is carried out for two different values of the water permeability, but the results are qualitatively the same: very narrow channels with low radii have transported fluids that are isotonic, 0.3 osmol; the wider the channel, the more hypertonic the transported osmolarity becomes. This conclusion one can also understand intuitively: the smaller the radius, the smaller the volume into which a given amount of solute is dumped, the higher is the concentration set up in the channel, hence the larger the osmotic gradient and water inflow. Figs. 12 and 13 suggest why epithelia tend to have long and narrow channels: the longer and the narrower the channel, the closer is the approach to osmotic equilibrium, and the more likely one is to have isotonic transport.

Fig. 14 depicts the relation between transported osmolarity and the permeability of the channel wall. The calculation is carried out for four different values of the solute diffusion coefficient, but all four curves are qualitatively similar: for very permeable

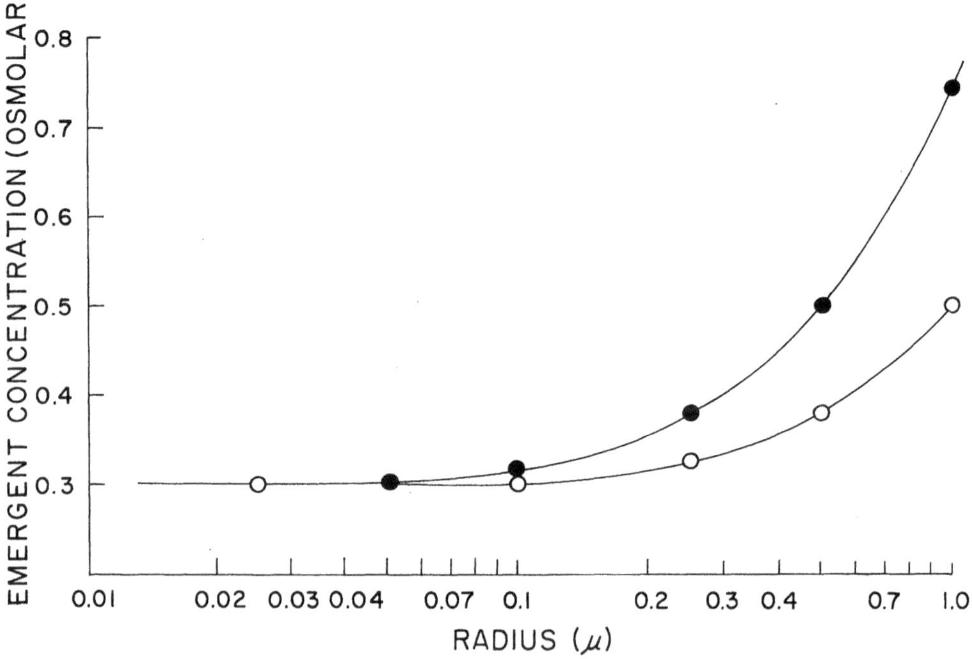

Fig. 13. The effect of varying channel radius upon the osmolarity of fluid produced by a standing-gradient flow system. L was held fixed at 100 μ, C_0 at 0.3 Osm, and D at 10^{-5} cm^2 per sec. P was held fixed at 2×10^{-5} (upper curve, solid circles) or at 4×10^{-5} (lower curve, open circles) cm per sec, Osm. From $x = 0$ to $x = 10$ μ the transport rate per unit channel length was held fixed at $\pi \times 10^{-11}$ milliosmols per cm, sec, independent of variations in r, by choosing N (the transport rate per unit wall area) as $\pi \times 10^{-11}/2\pi r$ milliosmols per cm^2, sec. At $x > 10$ μ, N was always zero. The abscissa is radius plotted on a logarithmic scale. Note that the lower the radius, the more nearly isotonic (0.3 Osm) is the emergent fluid. (After DIAMOND and BOSSERT, 1967).

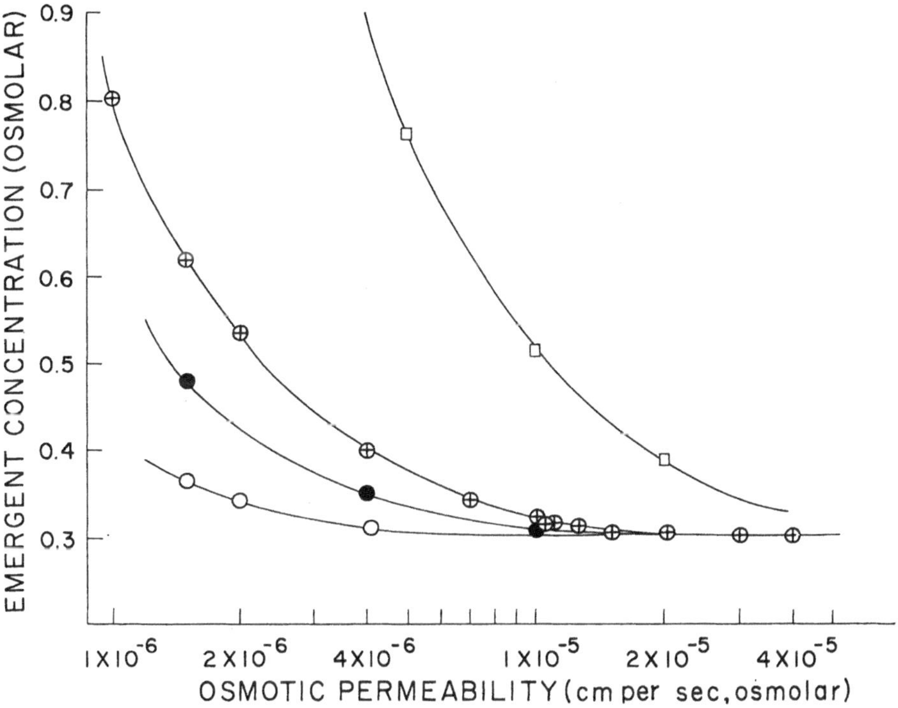

Fig. 14. The effect of varying channel water permeability upon the osmolarity of fluid produced by a standing-gradient flow system. L was held fixed at 100 μ, r at 0.05 μ, C_0 at 0.3 Osm, and N at 10^{-6} milliosmols per cm^2, sec for the range $0 < x < 10$ μ and zero for $x > 10$ μ. The abscissa is the osmotic water permeability plotted on a logarithmic scale. D was taken as 10^{-6} (○), 5×10^{-6} (●), 10^{-5} (⊕), or 5×10^{-5} (□) cm^2 per sec. Note that the higher the water permeability, the more nearly isotonic (0.3 Osm) is the emergent fluid. (After DIAMOND and BOSSERT, 1967).

channels the transported fluid is isotonic (0.3 osmol), and as the channel becomes less and less permeable, the transported fluid becomes progressively more and more hypertonic. The intuitive explanation is that the water inflow, hence the completeness of equilibration, for a given gradient is proportional to the water permeability.

Fig. 15 shows the effect of varying the site along the channel at which active solute transport takes place. When solute transport is confined to the bottom of the channel, the transported fluid is most nearly isotonic. When solute transport is extended over the whole channel, the transport becomes more and more hypertonic, the extent of this hypertonicity depending on values of other parameters such as water permeability. This suggests that, all other things being equal, isotonic equilibration is more efficient the more the pump is concentrated towards the bottom of the channel. Remembering that in gall bladder epithelial cells (Fig. 6) the density of mitochondria is highest towards the bottom of the channels (i. e., towards the luminal surface), one may interpret this in terms of efficiency of equilibration, if the distribution of mitochondria may be taken as indicative of the distribution of solute pumps.

Finally, the last figure (Fig. 16) shows perhaps the most interesting result of these calculations, the transported osmolarity as a function of transport rate. The calculation was carried out for three different values of the water permeability. For a very permeable channel ($P = 2 \times 10^{-5}$ cm/sec, Osm; points ◐ in Fig. 16) the transported fluid is isotonic (0.3 osmol) regardless of the transport rate. For a channel with lower water permeability ($P = 2 \times 10^{-6}$ cm/sec, Osm; points ● in Fig. 16) the transported fluid is hypertonic,

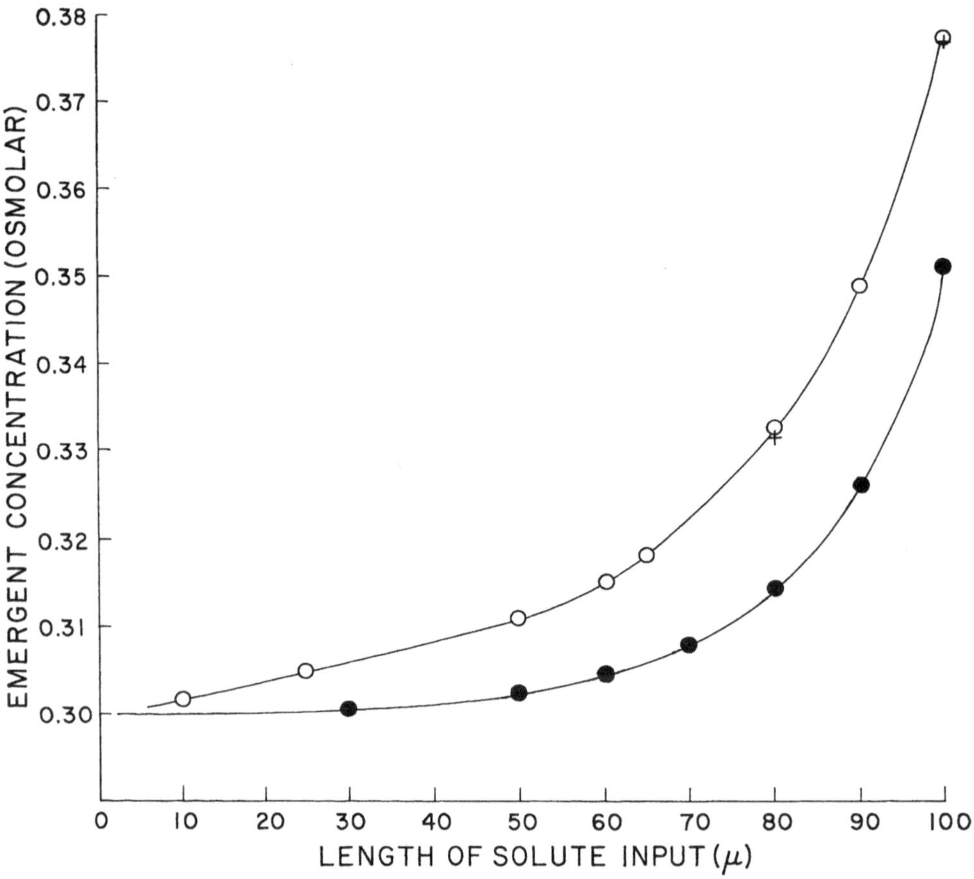

Fig. 15. The effect of solute transport site upon the osmolarity of fluid produced by a standing-gradient flow system. L was held fixed at 100 μ, r at 0.05 μ, C_0 at 0.3 Osm, and D at 10^{-5} cm² per sec. P was held at 2×10^{-5} (○ and +) or 4×10^{-5} (●) cm per sec, Osm. A given solute transport rate (N) held over a range of x from zero out to the value given on the abscissa, and N was zero for x greater than this value. The transport rate for the whole channel was held fixed at (2π rL) (10^{-8}) milliosmols per sec, by choosing N (transport rate per unit wall area) as (100) (10^{-8}) divided by the length of solute input, in milliosmols per cm², sec (○ and ●). In the two points marked by crosses N was ten times lower. Note that the shorter the length of solute input (i. e., the more the pump is concentrated towards the closed end of the channel), the more nearly isotonic (0.3 Osm) is the transported fluid. (After DIAMOND and BOSSERT, 1967.)

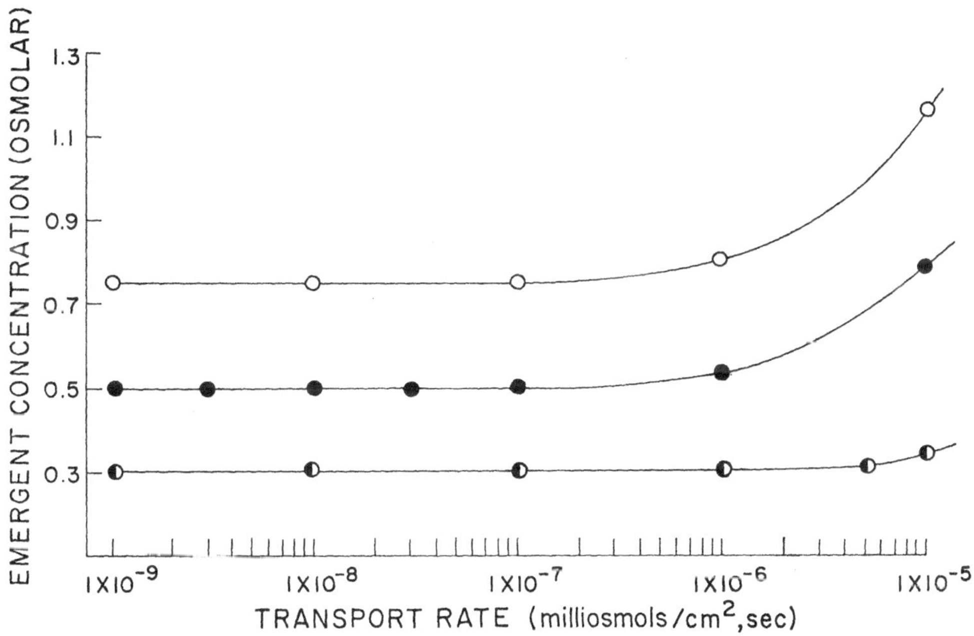

Fig. 16. The effect of varying solute transport rate upon the osmolarity of fluid produced by a standing-gradient flow system. L was held fixed at 100 μ, r at 0.05 μ, C_0 at 0.3 Osm, and D at 10^{-5} cm² per sec. P was held at 2×10^{-5} (◐), 2×10^{-6} (●), or 1×10^{-6} (○) cm per sec. The abscissa is transport rate plotted on a logarithmic scale. This value of transport rate holds in the range $0 < x < 10$ μ, and the rate is zero for $x > 10$ μ. Note that for any given value of the permeability P, the emergent concentration is virtually indepedent of transport rate as transport rate is decreased indefinitely below about 1×10^{-6} milliosmols/cm², sec. (After DIAMOND and BOSSERT, 1967.)

0.5 osmol. The interesting feature is that as the transport rate is lowered indefinitely, the hypertonicity remains the same, and the transported fluid does not approach isotonicity. Finally, when a still lower value is chosen for the water permeability ($P = 1 \times 10^{-6}$ cm/sec, Osm; points ○ in Fig. 16), the transported fluid is still more hypertonic (0.75 osmol), but again the osmolarity of the transported fluid is virtually independent of transport rate as transport rate is reduced indefinitely. The physiological interest of this slide is that it duplicates what has been a puzzling finding in hypertonically transporting organs such as the salt gland of birds and the distal tubule of the kidney. For instance, the salt gland of birds produces a hypertonic secretion, whose osmolarity Dr. K. SCHMIDT-NIELSEN (1960) found to be constant over a wide range of secretion rates. Similarly, Drs. L. DAVIS and B. SCHMIDT-NIELSEN (1967) showed that the hypertonic absorbate formed by the distal tubule of the crocodile had an osmolarity essentially independent of transport rate. I emphasize again that these findings follow inevitably from the geometry of the kind of systems we have been considering, if one accepts that the fluid in them is unstirred.

What is the meaning of these calculations? On the one hand, one can say that the physiology of water-to-solute coupling in epithelia is a geometrical consequence of epithelial ultrastructure. The peculiar rate dependence of osmolarity, and the formation of isotonic fluids, result from the presence of long and narrow dead-end channels with the particular lengths and radii found in epithelia. On the other hand, the reason why long and narrow dead-end channels consistently occur in fluid-transporting epithelia is to make possible the physiological goal of coupling water transport to solute transport. It has been customary to regard structures such as basal infoldings and microvilli as means of increasing surface area. This may be of importance, but, in addition, the geometry of these structures may be crucial in permitting water-to-solute coupling. One can make two kinds of predictions which hopefully will be tested in the next several years: 1. When adequate techniques are devised to localize the transepithelial solute pumps in epithelia, they will be found on basal infoldings and lateral spaces and microvilli. 2. When adequate techniques are devised to localize diffusable solutes such as sodium chloride, using techniques of rapid freezing to prevent solute translocation, it will be found that the lateral spaces and basal infoldings of the gall bladder and proximal tubule are hypertonic, with the osmolarity decreasing from the closed to the open end.

Let us summarize, then, these conclusions.

We have seen that a major function of epithelia such as the proximal tubule and gall bladder is the formation of specific isotonic transported fluids; that water transport is coupled to active solute transport; and that the coupling mechanism involves local osmotic equilibration within the epithelium. In the gall bladder correlated physiological and anatomical experiments show that this local osmotic equilibration takes place within the lateral intercellular spaces, which are long and narrow dead-end channels. Structures with a similar geometry are found in other fluid-transporting epithelia. All these structures may have a geometrical significance in permitting the establishment of standing osmotic gradients and hence the coupling of water transport to solute transport.

References

1. Berridge, M. J.: Urine formation by the Malpighian tubules of *Calliphora*. I. Cations. J. Exp. Biol. **48**, 159 (1968).
2. Case, R. M., A. A. Harper and T. Scratcherd: Water and electrolyte secretion by the perfused pancreas of the cat. J. Physiol. (London) **196**, 133 (1968).
3. Davis, L. E. and B. Schmidt-Nielsen: Ultrastructure of the crocodile kidney *(Crocodylus acutus)* with special reference to electrolyte and fluid transport. J. Morphol. **121**, 255 (1967).
4. Diamond, J. M.: The reabsorptive function of the gall-bladder. J. Physiol. (London) **161**, 442 (1962a).
5. Diamond, J. M.: The mechanism of solute transport by the gall-bladder. J. Physiol. (London) **161**, 474 (1962b).
6. Diamond, J. M.: The mechanism of water transport by the gall-bladder. J. Physiol. (London) **161**, 503 (1962c).
7. Diamond, J. M.: Transport of salt and water in rabbit and guinea pig gall bladder. J. Gen. Physiol. **48**, 1 (1964a).
8. Diamond, J. M.: The mechanism of isotonic water transport. J. Gen. Physiol. **48**, 15 (1964b).
9. Diamond, J. M. and W. H. Bossert: Standing-gradient osmotic flow. A mechanism for coupling of water and solute transport in epithelia. J. Gen. Physiol. **50**, 2061 (1967).
10. Diamond, J. M. and W. H. Bossert: Functional consequences of ultrastructural geometry in "backwards" fluid-transporting epithelia. J. Cell. Biol. **37**, 694 (1968).

11. DIAMOND, J. M. and J. McD. TORMEY: Studies on the structural basis of water transport across epithelial membranes. Federation Proc. **25,** 1458 (1966).
12. DIETSCHY, J. M.: Water and solute movement across the wall of the everted rabbit gall bladder. Gastroenterology **47,** 395 (1964).
13. KAYE, G. I., H. O. WHEELER, R. T. WHITLOCK and N. LANE: Fluid transport in the rabbit gall bladder: a combined physiological and electron microscopic study. J. Cell. Biol. **30,** 237 (1966).
14. LEE, J. S.: Gastroenterology, in press.
15. SCHMIDT-NIELSEN, K.: The salt-secreting gland of marine birds. Circulation **21,** 955 (1960).
16. TORMEY, J. McD. and J. M. DIAMOND: The ultrastructural route of fluid transport in rabbit gall bladder. J. Gen. Physiol. **50,** 2031 (1967).
17. WHEELER, H. O.: Transport of electrolytes and water across wall of rabbit gall bladder. Am. J. Physiol. **205,** 427 (1963).

HERMS: Dr. DIAMOND, does vasopressin also stimulate active sodium transport in the gall-bladder as it does e. g. in the frog skin or toad bladder and, if so, is the fluid reabsorbed also isotonic ?

DIAMOND: Vasopressin has no effect on transport in the gall-bladder. Other agents which affect the rate of sodium chloride transport in the gall-bladder do exist, but the fluid absorbed is isotonic under all conditions.

ULLRICH: Since you mentioned isotonic reabsorption in the kidney I want to ask you a question which arose from experiments we did recently. In these experiments on rats the lumen of a proximal tubule, as well as the surrounding capillaries were perfused with artificial solutions. The luminal perfusate was isotonic saline and the capillary perfusate contained 110 mEq/l saline and 70 mol/l raffinose. Both solutions contained 10^{-4} Ouabain, which is sufficient to block the active Na transport totally. Under these conditions, we observed an absorption of NaCl and water from the lumen which was of the same magnitude as the volume absorption in an unpoisoned tubule with Ringer's solution at both sites of the tubular wall. The absorption of NaCl and water in the Ouabain poisoned tubule was strictly isotonic. Since the standing gradient model for isotonic absorption contains an active transport mechanism which creates somewhere a local hypertonicity, I wonder how the isotonic absorption which was observed in our experiments could be explained when the Na pump was blocked. Do you think, that, besides yours, other models could account for isotonic fluid transport ?

DIAMOND: The identical phenomenon has been observed in the gall-bladder (J. Physiol. **161,** p. 511 and 517, 1962). When the pump is eliminated by metabolic poisons and a concentration gradient of sodium chloride is established so that sodium chloride moves passively down its concentration gradient, water accompanies the sodium chloride. Furthermore, the ratio of water to salt is approximately isotonic in the gall-bladder, just as you found in the kidney. There are two possible explanations for this finding. One possibility is that salt and water cross the cell membrane by the same channels and frictionally interact with each other in these channels, so that a molecule of salt drags water molecules with it. From estimates of the frictional coefficients the observed isotonic proportions are not at all unreasonable. The other possibility is that the coupling in this passive case does not involve frictional interactions within the cell membrane but instead involves local osmotic forces within the epithelium, as in the case of active salt transport: sodium chloride crossing the gall-bladder or kidney may pile up near the cell membranes and thus pull water across osmotically. One of these two explanations probably accounts for the coupling of water transport to passive salt fluxes in both the gall-bladder and the kidney.

MERTZ: Wird der aktive Transport von gelösten Bestandteilen in den Gallenblasenepithelien durch Diuretica gehemmt ?

DIAMOND: Ich habe keine Diuretica an der Gallenblase ausprobiert.

HOLZGREVE: I would like to ask Dr. DIAMOND whether his results can be used to exclude the existence of the Curran-MacIntosh double membrane model as an explanation for isotonic fluid reabsorption.

DIAMOND: The Curran-MacIntosh double-membrane model is really a local osmotic mechanism. What Curran and McIntosh showed experimentally is that when hypertonicity is established in the middle compartment of a three-compartment system, water fluxes between identical external bathing solutions may be observed. The differences between the double-membrane model and the standing-gradient model are ones which seem to be required by the more recent evidence concerning epithelial ultrastructure: namely, that the epithelial channels in which osmotic equilibration occurs are long and narrow, so that it is no longer plausible to assume that these channels are perfectly stirred; and that the basement "membrane" at the end of the channels is probably not a significant barrier to salt diffusion but that the length of the channels themselves is the barrier. If one takes into account these anatomical findings and does the calculation for unstirred channels, one obtains the predictions I've discussed.

THURAU: I would like to ask Dr. DIAMOND about the dead end of the "Sackgasse". In the proximal convolution of the kidney the net fluid reabsorption can be abolished by the intraluminal instillation of non-reabsorbable substance, e. g. mannitol. Under those conditions most of the data on permeabilities and bi-directional fluxes were established. Could you tell us whether the sodium concentration at the dead end will change when net fluid reabsorytion is zero ? If the technique of abolishing reabsorption interferes with local sodium concentrations, the data on passive transtubuıar fluxes may also be influenced.

DIAMOND: When one applies an opposing external osmotic gradient, fluid transport will stop only when the local osmotic forces within the spaces are equal and opposite to the external osmotic forces. Under these conditions I expect the salt concentration throughout the spaces, and especially at the dead end, to be higher. Some electrical observations on the gall-bladder suggest that the salt concentration in the spaces actually does rise when external osmotic gradients are applied.

Water Permeability of Different Nephron Segments in the Mammalian Kidney

K. J. ULLRICH

In order to characterize a membrane, it is of primary importance to know its permeability to water. This characteristic comprises the filtration permeability, Lp, and the diffusion permeability, P_{dH_2O} of the membrane. For the filtration permeability we may write: $Lp = \frac{Jv}{\Delta p} = \frac{Jv}{\Delta \pi}$ in which Jv is the total water flux, Δp is the hydrostatic pressure difference, and $\Delta \pi$ is the osmotic pressure difference.

For the diffusion permeability we may write $P_{dTHO} = \frac{J_{THO}}{\Delta C_{THO}}$ in which J_{THO} is the flux of tritiated water and ΔC_{THO} is the concentration difference of tritiated water.

In order to explain the variable absorption of fluid in the renal tubules during antidiuresis, water diuresis, hypercalcaemia and adrenal insufficiency, it is sufficient to know the filtration permeability alone. If, however, the diffusion permeability is also known, then the difference between diffusion and filtration permeability indicates the degree of isotope interaction (9). In the case of the flux of water through biological membranes, such an interaction is present in all instances (for ref. see Table 3). Explicit interactions are reasonably explained by "bulk-flow" of water through pores. Small degrees of interaction, however, do not necessitate the assumption of pores.

The experimental prerequisite necessary to measure the water permeability of the kidney tubules is the microperfusion method first applied by SONNENBERG and DEETJEN (25). With this method, superficial tubules of the kidney are perfused *in situ* by a micropump, and aliquot samples of the perfusate are withdrawn for analysis at variable distances from the infusion site. A great advance was made later by the method of BURG et al. (2) in which isolated kidney tubules are perfused *in vitro*. With this method it is possible to investigate all tubular segments and to vary the composition of the fluid bathing the outside of the tubules almost *ad libidum*. The last mentioned authors were the first to use perfusion rates in the range of $1 \cdot 10^{-3}$ µl/min, which is only one tenth of that used by previous investigators. Although several biological phenomena, such as the mode of action of antidiuretic hormone could be more easily investigated with the toad bladder or frog skin (6, 13, 16, 18), the microperfusion method as applied to the kidney has several advantages. The test substances under investigation have to pass only one cell layer and no connective tissue; therefore the influence of the unstirred layer is less problematic (12). Since the radius of the perfused tubules is only 8–10 µ the unstirred layer at the inner surface of the tubules could be neglected as well as the radial concentration profile within the tubule (10, 20). Using the BURG method there is an unstirred layer at the outside of the tubule which is dependent on the stirring system and therefore manageable by the experimenter. Using the SONNENBERG-DEETJEN method there is at the outside of the tubules a capillary network, in which the blood is in rapid movement. The assumption that in the latter case the outside concentration is the same everywhere and not different from the composition of the extracellular fluid is supported by the finding of CAPEK et al. (4) that in the proximal convolution $\frac{P_{^{14}C\ Urea}}{P_{Urea}}$ equals one. To calculate the permeability of ^{14}C labelled urea ($P_{^{14}C\ Urea}$) an outside concentration of zero was used in the calculation; to determine the permeability of unlabelled urea (P_{Urea}) the urea concentration within the systemic blood was used for the outside concentration.

The data for the filtration permeability summarized in Table 1 and 2, were evaluated by three different methods. With the first and second method the tubules were perfused *in situ* by solutions which contained the sodium "equilibrium concentration" i. e. those sodium concentrations at which the sodium net transport becomes zero (14). Raffinose or mannitol were added so that the perfusate was slightly hyper- or hypotonic with respect to the interstitial fluid. With the first method only the freezing points were determined and the filtration permeabilities were calculated with the simplifying assumption that the osmotic equilibration between the perfusate and the interstitial fluid takes

Table 1. Filtration coefficient in the *proximal convolution* of rats. The test solutions (tubular perfusates) contained NaCl and/or Raffinose or mannitol. This is indicated in the column "Test Solutions". The different test solutions used to get one Lp value are connected by brackets.

Experimental Condition	Lp 10^{-8} $cm^3/cm^2 \cdot sec \cdot cm\ H_2O$	Number of Perfusions	Test-Solutions NaCl mEq/l	Raffinose (R) Mannitol (M) in mmol/l	Reference
Antidiuresis	17.4	19	100	50 (R)	ULLRICH et al. (27)
			115	20 (M)	
Water diuresis (Diabetes insipidus)	15.8	18	100	160–180 (M)	
			120	140 (M)	
Antidiuresis + EDTA 20 meq/l in the perfusate	16.0	21	100	140 (M)	LASSITER et al. (17)
			110	30 (M)	
Antidiuresis + $CaCl_2$ 15 mEq/l in the perfusate	17.6	17	110	100 (M)	
			110	–	
Antidiuresis	19.2	17	100	50 (M)	STOLTE, et al. (26)
Adrenalectomy	20.9	16	100	20 (M)	
Antidiuresis	21.0*)	24	115 (R)–250 (R)		ULLRICH et al. (29)
	3.8*)	24	250 (R)–370 (R)		

*) These values are measured with method No. 3, all other values with method No. 1.

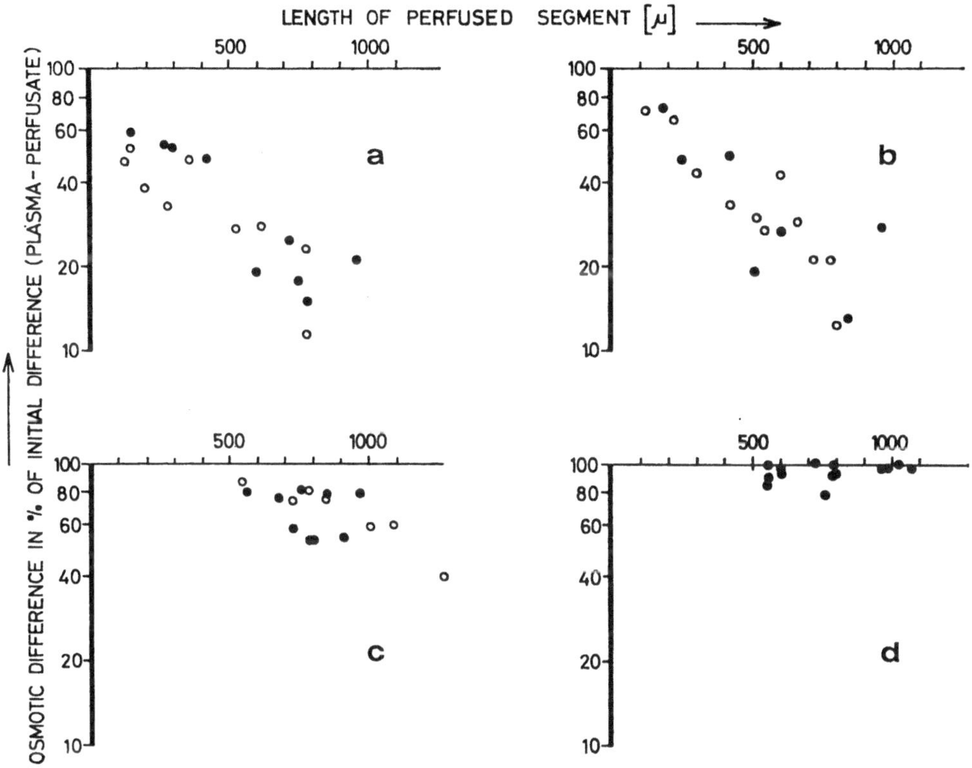

Fig. 1. Experimental data from which the filtration permeability is calculated. a) proximal convolution in antidiuresis, b) proximal convolution in water diuresis, c) distal convolution in antidiuresis, d) distal convolution in water diuresis. The difference of osmotic pressure between perfusate and plasma in percent of the initial difference is plotted versus the length of the perfused segment. Solid circles = perfusion with hypotonic, open circles with hypertonic solutions. The slope through the points corresponds to the filtration permeability (ULLRICH et al. 27).

place by water flux only (27). With the second method the water flux was explicitly evaluated by the change of the inulin concentration of the perfusate (26). With the third method the tubule was perfused with NaCl-free solutions of Raffinose of different osmolalities, and the water flux was calculated by the change of the inulin concentration (29). All values are related to a cylindrical volume having the same radius as the tubular lumen. This simplification was necessary since the real membrane area with brush border and basal infoldings cannot be measured with the necessary accuracy.

The filtration permeability of the *proximal convolution* (Table 1, Fig. 1) was found to be 17.4 and 19.2 $\cdot 10^{-8}$ $cm^3 \cdot cm^{-2} \cdot sec^{-1} \cdot cm\ H_2O^{-1}$ in the experimental series with the first method. A slightly higher value, namely 21.0, was found with the third method. The values obtained under different experimental conditions, for instance water diuresis (15.8), perfusion with high Ca^{++} concentration (17.6), with EDTA (16.0), and after adrenalectomy (20.9) do not deviate significantly from the corresponding control values.

Table 2. Filtration coefficient Lp in the distal convolution of rats*).

Experimental Conditions	Lp $\cdot 10^{-8}$ cm³/cm² $\cdot$ sec $\cdot$ cm H_2O	Number of Perfusions	Test Solutions NaCl mEq/l	Raffinose (R) Mannitol (M) in mmol/l	Reference
Antidiuresis	3.1	16	30 30	480 (M) 60 (M or R)	ULLRICH et al. (27)
Waterdiuresis (Diabetes insipidus)	1.5	14	30	—	
Antidiuresis	3.0	20	30 30	390 (M) 80 (M)	LASSITER et al. (17)
Antidiuresis + 15 mEq/l Ca^{++} in the perfusate	1.9	22	30 30	370 (M) 60 (M)	
Waterdiuresis (Diabetes insipidus)	1.84	14	30	—	ULLRICH et al. (28)
Waterdiuresis (Diabetes insipidus) + furosemide in the perfusate 50 mg%	2.27	11	30	—	
Antidiuresis	4.9 [2.7]	17 [12]	35 35	— 110 (M)	STOLTE, et al. (26)
Antidiuresis + Adrenalectomy	6.9 [5.1]	18 [16]	75 75	— 30 (M)	
Antidiuresis — Adrenalectomy + Cortisone	4.2 [3.2]	10 [7]	75 75	— 30 (M)	
Antidiuresis + Adrenalectomy + Dexamethasone	4.7 [2.1]	14 [7]	75	—	

*) The values in brackets [ ] are measured with method No. 2, all other values with method No. 1.

The data from different experimental series are also available for the *distal convolution*, namely 3.1; 3.0; 4.9 measured with method No. 1, and in addition $2.7 \cdot 10^{-8}$ cm³ $\cdot$ cm^{-2} $\cdot$ sec^{-1} $\cdot$ cm H_2O^{-1} measured with method No. 2 (Table 2 and Fig. 2). In water diuresis the filtration permeability was reduced to 1.5 and $1.8 \cdot 10^{-8}$ cm³ $\cdot$ cm^{-2} $\cdot$ sec^{-1} $\cdot$ cm H_2O^{-1}. These data are mean values. The lowest values found in water diuresis are smaller than $0.6 \cdot 10^{-8}$ cm³ cm^{-2} sec^{-1} cm H_2O. Perfusion of the distal convolution with a solution containing 15 m Eq/l Ca^{++} reduced the filtration permeability to values almost as small as in water diuresis. This fact explains the reduced concentrating ability of the mammalian kidney in hypercalcaemia. Also, the underlying defect for the delayed water excretion in adrenal insufficiency has been analyzed by STOLTE et al. (26). These authors showed that in adrenalectomized rats the filtration permeability of the distal convolution is higher than normal (Fig. 3). Steroids with predominant or exclusive glucocorticoid activity normalize the increased filtration permeability in a chronic experiment. In contrast to that it was not possible to explain on the basis of filtration permeability the well known effect of saluretic sulfonamides to reduce the water excretion in diabetes insipidus. Addition of furosemide to the perfusate does not change the distal filtration permeability significantly (28).

In Table 3 are listed the values of diffusion permeability of tritiated water measured in different nephron segments by PETERS et al. (21) and by GRANTHAM and BURG (11).

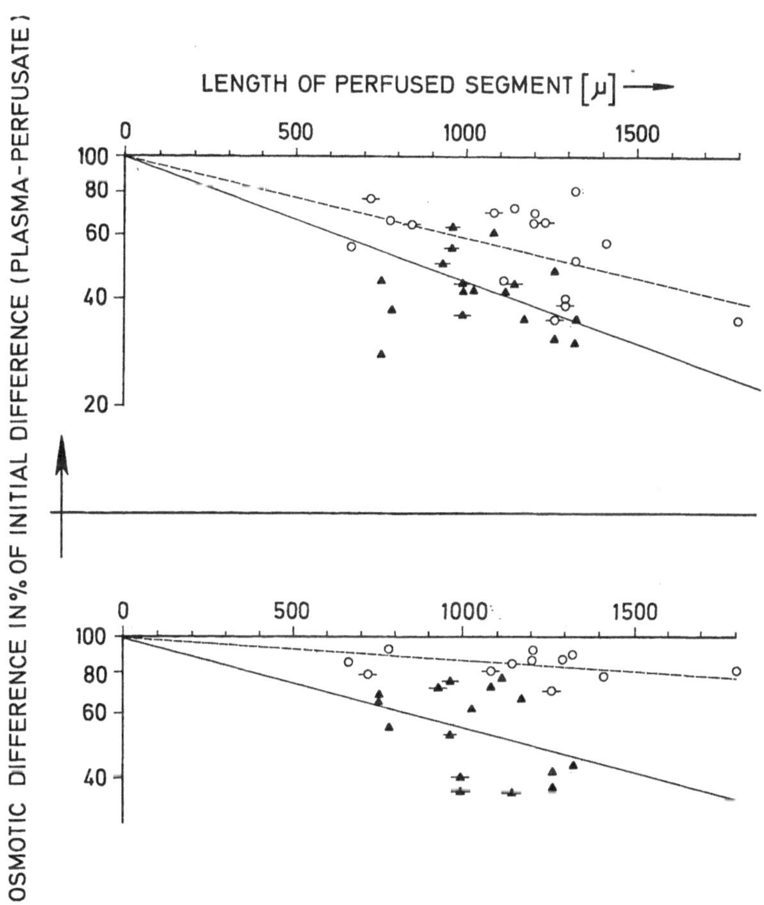

Fig. 2. Experimental data from distal tubular segments of intact rats (○) and adrenalectomized rats (▲) both in antidiuresis. Presentation as in Fig. 1. In the upper part osmotic difference has been calculated from cryoscopic measurements (method 1, compare text), in the lower part it has been calculated from the change of inulin concentration in the perfusate (method 2, compare text), (STOLTE et al. 26).

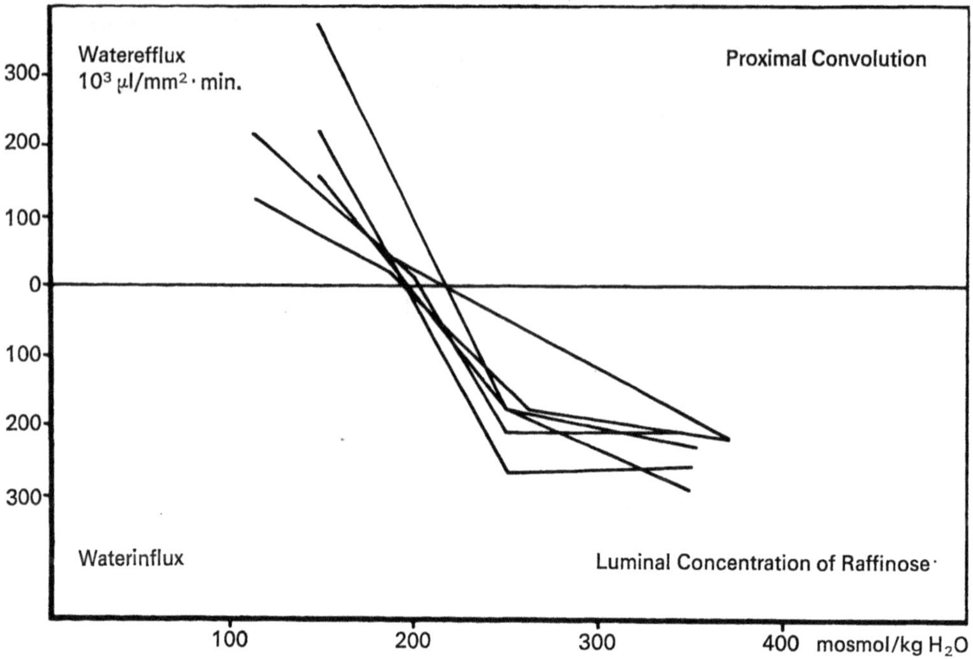

Fig. 3. Water influx resp. water efflux plotted against the concentration of Raffinose in the perfusate. The slope corresponds to the filtration permeability Lp. In the higher concentration range the permeability is lower than in the lower concentration range (ULLRICH et al. 29).

For comparison, the filtration permeabilities converted into the same dimension are also given. The values for diffusion permeability in the proximal and distal convolution deviate only slightly from each other. In the collecting ducts of the rabbit, however, it is approx. 70% smaller. The ratio filtration permeability/diffusion permeability is in all instances higher than 10, even higher than 70 in the proximal convolution. As already mentioned above these high ratios indicate in general isotope interaction and in the case of tubular cells they render likely the presence of pores (9).

Similar high ratios were seen also in other epithelial membranes (for ref. see Table 3). After administration of ADH the ratio becomes only slightly smaller in the collecting ducts, while they diminish considerably in the toad skin and toad bladder. This was interpreted to indicate that with decreasing pore radius, the bulk flow of water becomes more restricted than the diffusion of water.

In experiments where the proximal convolution was perfused with different solutions containing Raffinose it was observed that the transtubular water flux is not a linear function of the transtubular osmotic pressure difference, i. e. the filtration permeability is not constant (29). As shown in Fig. 3 it decreased with increasing osmolality of the perfusate. A similar non-linear osmosis was observed by BRODSKY and SCHILB (3) in the bladder of the turtle and by DIAMOND in the gall bladder of the rabbit.

The distal convolution seems to behave similarly. However, here the data show a larger scatter probably due to changing ADH production. Therefore the non-linearity of

Table 3. Filtration permeability (Lp) and diffusion permeability (P_d) in [cm/sec] and the ratio of both values for various biological membranes. To bring both permeabilities to the same dimension [cm · sec^{-1}] Lp [ml/cm^2 · sec (cm H_2O pressure)] has been multiplied with RT · $\bar{V}^{-1}$. The numerical conversion factor is 1.38 · 10^6 [cm H_2O pressure]. $\bar{V}$ = partial molal volume of water, R and T have their usual connotation.

		Filtration-permeability $Lp \frac{RT}{\bar{V}}$ [10^{-5}cm/sec]	Diffusion-permeability P_d [10^{-5}cm/sec]	Ratio $Lp \frac{RT}{\bar{V}} / P_d$	Author
Proximal Convolution	Antidiuresis	24000	346	70	ULLRICH et al. (27)
Distal Convolution (rat)	Antidiuresis	4100	284	14	PETERS et al. (21)
Collecting Duct (rabbit)	with ADH	2260	97.1	23	GRANTHAM, BURG (11)
In vitro	without ADH	690	37.8	18	
Toad Skin	with ADH	164	11	15	KOEFOED-JOHNSEN, USSING (16)
	without ADH	72	10	7	
Toad Bladder	with ADH	1930	16.9	115	HAYS, LEAF (13)
	without ADH	48	8.6	6	
Red Cell (human)		1278	530	2.4	SIDEL, SOLOMON (24) and PAGANELLI, SOLOMON (19)

osmosis could not be demonstrated with equal certainty as in the proximal convolution.

In order to explain the nonlinear osmosis, DIAMOND (8) suggested that waterfilled channels in the cell membrane behave as osmometers; SCHLÖGL (23) pointed out that membranes show a nonhomogenous swelling or shrinking when in contact with different solutions, and KEDEM and KATCHALSKY (15) stated that in a series array of charged membranes, which is what we apparently have in an epithelial layer, linear relations exist only if flows and forces approach zero.

When the filtration coefficient of the distal convolution is compared with the osmotic pressure difference and the water absorption under free flow conditions, it turns out that the osmotic pressure difference between the tubular fluid and the plasma is sufficient to provide the driving force for distal water absorption. In the proximal tubule, however, the situation is different. If the water absorption under free flow conditions is driven by the transtubular osmotic pressure gradient, the proximal tubular fluid would have to be at least 23 mosmol/l hypotonic to plasma, corresponding to a freezing point difference of 0.04 °C. This is certainly not the case: the freezing points of the proximal tubular fluid and plasma are equal. Similar conditions were observed in all organs in which isotonic fluid transport occurs: in the intestine, the gall bladder, the ciliary body, the tubules of Necturus, and the toad bladder (for ref. see 27). An explanation for this was offered by DIAMOND (7) with his theory of local osmosis and by CURRAN and MACINTOSH(5) with the double membrane model. We must also consider, however, the possibility of electroosmosis. But a comparison of the available data for water transport, electrical potential difference and experimental streaming potentials across the gall bladder shows that electroosmosis cannot be the mechanism of water transport since electroosmosis is several orders of magnitude too small and in the wrong direction (7).

Recently isotonic absorption from the proximal convolution could also be demonstrated when the active sodium outtransport was poisoned with 10^{-4} M Ouabain (22). In these experiments the lumen contained isotonic saline, while the peritubular capillaries were perfused with a solution of the same osmolality but with 70 mosmol/l Raffinose replacing 35 mmol/l NaCl. The observed isotonic outflux of NaCl and water was of the same magnitude as in the intact proximal tubule *in situ*.

Applying the principles of irreversible thermodynamics the isotonic absorption could be accounted for if a proper adjustment of the transport parameters namely filtration permeability, NaCl permeability, reflection coefficient for NaCl and water flux is made. The available parameters for the proximal convolution (1) fits the correspondent formulas for isotonic absorption fairly well. It is, however, unclear what mechanisms underly the adjustment of these transport parameters during isotonic absorption and what model is pertinent to the biological systems involved.

Since this talk had been given in June 1968, two papers on diffusion and filtration permeability of Henle's loop and medullary vasa recta of the rat have been published by MORGAN et al. (Am. J. Physiol. **214**, 574, 1968 and **215**, 108, 1968), while GRANTHAM and ORLOFF (J. Clin. Invest. **47**, 1154, 1968) reported on the effects of ADH, 3,5-AMP, theophyllin and prostaglandin E_1 on the water permeability of cortical collecting ducts of the rabbit.

References

1. BAUMANN, K., E. FRÖMTER und K. J. ULLRICH: Passiver Stofftransport durch Epithelzellschicht von Harnkanälchen. Berichte d. Bunsengesellschaft f. physik. Chemie Band 71, H. 8, 834-838 (1967). Verlag Chemie, GmbH, Weinheim.
2. BURG, M., J. GRANTHAM, M. ABRAMOW and J. ORLOFF: Preparation and study of fragments of single rabbit nephrons. Am. J. Physiol. **210**, 1293 (1966).
3. BRODSKY, W. A. and T. P. SCHILB: Osmotic properties of isolated turtle bladder. Am. J. Physiol. **208**, 46 (1965).
4. CAPEK, K., G. RUMRICH and K. J. ULLRICH: Permeabilität der kortikalen Tubulusabschnitte von Ratten für Harnstoff. Pflügers Arch. ges. Physiol. **290**, 237 (1966).
5. CURRAN, P. F. and J. R. MACINTOSH: A model system for biological water transport. Nature (Lond.) **193**, 347 (1962).
6. CURRAN, P. F., F. C. HERRERA and W. J. FLANIGAN: The effect of calcium and antidiuretic hormone on sodium transport across frog skin. II. Sites and mechanisms of action. J. gen. Physiol. **46**, 1011 (1963).
7. DIAMOND, J. M.: The mechanism of isotonic water absorption and secretion. 19th Symposium of the society for experimental biology. Swansea 1964. p .329.
8. DIAMOND, J. M.: Non-linear osmosis. J. Physiol. **183**, 58 (1966).
9. ESSIG, A.: Isotope interaction and "abnormal" flux ratios. A frictional model. J. theoret. Biol. **13**, 63 (1966).

10. FRIEDLÄNDER, S. K. and M. WALSER: Some aspects of flow and diffusion in the proximal tubule of the kidney. J. theoretical Biology **8**, 87 (1965).
11. GRANTHAM, J. J. and M. B. BURG: Effect of vasopressin and cyclic AMP on permeability of isolated collecting tubules. Am. J. Physiol. **211**, 255 (1966).
12. HANAI, T., D. A. HAYDON and W. R. REDWOOD: The water permeability of artificial bimolecular leaflets. A comparison of radio-tracer and osmotic methods. Annals. New York Academy of Sciences **137**, 403 (1966).
13. HAYS, R. M. and A. LEAF: Studies on the movement of water through the isolated toad bladder and its modification by vasopressin. J. Gen. Physiol. **45**, 905 (1962).
14. KASHGARIAN, M., H. STÖCKLE, C. W. GOTTSCHALK and K. J. ULLRICH: Transtubular electrochemical potentials of sodium and chloride in proximal and distal renal tubules of rats during antidiuresis and water diuresis (Diabetes insipidus). Pflügers Arch. ges. Physiol. **277**, 89 (1963).
15. KEDEM, O. and A. KATCHALSKY: Permeability of composite membranes. Part 3. – Series array of elements. Trans. Faraday Soc. **59**, 1941 (1963).
16. KOEFOED-JOHNSEN, V. and H. H. USSING: Contributions of diffusion and flow to the passage of D_2O through living membranes. Acta Physiol. Scand. **28**, 60 (1953).
17. LASSITER, W. E., A. FRICK, G. RUMRICH and K. J. ULLRICH: Influence of ionic calcium on the water permeability of proximal and distal tubules in the rat kidney. Pflügers Arch. ges. Physiol. **285**, 90 (1965).
18. LEAF, A. and R. M. HAYS: Permeability of the isolated toad bladder to solutes and its modification by vasopressin. J. Gen. Physiol. **45**, 921 (1962).
19. PAGANELLI, C. V. and A. K. SOLOMON: The rate of exchange of tritiated water across the human red cell membrane. J. Gen. Physiol. **41**, 259 (1957).
20. PASSOW, H.: Personal communication.
21. PETERS, R., K. BAUMANN und H. OELERT: Diffusion von Wasser im proximalen und distalen Konvolut der Rattenniere. Pflügers Arch. ges. Physiol. **294**, R 20 (1967).
22. SAUER, F., K. J. ULLRICH und G. RUMRICH: Unpublished data.
23. SCHLÖGL, R.: Stofftransport durch Membranen. Fortschritte der physik. Chemie 9. Dr. Dietrich Steinkopf Verlag, Darmstadt 1964.
24. SIDEL, V. W. and A. K. SOLOMON: Entrance of water into human red cells under an osmotic pressure gradient. Journ. Gen. Physiol., **41**, 243 (1957).
25. SONNENBERG, H. und P. DEETJEN: Methode zur Durchströmung einzelner Nephronabschnitte. Pflügers Arch. ges. Physiol. **278**, 669 (1964).
26. STOLTE, H., J. P. BRECHT, M. WIEDERHOLT und K. HIERHOLZER: Einfluß von Adrenalektomie und Glukocorticoiden auf die Wasserpermeabilität cortikaler Nephronabschnitte der Rattenniere. Pflügers Arch. ges. Physiol. **299**, 99, (1968).
27. ULLRICH, K. J., G. RUMRICH und G. FUCHS: Wasserpermeabilität und transtubulärer Wasserfluß cortikaler Nephronabschnitte bei verschiedenen Diuresezuständen. Pflügers Arch. ges. Physiol. **280**, 99 (1964).
28. ULLRICH, K. J., K. BAUMANN, K. LOESCHKE, G. RUMRICH and H. STOLTE: Micropuncture experiments with saluretic sulfonamides. Annals New York Academy of Sciences **139**, 416 (1966).
29. ULLRICH, K. J. and G. RUMRICH: Unpublished data.

Transport Characteristics of Isolated Perfused Proximal Tubules

M. B. BURG

Today I would like to report investigations of the transport properties of the proximal renal tubule. In order to study renal tubule function, we have been perfusing single fragments of renal tubules *in vitro* (1, 2). This method has several advantages over conventional micropuncture. First, more of the nephron is available for study. For example, it is possible to investigate directly the function of the pars recta of the proximal tubule, as well as the convoluted portion. Further, the composition of the fluid surrounding the tubule, as well as that perfusing it can be precisely controlled. Also, it is possible to analyze the tubule cells in the segment studied to determine the concentration or exchange of the transported substances or the amount of metabolic substrate.

This method has been used in the studies I am presenting today to investigate active fluid absorption, glomerulotubular balance, and electrical potential difference of the renal proximal tubule.

We chose the rabbit for our experiments since it is the only mammal from which we have found it technically feasible to dissect nephrons and study them in isolation. In the present studies fragments of single proximal tubules were dissected from rabbit kidneys and the rate of fluid absorption was measured *in vitro*. The first experiments I am going to describe were carried out to assess the rate of active fluid transport.

The arrangement used for perfusing isolated kidney tubules is shown in Fig. 1. Immediately after the rabbit had been killed a small piece of cortex was cut out of a kidney and placed in chilled, oxygenated rabbit serum. Then, a fragment of proximal convoluted tubule one to two mm long was dissected free hand using fine forceps and needles. Note that no enzyme or other maceration procedure was used. The dissected tubule was transferred to a bath of oxygenated rabbit serum at 37° C and perfused with ultrafiltrate of the same serum containing I^{131} albumin, as shown here. The direction of perfusion is from right to left. At the proximal end the tubule is positioned between concentric glass micropipets by suction and perfused through the inner pipet. By using microliter syringes on a Sage infusion pump controlled delivery at extremely slow rates is possible. The tubule fluid emerges from the distal end of the tubule under mineral oil and is collected at timed intervals of 5 to 15 minutes with a calibrated glass capillary; then, the volume of the collection and the concentration of I^{131} are measured. From these data the rate of fluid absorption and the perfusion rate are calculated for each period. Radioactivity in the bath solutions is also measured in order to test for leaks of perfusion fluid. The mean loss of I^{131} to the bath was less than 2% and cannot significantly affect the results.

It is difficult to estimate what the normal absorption rate should be for rabbit proximal tubules since there are no micropuncture studies reported. Under the conditions of our

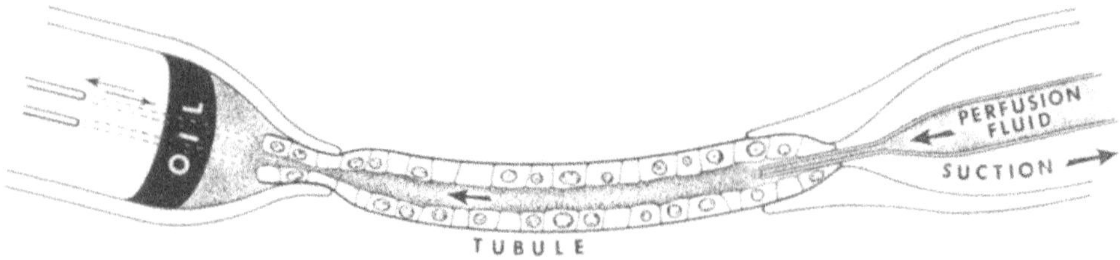

Fig. 1. Arrangement for perfusing kidney tubules.

experiments the mean rate of absorption during the first hour of perfusion was 1.18 nl min^{-1} mm^{-1} tubule length in forty tubules, as shown in Table 1. From reported clearance studies and glomerular counts, the glomerular filtration rate per nephron in rabbits this size can be estimated to be 15 nl min^{-1} (3). Micropuncture studies in other species have indicated that approximately one-half of the glomerular filtrate is absorbed in the accessible portion of the proximal tubule. A similar fraction of the glomerular filtrate would be absorbed in the rabbit proximal tubule at the absorption found in the present studies. Thus, the absorption rate found here is considered to be reasonably normal.

You will note that rabbit serum and ultrafiltrate were used in all these experiments. When artificial saline solutions were tested, the absorption rate was approximately half as great. Presumably, there are some factors in the serum other than the usual electrolytes necessary for preserving optimal function. We have not as yet tried systematically to identify these factors.

An incidental finding shown in Table 1 is that absorption by the straight portion of the proximal tubule is significantly less than that of the convoluted portion, .47 nl mm^{-1} tubule length min^{-1} compared to 1.18. It had not been possible previously to make this comparison directly since the straight portion does not approach the surface of the kidney and cannot be studied by micropuncture. However, a lower rate of absorption in the straight portion had been suspected. It had been calculated that if the higher rate of absorption measured in the accessible convoluted portion were to continue to the end of the proximal tubule, all or nearly all of the fluid would be absorbed, which is obviously not the case (4, 5, 6). This difference in absorption rates between the two segments of the tubule cannot be attributed to damage to the proximal straight tubule during dissection since in other experiments (by Dr. Bruce Tune at NIH) the opposite result was found for PAH secretion. With 20×10^{-6} M PAH in the bath secretion rate was approximately three times as great in the straight as in the convoluted portion of the

Table 1. Transport properties of rabbit proximal tubules.

	Convoluted portion	Straight portion
PAH secretion ($M\ mm^{-1}\ min^{-1} \times 10^{-15}$)	252 ± 22 (15)	790 ± 42 (15)
Water absorption ($nl\ mm^{-1}\ min^{-1}$)	$1.18 \pm .07$ (40)	$47. \pm .06$ (15)

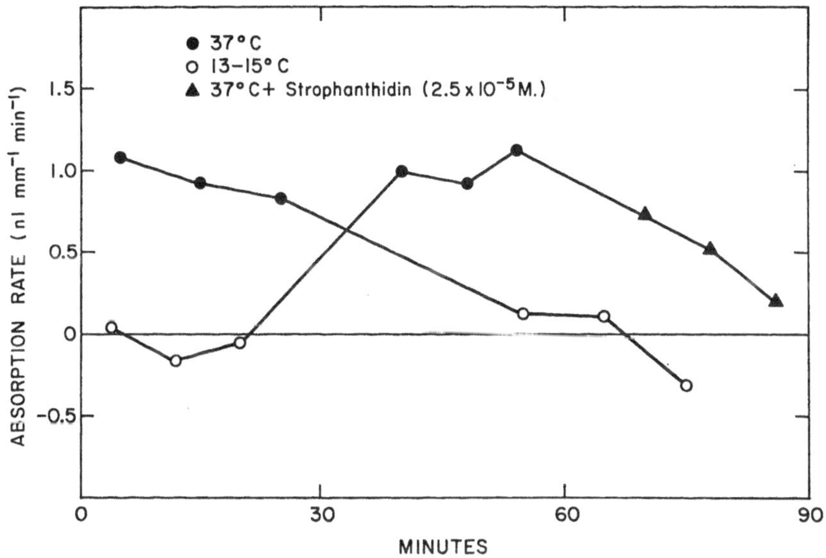

Fig. 2. Inhibition of fluid absorption in proximal convoluted tubules.

proximal tubule. From these results, it is apparent that straight and convoluted proximal tubules differ in their relative transport capacities for different substances.

In order to test whether the absorption measured *in vitro* is an active process comparable to that observed *in vivo*, the effect of inhibition was measured. On the ordinate of Fig. 2 is the absorption rate; on the abscissa the time after the start of perfusion. Two separate experiments are shown. In the first, starting at 37° absorption was approximately 1 nl min^{-1}. When the temperature was lowered to 13–15° C, absorption decreased to zero. In the other experiment the tubule was initially chilled and there was no absorption. When it was warmed to 37° absorption became normal. Then when the cardiotonic steroid strophanthidin, an inhibitor of Na transport, was added, absorption decreased again. These results confirm that this fluid absorption is active.

We next attempted to determine whether the contribution of the proximal convoluted tubule to glomerulotubular balance is intrinsic to that part of the tubule or whether there is an extrinsic regulating mechanism.

Krühoffer in 1950 reported that there is glomerulotubular balance in rabbit kidneys similar to other species (7). Following changes in filtration rate in the rabbit both the filtered load of Na and Na reabsorption change, minimizing alteration in urine sodium excretion. On the basis of his clearance studies, Krühoffer concluded that fractional absorption in the rabbit proximal tubule remained constant when filtration rate changed. In view of micropuncture studies in other species, it seems likely that his conclusion was correct, although micropuncture studies in the rabbit to confirm this directly have not been reported.

Using the method described here the tubules are removed from the kidney and any extrinsic regulating mechanism must have been disrupted. Therefore, if absorption were

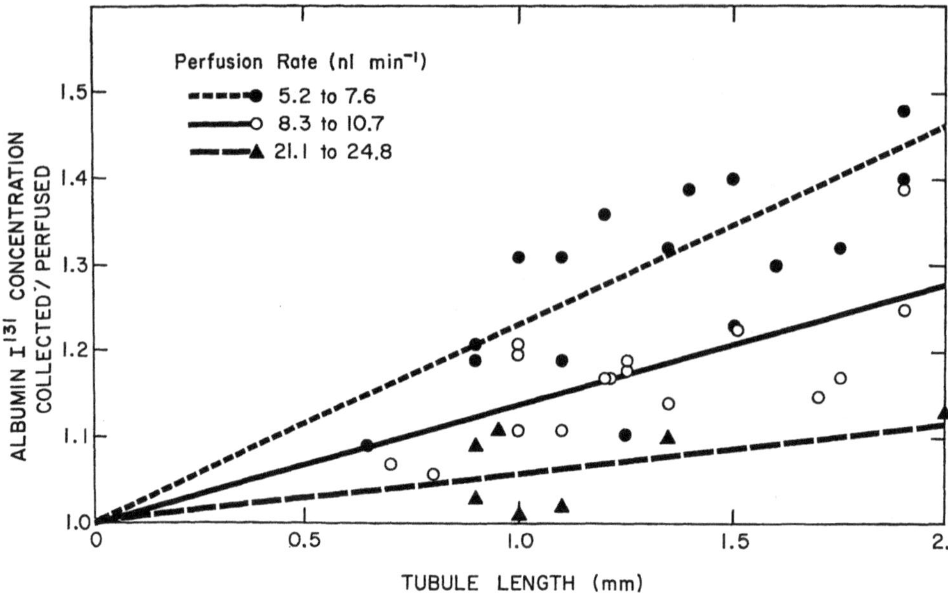

Fig. 3. Albumin I^{131} concentration ratio from isolated perfused proximal convoluted tubules.

to remain a constant fraction of perfusion rate (i. e., if glomerulotubular balance were to persist under these circumstances) the mechanism responsible must be intrinsic to the proximal tubule. If on the other hand, absorption were no longer directly related to perfusion rate, it could be inferred that an extrinsic regulating mechanism had been responsible for glomerulotubular balance *in vivo*.

When there is glomerulotubular balance *in vivo*, tubule to plasma inulin ratios are the same at a given point in the proximal tubule over a range of filtration rates. In the present experiments albumin I^{131} was used as a marker instead of inulin for the sake of convenience, and in Fig. 3 albumin ratios are shown on the ordinate plotted against the perfused length of tubule on the abscissa. These results are the individual control measurements on the 40 tubules which were summarized on the earlier figure. The data are arbitrarily divided into three groups depending on the perfusion rate. At any given perfusion rate the albumin ratio tended to be greater in the longer tubules, reflecting cumulative absorption with length. However, the ratio at a given length of tubule depended on the perfusion rate, being distinctly lower at highest perfusion rate (triangles) than at the middle rates (open circles) and slowest rates (closed circles). Therefore, in contrast to the findings *in vivo*, constant fractional absorption was not found at different perfusion rates.

In order to test this point further, experiments were performed in which a single tubule was perfused at different rates. Each tubule was perfused for two to four control collection periods at a slow rate, then for two to four periods at a faster rate, then at the slow rate again as an after control. In Table 2, the average absorption during rapid perfusion is compared to the average slower rate in the preceding and following periods. In 8 experiments, the average control perfusion rate was 8 nl per minute and the average

Table 2. Effect of flow rate on fluid absorption by proximal convoluted tubules.
Means of results for 8 experiments are shown except for tubule diameter which was measured in only the last 3 experiments. The mean of the differences in absorption between control and experimental periods (pairing the results from each tubule) is $+ .13 \pm .10$, $p > .2$.

	Control	Experimental
Perfusion rate (nl min^{-1})	8.	19.
Fraction Absorbed	.23	.11
Tubule diameter (μ)	21.	22.
Absorption (nl mm^{-1} min^{-1})	1.24	1.37

experimental rate was 19 nl per minute. The fraction of fluid absorbed fell from .23 to low flow at .11 at high flow. The fall in fractional absorption was approximately proportional to the increase in perfusion rate, so that there was no significant increase in absolute absorption at the higher perfusion rate. This means that there was essentially no glomerulotubular balance under these conditions.

Rector and his co-workers (8, 9) have ascribed altered fluid absorption in the proximal tubule *in vivo* under these conditions to changes in tubule volume rather than flow rate, finding that absorption increased as the square of tubule diameter. Therefore, it seemed important to measure tubule diameter in our experiments since if this had not changed the lack of change in absorption with flow might be explained. Our attempts to measure diameter through a dissecting microscope in the earliest of the experiments shown here were disappointing and we switched to a conventional single objective microscope for our photographs. Resolution was improved, but it was still difficult to identify the margin of the lumen, especially when the tubule was not distended. Empirically, it was found that use of a diffuse light source caused the luminal border to show up more clearly.

When adequate lighting was used it was found that there was essentially no change in tubule luminal diameter with the increase in perfusion rate. This method of measuring diameter was used for the last three studies shown here and the mean change in diameter was from 21 to 22 μ. Since the diameter was essentially unchanged in these studies, it still remained possible that the tubule diameter was the critical variable and that *had*

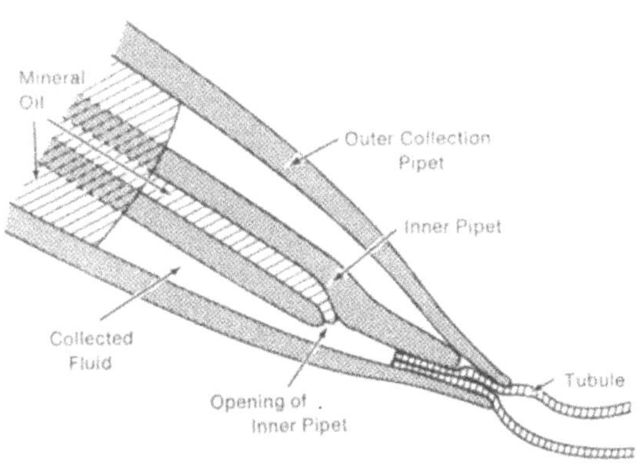

Fig. 4. Arrangement for increasing tubule diameter.

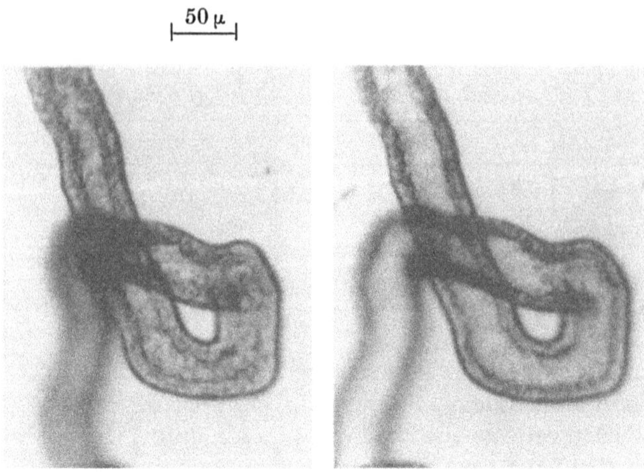

Fig. 5

Absorption: .96nl mm^{-1} min^{-1} .88nl mm^{-1} min^{-1}
Diameter: 18μ 27μ

this been altered, changes in absorption would have occurred. This possibility was tested in subsequent studies.

We found it possible to vary the tubule diameter at constant perfusion rate by changing outflow resistance with the apparatus shown in Fig. 4. This shows the pipet arrangement at the distal end of the tubule. As in the previous experiments, the tubule was held in a collecting pipet and the perfused fluid was allowed to accumulate under mineral oil. After a control period had been collected in this manner a special inner pipet shown here was inserted and its tip was used to compress the end of the tubule. The compression was adjusted until the desired degree of tubule distension was achieved, then the fluid which had accumulated under the oil during the period of adjustment was aspirated into the lumen of the special inner pipet and the timed collection began. After perfusing for a suitable period of time, the special inner pipet was rapidly removed and the sample was immediately collected using the usual calibrated pipet. With compression removed, the tubule diameter returned to the control value and an after control collection was made at the smaller tubule diameter. In this manner several alternate collections with small and large diameters could be made in a single tubule.

During each collection period the tubule was photographed and the luminal diameter was determined by measurements from prints enlarged to 400× total magnification. Measurements were made at the same location in each tubule during successive periods. In the experiment shown in Fig. 5, the tubule diameter at the point of measurement increased from 18 μ to 27 μ in successive periods at the same flow rate. However, the absorption rate remained essentially constant (.96 nl mm^{-1} min^{-1} in the control period compared to .88 nl mm^{-1} min^{-1} after distension).

A summary of the results of experiments with ten such tubules is shown in Table 3. In each experiment two or more control observations were compared to two or more alternating periods of tubule distension. The tubules were distended from a mean control diameter of 15 μ up to 26 μ diameter without any change in the perfusion rate of 9.6 nl

Table 3. Effect of luminal diameter on fluid absorption by proximal convoluted tubules. Mean of results for 10 experiments are shown. The mean of the differences in absorption between experimental and control periods (pairing the results from each tubule) is $+ .19 \pm .08$, $p = .05$. The mean of the differences in outside diameter is $+ 3.8 \pm .6$, $p < .05$.

	Control	Experimental	Ratio E/C
Tubule diameter (μ)			
Outside	50.2	54.0	1.07
Inside	15.	26.	1.73
Flow rate (nl min^{-1})	9.6	9.6	1.00
Absorption (nl mm^{-1} min^{-1})	1.00	1.19	1.19

min^{-1}. (Attempts to distend the tubule further usually resulted in completely blocking the outflow.) Absorption increased somewhat when the tubule was distended, the average increase being 19%. However, this was less than proportional to the increase in tubule diameter, whereas an increase proportional to the square of the diameter would be required were absorption proportional to tubule volume, as had been previously concluded by others.

This point is emphasized in Fig. 6 in which the average results from each of the 10 tubules are shown individually. On the ordinate is the fractional change in absorption, and on the abscissa is the fractional change in diameter. The diagonal line marked D indicates a change in absorption directly proportional to the diameter and the line marked D^2 shows a change proportional to the square of the diameter. In all experiments where absorption increased it was less than proportionate to the increase in tubule diameter.

GERTZ (10) originally proposed a causal relation between tubule volume and absorption rate on the basis of comparison of simultaneous measurements of transit time (T.) and inulin concentration ratio (TF/P) at a given point in the tubule and absorptive

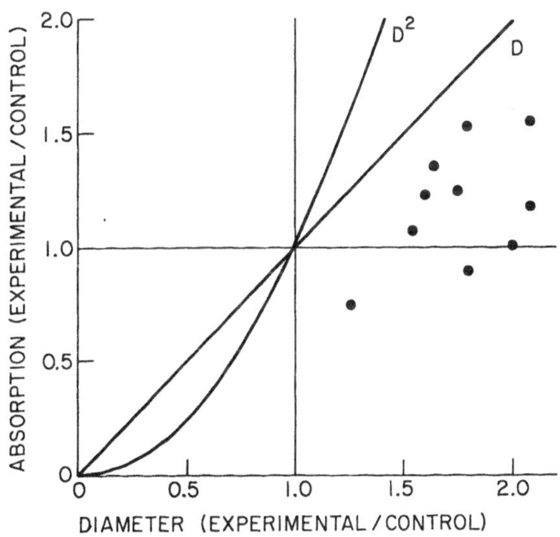

Fig. 6. Relation between diameter and fluid absorption rate in proximal convoluted tubules.

Table 4. Proximal tubule absorption rates and diameters in the rat.

$C/\pi r^2$	1. Free flow	$\frac{\ln (TF/P)}{T}$	3.54–5.76
	2. Split drop	$\frac{.693}{t^1/_2}$	3.99–5.22
C	3. Free flow	$\frac{\pi r^2 \ln (TF/P)}{T}$	1.33
nl mm^{-1} min^{-1}	4. Free flow	$\frac{V_L}{L}\left(1-\frac{P}{TF}\right)$	2.74–4.11
	5. Split drop	$\frac{\pi r^2\ .693}{t^1/_2}$	2.89–4.57
Diameter μ	6. Free flow 7. Split drop		19–25 28–37

half time using the split oil drop technique ($t_{1/2}$). The relationships as shown in Table 4 are:

$$\frac{\ln (TF/P)}{T} = \frac{C}{\pi r^2}$$

$$\frac{0.693}{t_{1/2}} = \frac{C}{\pi r^2}$$

where C is the reabsorptive rate per unit tubule length and r is the tubule radius. GERTZ found that $C/\pi r^2$ calculated from the separate experiments represented by these equations was the same. This has been confirmed by others, the values shown here being the range of those reported in the literature. In order to measure the $t_{1/2}$ the tubule must be filled with oil, distending it so that its observed radius is considerably greater than under free flow conditions, as shown at the bottom. For $C/\pi r^2$ to be constant despite the increase in radius, C must have increased in proportion to r^2. If it had not, $C/\pi r^2$ would have decreased enough for the difference to have been detected. The theoretic increase in C is shown in the middle where C has been calculated from $C/\pi r^2$ and r. Hence the theory is that absorptive rate is proportional to proximal tubule volume.

This interpretation of the results requires that C be less in free flow than with the split oil drop. In fact there is independent evidence that C is actually the same in the two situations and that the equality of $C/\pi r^2$ may therefore be fortuitous, a result of systematic errors in one or more of the measurements. Although GERTZ rejected this interpretation as being highly improbable, additional calculations suggest that it may actually be correct. C can be estimated independently for free flow from the relation shown:

$$C = \frac{V_L}{L}\left(\frac{TF}{P} - 1\right)$$

where V_L is the collection rate and L is the length of the tubule to the point at which TF/P inulin is measured. The reported values of C in free flow measured in this manner vary from 2.74 to 4.11 nl mm^{-1} min^{-1} compared to 2.89 to 4.57 based on measurements using the split drop technique. Thus, C measured by complete collections in free flow is approximately equal to that measured with split drop, despite the large difference in tubule radius, whereas using the transit time and TF/P inulin it had been concluded that C during free flow must be less because r was observed to be less. We believe that the value for fluid absorption measured by the complete collections in free flow is correct. Since it is equal to that measured with the split oil drop, despite the difference in tubule radius, we conclude that these studies show no causal relation between tubule volume and absorption rate.

Other evidence for the proposed relationship between tubule volume and absorption rate came from the effect of elevating ureteral pressure. Under these conditions, changes in tubule volume are dissociated from those in perfusion rate. Tubule volume increases while the perfusion rate is decreased. Therefore, if tubule volume is critical for the regulation of absorption rate, glomerulotubular balance should be disrupted, and absorption rate increased relative to perfusion rate. The actual results of studies by RECTOR and co-workers (8, 9) were that inulin TF/P (and presumably absorption) increased, suggesting that tubule volume is the primary factor controlling absorption. BRENNER, BENNETT, and BERLINER (11) have repeated the same experiments and have found essentially no change in TF/P inulin. They attributed the earlier result to technical inadequacy of the micropuncture method. When a sample of tubule fluid is aspirated by micropuncture during elevation of ureteral pressure, there may be reverse flow in the tubule causing fluid to arrive at the micropuncture site from more distal segments where inulin is more concentrated. Reflux of this nature may occur even when precautions are taken by placing an oil drop distal to the collecting pipet. Since contamination from more distal segments also results in a spurious elevation of measured filtration rate per nephron, gross contamination can be suspected if nephron filtration rate (V_O) is unreasonably high. Ureteral clamping should cause V_O to decrease since whole kidney GFR is decreased. However, in some studies V_O was found to increase, indicating contamination of the collected samples. When all results in which V_O *increased* more than 50% were excluded from consideration there was no increase in TF/P inulin during ureteral clamping and thus no increase in absorption. Actually there could have been a significant decrease in absorption which was not detected since the criterion used for selecting the data may not be sufficiently sensitive to exclude all contaminated samples.

Thus, the previous studies indicating a causal relation between tubule volume and absorption rate cannot be confirmed and another basis for glomerulotubular balance must be sought. In the present experiments we found that when proximal tubules are studied in isolation, there is little change in absorption as a function of perfusion rate. Therefore, the mechanism linking absorption and perfusion rate is disrupted when the proximal tubule is removed from the kidney, and must be extrinsic to the tubule.

LEYSSAC (12, 13, 14) has suggested one possible extrinsic factor. He proposed that changes in proximal tubule absorption associated with glomerulotubular balance are mediated by the effect of angiotensin released from the juxtaglomerular apparatus.

According to his view, one of the effects of angiotensin is directly to inhibit fluid absorption by the proximal tubule. We tested the effect of angiotensin on three tubules. Following two control periods, angiotensin (2.5 μgm ml^{-1}) was added to the bath during each of three experimental periods. Then the bath was changed several times to wash off the angiotensin and three additional periods were collected. The mean absorption rate without angiotensin during the initial and final periods was .95 nl mm^{-1} min^{-1}. In the presence of angiotensin absorption rate was .90 nl mm^{-1} min^{-1}. The difference was not statistically significant ($-.05 \pm .07$) when each experimental period was compared to the mean of the corresponding initial and final control periods. (There was also no significant difference comparing each experimental period to either the corresponding initial control periods or final control periods.)

Thus, even a high concentration of angiotensin in the bath surrounding the tubules is without an important effect on absorption. It had previously been shown by others that angiotensin within the proximal tubule lumen also does not affect Na absorption. These results are in disagreement with LEYSSAC's and suggest that there is no direct effect of angiotensin on fluid absorption in the proximal tubule.

None of the other current views are completely adequate to explain glomerulotubular balance. Even accepting that regulation of proximal reabsorption is not intrinsic to the tubule itself, the nature of the responsible extrinsic mechanism remains to be established.

I would now like to turn to studies measuring the electrical potential difference across proximal tubules.

Originally it had been found that the P. D. across the proximal convoluted tubule was approximately -20 mV (15), and on the basis of these measurements it was concluded that chloride (16) and potassium (17, 18) are transported actively in the proximal tubule. However, it has recently been shown by FRÖMTER and colleagues (20, 21) that there is no measurable P. D. across rat proximal tubule cells under ordinary conditions

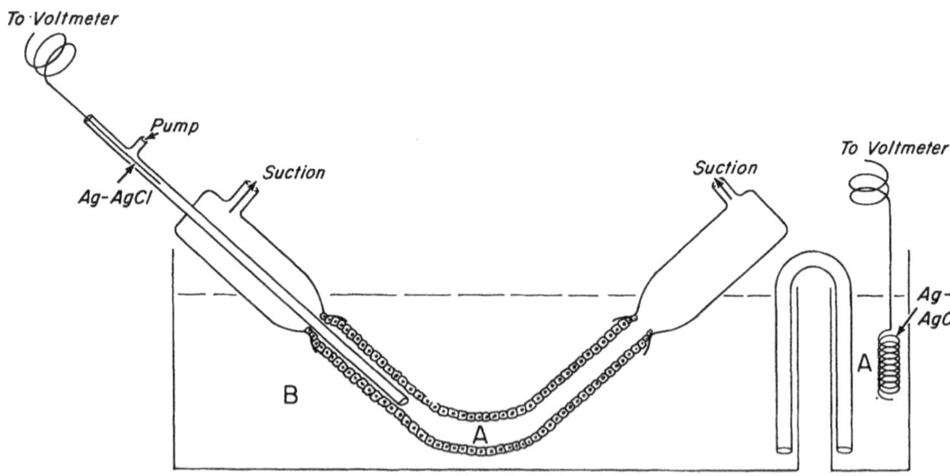

Fig. 7. Arrangement for measuring electrical potential difference across isolated perfused renal tubules.

in vivo. The previously recorded P. D.'s appear to have been intracellular potentials, since the tip of the recording pipet was most likely in the tubular cells rather than in the lumen, as intended.

In order to measure electric potential difference across isolated segments of proximal convoluted tubule the arrangement shown in Fig. 7 was used. The tip of the perfusion pipet within the tubule lumen was elongated, allowing it to be threaded down the lumen beyond the end of the outer pipet. An Ag-AgCl electrode was placed in the rear of the perfusion pipet and connected to the input of an electrometer. A second (reference) Ag-AgCl electrode served as ground. Both Ag-AgCl electrodes were immersed in identical solutions.

Electrical potential difference was measured in seven proximal convoluted tubules under conditions optimal for fluid absorption. The perfusing pipet was advanced as far as possible (usually approximately 200 μ) down the tubule lumen. Fig. 8 is a picture of

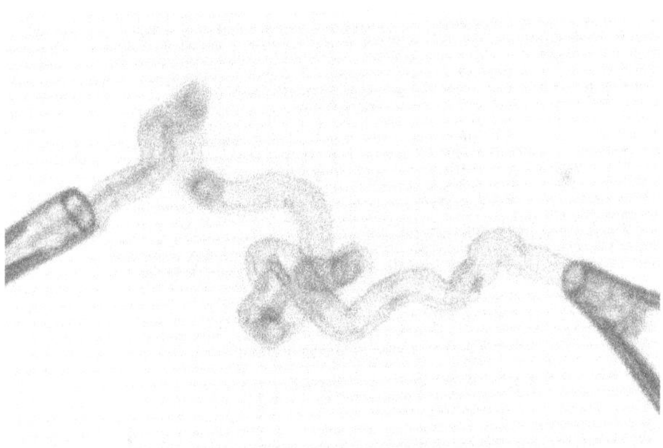

Fig. 8

a pipet being advanced. At this point it is approximately 150 μ down the lumen. It was not possible to advance any pipet more than 300 μ because of the convoluted shape of the tubules. However, if the length constant of the proximal tubule in the rabbit is as short as that previously reported in the rat (86 μ) (22), placement of the electrode (pipet) more than two length constants away from the "open" end should permit detection of a P. D. were it present.

Under these circumstances no measurable P. D. was recorded in 7 tubules during the first hour of perfusion (P. D. = -0.7 ± 0.6 SEM mV).

Thus, the absence of measurable P. D. has been confirmed in the present studies in which a perfusion pipet was used to measure P. D. Under these circumstances it can be ascertained with certainty that the pipet or electrode is within the tubule lumen. It is apparent that no P. D. normally exists in the proximal tubule and that previous conclusions concerning active chloride and potassium transport must be re-examined.

In summary, we have been attempting to characterize the mechanisms of salt and water transport using isolated perfused rabbit proximal tubules. In general the observed characteristics are consistent with those previously measured *in vivo* except that no evidence for glomerulotubular balance intrinsic to the tubule was found. It is hoped that additional studies with this preparation will help to elucidate further the nature of the transport mechanisms.

Note added in proof: Recently the method for measuring electrical P. D. has been improved by using a dielectric compound (Sylgard 184, Dow Corning Corp.) to insulate completely the tubule lumen from the bath. Using this improved method a small, but significant P. D. has been found (–3.8 ± .5 mV, 16 experiments).

References

1. Burg, M., J. Grantham, M. Abramow and J. Orloff: Preparation and study of fragments of single rabbit nephrons. Am. J. Physiol. **210,** 1293 (1966).
2. Grantham, J. and M. Burg: Effect of vasopressin and cyclic AMP on permeability of isolated collecting tubules. Am. J. Physiol. **211,** 255 (1966).
3. Strassberg, J., J. Paule, H. C. Gonick, M. H. Maxwell and C. R. Kleeman: The quantitative estimation of perfusible glomeruli and the collagen and non-collagen nitrogen of the normal kidney. Nephron. **4,** 384 (1967).
4. Gottschalk, C.: Renal tubular function: lessons from micropuncture. Harvey Lectures, Ser. 58, 99 (1963).
5. Giebisch, G. and E. Windhager: Renal tubular transfer of sodium, chloride, and potassium. Am. J. Med. **36,** 643 (1964).
6. Lassiter, W., C. Gottschalk and M. Mylle: Net transtubular movement of water and urea in saline diuresis. Am. J. Physiol. **204,** 669 (1964).
7. Kruhoffer, P.: Studies on water-electrolyte excretion and glomerular activity in the mammalian kidney. Rosenkilde and Bagger, Copenhagen (1950).
8. Rector, F., F. Brunner and D. Seldin: Mechanism of glomerulotubular balance. I. Effect of aortic constriction and elevated ureteropelvic pressure on glomerular filtration rate, fractional reabsorption, transit time, and tubular size in the proximal tubule of the rat. J. Clin. Invest. **45,** 590 (1966).
9. Brunner, F., F. Rector and D. Seldin: Mechanism of glomerulotubular balance. II. Regulation of proximal tubular reabsorption by tubular volume, as studied by stopped flow microperfusion. J. Clin. Invest. **45,** 603 (1966).
10. Gertz, K., J. Mangos, G. Braun and H. Pagel: On the glomerular tubular balance in the rat kidney. Arch. Ges. Physiol. **285,** 360 (1965).
11. Brenner, B., C. Bennett and R. Berliner: The relationship between glomerular filtration rate and sodium reabsorption by the proximal tubule of the rat nephron. J. Clin. Invest. **47,** 1358.
12. Leyssac, P.: The in vivo effect of angiotensin on the proximal tubular reabsorption of salt in rat kidneys. Acta Physiol. Scand. **62,** 436 (1964).
13. Leyssac, P.: The in vivo effect of angiotensin and noradrenaline on the proximal tubular reabsorption of salt in mammalian kidneys. Acta Physiol. Scand. **64,** 167 (1965).
14. Leyssac, P.: Dependence of glomerular filtration rate on proximal tubular reabsorption of salt. Acta Physiol. Scand. **58,** 236 (1963).
15. Windhager, E. and G. Giebisch: Electrophysiology of the nephron. Physiol. Rev. **45,** 214 (1965).
16. Kashgarian, M., Y. Warren and H. Levitin: Micropuncture study of proximal renal tubular chloride transport during hypercapnea in the rat. Am. J. Physiol. **209,** 655 (1965).
17. Bloomer, H., F. Rector and D. Seldin: The mechanism of potassium reabsorption in the proximal tubule of the rat. J. Clin. Invest. **42,** 277 (1963).
18. Marsh, D., K. Ullrich and G. Rumrich: Micropuncture analysis of the behavior of potassium ions in rat renal cortical tubules. Pflügers Archiv. **277,** 107 (1963).

19. WATSON, J., J. CLAPP and R. BERLINER: Micropuncture study of potassium concentration in proximal tubule of dog, rat, and necturus. J. Clin. Invest. **43**, 595.
20. FRÖMTER, E. and U. HEGEL: Transtubuläre Potentialdifferenzen an proximalen und distalen Tubuli der Rattenniere. Pflügers Archiv. **291**, 107 (1966).
21. FRÖMTER, E., T. WICK and U. HEGEL: Untersuchungen über die Ausspritzmethode zur Lokalisation der Mikroelektrodenspitze bei Potentialmessungen am proximalen Konvolut der Rattenniere. Pflügers Archiv. **294**, 265.
22. HEGEL, U., E. FRÖMTER and T. WICK: Der elektrische Wandwiderstand des proximalen Konvolutes der Rattenniere. Pflügers Archiv. **294**, 274.

GERTZ: You did not find a correlation between tubular diameter and reabsorption rate. Do you consider this lack of correlation to be a characteristic of the isolated tubule preparation, perfused with this artificial protein-containing fluid? Or do you claim that such a correlation is also absent in vivo?

BURG: We do not believe that the lack of glomerulotubular balance *in vitro* is due to a change in the function of the tubule itself, when it is dissected from the kidney. Rather we believe it is due to the absence of some other factor or factors extrinsic to the tubule and which induce balance *in vivo* by modifying tubule function. This factor(s) is left behind when the tubule is removed from the kidney thus disrupting glomerulotubular balance.

THOENES: Ihre Experimente an den isolierten Tubuli sind von großem Interesse, weil sie über die Funktion ausschließlich des Tubulusepithels, unbeeinflußt durch das Gefäßsystem, Aufschluß geben. Sie haben darauf hingewiesen, daß im gestreckten Teil des proximalen Tubulus, verglichen mit dem Konvolut, die resorptive Leistung niedrig und die sekretorische – jedenfalls für PAH – hoch ist, und dies erlaubt einen funktionsmorphologischen Rückschluß: im gestreckten Teil des proximalen Tubulus sind Verzahnung und Labyrinth sehr gering entwickelt, ebenfalls im Vergleich zum Konvolut. Man kann also sagen, daß im proximalen Nierentubulus die Labyrinth-Entwicklung mit reabsorptivem Transport korrespondiert, daß umgekehrt der sekretorische Transport aber von dem Labyrinth unabhängig ist.

The Regulation of Distal Tubular Potassium Transport*)**)

G. GIEBISCH, G. MALNIC

Dr. ROBERT BERLINER, in the introduction to his Harvey Lecture (1) on Renal Mechanisms for Potassium Excretion held in New York City on February 18, 1960, stated that this subject is one which had not yet been much illuminated by micropuncture studies. In the subsequent eight years, studies on the single nephron level have provided considerable insight into the tubular sites, into some of the cellular mechanisms of transport and into the factors controlling net transfer rates of this ion. Many of Dr. Berliner's inferences from 1960 have been conclusively proved to be correct. Some have undergone modifications.

If the concentration of potassium and the fraction remaining within the tubular lumen is measured along the mammalian nephron, a functional pattern emerges upon which there is general agreement. Most data are available for the rat nephron, although Dr. Berliner's group has undertaken studies on the dog (2, 3) and monkey (4). Dr. MOREL and his associates have studied potassium transport in several desert rodents (5). The pattern of concentration gradients along the nephron is also known for two amphibian species, *necturus* (6) and *amphiuma* (7).

I shall be brief concerning proximal data. Since the concentration of potassium in proximal tubule fluid remains about the same as in plasma or is only slightly less (2–6, 8, 9), the fractional reabsorption of potassium in the first 60% of the proximal tubule is similar to that of sodium and water; that is, some two thirds of the filtered potassium is reabsorbed along this nephron segment. It is of interest to note that this functional pattern is preserved in the presence of extreme variations in urinary excretion rates (9). It follows that modifications of the proximal tubular transport pattern do not – with the exception of brisk osmotic diuresis – contribute significantly to changes in the urinary potassium excretion (9).

It is not surprising that least is known about the handling of potassium by the loop of Henle. Three groups of investigators have found tubular fluid/plasma potassium ratios in the range of 3–5 at the tip of the loop (10, 11, 12) and it is therefore likely that some potassium, similar to urea, reenters the nephron at this site from the collecting ducts. Little is known about this process. It is doubtful whether it is of functional significance since by the time fluid has reached the distal tubule, tubular fluid/plasma potassium

*) Work carried out in the investigators' laboratories was supported by grants from the National Science Foundation and the American Heart Association.

**) Supported by Public Health Research Career Program Award 5-K6-AM-18 from the National Institute of Arthritis and Metabolic Diseases.

ratios are low, usually quite significantly below unity (2, 4, 5, 8, 9). The early distal tubule is the site along the nephron where, again, the amount of potassium relative to the amount that was filtered, is found to be fairly constant and independent of the urinary excretion. This would suggest that during free flow, the concentration of potassium in fluid from the distal tubule is independent of the fate of potassium in the proximal tubule and the loop of Henle.

It is the distal tubule and, to a considerably smaller extent, the collecting duct system which emerge as the most important nephron sites where potassium excretion rate is modulated. This is due to the fact that the fraction of potassium filtered which is commonly found in the early distal tubule varies but little, despite the fact that the urinary excretion rate might vary between 3 and 150% (9).

The view of BERLINER of a predominant role of the distal tubular system in regulating potassium transport has been directly confirmed. The few exceptions might be due to limitations of micropuncture techniques in that it is at present impossible to collect from the very beginning of the distal tubule.

A fairly comprehensive delineation of the range of distal tubular variation in potassium handling can be obtained by comparing the concentration of potassium and inulin in states of widely differing urinary excretion patterns. This is shown in Fig. 1. Distal tubular data in two extreme conditions demonstrate the great range of transport facilities of the distal tubular epithelium. On the left, data from a rat on a low dietary intake of potassium are shown. On the right, data are from a rat in which, by various manipulations, urinary potassium excretion was maximally stimulated. If we first look at the results obtained during dietary potassium deprivation, leading to a plasma potassium level of some 2.0 mEq/l and bicarbonate levels ranging from 35–40 mEq/l, it can be seen that early distal concentration ratios are significantly less than unity and, in absolute concentrations, less than 1 mEq/l. Distal transtubular concentration ratios tend to increase moderately as fluid passes along this nephron segment, but it is the collecting duct along which the highest potassium concentrations are achieved.

To evaluate these data in terms of transtubular net movement, potassium concentration ratios are divided by the corresponding inulin ratios. The lower graph on the left shows such ratios, that is, the amount of potassium relative to that which was filtered, plotted as a function of tubular length. Since the increase in inulin concentration ratios exceeded that for potassium, the slope is negative. This indicates that, in essence, the process of net reabsorption, manifest along the proximal tubule and the loop of Henle, continues along the distal tubule and the collecting duct. This leads to the very extensive removal of potassium from the urine, since only a mean of 3% of the filtered potassium is excreted.

On the right of Fig. 1 the results are shown of an experimental condition in which potassium excretion was maximally stimulated resulting in a mean potassium/inulin clearance ratio of 1.5. It can be seen that the potassium concentration again is quite low at the beginning of the distal tubule. However, in contrast to the situation described previously, it rises steeply along the distal tubule, reaching peak concentration ratios in excess of 10, corresponding to concentrations of some 80 mEq/l. The lower section summarizes the condition after correction for water movement. Inspection of early distal data indicates that some 80% of the filtered potassium has been reabsorbed by the time fluid reaches the early distal tubule. This could even be an underestimate of reabsorption, since it is impossible to collect from the very beginning of this tubular segment. However, in marked contrast to the state of potassium deprivation, massive distal tubular addition is evident. It can be calculated that a minimum of some 90% of urinary potassium may have entered the lumen by way of tubular secretory transfer. It follows that net influx of potassium across the distal tubules accounts almost exclusively for the excretory capacity of the kidney.

A comparison of the moiety of potassium present at the beginning of the distal tubule with that in the final urine permits an estimate of the extent to which urinary potassium is derived from distal nephron activity. Calculations indicate that a mean of 75% of urinary potassium can be accounted for by distal tubule secretion under non-diuretic control conditions. Higher fractions can be shown to be of distal secretory origin whenever potassium excretion is stimulated. As pointed out before, these are minimum values because the fluid from the first 20% of the distal tubular length, not being accessible for micropuncture, could have an even lower potassium content. There are only a few situations in which distal tubular secretion is absent. One of these is potassium deprivation, already shown. Another can be demonstrated after administration of a kaliopenic drug, Merck 870 (13). Free-flow micropuncture studies (prime: 1 mg/kg, sustaining infusion: 0.04 mg/kg/min) indicate the ability of this compound to suppress distal secretion completely. Thus, distal transtubular potassium concentration gradients frequently remain below unity all along the distal tubule. Interestingly, final urinary potassium concentrations are also low and it can be calculated that there is no significant secretory net transfer of potassium into the collecting ducts. In passing, it should be noted that the complete suppression of potassium secretion is not associated with any great modification of tubular sodium concentration at this site. The drug in the dose given is only a very mild diuretic in the rat.

Recently, two problems relating to tubular potassium transfer which have long attracted attention have come under direct investigation. They concern first, the nature of the role of intratubular sodium ions in distal potassium secretion and, secondly, the interrelationship between distal tubular hydrogen and potassium transport.

With respect to the first problem, the simultaneous measurement of transtubular concentration gradients and transport rates of both sodium and potassium has made it possible to assess their relationship under those conditions in which final urinary sodium excretion has been lowered and the rate of potassium excretion drastically curtailed. It has been suggested that under those conditions when low urinary sodium excretion compromises potassium appearance in the final urine tubular sodium reabsorption is almost complete prior to the site of potassium secretion, that is, by the time fluid reaches the early distal tubule. We have chosen two experimental conditions to put this thesis of a limited distal tubular sodium supply to the test. The first was dietary sodium depletion (9): rats maintained over several weeks on a low sodium diet excrete only $^1/_4$ of the potassium of control rats (9). Furthermore, such pretreatment prevents the urinary potassium loss normally observed after DOCA administration. Fig. 2 summarizes the pertinent data on sodium and potassium transport along the distal tubule. On the upper left, sodium -TF/P ratios are shown; below these, corresponding potassium data, obtained from analysis of the same collections, are summarized. Several points deserve comment.

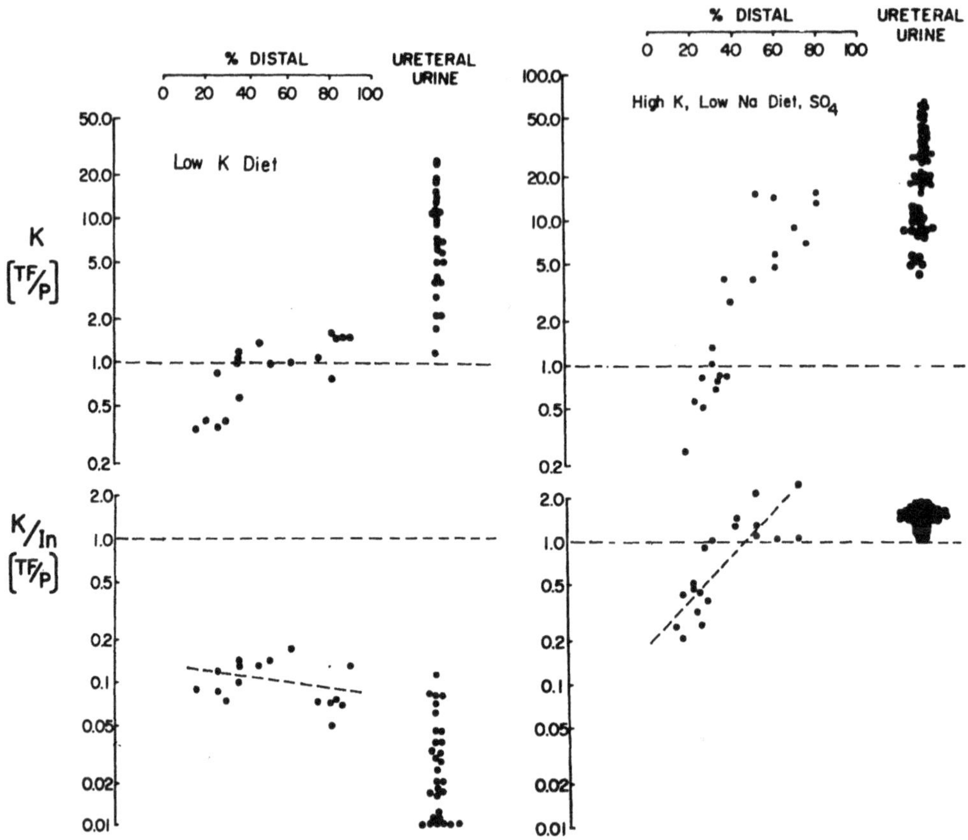

Fig. 1. Summary of distal tubular potassium and potassium/inulin concentration ratios. Left: Data from animals kept on a low K diet. Right: Data from animals in which potassium excretion was maximally stimulated by pretreatment with a high K low Na diet, and the intravenous administration of sodium sulfate, potassium chloride and dichlorphenamide (From ref. 8).

Despite the fact that final urinary sodium concentrations are quite low, considerably below values found in control animals, early distal tubular sodium concentrations are at least ten times that of potassium. Accordingly, as shown on the upper right, the fraction of filtered sodium entering the distal tubule still amounted to some 4–6%. It is apparent that the most dramatic drop in fractional sodium occurred along the collecting ducts. Thus, whereas the distal tubule is the main site of potassium secretion, it is the collecting duct where the lowest sodium concentrations and the almost complete sodium abstraction from the tubular contents are achieved. This dissociation of the main nephron site for potassium secretion and that for establishment of maximal sodium gradients and of sodium reabsorption is of obvious importance in evaluating the possibility of potassium secretory capacity being critically dependent upon the amounts of sodium available for exchange. If we consider the behavior of potassium, as shown on the lower right side of

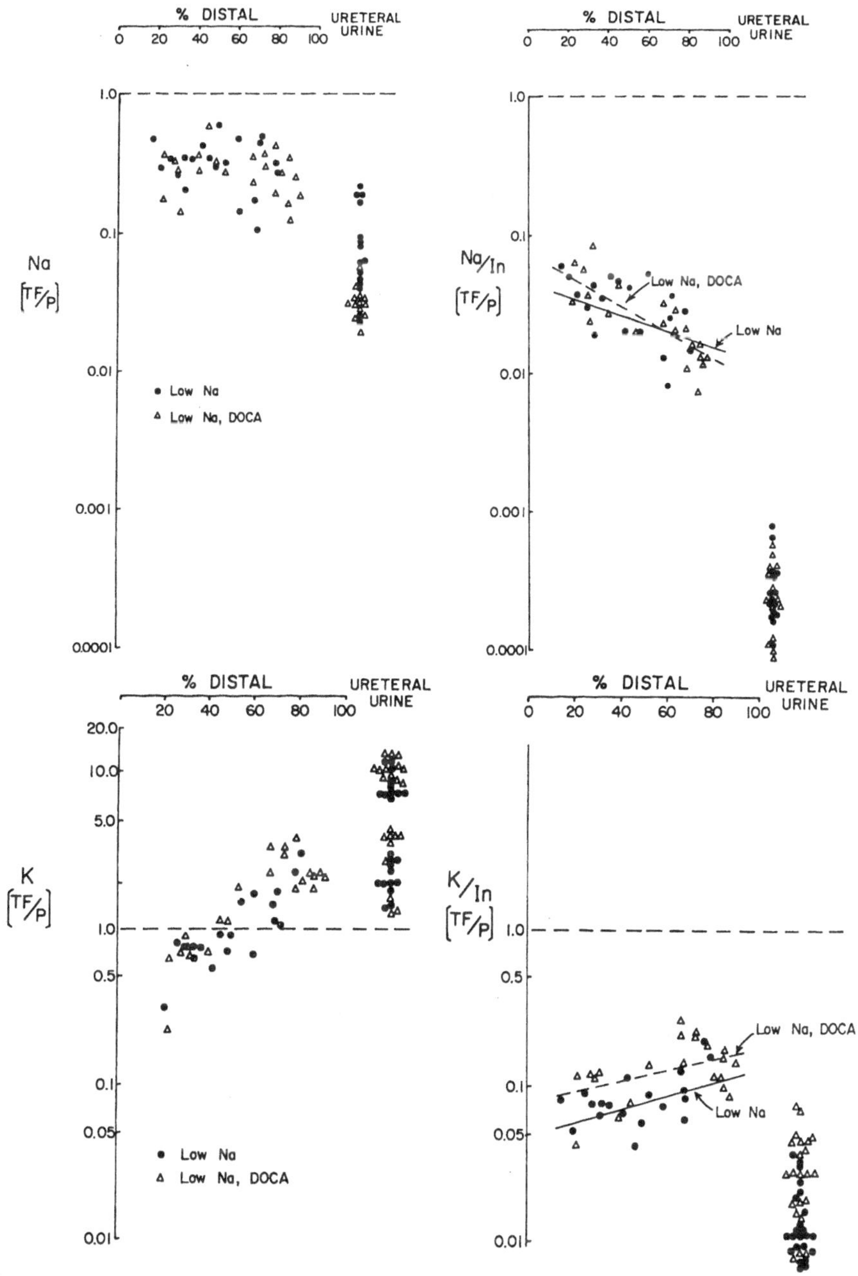

Fig. 2. Summary of distal tubular sodium and sodium/inulin concentration ratios (top) and of potassium and potassium/inulin concentration ratios (bottom). Animals were kept on a low sodium diet, one group pretreated with DOCA. (From ref. 9).

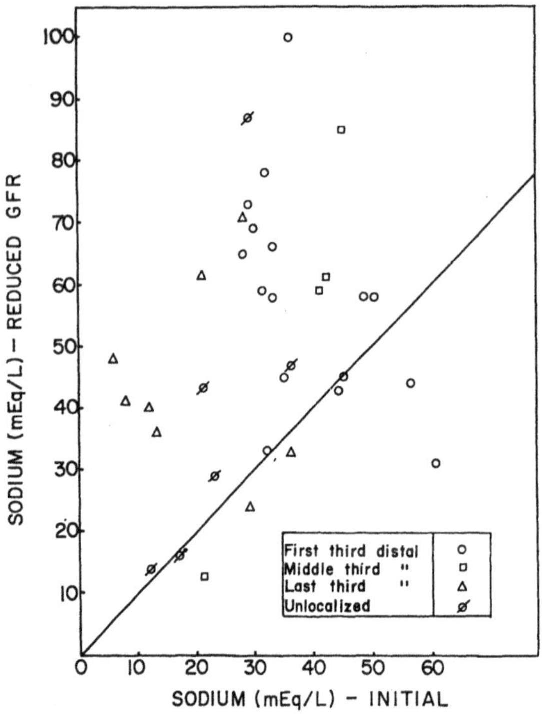

Fig. 3. Effect of acute reduction of filtration rate on distal tubular sodium concentration (From ref. 22).

Fig. 2, it becomes clear that it is not diminished secretion, but rather greatly enhanced reabsorption along the collecting ducts which is mainly responsible for the very low urinary excretion rates. We have concluded that reduced potassium excretion during sodium deprivation is not the consequence of, and cannot be related to enhanced sodium reabsorption proximal to the site of potassium secretion.

Results from studies in which tubular fluid samples were collected from the same distal location prior to and after an acute reduction in glomerular filtration rate, show the very same phenomenon. Some of the data are summarized in Fig. 3. They allow an assessment of the main sites at which modifications of tubular sodium transport occur when filtration rate is acutely reduced by application of a small silver clamp on the renal artery of the rat kidney. Mean filtration rate was reduced to 50% of control levels, urinary sodium excretion dropped sharply and potassium excretion similarly fell to low levels. Data on distal tubular sodium concentrations are shown in Fig. 3. On the abscissa, the sodium concentration prior to, and on the ordinate, the concentration in recollected samples from the same site after clamping are plotted. It is obvious that the majority of points fall above the line of equality. Obviously, the sodium concentration along the distal tubule increases after reduction in filtration rate, in all likelihood due to prolonged passage time through the loop and more complete water equilibration, as indicated by the increased inulin concentration ratios (not shown here) after clamping. Potassium data, similarly analyzed, show a similar behavior. Again, the fraction of sodium reabsorbed along the distal tubule greatly exceeds that of potassium secreted. Again, a reduced distal tubular supply of sodium is clearly not responsible for the dramatic suppression of potassium excretion. Rather it appears that a low sodium concentration in the final urine, due to more complete reabsorption along the collecting ducts, leads to curtailment of potassium excretion by increased reabsorption of potassium at that site and not, as previously postulated, by modification of the distal tubular secretory rate.

In collaboration with Dr. MALNIC and Miss MELLO AIRES we have also recently investigated the relationship between tubular hydrogen and potassium transport (14). In many experimental conditions, a reciprocal relationship between the excretion rates of these two cations has been established (1). To gain some insight into the nephron sites and some aspects of the mechanisms involved, we have carried out a number of free-flow studies in control rats made mildly diuretic by infusing 5% mannitol in isotonic saline, in rats receiving 5% sodium bicarbonate intravenously, and in animals either mechanically hyperventilated or breathing 15% CO_2. The effect of such variations in arterial pCO_2 and that of acute intravenous potassium chloride-loading was also studied in animals receiving the 5% sodium bicarbonate infusion. Such studies have been greatly aided by the development of an antimony electrode system by MALNIC and VIEIRA (23) permitting the measurement of instantaneous in situ pH and intratubular bicarbonate from the very same nephron site from which fluid is also withdrawn for the measurement of sodium, potassium and inulin.

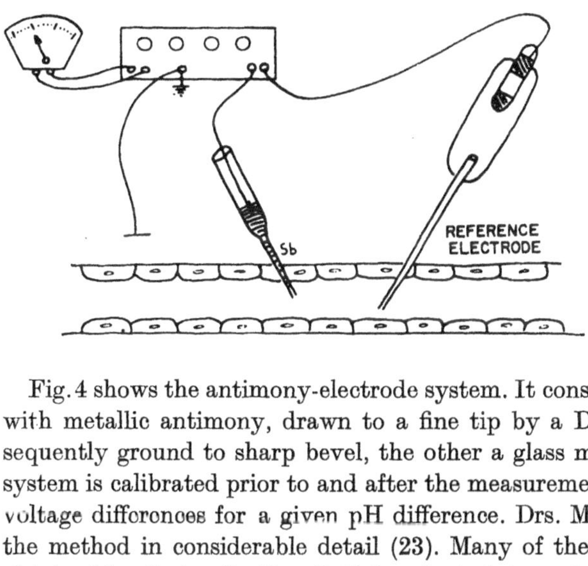

Fig. 4. Schematic drawing of pH-electrode assembly. "sb:" antimony electrode; reference electrode: Ling-Gerard type glass electrode.
(From ref. 23).

Fig. 4 shows the antimony-electrode system. It consists of two glass pipettes, one filled with metallic antimony, drawn to a fine tip by a DEFONBRUNE microforge and subsequently ground to sharp bevel, the other a glass microcapillary filled with KCl. The system is calibrated prior to and after the measurement, and found to give reproducible voltage differences for a given pH difference. Drs. MALNIC and VIEIRA have described the method in considerable detail (23). Many of the subsequently shown results were obtained by first collecting fluid for electrolyte and inulin analyses, and subsequently making the pH measurement at the same tubular site.

Fig. 5 summarizes estimates of distal tubular potassium secretion in the eight different experimental conditions studied. The data are presented in relation to plasma potassium levels. Since the fraction of potassium entering the distal tubule varies relatively little (averaging some 5%) late distal potassium/inulin ratios are a fair index of the secretory function of this nephron segment. Control animals, (C), at a plasma potassium level of

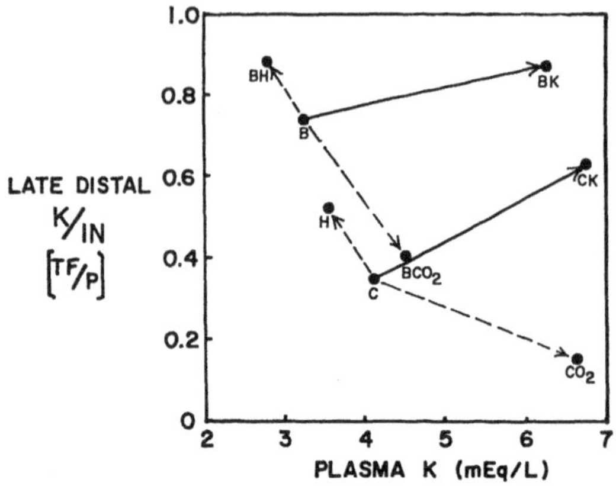

Fig. 5. Summary of distal tubular potassium secretion, plotted as function of the plasma-K level, during control conditions and during various acid-base disturbances. For details, see text.

4 mEq/l, have a mean ratio of 0.35. Three experimental conditions were superimposed upon the control state: first, respiratory acidosis (CO_2) leading to a significant drop in potassium secretion despite a sharp rise in plasma potassium. The latter is an extrarenal response due to the release of potassium from tissue upon acidifaction of the body fluids (15). Second, acute hyperventilation results in respiratory alkalosis and increases distal tubular secretion in the presence of a slight but significant fall in plasma potassium. Thirdly, intravenous administration of isosmotic potassium chloride (KCl) leads to both marked hyperkalemia and a powerful enhancement of distal potassium secretion. It is also apparent that acute loading with sodium bicarbonate (B), despite a drop in plasma potassium, stimulates distal secretion. Changes in pCO_2, symbolized by the points BCO_2 and BH, have effects similar to those observed under control conditions. Although starting from a different base line of secretory activity, breathing 15% CO_2 drops distal secretion, while further alkalinization by mechanical hyperventilation pushes the secretory activity of the distal tubular system to higher levels.

Acute potassium-loading (point BK) does lead to a further enhancement of distal potassium secretion, but compared to the effect of the same loading procedure under control conditions, it is evident that, superimposed on metabolic alkalosis in the bicarbonate-loaded animal, it is less efficient in its stimulatory effect on potassium secretion. There is some evidence that extracellular alkalinization leads both to intracellular alkalosis and an increase in cellular potassium content. If these results can be extended to cells of the distal tubule, the bicarbonate effect could be mediated by an increase in intracellular potassium. Provided that bicarbonate loading has indeed led to an increase in intracellular potassium the relatively small additional secretory response subsequent to potassium loading may mean that this maneuvre is less effective in further increasing intracellular potassium, and thus is also less effective in stimulating potassium secretion. Generally, these data are consistent with the thesis previously proposed, that it is the distal tubule where the most significant changes in potassium transport occur under the influence of acid-base alterations.

Data on distal tubular potassium secretion have also been evaluated as function of tubular in situ pH. In most instances, pH and potassium data were obtained from identical distal tubules. Two points should be noted. First, an increase in intratubular pH is generally associated with increasing potassium secretion rates. A second point of interest is the observation that at almost identical intratubular pH values breathing 15% CO_2 depresses distal potassium secretion. Increasing pCO_2 elevates the sodium-bicarbonate load by shifting sodium in exchange for hydrogen ions from cellular stores into the extracellular fluid. Thus, at high pCO_2 levels, a larger quantity of bicarbonate is filtered both in control and initially bicarbonate-loaded animals. Increasing pCO_2 enhances the rate of bicarbonate reabsorption – such that the rates of increased reabsorption balance the load increments and to stabilize intratubular pH at similar levels. It is safe to infer, however, that intracellular pH was more acid when the animal was breathing 15% CO_2. Thus, despite relative constancy of intratubular pH, potassium secretion is affected by changes in pCO_2. This underscores the importance of changes in intracellular hydrogen ion concentration as one additional regulatory factor in distal tubular potassium transfer: Increased intracellular acidity diminishes distal tubular secretion.

Our next subject of concern is a definition of the type of transport responsible for distal tubular potassium movement. The distal tubular epithelium has the unusual capacity of being able to effect either net reabsorption or net secretion of potassium. The latter is the more commonly observed mode of behavior, but we have seen that net reabsorption occurs in the state of low dietary potassium intake (8). In passing, we may note that in aquatic amphibian species like *Necturus* (6) or *Amphiuma* (7), extensive net reabsorption of potassium along the distal tubule is the normal state of affairs since these animals normally elaborate a virtually potassium- and sodium-free urine. Thus, in these species, as well as in perfused amphiuma kidneys (7), the potassium concentration declines progressively along the distal tubule.

Since there is general agreement that the distal tubular lumen is electrically negative with respect to the peritubular fluid (16), net reabsorptive movement occurs against an electrochemical gradient, suggesting, by the usual criteria, active movement out of the lumen. Our ideas concerning the mode of inward, that is, secretory movement into the lumen, that component of potassium transport which is most labile and most extensively modified by varying metabolic demands, have been influenced by the following observations.

First, an evaluation of the observed concentration ratios of potassium across the distal tubular epithelium with the measured electrical driving force indicates both in free-flow conditions and under steady-state conditions that the electrical potential difference is of adequate magnitude to account for the observed potassium concentration gradients. Such an interpretation emphasizes the role of the transepithelial electrical potential difference in *partly* determining the magnitude of the secretory process. It demands the demonstration that the electrical driving force is an effective factor in setting the extent of tubular potassium accumulation. Affirmative evidence has been obtained. Although we have recently carried out some electrical measurements of distal transepithelial conductance which indicate that electrical clamping of tubular segments might be feasible, we have not yet carried out such experiments and have had to rely on what might be called "chemical" clamping (25). It consists in the deposition of different solutions, known to alter the electrical potential difference, and observations of the effect upon the distribution of potassium ions. Fig. 6 summarizes data on distal transtubular potassium concentration ratios during perfusion with isosmotic sodium chloride, sodium sulfate and choline

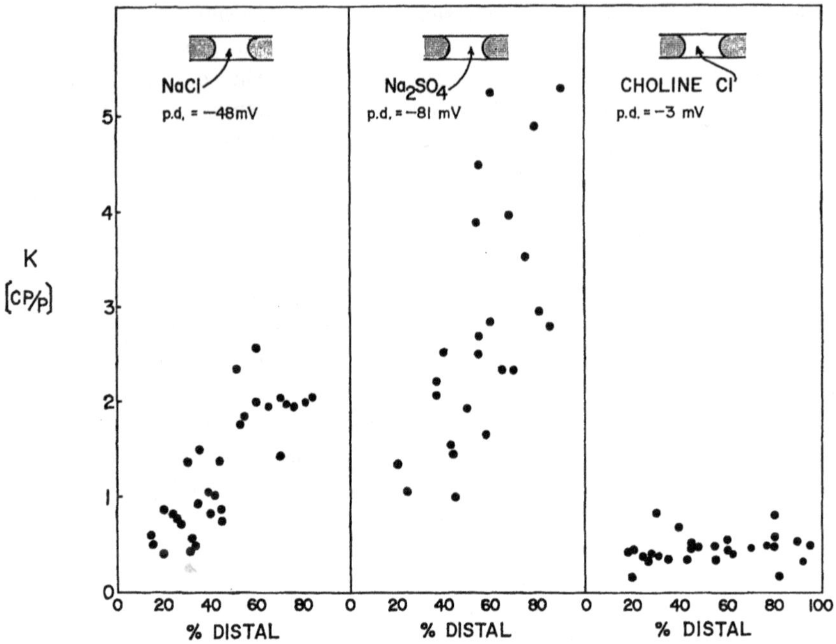

Fig. 6. Summary of distal transtubular concentration ratios during stationary perfusions with isosmotic NaCl, Na_2SO_4 and choline chloride. (From ref. 25).

chloride. It is clear that there are significant differences with respect to both electrical and chemical concentration gradients in the three series of experiments. Compared to isotonic sodium chloride perfusions, the electrical potential difference is significantly higher during sulfate perfusion. Concomitantly, steady-state concentration gradients for potassium ions are augmented along the whole distal nephron length. On the other hand, during perfusions with isotonic choline chloride, the transtubular potential difference is almost completely suppressed. This demonstrates that the presence of sodium ions is essential for the maintenance of a normal degree of intratubular negativity, and it also shows that absence of this potential difference prevents the development of normal transtubular movement of potassium ions. This is evident from the absence of increasing potassium concentrations along the nephron. It should be noted that in the almost complete absence of an electrical driving force, the transtubular concentration gradient for potassium is significantly less than one.

The observation which we have consistently made: intraluminal potassium concentrations lower than those expected from electrochemical equilibrium leads us to postulate that an activity reabsorptive movement of potassium prevents the tubular fluid from attaining the value expected from passive distribution according to the electrical potential gradient. Accordingly, there is no need to assume any specific active transport of potassium into the lumen.

A schematic presentation of some pertinent properties of such a distal tubule cell is given in Fig. 7. It incorporates the following characteristics: 1) a high intracellular

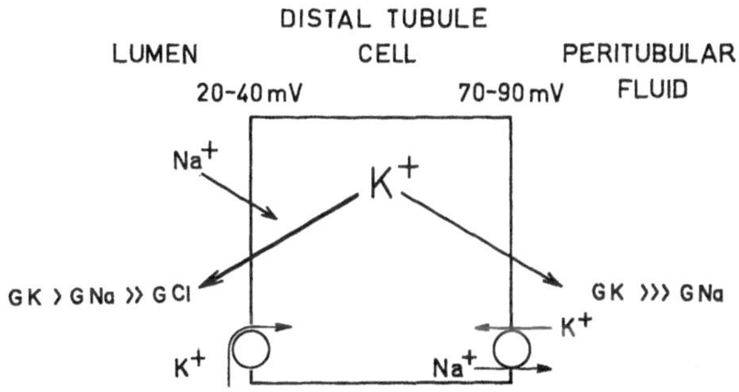

Fig. 7. Schematic presentation of some properties of distal tubule cells. (Modified from ref. 24).

potassium concentration maintained by a peritubular ion pump, effecting sodium extrusion and potassium accumulation. 2) Uneven electrical polarization such that the potential difference across the luminal cell membrane is significantly less than that across the peritubular membrane. This results in the overall transepithelial potential difference. We shall subsequently try to demonstrate that the differing electrical polarization is caused, at least in part, by differing passive permeability properties of the two cell membranes. Essentially, we believe that two parameters acting at the luminal cell border are significant factors in the regulation of potassium transport. One is the magnitude of the electrochemical potential gradient of potassium, that is the intracellular potassium concentration and the electrical potential difference. The other is the strength of the apparent electromotive force of the reabsorptive pump opposing passive leakage from the cell compartment into the tubular lumen. It should be noted that the arrangement of the reabsorptive potassium pump is not unusual; it merely represents the normal direction of active potassium movement, that is uphill transfer from the extracellular into the cellular compartment.

We have recently undertaken an extension of electrophysiological studies on the distal tubular epithelium of the rat, and I would like to discuss certain results which have a bearing on our topic, because they underscore the importance of differing properties of the luminal and peritubular cell membranes.

Fig. 8 gives a schematic survey of the types of experiments we have carried out (19, 20). Under A it is shown how single distal tubules can be perfused with different solutions. At the left, a double-barrelled perfusion-pipette is seen; at the right, a double-barrelled microelectrode is shown. Recording between the tubular lumen and the peritubular fluid pool yields the transepithelial potential difference. Injection of currents in the range of 10^{-8} ampere and assessment of the resulting voltage displacement gives an estimate of

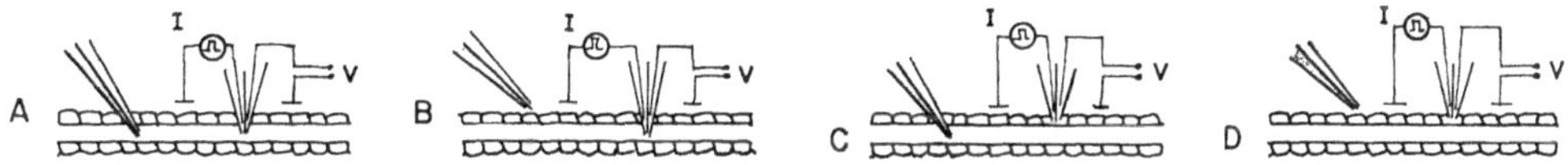

Fig. 8. Schematic presentation of methods of applying various perfusion fluids intratubularly and peritubularly. The double-barrelled micropipette contains two different fluids that can be ejected in an alternate fashion. Double-barrelled microelectrode can be placed either into the tubular lumen (A, B) or into a single distal tubular cell (C, D). One barrel of microelectrode is used to apply current (I), the other to measure potential differences.

the effective trans-epithelial resistance. Obviously, both potential differences and resistances can also be measured in the absence of perfusions, that is, under free-flow conditions in a wide range of experimental conditions.

In B), the same arrangement is shown, with one essential difference: here, the ionic environment not within the tubule, but on the peritubular side is changed by superfusion of the region, or by perfusion of single appropriately located peritubular capillaries. Such an approach yields information on the effects of peritubular ionic changes on the overall potential difference and on the respective resistance. C) shows an important arrangement of more recent origin. If a double-barrelled micropipette is placed into the interior of a single cell, the effect of intratubular ionic substitution upon the peritubular potential difference and resistance can be measured. In conjunction with arrangement A), such measurements allow one to pinpoint at which cell membrane a change in luminal ionic composition affects the overall potential difference. In addition, such measurements also permit an assessment of coupling between the two individual potential steps. Finally, as shown in D), it is similarly possible to measure the effect of peritubular ionic changes upon the potential step and apparent resistance across the cell membrane separating the cell interior from the peritubular fluid. This latter approach has also been extensively used in the amphibian kidney (18).

If the effectiveness of luminal or peritubular ionic substitutions is tested in its ability to change the transepithelial potential difference the following results are obtained (Fig. 9). Luminal substitution of 150 mEq/l sodium sulfate for potassium sulfate is

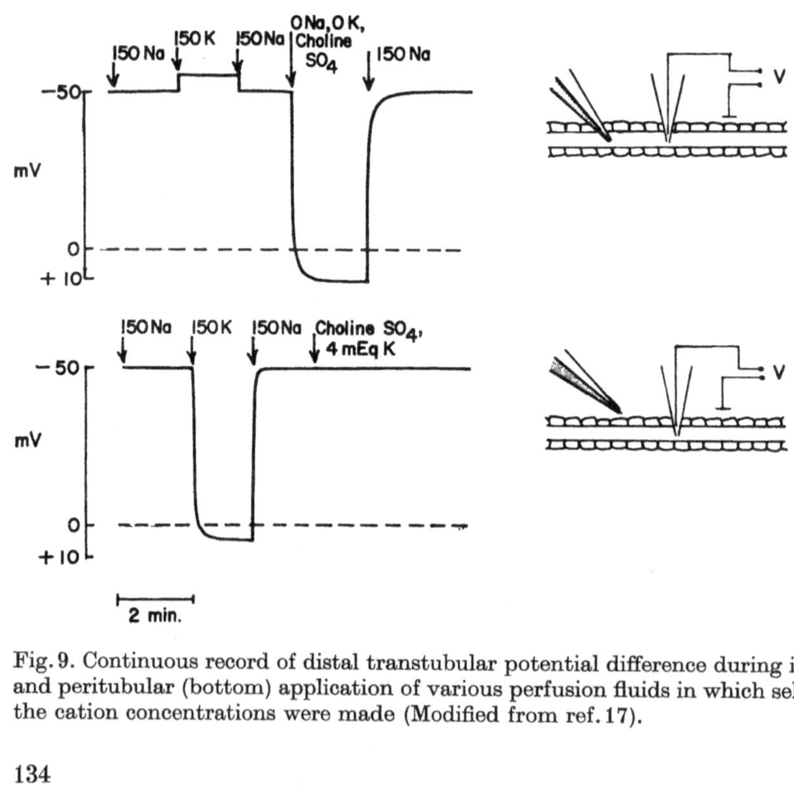

Fig. 9. Continuous record of distal transtubular potential difference during intratubular (top) and peritubular (bottom) application of various perfusion fluids in which selective changes in the cation concentrations were made (Modified from ref. 17).

relatively ineffective. Potassium substitution for sodium usually leads to a small increase in the observed potential difference. On the other hand, reducing both sodium and potassium, by substitution with choline sulfate, leads to a very dramatic drop in the potential difference. Frequently the lumen becomes positive with respect to the peritubular fluid. The effects are readily reversible as demonstrated by perfusing with solutions containing 150 mEq/l Na. In the lower part, the effect of peritubular ionic substitutions upon the transepithelial potential difference is shown. The control-level represents exposure to a solution containing sodium in about the normal concentration. In contrast to luminal effects, replacement of sodium by 150 mEq/l potassium drastically drops the potential difference, indicating a high sensitivity of the peritubular membrane to high potassium concentrations. It is this cell boundary then which presumably has a highly selective potassium permeability. On the other hand, it is rather insensitive to a selective reduction in sodium as shown by the effects of superfusion with a solution containing normal extracellular concentrations of potassium, but choline as the main cation.

As shown in Fig. 8 (C) the recording micropipette can also be placed intracellularly, recording the potential difference between cell inside and peritubular fluid. Now, the luminal reduction of potassium or of sodium is quite ineffective in changing the potential step. This is an important point. It demonstrates first that whatever changes one observes during luminal substitution upon the transepithelial potential difference are not due to simultaneous changes across the luminal *and* peritubular cell boundary, but solely to changes in the luminal potential step. Secondly, it shows the complete absence of electrical coupling by low resistance paths between luminal and peritubular cell membranes. This is in striking contrast to the behavior of the proximal tubular epithelium in Necturus where Dr. BOULPAEP demonstrated very effective interactions (19, 20).

Data on transepithelial conductances under conditions of various ionic substitutions have also been obtained. In conjunction with other electrophysiological data a description of some properties of the distal tubular epithelium has thus become possible. Compared to the proximal tubule and the collecting ducts, the distal tubular epithelium takes an intermediate position with respect to the magnitude of its specific resistance. Either from the input resistance and the dimensions, or from lambda, the space constant, which is about 400 mu, a specific resistance of some 300 ohm cm^2 can be derived. If we calculate, from the effective input resistance measured across the peritubular membrane and the cell dimension the specific resistance across the peritubular membrane, a value of some 20–30 ohm cm^2 obtains. Since this is about one-tenth of the total specific resistance, it is probably safe to conclude that the luminal cell membrane is normally limiting to ion movement, as its resistance is much higher. The current flowing when potassium is the main current – carrying ion species may thus allow the calculation of a potassium conductance, and, accordingly, that of a potassium current which is carried when a normal transtubular potential difference is present. A comparison of the potassium current flowing at –48 mV with the actually chemically measured potassium influx (from early and late distal TF/P potassium and inulin ratios) indicates that the distal transtubular potassium conductance is large enough to account for the observed transtubular secretion rates on the basis of passive diffusion alone.

Furthermore, some inferences on the relative permeability properties of luminal and peritubular cell membranes may be made on the basis both of the potential changes induced and the resistance changes achieved upon appropriate substitutions. It can be stated that the peritubular cell membrane is highly potassium-selective while the luminal membrane shows the highest conductance for potassium a lower one for sodium and a still significantly lower one for chloride. We were unable to observe any changes in potassium conductance when the lumen was perfused with solutions of either potassium bicarbonate or potassium phosphate such that pH was either 8.0 or 5.6. Thus, acute changes in luminal pH do not affect the potassium conductance.

Inspection of Fig. 7 may be helpful in summarizing the factors affecting potassium transport at the distal tubular level. The intracellular potassium concentration is normally high and its magnitude affects the electrochemical potential gradient favoring potassium entry into the distal tubular lumen. The concentration of potassium in the cell may be affected by agents acting on the peritubular pump (whether it is an exchange pump or not, is entirely unknown). These factors may be poisons such as ouabain, metabolic inhibitors, adrenal steroids. They may be factors such as dehydration which increases intracellular potassium concentration and is known to enhance potassium secretion. They may be changes in intracellular pH, alkalosis increasing and acidosis decreasing intracellular potassium concentration.

Asymmetrical cell polarization is another regulating factor and caused, as we have seen, by the different conductance properties of the two cell membranes. It is the relative unselectiveness of the luminal membrane which causes depolarization and thus promotes leakage down the concentration gradient as indicated by the left-hand arrow. Obviously the extent of this leakage depends on the magnitude of the electrical potential gradient. The latter is sensitive to the sodium concentration in the lumen. If the electrical potential difference across the collecting duct, as across the distal tubular epithelium, were also partly dependent upon the concentration of sodium ions, reabsorptive loss of potassium from this nephron segment might be expected whenever the sodium concentration and the electrical negativity are decreased along this tubular segment. As I have pointed out before, a survey of our data shows that potassium reabsorption along the collecting duct is most significantly demonstrable under those very conditions when sodium reabsorption is almost complete along this part of the nephron. It is thus possible that the coupling between sodium and potassium movement across the collecting duct may be mediated electrically.

Finally, the relative potassium conductance of the luminal cell membrane and the strength of the reabsorptive pump are important factors. The exact role of changes in the reabsorptive pumping rate for potassium ions is, at the moment, the most difficult variable to assess. An additional uncertainty here is the possibility that the rate of potassium transfer, either from lumen or from the peritubular fluid into the cell interior, also affects the intracellular potassium concentration. Such a change in intracellular potassium concentration could affect both the driving force for diffusion into the lumen as well as the concentration gradient against which potassium is pumped. Thus, a fall in intracellular potassium could lower luminal potassium, and distal secretion rate, by diminished downhill movement from cell to lumen as well as by more efficient inward (uphill) pumping. The relative contribution of these factors will have to await quantitative estimates of intracellular concentration changes of distal tubule cells, and measurements of individual flux components across the two cell boundaries.

References

1. BERLINER, R. W.: Harvey Lect. **55**, 141 (1961).
2. BENNET, C. M., J. R. CLAPP and R. W. BERLINER: Am. J. Physiol. **213**, 1254 (1967).
3. WATSON, J. F.: J. Clin. Invest. **45**, 1341 (1966).
4. BENNET, C. M., B. M. BRENNER and R. W. BERLINER: J. Clin. Invest. **47**, 203 (1968).
5. LECHENE, C., F. MOREL, M. GUINNEBAULT and C. DE ROUFFIGNAC: Nephron, in press.
6. BOTT, P. A.: Am. J. Physiol. **203**, 662 (1962).
7. WIEDERHOLT, M., J. SULLIVAN and G. GIEBISCH: (unpublished observations).
8. MALNIC, G., R. M. KLOSE and G. GIEBISCH: Am. J. Physiol. **206**, 674 (1964).
9. MALNIC, G., R. M. KLOSE and G. GIEBISCH: Am. J. Physiol. **211**, 529 (1966).
10. JAMISON, R. L.: Am. J. Physiol. **215**, 236 (1968).
11. MARSH, D. J. and S. SOLOMON: Am. J. Physiol. **208**, 1119 (1965).
12. GIEBISCH, G. and E. E. WINDHAGER: Am. J. Med. **36**, 643 (1964).
13. DUARTE, CH., F. CHOMETY and G. GIEBISCH: (unpublished observations).
14. MALNIC, G., M. MELLO-AIRES and G. GIEBISCH: Fed. Proc. **27**, 695 (1968).
15. GIEBISCH, G., L. BERGER and R. F. PITTS: J. Clin. Invest. **34**, 231 (1955).
16. WINDHAGER, E. E. and G. GIEBISCH: Physiol. Rev. **45**, 214 (1965).
17. GIEBISCH, G., G. MALNIC, R. M. KLOSE and E. WINDHAGER: Am. J. Physiol. **211**, 560 (1966).
18. SULLIVAN, W. J.: Am J. Physiol. **214**, 1096 (1968).
19. BOULPAEP, E. L.: In Transport und Funktion intracellulärer Elektrolyte, page 98, Urban und Schwarzenberg, München-Berlin-Wien (1967).
20. GIEBISCH, G.: J. Gen. Physiol. 51, part **2**, 315 (1968).
21. WINDHAGER, E. E., E. L. BOULPAEP and G. GIEBISCH: Proc. 3rd Int. Congr. Nephrol., Washington 1966, Vol. 1, p. **35** (1967) (Karger, Basel-New York).
22. LANDWEHR, D. M., J. SCHNERMANN, R. M. KLOSE and G. GIEBISCH: Am. J. Physiol., in press.
23. VIEIRA, F. L. and G. MALNIC: Am. J. Physiol. **214**, 710 (1968).
24. GIEBISCH, G., R. M. KLOSE and G. MALNIC: Bull. Swiss Acad. Med. **23**, 287 (1967).
25. MALNIC, G., R. M. KLOSE and G. GIEBISCH: Am. J. Physiol. **211**, 548 (1966).

BURG: I would like to comment on some related work in our own laboratory.

We have also been interested in measuring electrical characteristics and ion transport in the distal nephron. The studies involved isolated perfused rabbit cortical collecting tubules and were conducted in collaboration with Drs. GRANTHAM, HELMAN and ORLOFF at the National Institutes of Health.

As in the distal convoluted tubule, there is K secretion and Na reabsorption in the cortical collecting tubule. However, the nature of K transport appears to differ from distal tubules in that higher concentrations of K are achieved in the tubule fluid. Further, under the conditions of our experiments, we find no evidence of active K reabsorption.

A second point is that the amount of K secreted is similar to the amount of Na reabsorbed in the cortical collecting tubule. This is of interest in view of Dr. GIEBISCH's comment that the mechanism which limits K secretion when urine Na is low might reside in a portion of the nephron beyond the distal convoluted tubule.

Lastly, we have measured the electrical resistance of the cortical collecting tubule and have found values similar to those which Dr. GIEBISCH has just reported for the distal tubule.

THURAU: Yesterday we heard Dr. THOENES reporting on the histological structure of the distal tubule. He described two types of distal tubular cells. I would like to ask Dr. GIEBISCH whether or not he found evidence for the existence of different types of cells from his measurements of membrane potentials.

GIEBISCH: It is the second half of the distal tubule which is capable of variable potassium secretion. The first part of this nephron part (– to about 50% distal tubular length –) shows a more monotonous behaviour. Independent of the metabolic situation, transport rate of potassium varies but little along this part of the nephron. It might be added that the transtubular electrical conductance is not different when early and late distal tubular data are compared. This holds both for conditions in which normal tubular fluid or potassium sulphate only is present in the lumen.

Intracellular Action of Aldosterone on Sodium Transport

I. S. EDELMAN

Summary: Additional evidence has been presented in support of the inference that aldosterone regulates active sodium transport by an induction mechanism, initiated at the level of DNA-dependent RNA synthesis. FANESTIL's (7) recent results indicate that DNA synthesis is not involved in the process. The intermediate active product is an aldosterone-induced protein(s) (AIP) which is accumulated during the induction process. This conclusion is derived from the finding that cycloheximide (an inhibitor of ribosomal assembly of polypeptides) did *not* inhibit the substrate-dependent response of toad bladders pre-treated with aldosterone (Fig. 3). The induction hypothesis does not, of course, rule out the possibility that aldosterone might either directly or indirectly reduce the rate of degradation of an active intermediate protein. To assess this possibility we (10) pre-treated hemibladders with aldosterone and then inhibited protein synthesis in the continued presence and absence of aldosterone. A stabilizing effect of aldosterone on AIP should have shown up as a decreased rate of inhibition of sodium transport when aldosterone was added to the media (Fig. 5). No such effect was found. The alternative possibility was also considered that aldosterone might induce at the translational rather than the transcriptional level (10). If this were the case, the latent period should be taken up in accumulating threshold amounts of AIP and should depend on intact protein synthesis pathways. Contrary to this expectation, we found that the system was insensitive to cycloheximide during the latent period as revealed by the rapid response in sodium transport on removal of cycloheximide just before the end of the latent period (Fig. 4). These results led us to conclude that aldosterone initiates the induction mechanism at the level of DNA-dependent RNA synthesis.

As an approach to the problem of where and how aldosterone initiates the induction process a series of studies have been carried out on the binding of aldosterone to subcellular sites and binding proteins. Some information has been provided by radioautographs of the toad bladder. ^{3}H-Aldosterone was localized over the nuclear areas of the target epithelial cells but the inactive steroid, ^{3}H-progesterone, was distributed more evenly between the nuclear and cytoplasmic regions. The nuclear localization pattern also appeared to be specific for mineralocorticoids as 9α-fluorocortisol displaced ^{3}H-aldosterone from the nuclear areas significantly but estradiol-17β was without effect (Table 2). The possibility that the binding process is involved in the initiation of the induction process has been gaining credence. My colleagues and I (13, 18, 20) have extended the studies of binding of aldosterone in tissues to the adrenalectomized rat kidney. Differential and saturable binding to the nuclear fraction was observed. Recently, we succeeded in isolating and partially purifying aldosterone-binding proteins from renal nuclear and cytosol fractions. These tissue binding proteins are stereo-specific (Table 4) and show an impressive correlation between affinities for steroids and the mineralocorticoid potency of these steroids. Moreover, significantly higher aldosterone-binding activity was found in the epithelial tissues (kidney and duodenal mucosa) than in the parenchymal organs, spleen, liver and brain (Table 3). Further studies are underway on the relation of tissue steroid-binding proteins to physiological action.

From earlier studies on the rat kidney and the urinary bladder of the toad, *Bufo marinus*, it was inferred that aldosterone controls sodium transport by initiating a sequence of reactions which include stimulation of DNA-dependent RNA synthesis and *de novo* synthesis of proteins (1–6). In this communication, I will consider the following questions: 1. Does the action of aldosterone begin with an effect on RNA synthesis or is DNA synthesis involved as well? 2. Is the intermediate an accumulated aldosterone-induced protein (AIP) or does continued protein synthesis prevent the disappearance of a normal component that plays only a facultative role? 3. If AIP mediates the action of aldosterone, is the induction primarily transcriptional rather than translational? 4. Where in the cell and how does aldosterone initiate the induction process?

I. Role of RNA vs DNA Synthesis in the Action of Aldosterone

Impairment of RNA synthesis with actinomycin D inhibits the aldosterone-mediated increase in sodium transport in the isolated toad bladder at concentrations that do not depress the baseline rate of sodium transport or the response to vasopressin (1, 4, 5). The magnitude of inhibition of the effect on sodium transport is proportional to the effect on RNA synthesis (5). These results are summarized in Table 1. Note that the analogue

Table 1. Comparison of the effects of actinomycin D and 6-azauracil on RNA synthesis and aldosterone stimulation of active sodium transport.

No. of Pairs*)	Inhibitor	RNA Specific Activity+ (Inhibitor/Control)	scc Ratio**) (Inhibitor +Aldosterone/ Aldosterone)
4	Actinomycin D (5 μg/ml)	0.53 ± 0.052	0.59 ± 0.079
4	Actinomycin D (20 μg/ml)	0.33 ± 0.052	0.39 ± 0.094
8	6-Azauracil (1.31×10^{-3} M)	1.07 ± 0.21	0.94 ± 0.065

* No. of pairs refers to the studies of ^{3}H-uridine incorporation into RNA. +Specific activity of RNA (cpm/μg RNA) of the inhibitor-treated hemibladder divided by the specific activity of the paired control expressed as a mean ± SEM.

** The "scc ratio" denotes the fractional rise in short-circuit current (i. e., scc at 6 hr/scc at 0 time) of the hemibladders treated with the inhibitor plus aldosterone (7×10^{-7} M) divided by the fractional rise in short-circuit current of the hemibladders treated only with aldosterone (7×10^{-7} M). Mean ± SEM. Taken from FANESTIL and EDELMAN (5).

6-azauracil, which in other systems also inhibits RNA synthesis, had no effect on either the short-circuit current response to aldosterone or RNA synthesis. Recent findings of FANESTIL (7) indicate that the requirement for an intact pathway for nucleic acid synthesis is limited to RNA. He tested the effects of phleomycin and hydroxyurea, inhibitors of DNA synthesis, on the response of the toad bladder to aldosterone. These results are displayed in Fig. 1 and show no effect on the response to aldosterone. At these concentrations, FANESTIL (7) found that phleomycin inhibited incorporation of ^{3}H-thymidine into DNA by 25% and hydroxyurea inhibited incorporation by 62%, in the isolated toad bladder. The action of aldosterone, therefore, is selectively dependent on intact pathways for RNA synthesis. It is possible, however, that the requirement of intact pathways for RNA and protein synthesis involve the need for maintenance of normal levels of specific intracellular proteins but do not involve the accumulation of specifically-induced proteins.

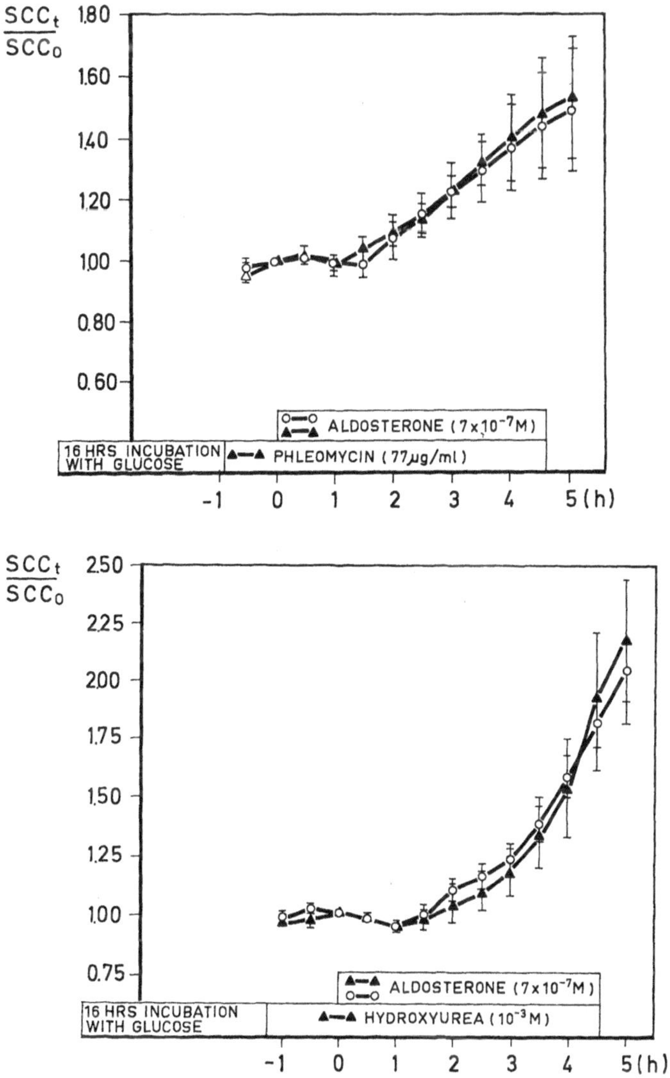

Fig. 1. scc_t/scc_0 is the short-circuit current at time "t" divided by that recorded at time zero. Vertical bars represent $\pm$ SEM. In the phleomycin experiments (upper half of the Figure) $scc_0 = 88 \pm 12$ µA (▲) and 104 ± 15 µA (○); n = 4 pairs. In the hydroxyurea experiments (lower half of the Figure) $scc_0 = 44 \pm 8$ µA (▲) and 42 ± 7 µA (○); n = 8 pairs. Reprinted from FANESTIL (7).

II. Accumulation of AIP in the Action of Aldosterone

As the identity of AIP has not been established, only indirect evidence has been obtained on its accumulation and role in the action of aldosterone. The argument we formulated was as follows: If aldosterone induces the formation and accumulation of AIP as an obligatory intermediate, then inhibitors of protein synthesis at the ribosomal level, such as cycloheximide, should not prevent the response in pre-induced toad bladders. To test this possibility, we took advantage of the substrate-dependence of the response to aldosterone. As shown in Fig. 2, substrate-depleted hemibladders are insensitive to

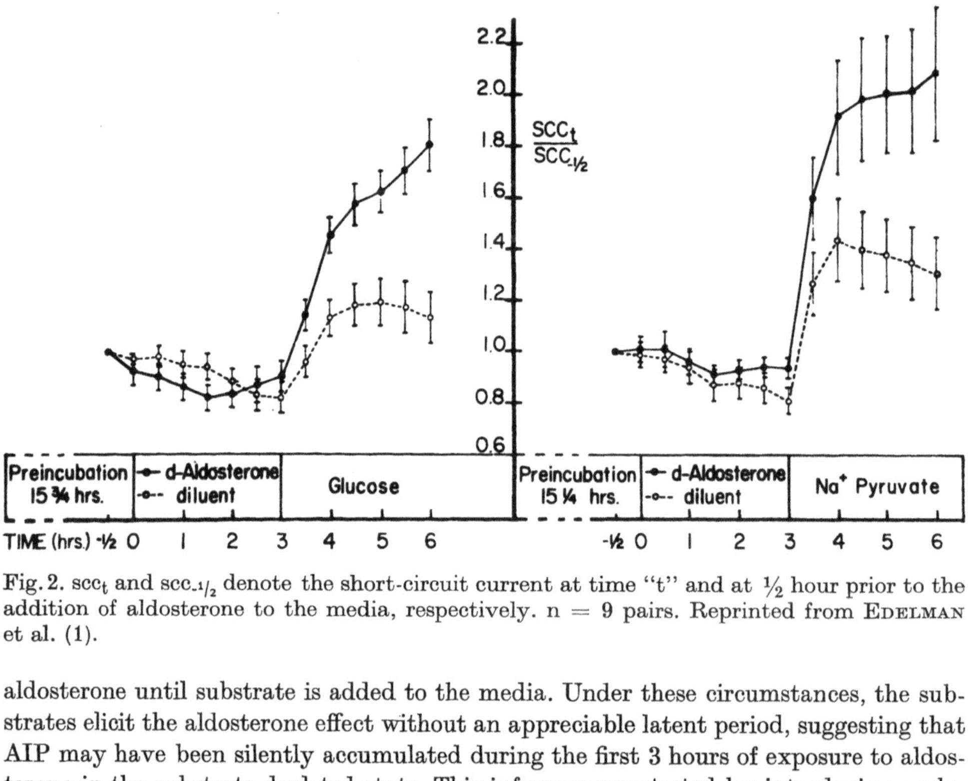

Fig. 2. scc_t and $scc_{-1/2}$ denote the short-circuit current at time "t" and at ½ hour prior to the addition of aldosterone to the media, respectively. n = 9 pairs. Reprinted from EDELMAN et al. (1).

aldosterone until substrate is added to the media. Under these circumstances, the substrates elicit the aldosterone effect without an appreciable latent period, suggesting that AIP may have been silently accumulated during the first 3 hours of exposure to aldosterone in the substrate-depleted state. This inference was tested by introducing cycloheximide into the media 30 minutes before adding pyruvate (Fig. 3). In earlier experiments, we found that at a concentration of 0.5 μg./ml, cycloheximide reduced the rate of protein synthesis to 37% of the control level and eliminated the sodium transport effect of aldosterone when the inhibitor was introduced at the same time as the steroid (5). As shown in Fig. 3, cycloheximide was added 3.5 hours after the addition of aldosterone to substrate-depleted hemibladders. Cycloheximide had no effect on the aldosterone-dependent response to pyruvate for 90 minutes (8). These results suggest that AIP accumulated during the first 3 hours of exposure to aldosterone and that inhibition of protein synthesis does not impair the expression of the biological activity of preformed AIP. It is pertinent to ask whether aldosterone induces by an action at the gene

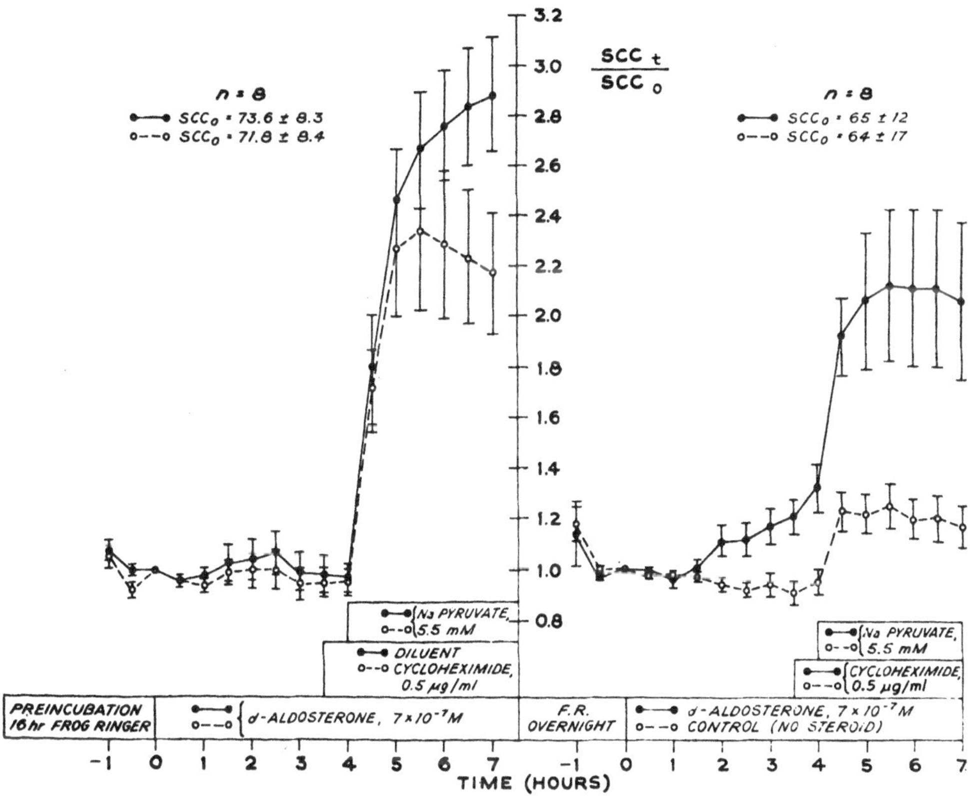

Fig. 3. See legend to Figure 1 for definitions. In the experiments on the left, both hemibladders received aldosterone and one of each pair (–○–) received cycloheximide. In the experiments on the right both hemibladders received cycloheximide and one of each pair (–●–) received aldosterone. Reprinted from FANESTIL et al. (8).

level or by stimulating protein synthesis at the ribosomal level or by stabilizing the intermediate protein being formed at a steady rate (i. e., preventing breakdown of AIP).

III. Genetic vs. Non-Genetic Induction by Aldosterone

To obtain information on the locus of action of aldosterone in the induction process, we turned our attention to the significance of the latent period. It is well-known that the response to aldosterone in mammalian as well as anuran systems is characterized by a latent period of from 45 to 90 min. CRABBÉ (9) noted that the latent period ($\sim$90 min) in the response of the toad bladder to aldosterone was not reduced by increasing amounts of steroid. He concluded that the latent period was determined by the time required to accumulate an active intermediate rather than slow diffusion of aldosterone into the tissue. From the standpoint of the induction hypothesis, the latent period could signify the time required for the acquisition of threshold amounts of AIP following either altered translational (or protein degradation) or transcriptional actions of the steroid. If the former were the case, inhibition of protein synthesis during the latent period would lengthen the latent period proportionally, as the action of the steroid would be exerted on the process of protein synthesis or breakdown directly. If, however, aldosterone stimulates RNA synthesis which in turn directs protein synthesis, the latent period could be devoted solely to the time required to generate threshold quantities of steroid-induced RNA. If this were the case, inhibition of protein synthesis solely during the latent period should not lengthen the latent period appreciably. The experiment designed to test these alternatives is shown in Fig. 4. In this study cycloheximide (0.5 μg/ml) was added at

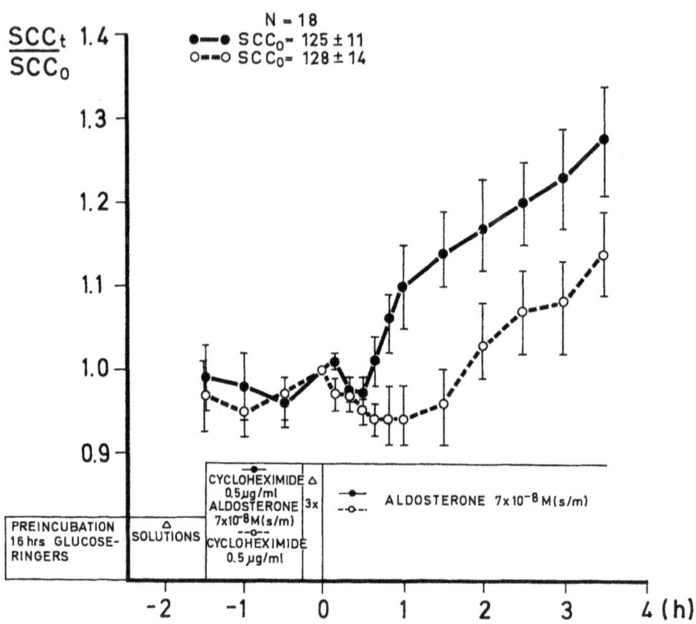

Fig. 4. See legend to Figure 1 for definitions. At t = −1.5 hr one of each pair of hemibladders (–●–) received cycloheximide, 0.5 μg/ml and aldosterone, 7×10^{-8} M, and the other (– – ○– –) was exposed only to cycloheximide, 0.5 μg/ml. At t = −15 min all solutions were removed and replaced with glucose-Ringer's solution. The solutions were changed three times in 15 min. At t = ○, all solutions were fortified with aldosterone, 7×10^{-8} M. Taken from HERMAN and EDELMAN (23).

time zero to both hemibladders, one of which was also exposed to aldosterone. After 75 minutes, the media were removed and both hemibladders exposed to aldosterone. In the control hemibladders, pre-treatment with cycloheximide had no effect on the subsequent response to aldosterone as indicated by the usual latent period of 90 min. Moreover, the simultaneous addition of cycloheximide and aldosterone followed by removal of cycloheximide at the end of the normal latent period did not lengthen this period appreciably. These results indicate that the latent period is not devoted to events at the ribosomal level and may, therefore, represent the time required for the formation of steroid-dependent RNA. These results also tend to contradict the possibility that aldosterone reduces the rate of degradation of AIP. As a further test of this inference, LAHAV and I (10) studied the effect of aldosterone on the reversal of the response to aldosterone produced by cycloheximide. The design of the experiment was as follows: Pairs of hemibladders were preincubated in glucose-Ringer's solution for six hours and then exposed to aldosterone, 7×10^{-8} M, for an additional eight hours. At this time, all of the hemibladders showed a maximum response to aldosterone. The solutions were removed and replaced three times with steroid-free Ringer's solution to eliminate virtually all of the aldosterone from the system. One of each pair of hemibladders was exposed to cycloheximide (0.5 μg/ml) and aldosterone (7×10^{-8} M) and the other to cycloheximide alone. At this concentration, cycloheximide completely inhibits the response to aldosterone, presumably because of inhibition of the formation of AIP. If aldosterone either directly or indirectly slows the degradation of AIP this should be revealed by a slower rate of decay in short-circuit current despite the presence of cycloheximide. The results shown in Fig. 5 give no indication of an effect of aldosterone on the rate of degradation of AIP.

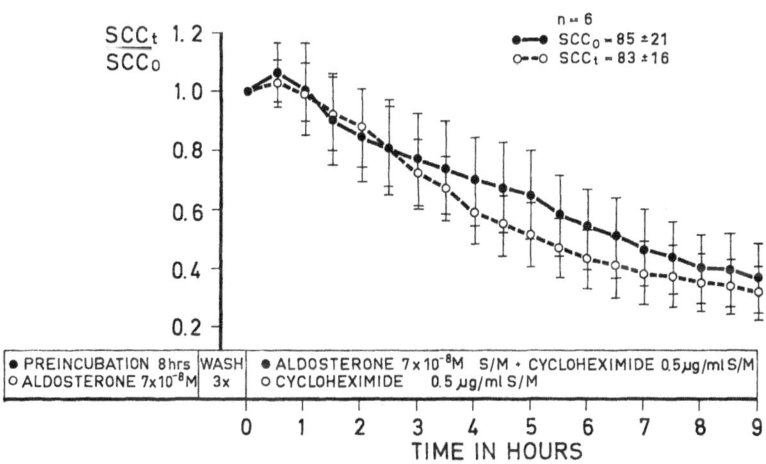

Fig. 5. See legend to Figure 1 for definitions. Pairs of hemibladders were incubated in aldosterone (7×10^{-8} M) for 8 hours and then all solutions were removed and replaced 3 times with steroid-free glucose-Ringer's. At t = ○, one of each pair (–●–) was incubated in aldosterone, 7×10^{-8} M, and cycloheximide 0.5 μg/ml, and the other (– – ○– –) in cycloheximide, 0.5 μg/ml, alone. Taken from LAHAV and EDELMAN (10).

The evidence summarized above supports the inference that aldosterone activates DNA-dependent RNA synthesis and that this in turn leads to enhanced synthesis of steroid-specific proteins (AIP) which regulate sodium transport in proportion to the increase in local amounts of AIP. No effect of aldosterone is apparent on either translational control of synthesis of AIP or on rates of degradation of AIP. As an approach to the understanding of the process of initiation of the induction mechanism by aldosterone, my colleagues and I have been studying the interaction of aldosterone with specific components in target tissues.

IV. Site of Initial Action of Aldosterone in Target Tissues

The first clue to the possible subcellular site of action of aldosterone was provided by radioautographs of the toad bladder (1, 3). ^{3}H-aldosterone was concentrated over the nuclei of the epithelial cells. This distribution contrasted with that of the inactive steroid, ^{3}H-progesterone, which was randomly distributed between the nuclear and cytoplasmic regions (3). Recently, R. BOGOROCH (11) extended these studies by testing the relative effects of the active mineralocorticoid, 9α-fluorocortisol and the inactive steroid, estradiol-17β, on the localization of ^{3}H-aldosterone. Her results are summarized in Table 2 and indicate that 9α-fluorocortisol displaced aldosterone from most of the

Table 2. Distribution of ^{3}H-Aldosterone in Toad Bladder Epithelial Cells*).

Competing Steroid	Concentration	Grain Counts	
	$\times 10^8$ Molar	nucleus	cytoplasm
None	—	5	2
Estradiol-17β	600	5	2
9α-fluorococortisol	600	2	1

* ^{3}H-aldosterone was added to all media at a concentration of 6×10^{-8} M. These results are summarized from BOGOROCH (11).

nuclear binding sites, whereas estradiol-17β was without effect. Additional evidence of a mineralocorticoid specific binding mechanism in the toad bladder has been obtained by SHARP et al. (12) who determined the ability of a variety of steroids to displace ^{3}H-aldosterone. Except for progesterone, they found a positive correlation between mineralocorticoid activity and displacing potency. The correlation between nuclear localization of steroids and mineralocorticoid potency has been extended in studies on adrenalectomized rats (13). Within physiological plasma concentrations, only the nuclear fraction of renal homogenates gave saturation kinetics in the uptake of ^{3}H-aldosterone. Moreover, at plasma aldosterone concentrations below that needed to produce maximum urinary sodium retention, the nuclear fraction contained the highest concentration of ^{3}H-aldosterone compared to that of the cytosol, mitochondrial and microsomal fractions. In competition studies, nuclear uptake of ^{3}H-aldosterone was reduced to less than 10% of the control value by 75-fold greater quantities of 9 α-fluorocortisol. In contrast, 6 α-methylprednisolone and estradiol-17β (steroids with little or no effect on urinary excretion of sodium) had no effect on renal nuclear uptake of ^{3}H-aldosterone. In the other cell fractions (mitochondrial, microsomal and cytosol) none of the steroids tested altered the uptake of ^{3}H-aldosterone. Evidence was also obtained that the nuclear binding mechanism involved the formation of steroid: protein complexes. Incubation of pre-labeled renal nuclei with broad spectrum proteolytic enzymes accelerated the release of ^{3}H-aldosterone whereas DNase, RNase, lipase, phospholipase D and neuraminadase had no effect. Similar results have been obtained in studies on the binding of estradiol to the nuclear myofibrillar fraction of the rat uterus supporting the inference that most if not all of the binding mechanism consists of specific binding proteins (14).

My colleagues and I have also tried to clarify or define the site and nature of the aldosterone-initiated induction mechanism by attempting to isolate and purify the tissue-binding substances and to explore the possible role of these binding substances in initiating the physiological response. An explanation of how such steroid: protein complexes might lead to specific functional outputs has been suggested by MONOD et al. (15). They proposed that the binding of small molecules (e. g., hormones) to allosteric sites could result in conformational changes in the protein that would produce profound changes in function. For two systems, cortisol acting on the liver and ecdysone on the immature insect, it has been postulated that the interaction of the steroid and its receptor might stimulate transcription by derepression at the gene level (16, 17).

HERMAN, FIMOGNARI and I (18) recently succeeded in isolating and partially purifying aldosterone: protein complexes extracted from renal nuclear and cytosol fractions obtained from adrenalectomized rats. Purified renal nuclear fractions were prepared by centrifugation in 2.2 M sucrose – 3 mM $CaCl_2$ and were then extracted in 0.1 M tris-$CaCl_2$ buffer solutions for 10 min at 0° C. The nuclear pellets were sedimented and the tris extracts recovered and assayed for free and bound ^{3}H-aldosterone. The extracts contained 81% of the total nuclear ^{3}H-aldosterone content and 65% of the extractable activity proved to be bound to macromolecules. Steroid: polymer complexes were isolated both by precipitation in 50% $(NH_4)_2SO_4$ and by column chromatography on G-50 and G-75 Sephadex. Chemical analysis of the tris extracts revealed that the predominant macromolecular species were proteins as no DNA and only minute quantities of RNA were found. To carry the analysis of the binding species one step further, we tested the effect of a variety of hydrolases on the binding of aldosterone. Tris-$CaCl_2$ extracts of purified renal nuclear fractions obtained from adrenalectomized rats were incubated with the hydrolases for 10 min at 20° C and bound ^{3}H-aldosterone isolated by precipitation in 50% $(NH_4)_2SO_4$. DNase, RNase and trypsin had no effect on the recovery of bound ^{3}H-aldosterone. Pronase and chymotrypsin (broad spectrum proteolytic enzymes), however, liberated 50% and 65% of the bound ^{3}H-aldosterone, respectively. Further evidence that the renal nuclear binding substances are proteins was obtained with the sulfhydryl reagents pHMB and S-β aminoethyl thiourea (AET). Treatment of renal nuclear extracts with pHMB or AET destroyed virtually all of the binding activity indicating that intact SH groups of cysteine or methionine residues are necessary for steroid binding activity.

The availability of methods for quantifying the formation of aldosterone: protein complexes enabled us to compare the binding process in various organs and tissues. Differentiation of target tissues that are specialized for transepithelial sodium transport should correlate with the development of the binding mechanism. Thus, SULYA et al. (19) found that 60–90 minutes after i.v. administration, ^{3}H-aldosterone was preferentially accumulated by rat kidney and duodenal mucosa, tissues with known responsiveness to mineralocorticoids compared to a variety of other tissues. SWANECK, HIGHLAND and I (20) have extended these observations by determining the relative aldosterone-binding capacity of nuclear and cytosol fractions of kidney, duodenal mucosa, spleen, liver and brain in adrenalectomized rats. The results of these experiments are given in Table 3. The kidney and duodenal mucosa had the highest nuclear and cytosol binding activity. The spleen, liver and brain had very little aldosterone-binding protein in the cytosol

Table 3. Comparsion of Aldosterone-Binding Proteins in Various Tissues of Adrenalectomized Rats*)

No. of Rats	Tissue	Bound ^{3}H-Aldosterone (moles $\times$ 10^{14}/mgm protein)		
		Purified Nuclei	Nuclear Extract	Cytosol
7	Kidney	2.5 ± 0.3	11.5 ± 2.2	2.2 ± 0.4
7	Duodenal Mucosa	2.8 ± 0.7	5.9 ± 1.7	3.7 ± 1.2
8	Spleen	1.3 ± 0.2	4.4 ± 0.7	0.3 ± 0.1
8	Liver	0.9 ± 0.2	1.6 ± 0.3	0.04 ± 0.001
5	Brain	1.4 ± 0.3	1.5 ± 0.2	0.3 ± 0.04

*) All results are given as mean $\pm$ SEM. The purified nuclei were prepared by centrifugation through 2.2 M sucrose-3 mM $CaCl_2$. The nuclear extracts were prepared by eluting purified nuclear fractions in 0.1 M Tris-3 mM $CaCl_2$ for 10 min at 0° C, sedimenting the nuclei and precipitating bound ^{3}H-aldosterone in 50% $(NH_4)_2SO_4$. Cytosol fractions ($10^5 \times g$ supernatants) were passed through G-50 Sephadex columns. The bound ^{3}H-aldosterone was eluted in the external volume of the column coincidentally with the protein in each sample. Taken from SWANECK et al. (20).

fractions but significant binding was obtained in the nuclear fractions and the $(NH_4)_2SO_4$ precipitates of the nuclear extracts. Thus, the distinction in aldosterone-specific uptake by surface epithelial versus parenchymal cells is not absolute. There is no evidence, however, that the cells of liver, spleen and brain possess a mechanism for responding to steroid-binding with an effect on sodium transport. In the case of estrogens, the correlation between sensitivity to the hormone and tissue binding appears to be pronounced. JENSEN and JACOBSON (21) reported that ^{3}H-estradiol-17β was preferentially bound to the target tissues, uterus and vagina, but rapidly cleared from the liver and other estrogen-insensitive tissues.

As shown in Table 3, significant aldosterone binding activity is found in the renal cytosol as well as the nuclear fractions. HERMAN et al. (18) identified the cytosol binding substances as proteins by the following criteria: 1. Dissociation of the ^{3}H-aldosterone complexes by wide spectrum proteolytic enzymes (i. e., pronase and chymotrypsin) but not by nucleases, lipase or phospholipase. 2. Loss of binding activity on incubation of cytosol fractions with pHMB. It is reasonable to consider the possibility that the formation of aldosterone:protein complexes is directly involved in the initiation of the action on sodium transport. Binding *per se*, however, does not imply a direct physiological action. An alternative possibility is that tissue binding of aldosterone may provide a storage mechanism that regulates intracellular concentrations of the free hormone in the target tissues during periods of falling hormonal concentrations in the circulation, in the same sense that myoglobin preserves intracellular O_2 tensions during anoxia. Although no direct means is yet available for defining the physiological role of tissue aldosterone-binding proteins, we have explored the possible relevance of this mechanism to action on Na^+ transport by assessing the relative affinities of a variety of steroids for the aldosterone-binding sites. In the adrenalectomized rat, the relative mineralocorticoid potencies were found to be in the order: aldosterone $>$ 9α-fluorocortisol $>$ DOC $>$ 6α-methylprednisolone $\geq$ 17α-isoaldosterone $=$ estradiol-17β $=$ no steroid (6, 22). HERMAN et al. (18) determined the ability of these steroids to displace ^{3}H-aldosterone from binding proteins isolated from renal nuclear and cytosol fractions. We found that at dose ratios of ~75:1, the competing steroids displaced ^{3}H-aldosterone from both nuclear and cytosol complexes in the order: 9α-fluorocortisol > DOC > 6α-methylprednisolone > estradiol-17β = no steroid. There was, therefore, a striking correlation between potency as a mineralocorticoid and affinity for aldosterone binding sites. An even more stringent test of the correlation between binding and physiological action was found in studies with the stereoisomer, 17α-isoaldosterone. This isomer has been found to be devoid of activity on the rates of urinary Na^+ and K^+ excretion in adrenalectomized rats in doses of 1 μg/150 g rat. This dose is 5 times that needed to produce a maximal effect on urinary electrolytes with aldosterone (22). Tris-$CaCl_2$ extracts of crude renal nuclear fractions were prepared from untreated adrenalectomized rats and incubated for 2.5 hrs at 0° C with 5.9×10^{-10} M ^{3}H-aldosterone. Aliquots of these incubates were treated with either d-aldosterone or 17α-isoaldosterone at concentrations of 5×10^{-9} M. Bound ^{3}H-aldosterone was then isolated by chromatography on G-50 Sephadex. As indicated in Table 4, d-aldosterone reduced the binding of ^{3}H-aldosterone by 60% but

Table 4. In Vitro 17-Isoaldosterone and Unlabeled Aldosterone Competition for ^{3}H-Aldosterone Binding Sites in Nuclear Extracts*)

Steroid	Concentration ($M \times 10^{-9}$)	Bound ^{3}H-Aldosterone (% of control)
None	—	100
Unlabeled aldosterone	5.9	40.8
Isoaldosterone	5.9	109.2

*) Mean of 3 experiments. Tris-$CaCl_2$ extracts of crude nuclear fractions were incubated with 5.9×10^{-10} M ^{3}H-aldosterone for 2.5 hours alone or with an additional steroid. ^{3}H-aldosterone complexes were isolated by G-50 Sephadex chromatography. Nine aliquots from a single pool of kidneys obtained from 9 donor rats were used. Reprinted from HERMAN et al. (18).

17α-isoaldosterone had no effect on the recovery of ^{3}H-aldosterone:protein complexes. Additional evidence that the stereoisomer is unable to bind to aldosterone-specific sites was obtained with ^{14}C-17α-isoaldosterone. At a concentration of 2.9×10^{-8} M in the external medium, no steroid:protein complexes were formed in tris-$CaCl_2$ extracts of crude renal nuclear fractions prepared from adrenalectomized rats (18). Additional evidence has been obtained that the ^{3}H-aldosterone binding mechanism involves aldosterone-specific, saturable binding, *in vivo* (23). Adrenalectomized rats were injected with 2.6×10^{-10} moles of ^{3}H-aldosterone and either no additional d-aldosterone or 10 times (2.6×10^{-9} moles) or 100 times (2.6×10^{-8} moles) of d-aldosterone. Purified nuclear fractions and 50% $(NH_4)_2SO_4$ precipitates of tris-$CaCl_2$ extracts of the nuclear fractions were then prepared. The results in Table 5 show that at a 10:1 concentration ratio, ~80% of the ^{3}H-aldosterone is displaced from binding to nuclear binding proteins [i. e., the $(NH_4)_2SO_4$ precipitable activity] and at a 100:1 concentration ratio ~95% is displaced. The results indicate, therefore, that renal nuclear uptake is specific for aldosterone and related mineralocorticoids. Moreover, HERMAN et al. (18) found that

Table 5. Competition for ³H-Aldosterone Binding Sites by d-Aldosterone in Renal Nuclei*).

Fraction	*d-Aldosterone* Moles injected	*Specific Activity* Moles $\times 10^{14}$/mgm protein	% *Bound*
Purified Nuclei	0	4.3 ± 0.3	100
Purified Nuclei	2.6×10^{-9}	1.1 ± 0.2	25.5
Purified Nuclei	2.6×10^{-8}	0.41 ± 0.06	9.5
50% $(NH_4)_2SO_4$	0	18.4 ± 1.1	100
50% $(NH_4)_2SO_4$	2.6×10^{-9}	3.9 ± 0.3	21.1
50% $(NH_4)_2SO_4$	2.6×10^{-8}	0.97 ± 0.06	5.3

*) Results are given as mean ± SEM. All rats were injected with 2.6×10^{-10} moles of ^{3}H-aldosterone with or without added d-aldosterone. The rats were killed 30 minutes after injection. Results are from HERMAN and EDELMAN (23.)

spirolactone inhibited the formation of ^{3}H-aldosterone-protein complexes *in vitro*, in both renal nuclear and cytosol fractions and that the degree of inhibition correlated weel with the known effects of spirolactone on mineralocorticoid action, *in vivo*. It appears, therefore, that we have isolated and partially purified renal nuclear and cytosol proteins which have many of the properties to be expected of the specific mineralocorticoid receptors. It is not yet possible to define the number of such receptors or their roles in the physiological process. Indeed, the striking similarity in the relative affinities of a variety of steroids (9α-fluorocortisol, DOC, 6α-methylprednisolone, estradiol-17β and spirolactone) for the aldosterone-binding protein found in the nuclear and cytosol fractions suggests that the binding protein may be the same in both fractions. This raises the possibility that *in vivo* the binding mechanism as well as initiation of the physiological process is located solely in the nucleus. The definition of the role of specific aldosterone-binding proteins in mineralocorticoid action will depend on purification of the binding proteins and an analysis of their relationship to RNA synthesis.

References

1. EDELMAN, I. S., R. BOGOROCH and G. A. PORTER: *Proc. Nat. Acad. Sci.*, **50**, 1169 (1963).
2. WILLIAMSON, H. E.: *Biochem. Pharmacol.*, **12**, 1449 (1963).
3. PORTER, G. A., R. BOGOROCH and I. S. EDELMAN: *Proc. Nat. Acad. Sci.*, **52**, 1326 (1964).
4. CRABBÉ, J. and P. DEWEER: *Nature*, **202**, 298 (1964).
5. FANESTIL, D. D. and I. S. EDELMAN: *Federation Proc.*, **25**, 912 (1966).
6. FIMOGNARI, G. M., D. D. FANESTIL and I. S. EDELMAN: *Am. J. Physiol.* **213**, 954 (1967).
7. FANESTIL, D. D.: *Life Sciences*, **7**, 191 (1968).
8. FANESTIL, D. D., T. S. HERMAN, G. M. FIMOGNARI and I. S. EDELMAN: International Symposium on Regulatory Functions of Biological Membranes, Helsinki, Finland. *Biochim. Biophys. Acta*, Library Series, Vol. II Elsevier Publ. Co. 1968, p. 177.
9. CRABBÉ, J.: The Sodium-Retaining Action of Aldosterone. Presses Acad. Europ. S. C. Editions Arscia, Brussels, 1963.
10. LAHAV, M. and I. S. EDELMAN: Unpublished observations.

11. BOGOROCH, R.: Symposium on High Resolution Autoradiography of Diffusible Substances. Academic Press N. Y., L. J. ROTH and W. STUMPF, Editors. In press.
12. SHARP, G. W. G., C. L. KOMACK and A. LEAF: *J. Clin. Invest.*, **45,** 450 (1966).
13. FANESTIL, D. D. and I. S. EDELMAN: *Proc. Nat. Acad. Sci.*, **56,** 872 (1966).
14. NOTEBOOM, W. D. and J. GORSKI: *Arch. Biochem. and Biophys.*, **III,** 559 (1965).
15. MONOD, J., J. P. CHANGEUX and F. JACOB: *J. Mol. Biol.*, **6,** 306 (1963).
16. DAHMUS, M. E. and J. BONNER: *Proc. Nat. Acad. Sci.* (U. S.) **54,** 1370 (1965).
17. SEKERIS, C. E. and P. KARLSON: *Arch. Biochem. and Biophys.*, **105,** 483 (1964).
18. HERMAN, T. S., G. M. FIMOGNARI and I. S. EDELMAN: *J. Biol. Chem.*, **243,** 3849 (1968).
19. SULYA, L. L., C. S. McCAA, V. H. READ and D. BOMMER: *Nature*, **200,** 788 (1963).
20. SWANECK, G., E. HIGHLAND and I. S. EDELMAN: Unpublished observations.
21. JENSEN, E. V. and H. I. JACOBSON: In Recent Progress in Hormone Research, Vol. 18, p. 387, Ed. G. PINCUS, Academic Press, N. Y. (1962).
22. HIGHLAND, E. and I. S. EDELMAN: Unpublished observations.
23. HERMAN, T. S. and I. S. EDELMAN: Unpublished observations.

CRABBÉ: Dr. EDELMAN, let me tell you first what I think of the paper: "bravo!" Certainly, this is internationally understood. I am happy about these data you reported about cycloheximide; recently we have carried out an experiment much along the lines you have suggested here, namely: incubation of toad bladder in the presence of aldosterone on the one hand and of cycloheximide on the other hand, and then removal of cycloheximide after the latency period. This enabled us, as you actually have presented already, to unmask the effect of aldosterone almost immediately; so we would come to the same conclusion in that most of the latency period probably results from the time it takes aldosterone to stimulate ribonucleic acid synthesis, rather than protein synthesis.

May I now ask you a small question? I was a bit surprised about your statement that the small intestine is a target for aldosterone; I would be interested in the experimental evidence for this. And the corollary to this question: did you look at the extent of labelling of colonic mucosa with aldosterone, since this preparation is a well-known target for aldosterone action?

EDELMAN: Some evidence that duodenal mucosa is a target tissue for aldosterone has been summarized by SULYA, L. L. et al. (Nature, 200:788, 1963). I agree that there is more extensive evidence that colonic mucosa responds to aldosterone but we have not yet studied binding of ^{3}H-aldosterone to subcellular or isolated receptors in this target tissue.

GROSS: I have two questions. Firstly: In your nuclear fraction you had nuclei from the entire kidney, I assume. So you could not differentiate between nuclei from cells in which aldosterone may be of significance or not. Would it not be possible to study the attachment to the nuclei more specifically by means of autoradiographic techniques? Secondly: Did you also try analogues to aldosterone, not only 9-αfluoro-cortisol, but also desoyxcorticosterone and did it do the same as 9-αfluoro-cortisol?

EDELMAN: We have tried 9-αfluoro-cortisol, desoxycorticosterone, 6-αmethyl-prednisolone, estradiol, spironolactone and 17αisoaldosterone. And in all cases the competitive relationship is proportional to the physiological action. As far as the question of heterogeneity is concerned, we were relying to some extent on Dr. HIERHOLZER's findings indicating that aldosterone acts at both the proximal and distal levels of the kidney. R. BOGOROCH has prepared radioautographs of the rat kidney and found significant radioactivity in the nuclei at all levels of the kidney: collecting ducts, distal tubule and proximal tubule. Thus, our results tend, in turn, to support those of HIERHOLZER and his colleagues.

Leaf: We looked at the specificity of binding of aldosterone in several tissues of the toad. By specific binding I refer to the displaceable binding of aldosterone by the tissue. The tissue is incubated 60 minutes with tritium labeled aldosterone of high specific activity but a low total concentration (10^{-11} to 10^{-9} M, generally). A thousand fold excess of unlabeled aldosterone is then added and the decrease in the amount of radioactive aldosterone in the tissue assayed. This is our measure of the reversible binding or displaceable binding capacity of the tissue. When muscle, heart, lung, serosa and urinary bladder of the toad were examined, only the bladder showed such reversible binding capacity. This we regard as consistent with the fact that of the tissues tested only the bladder responds physiologically to the action of aldosterone. Thus, I wonder at the meaning of the binding you obtain in rat liver and spleen. Perhaps this is related to the glucocorticoid effect which aldosterone is known to possess.

I would like to add that Dr. Sharp has been examining the binding of aldosterone in the nuclei from scraped mucosal epithelial cells in the toad bladder and confirms what Dr. Edelman has demonstrated in the rat kidney. So I think the findings are specific to the cells involved in the active sodium transport which is stimulated by aldosterone.

Edelman: Although my associates and I have not studied binding of aldosterone to receptors in the toad bladder, G. Porter (personal communication) has obtained steroid protein complexes from toad bladder epithelial cells with a similar extraction procedure to ours. The radioactivity bound to nuclear and cytosol proteins of rat liver, spleen and brain represents unmetabolized aldosterone by extraction and chromatography. I did not mean to suggest that the extra-renal binding mechanisms imply an action of aldosterone on active sodium transport in these tissues (i. e. liver, spleen and brain). Separate experiments are needed to establish the physiological role of the binding system in extra-renal as well as in the epithelial tissues. Certainly, glucocorticoid effects may be involved.

Intrarenal Action of Steroid Hormones on Sodium Transport

Intrarenale Wirkung von Steroidhormonen auf den Natriumtransport*)

K. HIERHOLZER

Summary: In the kidneys of adrenalectomized rats we have analyzed Na^+ transport using various micropuncture techniques.

In the *proximal* as well as in the *distal* convolution of surface tubules an impairment of the local Na^+ reabsorptive capacity has been observed, using the split oil droplet method.

However, in the *proximal* convolution fractional reabsorption was found to be normal or even slightly elevated.

Only in the *distal* convolution the intraluminal Na^+ concentration increased both in free flow and in steady state – in the proximal convolution, no such change was observed, indicating that both *outward transport* and *back leakage* of NaCl is affected in adrenalectomy.

The impairment of local NaCl transport could be reversed by small doses of d-aldosterone after a typical delay time. The effects could be suppressed by actinomycin D.

Dexamethasone had no apparent mineralocorticoid effect, but Cortison normalized renal Na^+ reabsorption in high doses.

Seit den Untersuchungen von Loeb (1932/33) ist bekannt, daß ein Ausfall der NNR-Funktion zu einem Verlust von Natriumchlorid und Natriumbikarbonat führt, welcher mit einer Retention von Kalium einhergeht. Diese Störung der Mineralbilanz ist durch eine Störung der Nierenfunktion bedingt, und sie kann durch Aldosteron aufgehoben werden, wobei kleinste Dosen allerdings zunächst nur die tubuläre Resorption von Na^+ steigern ohne die K^+-Ausscheidung zu beeinflussen. Da die Wirkung von Aldosteron auf die Na^+-Resorption durch Actinomycin D unterdrückt werden kann, neigt man zu der Ansicht, daß Aldosteron seine Wirkung auf den Na^+-Transport über einen Eingriff in die DNA-abhängige messenger-RNA-Synthese ausübt.

Welche Vorgänge in der Niere verursachen die für die NNR-Insuffizienz charakteristischen Na^+-Verluste? Wo ist die Transportstörung lokalisiert, d. h. welche Segmente des Nephrons sind betroffen und was ist der Mechanismus – welches sind die Mechanismen – der tubulären Resorptionshemmung?

Es bedarf keiner Begründung, daß die Beantwortung dieser Fragen die Voraussetzung darstellt für die Analyse der intrarenalen Wirkung von Steroidhormonen auf den Natriumtransport. Ich möchte deshalb zuerst die Veränderungen beschreiben, die durch bilaterale Adrenalektomie ausgelöst werden. Nach dem vorangegangenen biochemischen Referat werde ich mich vor allem auf die *physiologischen* Meßgrößen konzentrieren.

Wegen der recht erheblichen Speziesunterschiede sowohl der normalen Nierenfunktion als auch der Ausfallerscheinungen, ist es notwendig zu betonen, daß die experimentellen Untersuchungen, über die ich im folgenden berichte, an Albinoratten durchgeführt wurden. Auf Ausnahmen werde ich ausdrücklich hinweisen.

*) Mit Unterstützung durch die Deutsche Forschungsgemeinschaft.

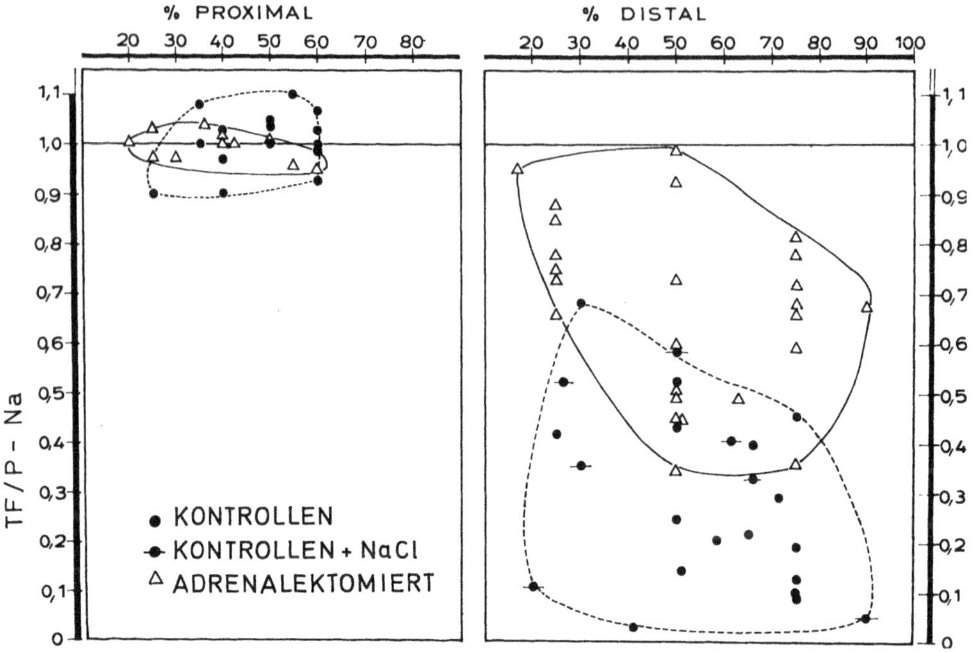

Abb. 1. TF/P-Na⁺-Quotienten in Abhängigkeit von der Punktionsstelle im proximalen und distalen Tubulus bei freiem Fluß (HIERHOLZER, 1965).

I. Änderungen der Na^+-Resorption in der Niere adrenalektomierter Ratten

Zur Frage der Lokalisation der Na^+-Resorptionshemmung im Nephron liegen eine große Zahl von klinischen (GOLDSMITH et al., 1961; CRABBÉ, 1962; SONNENBLICK et al., 1961; YUNIS et al., 1964; JICK et al., 1965) und tierexperimentellen Untersuchungen vor (NICHOLSON, 1957; VANDER et al., 1958; WILLIAMSON et al., 1961; DE LIMA und LOCKETT, 1963; MCEVOY et al., 1965), in denen Clearance- und Stopflow-Methoden angewandt wurden. Ihre Resultate waren recht uneinheitlich; die meisten Ergebnisse deuteten auf eine teilweise Hemmung der Na^+-Resorption in distalen Nephronsegmenten am Ort der fakultativen Na^+-Resorption hin. Für diese Annahme spricht auch die Tatsache, daß nach bilateraler Adrenalektomie nicht die gesamte tubuläre Na^+-Resorption, sondern bilanzmäßig gesehen, nur ein sehr geringer, scheinbar zu vernachlässigender Prozentsatz, gehemmt ist. Nach ROEMMELT, SARTORIUS und PITTS (1949) werden beim Hund nach Ausfall der NNR-Funktion nur 80 mÄq Na^+/min ausgeschieden; das sind ca. 2% der filtrierten Na-Ionen. Prinzipiell die gleichen Verhältnisse bestehen beim Menschen (AUGUST et al., 1959) und bei der Ratte.

Für eine *distale* Hemmung der Na^+-Resorption sprachen auch die ersten Ergebnisse, die wir in Zusammenarbeit mit WINDHAGER und GIEBISCH an adrenalektomierten Ratten erhielten (HIERHOLZER et al., 1965)*). Wie in Abb. 1 dargestellt, ließ sich aus den

*) Alle Tiere waren mindestens eine Woche vor dem Punktionsversuch adrenalektomiert worden. Sie wiesen die typischen Elektrolytveränderungen des Plasmas und des Urins und die typischen Störungen der Wasserausscheidungsfähigkeit auf.

durch Freiflußpunktionen proximaler Tubuli gewonnenen Flüssigkeitsproben kein Unterschied zwischen den Na^+-Konzentrationsquotienten adrenalektomierter und intakter Ratten nachweisen. Im distalen Tubulus dagegen waren die an adrenalektomierten Ratten gewonnenen Werte (Mittelwert = 0,68) deutlich höher als die Kontrollwerte (Mittelwert = 0,33).

Auch in stationären Mikroperfusionsexperimenten*) erhielten wir vergleichbare Befunde: d. h. keinen Unterschied der proximalen Ergebnisse, jedoch erhöhte intraluminale Na^+-Konzentrationen im distalen Konvolut adrenalektomierter Ratten (Abb. 2). Dies bedeutet, daß die distalen Tubulusepithelzellen nach Adrenalektomie Na^+ nur gegen eine sehr geringe Konzentrationsdifferenz resorbieren können.

Auch der K^+-Transport des distalen Konvolutes ist nach Adrenalektomie gestört. Die Abb. 3 zeigt transtubuläre Konzentrationsquotienten im stationären Zustand. Der bei intakten Tieren beobachtete Anstieg der intraluminalen K^+-Konzentration in der 2. Hälfte des distalen Tubulus blieb bei adrenalektomierten Tieren aus.

Die Tatsache, daß bei Freiflußpunktionen die Na^+-Konzentration der Tubulusflüssigkeit bereits am Anfang des punktierten distalen Konvolutes erhöht war (Abb. 1), ist außerdem ein Hinweis dafür, daß auch die Na^+-Resorption in der aufsteigenden Henleschen Schleife nach Ausfall der NNR-Funktion beeinträchtigt ist. Dafür spricht auch

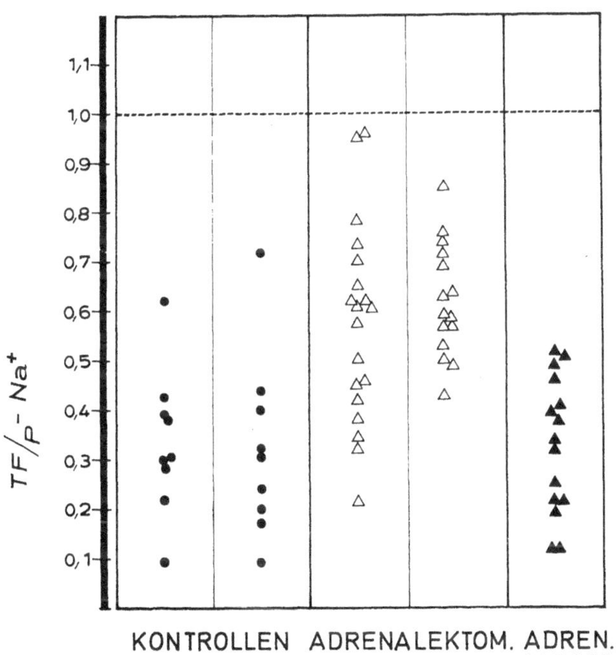

Abb. 2. TF/P-Na^+ im steady state. Distaler Tubulus (HIERHOLZER, 1965).

*) Nach der Methode von SHIPP et al. (1958), wurde eine Testlösung, die NaCl und Mannit (bzw. Polyaethylenglycol) enthielt, in das Tubuluslumen injiziert und nach 60 min wieder reaspiriert.

die Beobachtung, daß nebenniereninsuffiziente Menschen und Tiere eine Einschränkung der Konzentrierfähigkeit aufweisen (Kottke et al., 1942; Reforzo-Membrives et al., 1945; Robson, 1961; Goldsmith et al., 1961; Sigler et al., 1965). Wir haben damit eine Reihe von Befunden, die eine distale Lokalisation der renalen Transporthemmung belegen. Hierzu sind auch die von Cortney (1966) an adrenalektomierten Ratten in Mannit-Diurese erhobenen Befunde zu rechnen. Für eine proximale Hemmung ergab sich dagegen bisher kein Hinweis; jedenfalls nicht aus Messungen der intraluminalen Konzentrationen von Na^+ und K^+.

Es stellt sich natürlich die Frage, ob eine *proximale* Hemmung der Na^+-Resorption überhaupt erwartet werden kann. Dagegen scheint die Beobachtung zu sprechen, daß bei adrenalektomierten Tieren nur 2–3% der filtrierten Na-Ionen ausgeschieden werden. Dafür spricht u. E., daß die Steuerung der transzellulären Na^+-Resorption durch NNR-Steroide ein Prinzip darstellt, welches an sehr vielen Organen und tubulären Strukturen nachgewiesen wurde. Das proximale Konvolut würde also eine sehr bemerkenswerte Ausnahme darstellen.

Daß die Na^+-Resorption im proximalen Konvolut adrenalektomierter Ratten gehemmt ist, zeigt sich, wenn man die Flüssigkeits- und Na^+-Resorption mit der von Gertz (1963) angegebenen, photographischen Methode*) mißt.

Die Ergebnisse sind in der Abb. 4 zusammengefaßt. Trägt man die relative Volumenabnahme (V/V_0) halblogarithmisch gegen die Zeit auf, so erhält man Geraden, deren

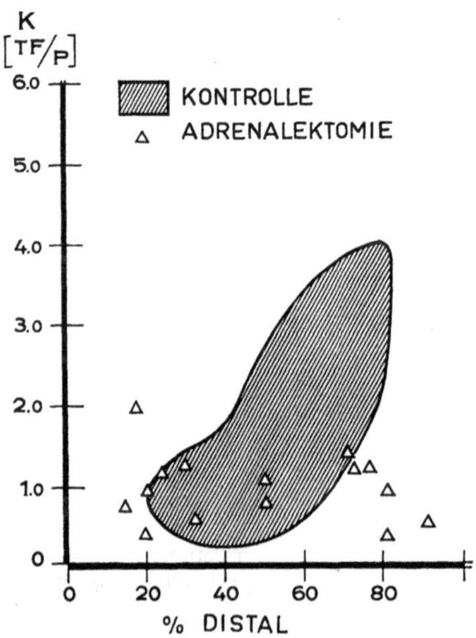

Abb. 3. TF/P-K^+ im steady state. Distaler Tubulus (Hierholzer et al., 1965).

*) Eine isotone NaCl-Lösung wird zwischen 2 gefärbte Öltropfen in das Tubuluslumen injiziert und anschließend die Volumenabnahme der Testlösung photographisch registriert.

Neigung proportional der transtubulären Resorptionsrate von Na^+ ist. Die geringere Neigung der Geraden im proximalen und distalen Konvolut adrenalektomierter Ratten weist also auf eine Verlangsamung des Resorptionsvorganges hin. Dieser Befund ist unabhängig von der Bikarbonatkonzentration des Plasmas (Abb. 5), d. h. die mit der Methode des gespaltenen Öltropfens gemessene Resorptionsverzögerung adrenalektomierter Ratten ist nicht bedingt durch die in der Nebenniereninsuffizienz bestehende hyperkaliämische metabolische Azidose. In der Abb. 6 sind die aus den Halbwertzeiten der Flüssigkeitsresorption berechneten transtubulären Na^+-Ströme verschiedener Tiergruppen dargestellt. Auf die Hormonbefunde wird später eingegangen.

Eine weitere Beobachtung war die, daß bei adrenalektomierten Tieren, die mit der Lissamingrünmethode gemessene proximale Passagezeit (STEINHAUSEN 1963) von im Mittel 8,6 sec bei Kontrolltieren auf 21 sec verlängert war. Dies ist deshalb von Bedeutung, weil die prozentuale Flüssigkeitsresorption bei freiem Fluß nicht nur von der lokalen Transportaktivität des Epithels, sondern auch von der Kontaktzeit zwischen Tubulusflüssigkeit und Epithel bestimmt wird und aus Halbwertzeit und Passagezeit nach einem von GERTZ et al., (1965) angegebenen Verfahren graphisch ermittelt bzw. errechnet werden kann. Man hat damit neben der Messung der Inulinkonzentration ein zweites Verfahren zur Bestimmung der prozentualen Flüssigkeitsresorption.

Die Ergebnisse, die wir mit dieser Methode erhielten, sind in der Abb. 7 dargestellt. Es zeigte sich, daß die Resorption am Ende des proximalen Konvolutes adrenalektomierter Ratten sogar etwas zunimmt, obwohl die lokale Ausstromrate erniedrigt ist. Die Verhältnisse werden durch das in Abb. 8 wiedergegebene Schema verdeutlicht. Prinzipiell die gleichen Unterschiede erhielt WIEDERHOLT (1968) durch Messung der Inulinkonzentration: TF/P Inulin am Ende des proximalen Konvolutes betrug bei Kontrollratten 3,02 und bei adrenalektomierten Ratten 4,7.

Wir haben hier eine sehr typische Eigenschaft des proximalen Konvolutes vor uns, sich bei Hemmung des Na^+-Resorptionsvorganges durch Erweiterung so anzupassen, daß die lineare Strömungsgeschwindigkeit abnimmt und die Konstanz der prozentualen Flüssigkeitsresorption erhalten bleibt. Ähnliche Beobachtungen machte man auch nach der Verabreichung von Diuretica (RECTOR et al., 1967) und nach Ca^{++}-Infusionen (FÜLLGRAF et al., 1967).

Durchströmt man proximale Nephronsegmente von intakten und adrenalektomierten Ratten in Mikroperfusionsexperimenten mit der gleichen Stromstärke, so beobachtet man bei adrenalektomierten Ratten eine Abnahme der prozentualen Flüssigkeitsresorption (STOLTE et al., 1966).

Zusammenfassend läßt sich also feststellen, daß die Hemmung der lokalen Na^+-Resorptionsrate des Tubulusepithels nach bilateraler Adrenalektomie nicht auf den distalen Tubulus beschränkt ist, sondern auch im proximalen Konvolut nachgewiesen werden konnte – allerdings mit der Einschränkung, daß die verminderte Resorptionskapazität im proximalen Konvolut durch eine verlängerte Verweilzeit so kompensiert wird, daß bei freiem Fluß eine normale oder leicht gesteigerte prozentuale Flüssigkeitsresorption erfolgt. Steroide können demnach den intrarenalen Na^+-Transport auf zweierlei Art beeinflussen: indem sie auf den lokalen Resorptionsmechanismus einwirken oder aber indem sie die glomeruläre Filtrationsrate und die Strömungsgeschwindigkeit der Tubulusflüssigkeit verändern.

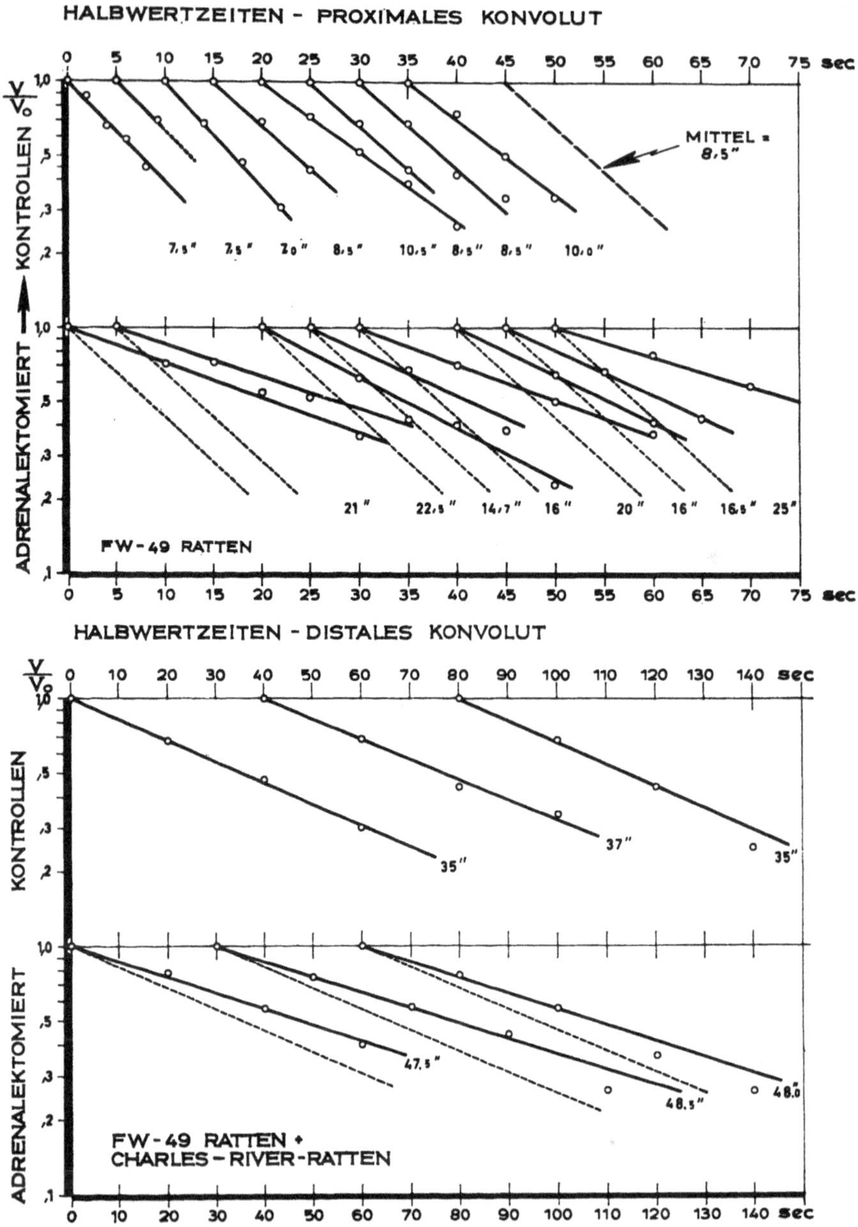

Abb. 4. Volumenabnahme einer intratubulär injizierten isotonen NaCl-Lösung. Oben: *proximales Konvolut*. Einzelversuche an 8 intakten und 8 adrenalektomierten Ratten. Unten: *distales Konvolut*. Einzelversuche an 3 intakten und 3 adrenalektomierten Ratten. Ordninate: V/V_0 (Logarithmischer Maßstab.) V_0 = Anfangsvolumen der injizierten NaCl-Lösung bei Beginn der photographischen Messungen. V = im Lumen verbliebenes Volumen nach verschiedenen auf der Abszisse angegebenen Zeitintervallen. Jede Gerade stellt einen Versuch dar und verbindet Mittelwerte von je 10–15 Einzelmessungen an verschiedenen Tubuli der glei-

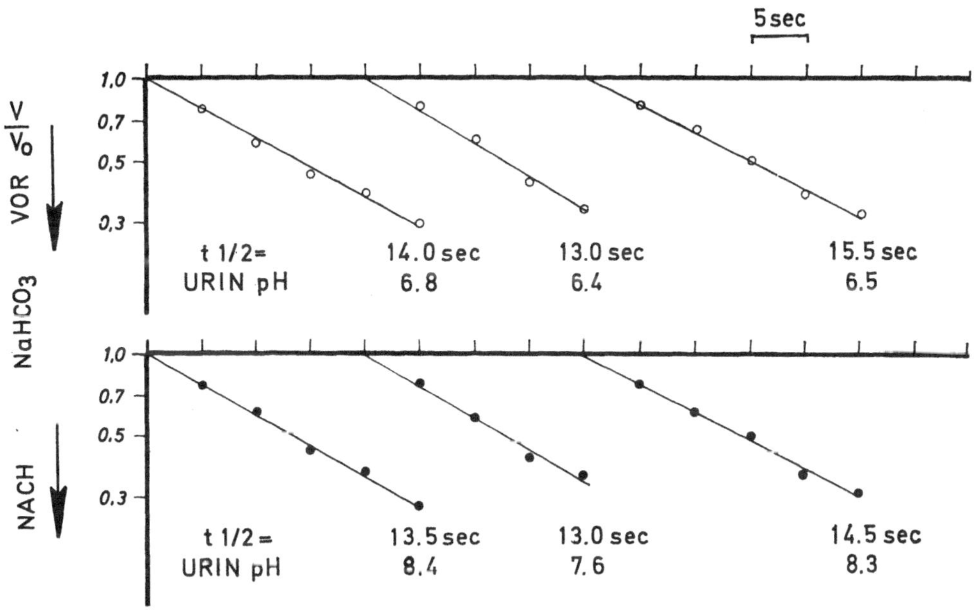

Abb. 5. Halbwertzeiten der Flüssigkeitsresorption im proximalen Konvolut adrenalektomierter Ratten vor und nach i. v. Infusion von isotoner $NaHCO_3$-Lösung (6 ml/Stunde) (WIEDERHOLT und HIERHOLZER, unveröffentlicht).

II. Intrarenale Wirkung von Steroidhormonen

Um den Einfluß von NNR-Steroiden auf den intrarenalen Na^+-Transport zu analysieren, verwandten wir *d-Aldosteron* als Mineralocorticoid, das synthetische *Dexamethason* als Glucocorticoid und *Cortison*, welches in der verwandten Dosierung eine Mittelstellung einnimmt*).

*) In den vorliegenden Experimenten verwandten wir folgende Hormone:

1. d-Aldosteron in wäßriger Lösung (»Aldocorten-CIBA«): 0,125 µg/100 g Körpergewicht i. v. + 7,5 µg/100 g Körpergewicht subcutan als einmalige Dosis.
2. d-Aldosteron-TMA in öliger Lösung (»CIBA«): 7,5 µg/100 g Körpergewicht und 24 Std. i. m., 3–5 Tage lang.
3. Cortison-Kristallsuspension (»Cortison-Hoechst«): 2,5 mg/100 g Körpergewicht i. m. als einmalige Dosis oder 2,5 mg/100 g Körpergewicht und 24 Std. i. m., 3–5 Tage lang.
4. Dexamethason (»Dexa-Scheroson«): 50 µg/100 g Körpergewicht i. m. als einmalige Dosis oder 50 µg/100 g Körpergewicht und 24 Std. i. m., 3–5 Tage lang.

Forts. Abb. 4.

chen Niere. Die in der Abbildung enthaltenen Zahlen geben die Halbwertzeiten der Flüssigkeitsresorption wieder. Die geringere Neigung der Resorptionsgeraden bei adrenalektomierten Tieren ist ein Maß für die verzögerte Flüssigkeitsresorption. (Die gestrichelten Linien in der unteren Bildhälfte geben zum Vergleich die mittlere Resorptionsgerade von intakten Kontrolltieren wieder. Methode nach GERTZ [23]). (HIERHOLZER et al., 1966).

PROXIMAL	Φ FLÜSSIGKEIT $\times 10^{-4}$ mm³/mm²·sec	Φ Na $\times 10^{-5}$ µeq/mm²·sec	
KONTROLLE	6.2	8.9 ± 0.3	$P < 0.001$
ADRENAL-EKTOMIERT	3.3	4.5 ± 0.2	
DISTAL			
KONTROLLE	1.2	1.7 ± 0.1	$P < 0.001$
ADRENAL-EKTOMIERT	0.8	1.2 ± 0.1	

Abb. 6. Transtubuläre Ströme von Flüssigkeit ($\varnothing_W$) und Natrium ($\varnothing_{Na}$) aus dem proximalen und distalen Konvolut (Lumen → Blut) (HIERHOLZER et al., 1966).

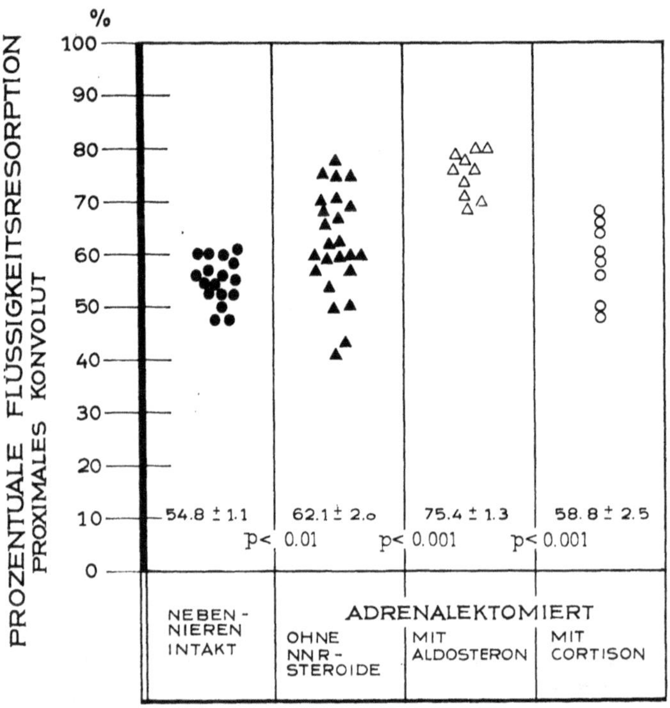

Abb. 7 (Einzelheiten siehe Text).

Aldosteron

Die Wirkung von d-Aldosteron wurde am proximalen und distalen Konvolut untersucht. Die intravenös verabreichte Dosis in den akuten Experimenten entsprach etwa der Menge, die normalerweise in 1–2 Stunden endogen sezerniert wird. Durch sie wurde nach einer Latenzzeit von ca. 45–60 min die intraluminale Na^+-Gleichgewichtskonzentration normalisiert (Abb. 2). Die Wirkung von d-Aldosteron auf die Halbwertzeit der lokalen Flüssigkeitsresorption bei akuter und chronischer Verabreichung ist in der Abb. 9 dargestellt. Sowohl im proximalen als auch im distalen Konvolut beobachten wir eine Normalisierung von t $^1/_2$. Der Blutdruck, die glomeruläre Filtrationsrate und die proximale Passagezeit blieben dagegen unbeeinflußt.

Es wurde bereits darauf hingewiesen, daß Actinomycin D an isolierten Membranen [EDELMAN et al., (1963); CRABBÉ und DE WEER, (1964); SHARP und LEAF, (1966)] und an der Niere [WILLIAMSON, (1963)] das Einsetzen der Aldosteronwirkung verhindert. Daß dies auch für die am proximalen und distalen Konvolut beobachteten Aldosteronwirkungen zutrifft, zeigt die Abb. 10, die einer Arbeit von WIEDERHOLT (1966) entnommen ist. Bei Kontrollratten und bei aldosteronbehandelten, adrenalektomierten Ratten wurde ein Anteil der Na^+-Resorptionsrate durch Actinomycin D gehemmt, der so groß ist wie der durch Aldosteron regulierte Anteil. Bei nicht substituierten, adrenalektomierten Ratten löste Actinomycin D keinen Effekt aus. Wie an isolierten Membranen läßt sich also die transtubuläre Na^+-Resorption trennen in einen steroidgesteuerten Anteil und

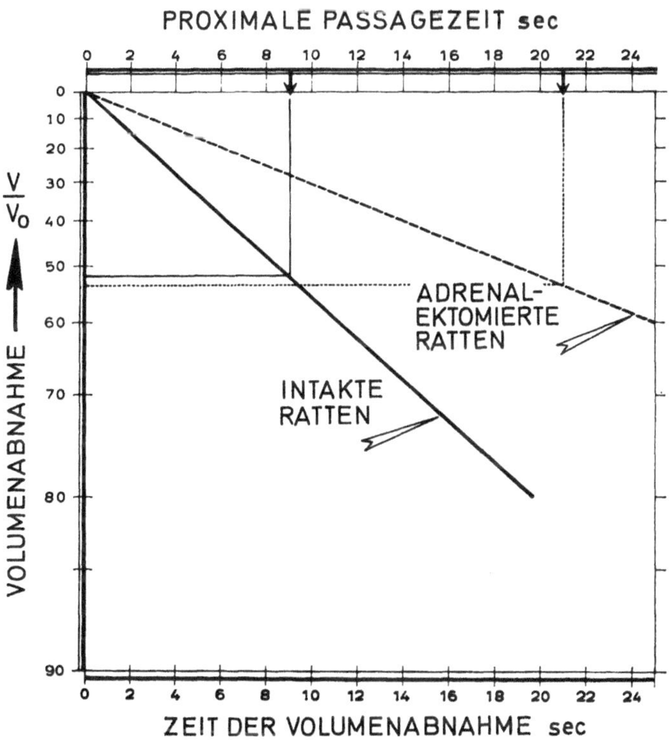

Abb. 8. Graphische Ermittlung der prozentualen Flüssigkeitsresorption im proximalen Konvolut aus dem Verlauf der Resorptionsgeraden und der proximalen Passagezeit. a Mittelwerte intakter; b adrenalektomierter Ratten.

Ordinate: $(1 - \frac{V}{V_0}) \cdot 100$

Verbindet man die Passagezeit (Abszisse) mit der Resorptionsgeraden, so ergibt der dazugehörige Ordinatenwert die prozentuale Flüssigkeits- und Na^+-Resorption im proximalen Konvolut.

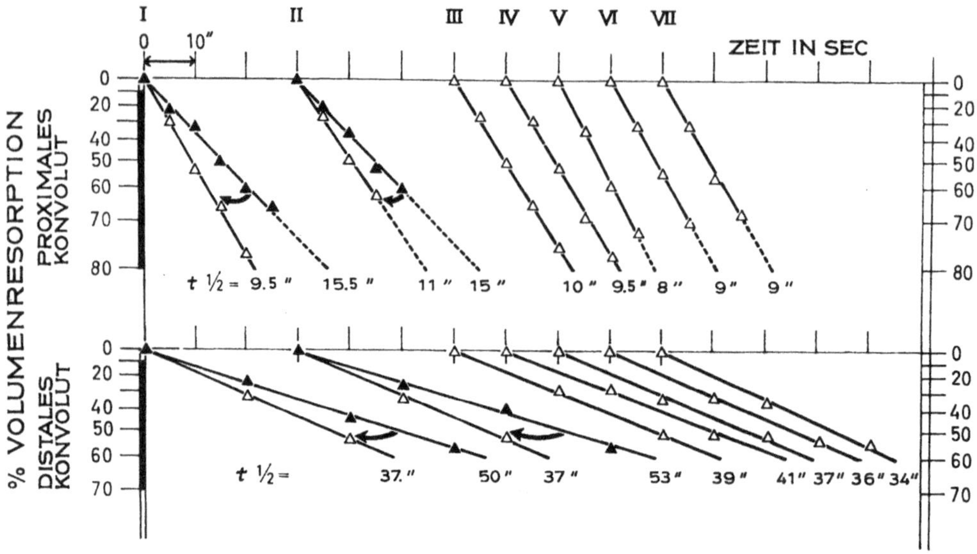

Abb. 9. Normalisierung der %Volumenresorption aus dem proximalen und distalen Konvolut adrenalektomierter Ratten durch d-Aldosteron. ▲ vor Aldosteron; △ nach Aldosteron; I, II akute Hormongabe; III-VII chronische Hormongabe.

einen von Aldosteron nicht beeinflußten, basalen Anteil. Letzterer wird unserer Erfahrung nach durch das Antibioticum nicht beeinflußt, obwohl Actinomycin D im Homogenat nicht substituierter adrenalektomierter Ratten die in-vitro Inkorporation von ^{3}H-Orotat in die Zellkernfraktion hemmt [Fimognari et al., (1967)]. Bemerkenswert ist überdies, daß nach den von Wiederholt (1966) vorgelegten Daten Actinomycin die Wirkung von Aldosteron unterbricht, und zwar mit einer Latenzzeit, die der an der Krötenblase gemessenen entspricht [Sharp und Leaf, (1966)]. Ludenz et al., (1967) fanden, ebenfalls an der Ratte, im Gegensatz dazu keinen Effekt von Actinomycin D auf die Aldosteronwirkung, wenn das Antibioticum 15 bis 40 min nach dem Steroid verabreicht wurde. Eine Erklärung dieser unterschiedlichen Befunde läßt sich aus den Versuchsprotokollen nicht ableiten.

Die Wirkung von Aldosteron am proximalen und distalen Konvolut der Rattenniere konnte also mit physiologisch niedrigen Dosen und nach der typischen Latenzzeit von ca. 45 bis 60 min ausgelöst und durch Actinomycin D aufgehoben werden.

Cortison

Cortison verabreichten wir in einer Dosierung, welche die bei adrenalektomierten Ratten verzögerte Wasserausscheidung normalisiert und sowohl glucocorticoide als auch mineralocorticoide Wirkungen auslöst. Wie aus Abb. 11 hervorgeht, waren die Ergebnisse im proximalen und distalen Konvolut den durch Aldosteron erzielten Befunden vergleichbar. Im Gegensatz zu den Aldosteronversuchen beobachteten wir nach Cortison jedoch einen Anstieg des vorher erniedrigten Blutdruckes auf Normalwerte. Parallel dazu normalisierten sich die glomeruläre Filtrationsrate und die proximale Passagezeit.

Dexamethason

Das vorwiegend glucocorticoide Dexamethason [ARTH et al., (1958); WETTSTEIN, (1960)] hatte bei einer äquivalent hohen Dosierung keinen Einfluß auf die lokale Flüssigkeitsresorption im proximalen und distalen Konvolut. Auch nach 3–5tägiger Verabreichung blieb die proximale Halbwertzeit unverändert, während der Blutdruck und die proximale Passagezeit auf normale Werte anstiegen. Im distalen Konvolut zeigte sich nach wiederholter Dexamethasoninjektion über 3–5 Tage eine deutliche Verlängerung der Halbwert-

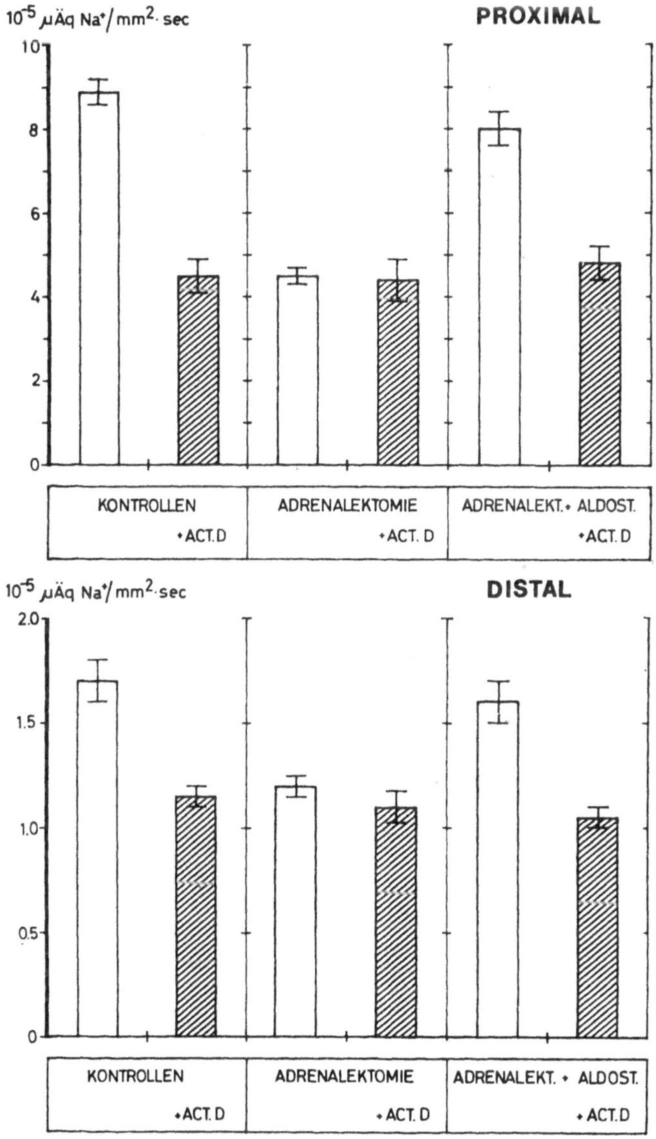

Abb. 10. Wirkung von Actinomycin D (200 µg/kg K. G.) auf den transtubulären Netto-Na^+-Ausstrom aus dem proximalen und distalen Konvolut. Mittelwerte von 30–60 Messungen an je 3 Ratten (± S. E.) Methode des gespaltenen Öltropfens. (WIEDERHOLT und HIERHOLZER, 1968).

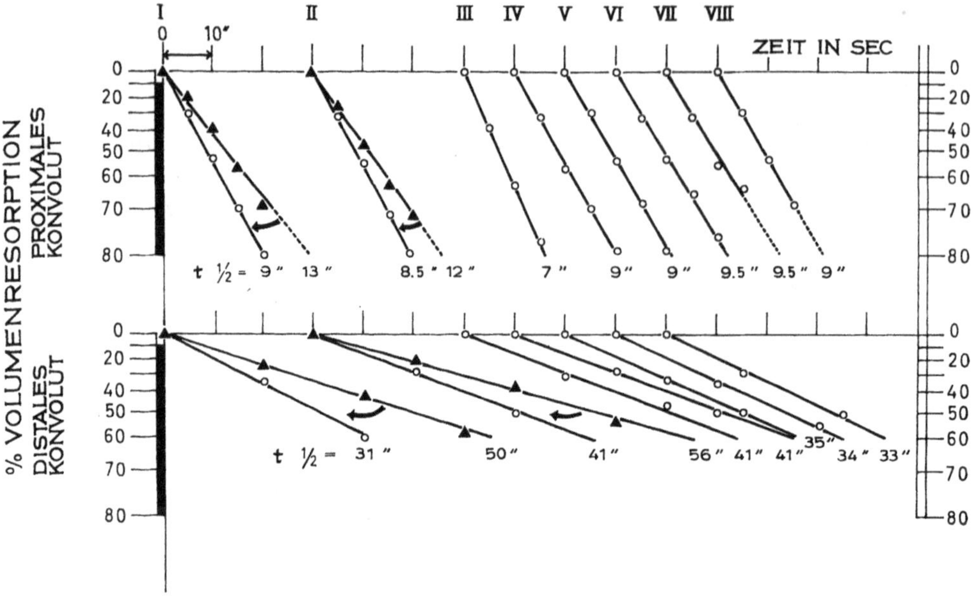

Abb. 11. Normalisierung der %Volumenresorption aus dem proximalen und distalen Konvolut adrenalektomierter Ratten durch Cortison. ▲ vor Cortison; ○ nach Cortison; I, II akute Hormongabe; III-VIII chronische Hormongabe.

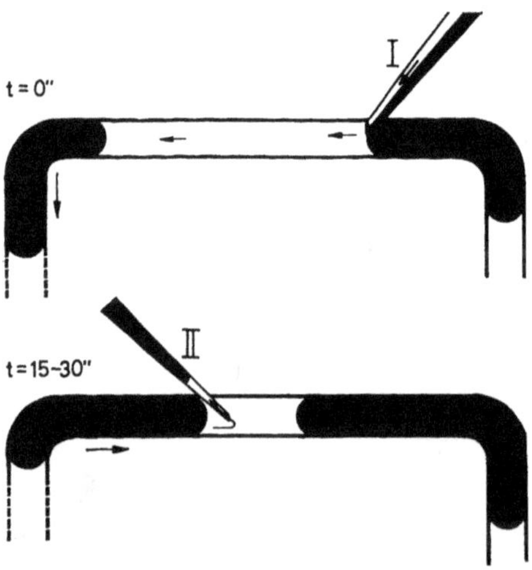

	TF/P-NA		TF/P-OSMOL	
	Kon-trollen	Adrex.+ Dexam	Kon-trollen	Adrex.+ Dexam
Proximal	1.00	0.98	1.04	0.99
Distal	1.03	0.55	0.99	0.78

Abb. 12. Reaspiration von intraluminal injizierter Kochsalzlösung. (Wiederholt und Wiederholt, 1968).

zeit. Wie Reaspirationsversuche ergeben haben [WIEDERHOLT, (1968)], liegt die Ursache hierfür in einer verminderten Wasserpermeabilität; diese bedingt es, daß die Na^+-Resorption bei der Methode des gespaltenen Öltropfens hyperton verläuft und im Lumen eine hypotone Lösung zurückbleibt (Abb. 12).

Die eben besprochenen Befunde sind zusammengefaßt in 2 Abbildungen. Abb. 13 zeigt, daß verschiedene NNR-Steroide den lokalen Na^+-Resorptionsvorgang in unterschiedlicher Weise beeinflussen: Aldosteron und Cortison normalisieren den Na^+-Transport, Dexamethason hat keine direkte Wirkung. Hiervon zu unterscheiden ist die *prozentuale Resorption* von Ultrafiltrat im proximalen Konvolut bei freiem Fluß, die – wie wir diskutiert haben – durch die Parameter Halbwertzeit und Passagezeit bestimmt wird. Die Verhältnisse sind in Abb. 14 zusammengefaßt. Nicht substituierte adrenalektomierte Tiere haben eine normale oder eine leicht gesteigerte Flüssigkeitsresorption. Aldosteron, welches nur die Transportleistung der Zellen, nicht aber Blutdruck und Passagezeit normalisiert, steigert die prozentuale Flüssigkeitsresorption (im Mittel von 62,1% auf

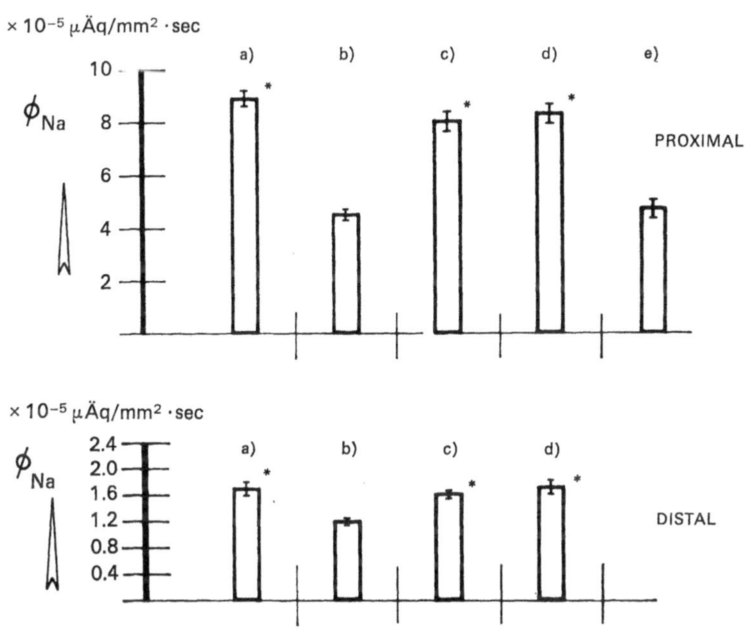

Abb. 13. Die Wirkung von Corticosteroiden auf den transtubulären Na^+-Ausstrom ($\varnothing_{Na^+}$) aus dem proximalen und distalen Konvolut von a) Kontrollratten mit intakten Nebennieren, b) adrenalektomierten Ratten ohne Hormonsubstitution, c) adrenalektomierten Ratten mit Aldosteron, d) adrenalektomierten Ratten mit Cortison und e) adrenalektomierten Ratten mit Dexamethason. Zur Bildung der Mittelwerte ($\pm$ S.E.) wurden die Befunde nach einmaliger Hormonverabreichung (0,125 μg d-Aldosteron bzw. 2,5 mg Cortison/100 g Körpergewicht) und die Befunde nach 3–5tägiger Hormonverabreichung (7,5 μg d-Aldosteron bzw. 2,5 mg Cortison bzw. 50 μg Dexamethason/100 g Körpergewicht und 24 Std.) zusammengefaßt. Werte für Kontrollratten und adrenalektomierte Ratten ohne Hormonsubstitution. Die mit * bezeichneten Mittelwerte sind gegenüber den Mittelwerten von adrenalektomierten Ratten ohne Hormonsubstitution signifikant unterschiedlich ($P < 0{,}001$). (WIEDERHOLT et al. 1966).

75,4%). Hat ein Steroid dagegen keine mineralocorticoide Aktivität, steigert es aber den Blutdruck und normalisiert es die Passagezeit, so ist – wie bei Dexamethason beobachtet – eine Abnahme der prozentualen Freiflußresorption zu erwarten.

Nur nach Verabreichung relativ hoher Dosen von Cortison war in den vorliegenden Versuchen sowohl eine Normalisierung der Halbwertzeit als auch gleichzeitig eine durch Blutdruckanstieg bedingte Verkürzung der Passagezeit zu beobachten. Die mittlere prozentuale Resorption im proximalen Konvolut war nach Cortisonverabreichung mit 58,8% deshalb nicht signifikant verschieden von Kontrollwerten.

Ich möchte die Besprechung der Hormonwirkung abschließen mit einigen Hinweisen auf eine proximale Wirkung von Aldosteron, die in letzter Zeit publiziert wurden, und die unsere Befunde stützen. STUMPE und OCHWADT (1967) beobachteten im proximalen Konvolut von chronisch kochsalzreich ernährten Ratten mit vermutlich erniedrigter

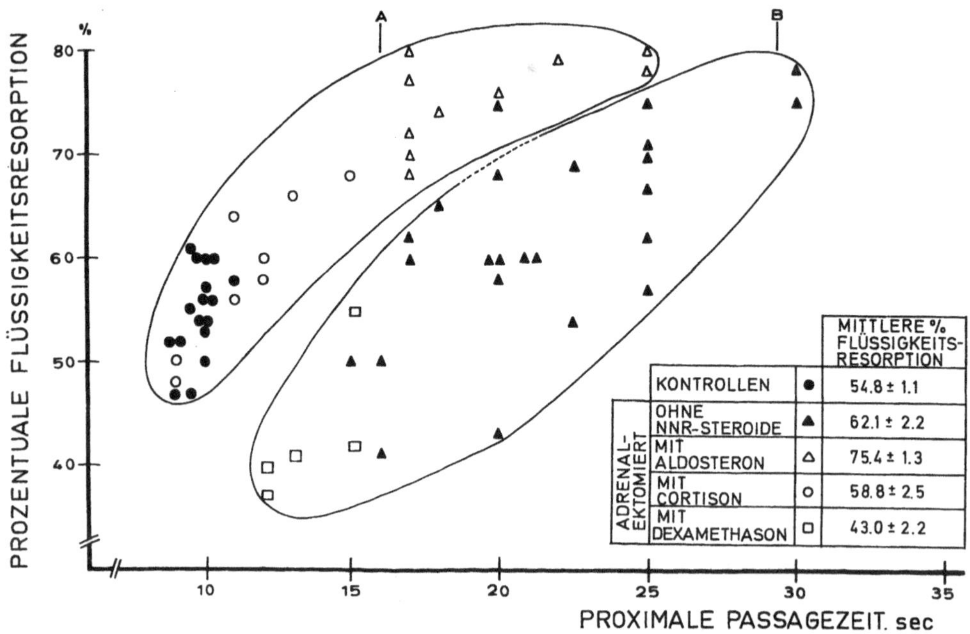

Abb. 14. Die Wirkung von Nebennierenrindensteroiden auf die Beziehung zwischen prozentualer Flüssigkeitsresorption und proximaler Passagezeit. Die prozentuale Flüssigkeitsresorption wurde aus der relativen Volumenabnahme einer intratubulär zwischen zwei Ölsäulen injizierten NaCl-Lösung und aus der proximalen Passagezeit berechnet (13). Jedes Symbol gibt den Mittelwert eines Tieres an. Werte für Kontrollratten und adrenalektomierte Ratten ohne Hormonsubstitution aus (18). Die mittlere prozentuale Flüssigkeitsresorption zwischen Kontrollratten und adrenalektomierten Ratten ohne Hormonsubstitution ($P<0{,}01$) und zwischen adrenalektomierten Ratten ohne Hormonsubstitution und adrenalektomierten Ratten mit Aldosteron ($P<0{,}001$) ist signifikant unterschiedlich. Alle Einzelwerte, bei denen die lokale Transportrate normal (Kontrollratten) oder normalisiert war (adrenalektomierte Ratten mit Aldosteron oder Cortison), sind als Gruppe A zusammengefaßt. Alle Einzelwerte, bei denen die lokale Transportkapazität gehemmt war (adrenalektomierte Ratten ohne Hormonsubstitution und adrenalektomierte Ratten mit Dexamethason), sind als Gruppe B zusammengefaßt (WIEDERHOLT et. al. 1966).

Aldosteronsekretion eine verminderte lokale Na^+-Resorptionsrate, die durch kleine Dosen von Aldosteron normalisiert werden konnte. Ähnliches beobachteten CAPEK et al., (1968) an 20 Tage alten Ratten. Nach in vitro Studien von KRAUS und POPP (1967) ist bei diesen Tieren die postnatale Entwicklung der Aldosteronproduktion noch nicht abgeschlossen. Dementsprechend war die Halbwertszeit der Flüssigkeitsresorption im proximalen Konvolut deutlich erniedrigt und stieg erst nach Aldosterongabe (25 μg/100 g Körpergewicht) auf den Wert erwachsener Ratten an. Ebenso wie bei unseren Versuchen blieb die Passagezeit dabei unverändert, so daß unter der Einwirkung von Aldosteron ein Anstieg der proximalen Freiflußresorption auftrat. Schließlich sei noch darauf hingewiesen, daß DLOUHA et al., (1968) bei Teleostiern (Myoxocephalus Scorpius) einen durch Aldosteron ausgelösten Anstieg des U/P-Natriumquotienten beobachteten, obwohl die Nieren dieser Fische keine distalen Tubuli besitzen und praktisch nur aus proximalen Tubuli bestehen.

III. Mechanismus der Na^+-Transporthemmung in der Niere adrenalektomierter Ratten

Abschließend möchte ich die Frage diskutieren, ob sich auf Grund der bisher vorliegenden Befunde etwas über den Mechanismus der Natriumtransporthemmung aussagen läßt. Wir haben zur Charakterisierung des Natriumtransportes a) die Nettonatriumresorption und b) die intraluminale Na^+-Gleichgewichtskonzentration gemessen und sowohl im proximalen als auch im distalen Konvolut Abweichungen von der Norm gefunden. Beide Segmente unterliegen also dem eingangs erwähnten Prinzip der Steuerung des transepithelialen Natriumtransportes durch Nebennierenrindensteroide, offenbar aber in quantitativ und qualitativ unterschiedlicher Weise. Da wir bisher nicht über die notwendigen Meßwerte verfügen, um die USSINGschen Flußgleichungen auf die Vorgänge an der luminalen und basalen Zellseite anwenden zu können, gehe ich bei der folgenden Diskussion von der einfachsten Modellvorstellung aus, welche die epitheliale Tubuluswand als ein Pump/Leck-System ansieht, wobei der Nettoausfluß durch die Mantelfläche sich zusammensetzt aus einem aktiven Ausfluß und einem passiven Rückfluß. Dabei sei zunächst offen, ob der passive Rückfluß von Na^+ ins Tubuluslumen durch den aktiven Transportweg oder – wie man vermutet – parallel dazu erfolgt. Eine Hemmung der Pumpe – z. B. durch Wegfall der NNR-Steroide – hätte eine Abnahme der Nettonatriumresorptionsrate zur Folge. Außerdem müßte bei Vorhandensein eines Leckes die transtubuläre Na^+-Konzentrationsdifferenz im stationären Zustand vermindert sein, d. h. die intraluminale Na^+-Konzentration ansteigen. Beide Ergebnisse erhielten wir im distalen Konvolut. Die distalen Befunde lassen sich also zwanglos als Hemmung des aktiven Transportmechanismus für Na^+ interpretieren.

Auch im proximalen Konvolut adrenalektomierter Ratten war, wie wir gezeigt haben, die Natriumausstromrate vermindert. Im Gegensatz zu distal war jedoch die transtubuläre Konzentrationsdifferenz im stationären Zustand gegenüber Kontrollwerten unverändert. Diese Befunde können nicht allein durch eine Hemmung des aktiven Na^+-Transportsystems verursacht sein, weil diese, analog zu distal, zum Anstieg der intraluminalen Gleichgewichtskonzentration führen müßte. Auch eine primäre Hemmung der Na^+-Permeabilität an der luminalen Zellseite könnte unsere Befunde nicht oder höchstens bei sehr unwahrscheinlichen Zusatzannahmen erklären. Die einfachste Hypothese ist die, daß im proximalen Konvolut nicht nur der Austransport von Na^+ aus dem Lumen ins

Interstitium, sondern auch der Rückstrom von Na^+ ins Lumen erschwert ist, d. h. die effektive Wandpermeabilität für Na^+ abnimmt.

Wir haben versucht, in Mikroperfusionsexperimenten das Tubuluslumen mit NaCl-freier Testlösung zu durchströmen und aus dem Anstieg der Na^+-Konzentration die effekte Na^+-Permeabilität zu berechnen. Die Störfaktoren innerhalb des Systems waren bei diesen Versuchen jedoch so groß, daß es bisher nicht gelungen ist, Unterschiede zwischen intakten und adrenalektomierten Tieren zu sichern.

Deshalb wurde in letzter Zeit auf eine andere Art versucht, Hinweise auf Permeabilitätsänderungen zu erhalten. Dabei gingen wir von folgender Überlegung aus:

In einem Tubulussegment findet unter den Bedingungen der stopped-flow Mikroperfusion ein allmählicher Abfall der intraluminalen Na^+-Konzentration auf die Na^+-Gleichgewichtskonzentration statt. Der exponentielle Verlauf wird charakterisiert durch die erreichte Endkonzentration (= Gleichgewichtskonzentration) und durch die Einstellzeit. Wird in einem solchen System der aktive Austransport und der passive Rückstrom um den gleichen Prozentsatz, z. B. auf die Hälfte erniedrigt, so bleibt die Gleichgewichtskonzentration unverändert. Die Einstellzeit t nimmt jedoch zu, d. h. die Exponentialkurve der Konzentrationsänderung verläuft flacher. Eine unterschiedliche Einstellzeit der Gleichgewichtskonzentration bei intakten und adrenalektomierten Ratten könnte uns bisher entgangen sein, da wir bei der Messung der Gleichgewichtskonzentration eine Zeitperiode von 60 oder mehr sec abgewartet haben.

Wir untersuchten deshalb in zwei weiteren Versuchsserien den Zeitgang der intraluminalen Na^+-Konzentrationsabnahme [Stolte et al., (1969)]. Es zeigte sich, daß bei gleicher Kontaktzeit bei adrenalektomierten Ratten eine geringere transtubuläre Konzentrationsdifferenz aufgebaut wird. In weiteren Versuchen wurden intratubulär injizierte Mannit-Tropfen bereits nach ca. 30 sec reaspiriert. Auch hier wiesen die adrenalektomierten Tiere eine geringere Konzentrationsdifferenz auf. Aus diesen Befunden ist auf eine Abnahme der effektiven Wandpermeabilität für Na^+ im proximalen Konvolut adrenalektomierter Ratten zu schließen.

Literatur

1. Arth, G. E., D. B. R. Johnston, J. Fried, D. R. Hoff, L. H. Sarett, R. H. Silber, H. C. Stoerk and C. A. Winter: 16α-Methyl analogs of cortisone, a new group of antiflammatory steroids. 9α-Haloderivates. J. amer. chem. Soc. **80**, 3161 (1958).
2. Arth, G. E., D. B. R. Johnston, J. Fried, W. W. Spooncer, D. R. Hoff, L. H. Sarett: 16α-Methylated analogs of cortisone. A new group of antiflammatory steroids. J. amer. chem. Soc. **80**, 3160 (1958).
3. August, J. T. and D. H. Nelson: The dual action of aldosterone on renal sodium reabsorption in normal subjects. Clin. Res. **7**, 274 (1959).
4. Capek, K., J. Fernandez und H. Dlouha: Natriumresorption im proximalen Konvolut der jungen Rattenniere. Pflügers Arch. ges. Physiol. **300**, 24 (1968).
5. Cortney, M. A.: Renal tubular transfer of sodium, potassium, and water in adrenalectomized rats. Physiologist **9**, 158 (1966).
6. Crabbé, J.: The role of aldosterone in the renal concentration mechanism in man. Clin. Sci. **23**, 39 (1962).
7. Crabbé, J. and P. De Weer: Action of aldosterone on the bladder and skin of the toad. Nature Lond. **202**, 298 (1964).

8. DLOUHA, H., V. F. VASILJEVA, T. V. KRESTINSKAJA and K. P. VOROBJEVA: The tubular reabsorption of sodium in the Marine Teleost. *In: Abstracts of Papers* for the VIth Conf. of European Comparative Endocrinologists, Carlsbad **43** (1967).
9. EDELMAN, I. S., R. BOGOROCH and G. A. PORTER: On the mechanism of action of aldosterone on sodium transport: the role of protein synthesis. Proc. nat. Acad. Sci. **50,** 1169 (1963).
10. FIMOGNARI, G. M., D. D. FANESTIL and I. S. EDELMAN: Induction of RNA and protein synthesis in the action of aldosterone in the rat. Amer. J. Physiol. **213,** 954 (1967).
11. FÜLGRAFF, G. und O. HEIDENREICH: Mikropunktionsuntersuchungen über die Wirkung von Calciumionen auf die Resorptionskapazität und auf die prozentuale Resorption im proximalen Konvolut von Ratten. Naun.-Schm. Arch. Pharmakol. + exp. Pathol. **258,** 440 (1967).
12. FÜLGRAFF, G., O. HEIDENREICH und H. LAAFF: Über die diuretische Wirkung von Calciumionen beim Hund. Naun.-Schm. Arch. Pharmakol. u. exp. Pathol. **257,** 372 (1967).
13. GERTZ, K. H.: Transtubuläre Natriumchloridflüsse und Permeabilität für Nichtelektrolyte im proximalen und distalen Konvolut der Rattenniere. Pflüg. Arch. ges. Physiol. **276,** 336 (1963).
14. GERTZ, K. H., J. A. MANGOS, G. BRAUN and H. D. PAGEL: On the glomerular tubular balance in the rat kidney. Pflüg. Arch. ges. Physiol. **285,** 360 (1965).
15. GOLDSMITH, C., H. K. BEASLEY, P. J. WHALLEY, F. C. RECTOR, Jr. and D. W. SELDIN: The effect of salt deprivation on the urinary concentrating mechanism in the dog. J. clin. Invest. **40,** 2043 (1961).
16. HIERHOLZER, K.: Analyse der Natrium-Transportstörung in der Niere adrenalektomierter Ratten. Untersuchungen am Einzelnephron. Habilitationsschrift Berlin 1964.
17. HIERHOLZER, K., M. WIEDERHOLT, H. HOLZGREVE, G. GIEBISCH, R. M. KLOSE and E. E. WINDHAGER: Micropuncture study of renal transtubular concentration gradients of sodium and potassium in adrenalectomized rats. Pflüg. Arch. ges. Physiol. **285,** 193 (1965).
18. HIERHOLZER, K., M. WIEDERHOLT und H. STOLTE: Hemmung der Natriumresorption im proximalen und distalen Konvolut adrenalektomierter Ratten. Pflüg. Arch. ges. Physiol. **291,** 43 (1966).
19. JICK, H., J. G. SNYDER, E. W. MOORE and R. S. MORRISON: The effect of aldosterone and glucocorticoid on free water reabsorption. Clin. Sci. **29,** 25 (1965).
20. KOTTKE, F. J., C. F. CODE and E. H. WOOD: Urine dilution and concentration tests in adrenalectomized dogs. Amer. J. Physiol. **136,** 229 (1942).
21. KRAUS, M. and M. POPP: Determination of small amounts of aldosterone and corticosterone in the incubation medium of the adrenal gland of rats. Physiol. Bohemoslov. **13,** 457 (1964).
22. DE LIMA, T. and M. F. LOCKETT: An investigation of the actions of aldosterone on perfused cat kidneys, by ureteric stop-flow analysis. Arch. int. Physiol. Biochem. **71,** 83 (1963).
23. LOEB, R. F.: Chemical changes in the blood in Addisons disease. Sci. **76,** 420 (1932).
24. LOEB, R. F.: Effect of sodium chloride in treatment of a patient with Addisons disease. Proc. Soc. exp. Biol. Med. **30,** 808 (1933).
25. LUDENS, J. H., J. B. HOOK and H. E. WILLIAMSON: Lack of effect of actinomycin D on aldosterone induced antinatriuresis when administered after the hormone. Proc. Soc. exp. Biol. Med. **124,** 539 (1967).
26. MCEVOY, J., G. HOLLMANN und G. SENFT: Einfluß von Mineralocorticoiden auf die tubuläre Rückgewinnung von Na-Ionen. Naun.-Schm. Arch. exp. Pathol. u. Pharmacol. **250,** 318 (1965).
27. NICHOLSON, T. F.: A comparsion of the effects of proximal and distal tubular damage on the action of desoxycorticosterone and aldosterone. Canad. J. Biochem. Physiol. **35,** 641 (1957).
28. RECTOR, F. C., Jr., J. C. SELLMAN, M. MARTINEZ-MALDONADO and D. W. SELDIN: The mechanism of suppression of proximal tubular reabsorption by saline infusions. J. clin. Invest. **46,** 47 (1967).

29. Reforzo-Membrives, J., M. H. Power and R. J. Keppler: Studies on the renal excretion of water and electrolytes in cases of Addisons disease. J. clin. Endocrin. **5,** 76 (1945).
30. Robson, J. S.: Water and electrolyte metabolism. Ed. by: C. P. Stewart and T. Strengers pp. 109 (1961). Elsevier, Amsterdam.
31. Roemmelt, J. C., O. W. Sartorius and R. F. Pitts: Excretion and reabsorption of sodium and water in the adrenalectomized dogs. Amer. J. Physiol. **159,** 124 (1949).
32. Sharp, G. W. G. and A. Leaf: Mechanism of action of aldosterone. Physiol. Rev. **46,** 593 (1966).
33. Shipp, J. C., I. B. Hanenson, E. E. Windhager, H. J. Schatzmann, G. Whittembury, H. Yoshimura and A. K. Solomon: Single proximal tubules of the necturus kidney. Methods for micropuncture and microperfusion. Amer. J. Physiol. **195,** 563 (1958).
34. Sigler, M. H., J. N. Forrest, Jr. and J. R. Elkinton: Renal concentrating ability in the adrenalectomized rat. Clin. Sci. **28,** 29 (1965).
35. Sonnenblick, E. H., P. J. Cannon and J. H. Larach: The nature of the action of intravenous aldosterone: evidence for a role of the hormone in urinary dilution. J. clin. Invest. **40,** 903 (1961).
36. Steinhausen, M.: Eine Methode zur Differenzierung proximaler und distaler Tubuli der Nierenrinde von Ratten in vivo und ihre Anwendung zur Bestimmung tubulärer Strömungsgeschwindigkeiten. Pflüg. Arch. ges. Physiol. **277,** 23 (1963).
37. Stolte, H., M. Wiederholt und K. Hierholzer: Resorptionshemmung im proximalen Konvolut der Säugetierniere nach Adrenalektomie und ihre Beeinflussung durch Steroidhormone. Aktuelle Probleme der Nephrologie. Hrsg. F. Krück, Springer-Verlag, Berlin-Heidelberg-New York, S. 521 (1966).
38. Stolte, H., J. P. Brecht, M. Wiederholt und K. Hierholzer: Einfluß von Adrenalektomie und Glucocorticoiden auf die Wasserpermeabilität kortikaler Nephronabschnitte der Rattenniere. Pflüg. Arch ges. Physiol. **299,** 99 (1968).
38a. Stolte, H., N. De Santo and K. Hierholzer: The effect of adrenalectomy on the development of proximal and distal transtubular concentration gradients for sodium. Proc. IVth Internat. Congr. Nephrol., Stockholm (1969) in preparation.
39. Stumpe, K. O. und B. Ochwadt: Resorptionskapazität des proximalen Tubulus unter chronischer isotonischer Kochsalzbeladung. Pflüg. Arch. ges. Physiol. **294,** R 19 (1967).
40. Vander, A. J., R. L. Malvin, W. S. Wilde, J. Lapides, L. P. Sullivan and V. M. McMurray: Effects of adrenalectomy and aldosterone on proximal and distal tubular sodium reabsorption. Proc. Soc. exp. Biol. and Med. **99,** 323 (1958).
41. Wettstein, A.: Nebennierenrindenhormone und ihre Derivate. Mschr. Kinderheilk. **108,** 164 (1960).
42. Wiederholt, M., K. Hierholzer und J. P. Brecht: Die Wirkung von Aldosteron und Cortison auf den tubulären Na^+-Transport adrenalektomierter Ratten. Pflüg. Arch. **283,** R 71 (1965).
43. Wiederholt, M., H. Stolte, J. P. Brecht und K. Hierholzer: Mikropunktionsuntersuchungen über den Einfluß von Aldosteron, Cortison und Dexamethason auf die renale Natriumresorption adrenalektomierter Ratten. Pflüg. Arch. **292,** 316 (1966).
44. Wiederholt, M.: Mikropunktionsuntersuchungen am proximalen und distalen Konvolut der Rattenniere über den Einfluß von Actinomycin D auf den mineralocorticoidabhängigen Na^+-Transport. Pflüg. Arch. **292,** 334 (1966).
45. Wiederholt, M. und K. Hierholzer: Wirkung von Actinomycin D auf den transepithelialen Na^+-Transport. V. Symposion der Ges. für Nephrologie, Lausanne 1967 (im Druck).
46. Wiederholt, M. und B. Wiederholt: Der Einfluß von Dexamethason auf die Wasser- und Elektrolytausscheidung adrenalektomierter Ratten. Pflüg. Arch. ges. Physiol. **302,** 57 (1968).
47. Williamson, H. E., T. W. Skulan and F. E. Shideman: Effects of adrenalectomy and desoxycorticosterone on stop-flow patterns of sodium and potassium in the rat. J. Pharmacol. exp. Ther. **131,** 49 (1961).

48. WILLIAMSON, H. E.: Mechanism of the antinatriuretic action of aldosterone. Biochem. Pharmacol. **12**, 1449 (1963).
49. YUNIS, S. L., D. D. BERCOVITCH, R. M. STEIN, M. F. LEVITT and M. H. GOLDSTEIN: Renal tubular effects of hydrocortisone and aldosterone in normal hydropenic man: Comment on sites of action. J. clin. Invest. **43**, 1668 (1964).

GROSS: I was somewhat surprised at your finding that you could not restitute the passage time in the proximal tubule by dexamethasone and I wonder, whether you have studied dose-response curves and also what actual doses you gave of dexamethasone as compared with cortisone. And my second question: do you have any explanation for the insufficiency of the kidney of the adrenalectomized animal to eliminate urea?

HIERHOLZER: Well, as to the first point, I demonstrated (slide 14) that dexamethasone did, indeed, shorten proximal passage time. We have not studied dose response curves in these experiments, which are rather difficult from a technical point of view.

Cortisone was administered in the dose used by PETERS (1959) i. e. 2,5 mg/100 g 24 h. The dose of dexamethasone used was 50 µg/100 g · 24 h. This is equivalent to the cortisone dose according to the dose equivalents given by HÜBENER and STAIB (1965).

GROSS: I wonder whether with lower doses of dexamethasone you would have found a response similar to the one obtained with cortisone.

HIERHOLZER: I would expect quite the opposite result. If we increase the dose of dexamethasone we must come into a range where, as with any steroid, dexamethasone would exert some mineral corticoid activity.

DEETJEN: Herr HIERHOLZER, Sie sagten, daß die Permeabilität für Kochsalz bei Adrenalektomie herabgesetzt ist. Haben Sie, um das zu bestätigen, auch einmal mit Na^+-freier Lösung Tubuli perfundiert und den Na^+-Einstrom gemessen?

HIERHOLZER: Ja, das haben wir versucht und zwar in Mikroperfusionsexperimenten. Wir haben jedoch weder im proximalen noch im distalen Konvolut einen signifikanten Unterschied zwischen beiden Tiergruppen gefunden: dieses negative Ergebnis war durch die große Streuung der Einzelwerte bedingt.

DEETJEN: Muß dieser merkwürdige Befund, daß unter der Adrenalektomie die proximale Passagezeit verlängert ist, das TF/P-Inulin endproximal aber gleichbleibt, nicht bedeuten, daß irgendwann einmal der intratubuläre Druck erhöht gewesen ist und den Tubulus dilatiert hat? Oder haben Sie eine andere Vorstellung, welches die treibende Kraft gewesen sein kann, die zu der Dilatation geführt hat?

HIERHOLZER: Es ist nicht notwendig und m. E. auch nicht wahrscheinlich, daß der intratubuläre hydrostatische Druck angestiegen ist. Näherliegend ist die Annahme, daß die proximale Tubuluswand 6–8 Tage nach der Adrenalektomie andere mechanische Eigenschaften besitzt als vorher, d. h. eine andere Druck-Volumen-Charakteristik existiert. Außerdem muß man berücksichtigen, daß bei adrenalektomierten Ratten unter unseren Versuchs-Bedingungen die glomeruläre Filtrationsrate erniedrigt ist.

OCHWADT: Herr HIERHOLZER, da Sie die Arbeit von Herrn Dr. STUMPE und mir erwähnt haben, möchte ich einen kurzen Kommentar dazu geben. Es ist richtig, daß die chronisch mit Kochsalz beladenen Ratten genau dieselbe Verlängerung der Halbwertzeit im proximalen Tubulus zeigten, wie Ihre adrenalektomierten Tiere. Bei diesen chronisch mit Kochsalz belasteten Tieren waren das Glomerulumfiltrat und die Passagezeit im proximalen Tubulus aber normal und deshalb war die fraktionelle Resorption im proximalen Tubulus niedriger, und zwar ungefähr um 10%. Nun scheidet eine solche Ratte nicht 10% ihres gefilterten Kochsalzes aus, sondern nur 1%. Das bedeutet also, daß bei der kochsalz-belasteten Ratte der proximale Tubulus fraktionell weniger resorbiert und daß distalere Tubulusabschnitte, damit meine ich die Henle'sche Schleife, den distalen Tubulus und das Sammelrohr, insgesamt fraktionell mehr resorbieren müssen.

HIERHOLZER: Die Befunde, die Sie nennen, sind zu erwarten, wenn man annimmt, daß bei Ihren Tieren *nur* die Aldosteronsekretion vermindert ist. Im Grunde entspricht dies den Daten, die wir bei adrenalektomierten Ratten nach Dexamethasonverabreichung erhalten haben. Auch hier war bei verlängerter Halbwertzeit die Passagezeit normal.

KRÜCK: Dr. PITTS hat früher angegeben, daß 2% der fraktionalen tubulären Natrium-Reabsorption unter dem Einfluß der Nebennierenrinden-Steroide stehen. Hat diese Zahl aufgrund Ihrer Untersuchungen auch heute noch Gültigkeit oder muß sie korrigiert werden?

HIERHOLZER: Es gibt keinen Grund an den von Professor PITTS am Hund erhobenen Daten zu zweifeln. Nach den Untersuchungen von AUGUST et al. (1959) und nach unseren eigenen Erfahrungen bestehen die gleichen Verhältnisse auch beim Menschen und bei der Ratte.

Intrarenal Action of Angiotensin*)

K. THURAU

Summary: In those nephrons, whose long loops of HENLE do not participate in the counter-current system, that is to say in approximately 80% of the entire nephron population, the magnitude of the filtered sodium load is adjusted to the tubular reabsorptive capacity. This is made possible by the fact that the velocity of angiotensin formation and hence the degree of constriction of the afferent arteriole is regulated by the sodium concentration at the macula densa site. This servo-mechanism operates at the level of each nephron unit. The potency of this control mechanism for single nephron sodium load is enhanced when total body sodium is low and reduced when dietary salt is high. This hypothesis relegates angiotensin to the role of a sodium conserving agent. This is consistent with the generally accepted view that angiotensin *per se* stimulates the release of aldosterone. Accordingly, then, angiotensin exerts a control of sodium excretion at the glomerular site while aldosterone exerts its influence at the level of the tubular epithelium.

For the last three decades it has been a consistent belief that angiotensin I is a vaso-active substance. This vaso-active function of angiotensin was at first primarily considered in the patho-physiological context generated by the GOLDBLATT experiments. This concept has been recently questioned in view of the demonstration of GROSS et al. (7) that systemic blood pressure and renin activity are not necessarily correlated. In addition, they found evidence that the renin angiotensin system may participate in the maintenance of sodium balance. Furthermore, the fact that the angiotensin forming enzyme, renin, is located in the juxtaglomerular apparatus of the kidney led to the belief that angiotensin may play a role in tubular sodium transport. This view seems to be supported by the finding of several investigators (Lit. see 18) that the injection of synthetic angiotensin-amide in the rat is followed by an increase in urinary sodium excretion, suggesting, of course, an inhibitory effect upon tubular sodium reabsorption.

I would like to discuss now some studies on the intrarenal action of angiotensin which have been carried out in the last years in collaboration with Drs. SCHNERMANN, DAHLHEIM, HORSTER, NAGEL and WAHL (6, 9, 10, 13, 14, 16, 17, 19, 21). The concept of an inhibitory action of angiotensin on tubular sodium reabsorption has been favoured by LEYSSAC (11). As a means of measuring proximal tubular sodium reabsorption LEYSSAC observed the time required for reabsorption of all the tubular fluid after the abrupt cessation of glomerular filtration by renal artery clamping. This so-called occlusion time is shortened when sodium reabsorption proceeds at a high rate and is lengthened when sodium reabsorption is inhibited. After the i. v. injection of angiotensin-amide he

*) The work referred to herein of the author and his associates has been generously supported by the U.S. Department of the Army through its European Research Office and the Deutsche Forschungsgemeinschaft.

observed a prolongation of the occlusion time and accepted this as evidence for an inhibitory effect of angiotensin on proximal tubular sodium reabsorption.

In order to establish whether this method validly reflects reabsorptive activity we repeated these experiments with quantitative control of several tubular parameters (21).

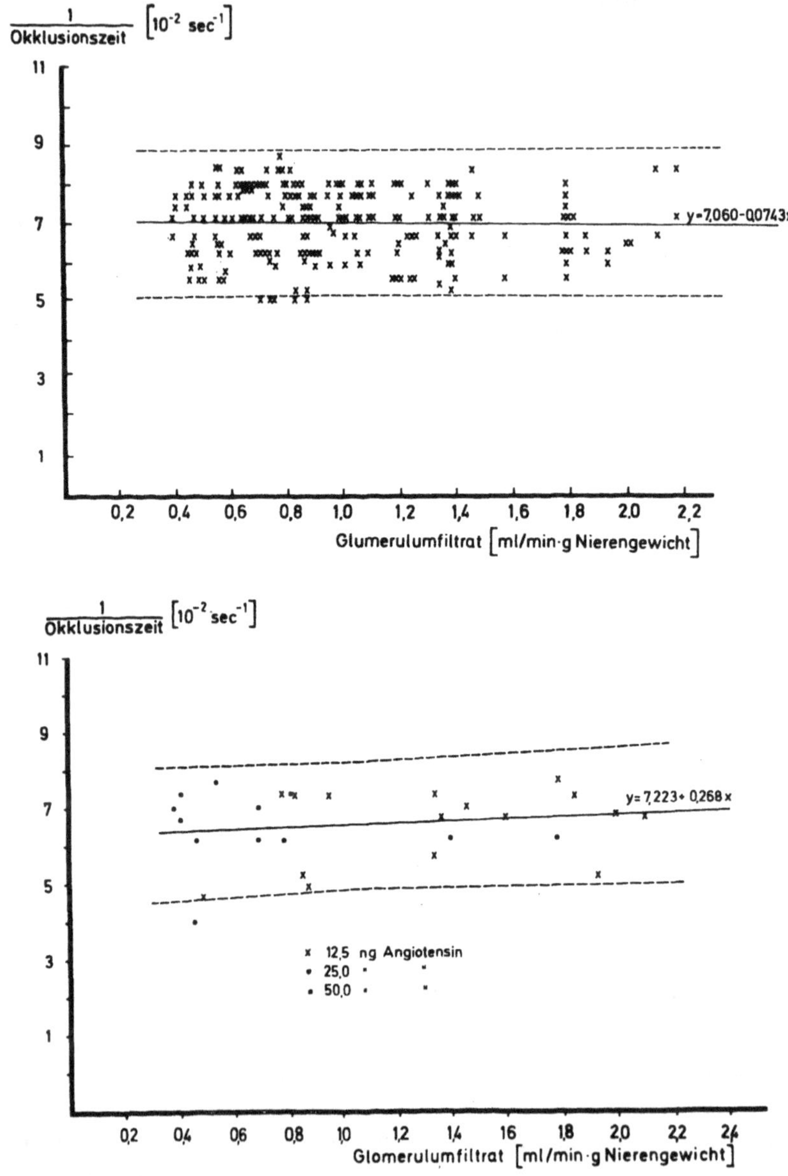

Fig. 1. Correlation between the reciprocal of the occlusion time of superficial proximal tubules in the rat kidney and glomerular filtration rate. Top: Control group. Bottom: After injection of 12.5, 25, and 50×10^{-9} g angiotensin-amide. [Data from WAHL, NAGEL, FISCHBACH and THURAU (21)].

Fig. 1 summarizes the results which led to two conclusions: a) occlusion time is independent of GFR, and b) occlusion time is not influenced by angiotensin administration.

In other experiments (10) we clearly demonstrated that the intratubular instillation of angiotensin-amide as well as the peritubular application of angiotensin does not alter the reabsorptive capacity in split-droplet experiments (Fig. 2 and 3). On the basis of perfusion experiments of the isolated rabbit renal tubule the same conclusions were drawn by Dr. BURG, as we heard yesterday.

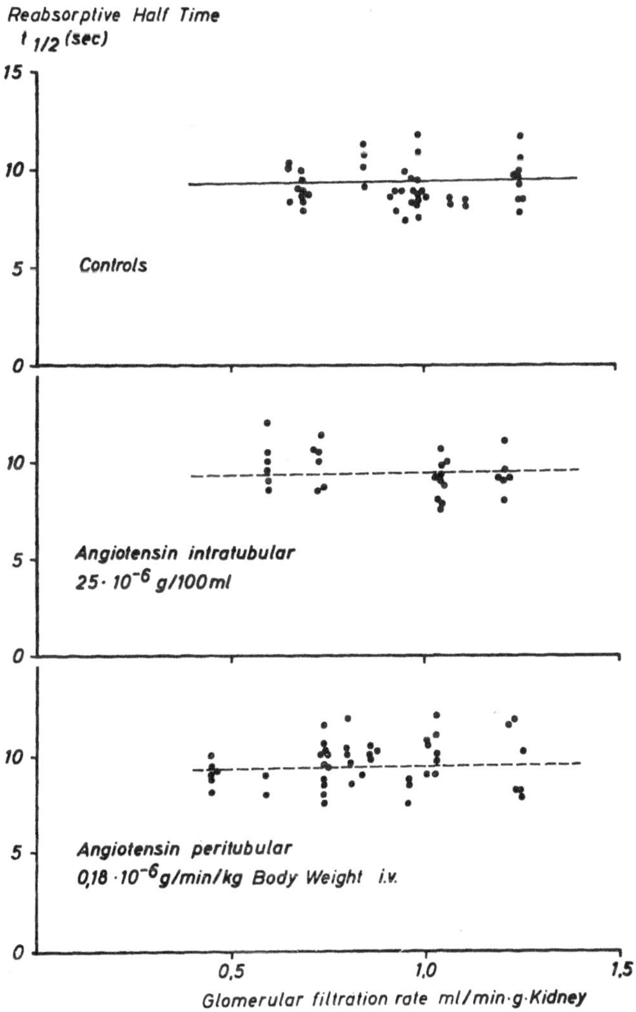

Fig. 2. Half time reabsorption of isotonic saline in the proximal convolution of the rat kidney undergoing spontaneous variations of GFR, and at elevated angiotensin concentrations, using the split oil droplet method of GERTZ. The broken lines duplicate the regression line obtained in the control group [Data from HORSTER, NAGEL, THURAU and SCHNERMANN (10)].

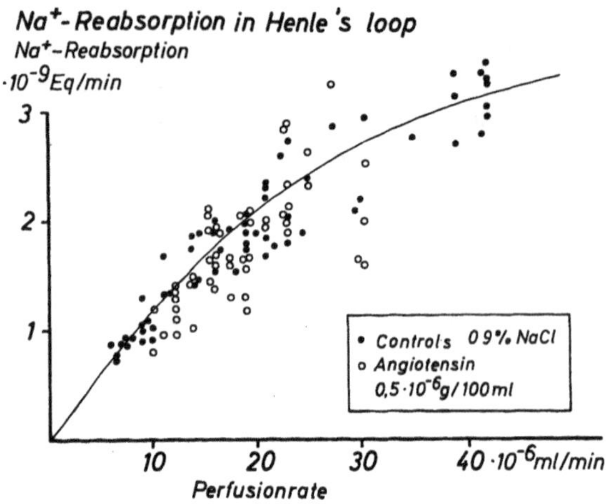

Fig. 3. Correlation between net sodium reabsorption in Henle's loop and perfusion rate (microperfusion experiments) before and after the inclusion of angiotensin into the perfusion fluid [Data from HORSTER, NAGEL, THURAU and SCHNERMANN (10)].

Since it is generally accepted that renal renin content is increased by a low sodium diet it is reasonable to anticipate a changed angiotensin activity. If there is any significant effect of angiotensin on the proximal sodium reabsorption it is to be expected that this would be manifest in the micropuncture measurement of tubular parameters. Accordingly, under a low salt diet with high renal renin contents one would expect, following the concept of LEYSSAC (11), a reduced reabsorptive capacity. Table 1 summarizes our results

Table 1. Endproximal TF/P_{In} and proximal tubular passage time in low and high sodium groups [from HORSTER and THURAU (9)].

	Low sodium	High sodium
TF/P_{In}	2.36 ± 0.36 (n = 49)	2.31 ± 0.28 (n = 28)
Passage time (sec)	9.8 ± 1.0 (n = 38)	9.6 ± 1.1 (n = 40)

from micropuncture experiments on the proximal convolution of rats kept on high or low sodium diet (9). In both groups of animals late proximal TF/P inulin and proximal tubular passage time (T) are essentially the same. From these data it appears that the reabsorptive capacity for the proximal convolution (K) in both groups is identical. This fact may be stated in equation form as follows:

$$K = \frac{C}{2\pi r^2 \cdot l} \tag{1}$$

$$C = \dot{V}_0 \cdot 1\text{-}P/TF \tag{2}$$

$$2\pi r^2 \cdot l = \dot{V}_0 \cdot (1 + P/TF) \cdot T \tag{3}$$

where: $\dot{V}_0$ = single nephron filtration rate, T = proximal tubular passage time, K = reabsorptive capacity, C = reabsorptive rate, r = inner tubular radius, l = proximal tubular length up to puncture site. Substituting Equations (2) and (3) in Equation (1):

$$K = \frac{\dot{V}_0 \cdot (1 - P/TF)}{\dot{V}_0 \cdot (1 + P/TF) \cdot T} \quad (4a)$$

$$= \frac{1 - P/TF}{(1 + P/TF) \cdot T} \quad (4b)$$

Since the values of P/TF and T in both groups are unchanged, equation (4b) states that the reabsorptive capacity (K) is the same in high and low salt groups. This result is entirely consistent with the observations of HAYSLETT et al. (8) who found transit time and reabsorptive half-time to be unchanged in sodium deficient and chronically salt-loaded rats. However, STUMPE and OCHWADT (15) found fractional proximal reabsorption to be reduced by chronic salt loading and subsequently restored to normal values by aldosterone administration.

Less clear are the data on the effect of angiotensin upon sodium reabsorption in the distal convolution. On the basis of stop-flow analyses VANDER (20) postulated a distal tubular inhibitory effect. However, it must be noted that this conclusion was based on an increase in sodium concentration of only 4 mEq/l in the distal tubular stop flow sample. Indeed, at best, stop flow data in this order of magnitude are difficult to interpret. Furthermore, data obtained in frog skin, toad skin and toad bladder (1, 5, 12) uniformly deny an inhibitory effect of angiotensin on sodium transport. In addition BONTING et al. (2) were unable to demonstrate an effect of angiotensin upon the Na-K activated ATPase of kidney homogenates. Finally, to the momentary relief but lasting terror of various investigators, MCAFEE and LOCKE (12) indeed did show an angiotensin influence on the sodium transport in the frog skin. However, sodium transport was shown to be enhanced rather than inhibited.

In summary, then, I feel that to date there are no conclusive data demonstrating an inhibitory effect of angiotensin upon tubular sodium reabsorption.

Before I proceed to outline our concept of the intrarenal function of angiotensin I would like to briefly comment on the method commonly used to simulate the intrarenal mechanisms associated with naturally occurring angiotensin by the intravascular injection of synthetic angiotensin-amide. In essence, two important limitations must be considered. Firstly, on the basis of our enzymatic studies on the renin-angiotensin system (6, 13) it appears that the degradation of natural and synthetical angiotensin by angiotensinase involves different processes. This follows from inspection of Fig. 4 which demonstrates that natural angiotensin II is degradated by angiotensinase at a much slower rate than synthetic angiotensin-amide.

The second limitation stems from the intrarenal profile of renin distribution. From the work of BROWN et al. (3) it is known that the juxtaglomerular apparatus associated with superficial glomeruli contains a high renin activity and the deeper the location of the nephron within the renal cortex the smaller the renin content of its juxtaglomerular apparatus. Clearly, then, the injection of synthetic angiotensin-amide would be expected to have a uniform influence among the different nephrons in the renal cortex, whereas the natural phenomenon appears to have an inherent concentration distribution. Accordingly, the events following the exogenous administration of synthetic angiotensin-amide may have little relation to *in vivo* mechanisms.

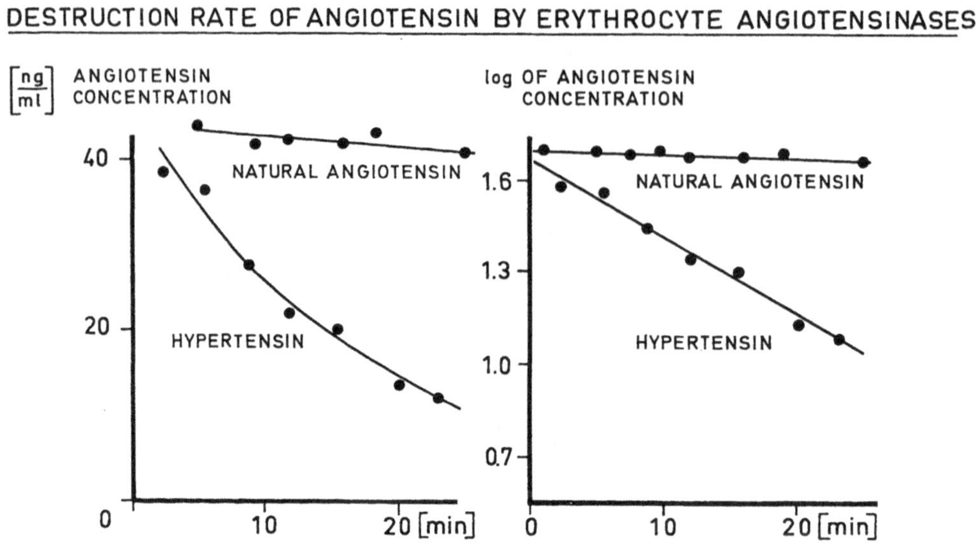

Fig. 4. Degradation of natural and synthetical angiotensin by erythrocyte angiotensinase [Data from DAHLHEIM and PETSCHAUER, unpublished).

With this in mind we have felt compelled to turn to other methods for the study of the physiological function of the renin-angiotensin system. We should note at the outset that any hypothesis concerning the function of the renin-angiotensin system must be related to the juxtaglomerular apparatus, in which the enzyme renin is formed. According to the laws of enzyme kinetics it is to be expected that the highest velocity of angiotensin formation occurs in regions where the concentration of the enzyme is also highest. This is true for the area of the juxtaglomerular apparatus. It is obvious, then, that studies measuring the concentration of renin in mixed renal venous blood probably have little relevance to the way in which natural angiotensin is formed within the kidney.

In order to obtain direct evidence concerning the function of the juxtaglomerular apparatus, several years ago we carried out micropuncture studies (14, 16, 17, 19) which suggested a mechanism whereby angiotensin could participate in the intrarenal control of sodium excretion. These experinents supported the view that by means of vasoconstriction of the afferent arteriole, released angiotensin can reduce the magnitude of the filtered sodium. The triggering of this system must be viewed in the light of the following experimental data:

In micropuncture experiments it was shown that an increase in the sodium concentration in the macula densa segment was immediately followed by a decrease in the filtration rate of the same nephron. Since the juxtaglomerular apparatus is the only point of contact of the punctured distal tubule with the glomerulus, and in view of the fact that this effect was largely diminished in high salt (renin-poor) kidneys, we postulated that the secretion of renin, and thereby the local formation of angiotensin, is regulated by the sodium concentration of the tubular fluid or of the reabsorbate in the macula densa segment.

With this triggering mechanism it is quite plausible that the glomerular delivery of sodium can be adjusted to the reabsorptive capacity of the tubule, which, in other words, is glomerulo-tubular balance. The consequences of this regulatory mechanism, namely a decrease in filtrate in the face of high sodium concentration at the macula densa site, can

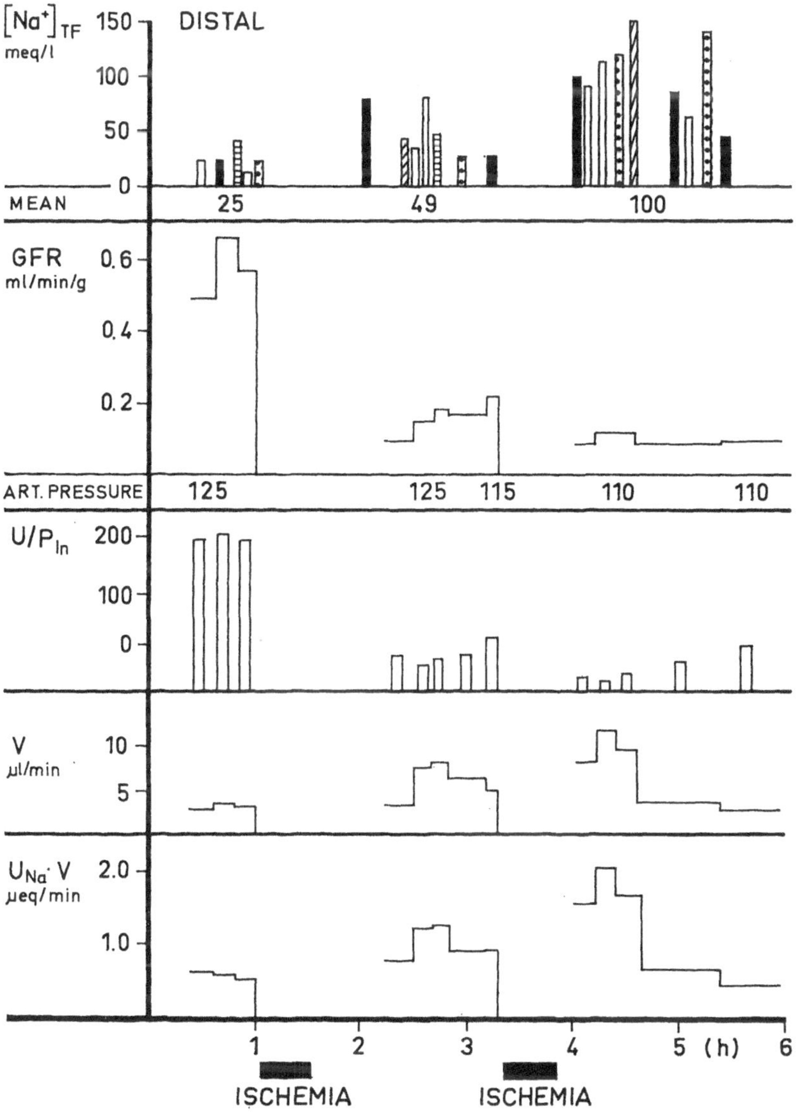

Fig. 5. Early distal sodium concentration, glomerular filtration rate and excretory function in the rat kidney before and after two ischemic periods. Early distal sodium concentration obtained in an individual nephron by the repuncture technique marked by the same symbols [Data from SCHNERMANN, NAGEL and THURAU (14)].

be well demonstrated during the administration of several diuretics (17) or in the kidney following temporary ischemia (14) as shown in Fig. 5.

This concept should be modified in the light of the fact that renin content in the juxtaglomerular apparatus is dependent upon dietary salt intake. Accordingly, we further postulate that the response of the feedback mechanism upon single nephron GFR following a given sodium stimulus to the macula densa is modulated by the renin stores of the juxtaglomerular apparatus of that nephron. This concept is further strengthened by the following observations. In the rat kidney it is possible to determine simultaneously the single nephron GFR of cortical (superficial) and juxtamedullary nephrons by micropuncture techniques. The comparison of the filtrates of these two nephron types (see Table 2 and Fig. 6) indicates that the magnitudes of superficial and juxtamedullary filtrates are dependent upon the salt intake; in rats on a high salt diet the superficial and juxtamedullary filtrates are higher and lower, respectively, than in rats on a low salt

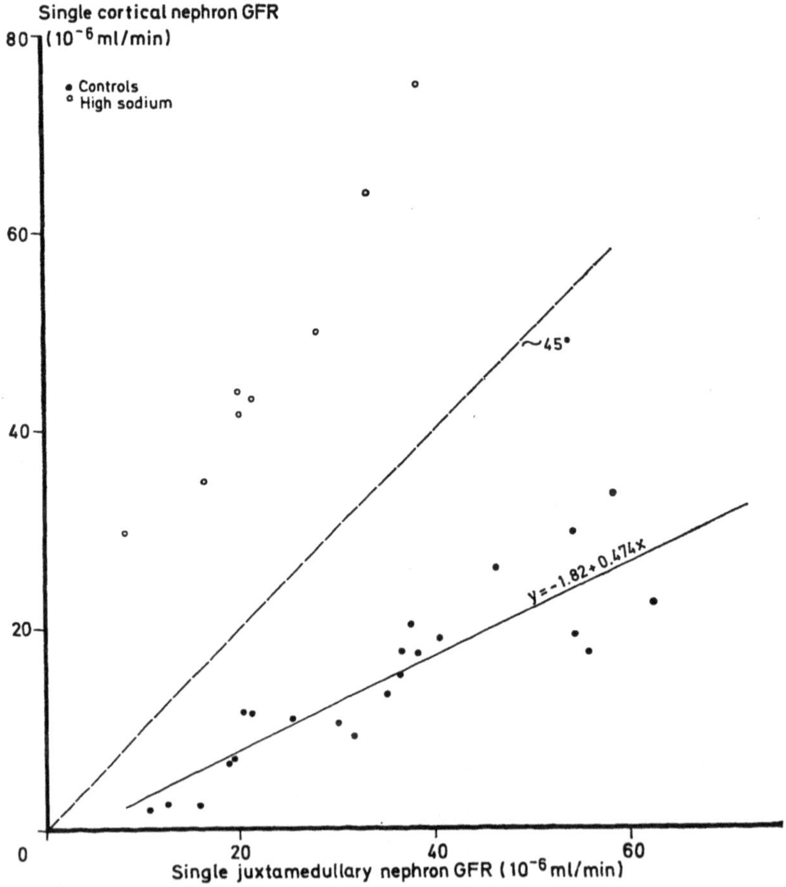

Fig. 6. Correlation between simultaneously determined single superficial and single juxtamedullary nephron filtration rates in rats kept on high (o) and low (·) sodium chloride diet [Data from HORSTER and THURAU (9)].

Table 2. Single nephron GRF's during low and high sodium diet (10^{-6} ml/min · gKW) [from Horster and Thurau (9)].

	Low sodium	High sodium
Superficial	23.5±6.4 (n = 59)	38.1±11.3 (n = 28)
Juxtamedullary	58.2±13.6 (n = 26)	16.5±6.6 (n = 15)
Total kidney GFR (ml/min · gKW)	0.94±0.16 (n = 26)	1.01±0.24 (n = 15)

diet. During high sodium diet superficial single GFR increased by 62% when compared to low sodium diet. Yet, total kidney filtrate was increased by only 9.3%, since single juxtamedullary GFR is reduced simultaneously to less than half. A mathematical analysis of these data reveals that appr. 80% of all nephrons are of the superficial type and the remainder of the juxtamedullary type. This pattern of distribution based on functional data is in close agreement with data based on histological analyses (Lit. see 9).

In the above mentioned study of Brown et al. (3) it was demonstrated that superficial juxtaglomerular apparatuses contain high renin concentrations, whereas the juxtaglomerular apparatuses of juxtamedullary glomeruli are almost free of renin. This pattern of renin distribution is consistent with our findings of a low superficial and a high juxtamedullary GFR in non-salt-loaded rats. Furthermore, it was shown (7, 4) that renal content of renin is diminished at high salt intake. Since renin primarily is distributed among superficial juxtaglomerular apparatuses, it is expected that a decrease in renin content due to salt intake takes place primarily in the superficial juxtaglomerular apparatus. This decrease in superficial renin concentration would be in accordance with the observed increase in single superficial GFR's during high salt intake. Whether or not the decrease in single juxtamedullary GFR's during high salt intake corresponds with an intrarenal redistribution of renin activity remains unknown. To answer this question, renin activity in single juxtaglomerular apparatuses during high sodium chloride intake would have to be analyzed.

References

1. Barbour, B. H., J. R. Gill and F. C. Bartter: Proc. Exptl. Biol. Med. **116,** 806 (1964).
2. Bonting, S. L., M. R. Canady and N. M. Hawkins: Biochem. Biophys. Acta, **82,** 427–429 (1964).
3. Brown, J. J., D. L. Davies, A. F. Lever, R. A. Parker and J. I. S. Robertson: J. Physiol. (London) **176,** 418 (1965).
4. Cockett, A. T. K., R. S. Moore, M. Kazmin and A. P. Roberts: J. Urol. (Baltimore) **97,** 168 (1967).
5. Coviello, A. and J. Crabbé: Biochem. Pharmacol. **14,** 1739 (1965).
6. Dahlheim, H., P. Weber, I. Herold and K. Thurau: Pflügers Arch. ges. Physiol. **298,** 131 (1967).
7. Gross, F., G. Schaechtelin, H. Brunner and G. Peters: Canad. med. Ass. J. **90,** 258 (1964).

8. HAYSLETT, J. P., M. KASHGARIAN and F. H. EPSTEIN: J. clin. Invest. **46**, 1254 (1967).
9. HORSTER, M. and K. THURAU: Pflügers Arch. ges. Physiol. **301**, 162 (1968).
10. HORSTER, M., W. NAGEL, J. SCHNERMANN und K. THURAU: Pflügers Arch. ges. Physiol. **292**, 118–128 (1966).
11. LEYSSAC, P. P.: Acta Physiol. Scand. 70, Suppl. **291**, 152 pp. (1966).
12. MCAFEE, R. D. and W. LOCKE: Endocrinology **18**, 1301 (1967).
13. PETSCHAUER, K., H. DAHLHEIM und K. THURAU: Pflügers Arch. ges. Physiol. **300**, 38 (1968).
14. SCHNERMANN, J., W. NAGEL und K. THURAU: Pflügers Arch. ges. Physiol. **287**, 296–310 (1966).
15. STUMPE, K. O. und B. OCHWADT: Pflügers Arch. ges. Physiol. **300**, 148 (1968).
16. THURAU, K. und J. SCHNERMANN: Klin. Wochschr. **43**, 410–413 (1965).
17. THURAU, K.: Ann. N. Y. Acad. Sci. **139**, 388 (1966).
18. THURAU, K., H. VALTIN and J. SCHNERMANN: Ann. Rev. Physiol. **30**, 441 (1968).
19. THURAU, K., J. SCHNERMANN, W. NAGEL, M. HORSTER and M. WAHL: Circ. Res. **20/21**, Suppl. II, 79 (1967).
20. VANDER, A. J.: Am. J. Physiol. **205**, 133 (1963).
21. WAHL, M., W. NAGEL, H. FISCHBACH and K. THURAU: Pflügers Arch. ges. Physiol. **298**, 141 (1967).

GROSS: I could not agree more with Dr. THURAU when he said that the effects of exogenous angiotensin do not correspond to what may happen in the kidney with endogenous angiotensin either formed or released there. But I think you should have gone one step further. So far, it is unknown where the renin substrate-reaction takes place and where angiotensin is liberated. Does this occur in the juxtaglomerular cells where renin is stored or does this occur in the plasma? Nobody knows exactly what is going on. In addition, it is highly probable that the renin-angiotensin system, as we consider it today, is much more complicated and various other factors may play a role in that enzyme-substrate system.

When you mentioned the profile of renin distribution in the kidney, you have given only part of the story. You have referred to the normal kidney, but after a GOLDBLATT clamp has been placed on the renal artery the renin content of the deep glomeruli increases to similar values as in the superficial glomeruli. During sodium loading, the renin content of the superficial glomeruli falls to values similar to those normally found in the deep glomeruli. Now, when you say that angiotensin may play a role in the adjustment of the nephra to the actual sodium load, I wonder whether you have considered this for acute or chronic experiments. Changes in renin content generally need about 1 to 2 weeks to become demonstrable. It may certainly be that the release of renin from the juxtaglomerular cells is not directly correlated to the stores found in the juxtaglomerular cells, and it may be that the secretory capacity of glomeruli is high enough to react to acute changes of sodium load, but it is unknown where changes in sodium load are really perceived. The macula densa is a very suggestive place for a receptor area but, as you and others, too, have demonstrated, it is highly improbable that changes in sodium concentration at the macula densa affect directly the release of renin. Therefore, it must be some other mechanism and I wonder what eliciting stimulus you consider important and where this eliciting stimulus might be perceived.

THURAU: Let me first comment on the last point you raised. I agree that the sodium concentration in the tubular fluid *per se* at the macula densa site may not be the direct releasing factor for renin. Nevertheless, to my knowledge this possibility has not yet been disproven as you suggest. The sodium concentration might be the stimulus for another releasing factor(s). The great unknown in this feedback mechanism is the function of the macula densa cells, which histologically differ very much from the adjacent tubular cells. As long as we do not know their function, any hypothesis about the details of the releasing mechanisms must be highly speculative. The data I showed you about the intrarenal distribution of single nephron filtration rates and their adjustment to dietary sodium load were obtained in animals kept on high or low sodium diet for at least 3 weeks. Therefore, I would consider this to be a chronic experiment. We have not yet done experiments on low sodium rats acutely loaded with saline. But it is well known from micropuncture work that superficial single nephron filtrate increases during saline loading. Also, it is known that renin release into the renal venous blood can be acutely changed by saline infusion (BUNAG, PAGE and MCCUBBIN, Am. J. Physiol. **211,** 1383, 1966).

GROSS: I agree fully with your hypothesis in so far as renin may contribute to the renal excretory mechanisms.

OCHWADT: Dr. THURAU, I fully agree that there is no definite proof that angiotensin acts directly on renal sodium reabsorption. However, I should like to mention a few findings from our laboratory which do suggest an effect on the distal sodium concentration. In one set of experiments, we infused in normal rats angiotensin in an amount which did not lower the glomerular filtration rate. Before and during this infusion, sodium and inulin TF/P-ratios in the distal tubule were determined by means of the recollection method. The slide shows the results from 9 preliminary experiments (Fig. 1). In spite of the relative large scatter of the values, one certainly gets the impression that the sodium concentration in the distal tubule increases during the infusion of angiotensin. I may mention that the TF/P inulin-ratio in these samples did not change.

The second line of evidence comes from rats with experimental renal hypertension. In those rats, we put a GOLDBLATT-clip on one renal artery, leaving the other kidney untouched. Now, in the untouched kidney, the course of the sodium TF/P-ratio along the distal tubule was

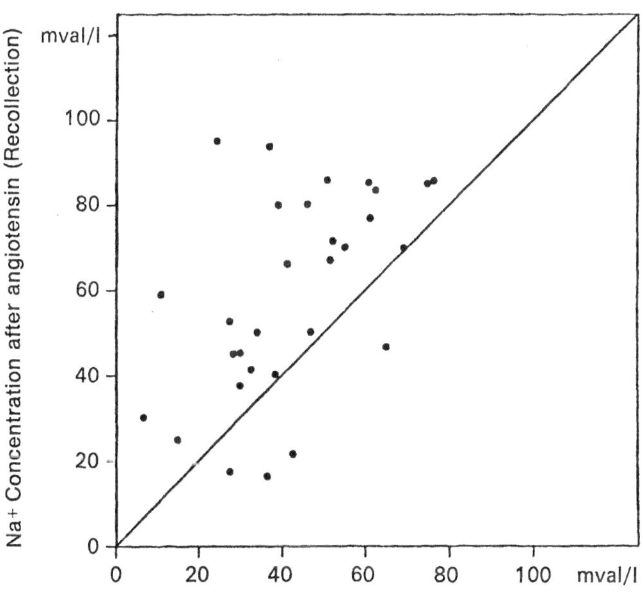

Fig. 1. Distal tubular fluid sodium concentration before and during the infusion of angiotensin (recollection-method).

quite normal. In the clipped kidney, however, sodium TF/P-ratio did not decrease towards the end of the distal tubule but remained high. As shown by GROSS, such a clipped kidney contains much more renin than normal. GROSS has also shown that the renin content of the clipped kidney becomes normal when untouched kidney is removed. Under those conditions, the sodium TF/P-ratio along the distal tubule also becomes normal. There seems to be a correspondence between the renin content of the kidney and of the sodium concentration in the distal tubule. Well, I do not, as I said, regard this as proof but I wouldn't be surprised if we find in the future a direct effect of angiotensin on the sodium transport mechanism in the distal tubule.

Finally, it may be of interest that the single nephron filtrate per g kidney does not differ significantly from normal in both the clipped and in the untouched kidney in spite of the fact that the renin content of such kidneys is very different.

THURAU: It is rather difficult to assume an inhibitory effect of angiotensin on sodium reabsorption within the framework of our understanding of the renin-angiotensin system. It is widely accepted that renin and angiotensin activity are elevated during sodium depletion, i. e. when sodium conserving mechanisms are stimulated. In this situation, then, an inhibition of tubular sodium reabsorption would be implausible. There is another observation which hardly goes along with an inhibitory function of angiotensin. In many patients with unilateral renal artery stenosis investigators employing ureteral catheterization (Howard-test) often reveal a decreased urinary sodium concentration on the affected side.

BOHLE: Herr THURAU, ich möchte Sie darauf aufmerksam machen, daß EDUARDS (Anat. Rec. **125,** 521, 1956) gezeigt hat, daß die Vasa efferentia der juxtamedullären Glomerula überwiegend weitere Lichtungen besitzen als die der übrigen Nierenrinde. Außerdem wird von EDUARDS angegeben, daß die Wände der medullären efferenten Arteriolen insgesamt muskelstärker als die Vasa efferentia der gesamten übrigen Nierenrinde sind. EDUARDS nimmt an, daß, wenn die genannten Gefäße nicht so muskelstark wären, die Nierenrindendurchblutung unter normalen Bedingungen nicht garantiert sei. 2. Die das akute Nierenversagen kennzeichnende Funktionsstörung wird für uns am einfachsten erklärbar, wenn Macula densa und juxtaglomerulärer Apparat in der von Ihnen und SCHNERMANN angegebenen Weise funktionieren.

THURAU: Zu einem ähnlichen Ergebnis über die Verteilung der Gefäßmuskulatur in den Arteriolen oberflächlicher und juxtamedullärer Glomerula ist kürzlich auch MOFFAT (J. Ultrastructure Res. **19,** 532, 1967) gekommen. Auch er zeigte, daß die efferenten Arteriolen der juxtamedullären Glomerula viel muskelreicher sind als die der superfiziellen Glomerula. Außerdem scheinen Unterschiede in der sympathischen und parasympathischen Innervation zu bestehen. Das läßt nicht nur eine Besonderheit in der Regulation der Markdurchblutung vermuten, sondern auch in der Regulation des Filtrates derjenigen Nephrone, die mit ihren langen dünnen Schleifen am Konzentrierungsmechanismus beteiligt sind.

GESSLER: Wenn die Pathogenese des akuten Nierenversagens zur Sprache kommt, möchte ich feststellen, daß auch Volumenveränderungen bei seiner Entstehung eine Rolle spielen dürften. Nach Befunden, die wir kürzlich erhoben, ergibt sich bei salzverarmten und dehydrierten Ratten ein wesentlich schwererer Verlauf der experimentellen Anurie. Während eine Hämatinvergiftung ohne Salzverarmung oder Wasserentzug erst bei Blutdrucksenkung auf 70 mm Hg und darunter zur Anurie führt, tritt diese bei isotoner oder hypotoner Dehydration bereits bei einem Blutdruck von 100 mm Hg auf. Nach diesen Befunden nehmen wir an, daß bei der Pathogenese der akuten Anurie neben dem von Herrn THURAU angeführten Rückkoppelungsmechanismus durch Osmo- oder Chemorezeptoren auch Volumenrezeptoren eine Rolle spielen.

The Effect of Angiotensin upon Blood Pressure Dependent Increases of Na-Excretion in Essential Hypertension

Über die Beeinflussung der blutdruckabhängigen Zunahme der Natriumausscheidung bei essentieller Hypertonie durch Angiotensin*)

W. SCHOEPPE

Summary: Following infusion of isotonic saline, sodium excretion in patients with essential hypertension increases with mean arterial blood pressure. Angiotensin applicated in a rate to increase mean arterial blood pressure by an average of 20 mm Hg causes a decrease in sodium excretion compared to control values. However the correlation between mean arterial blood pressure and sodium excretion is preserved.

The same correlation between mean arterial blood pressure and sodium excretion exists when urinary sodium output increases up to tenfold following a single dose of furosemide. Again, angiotensin causes only an overall reduction of sodium excretion without affecting the correlation between mean arterial blood pressure and urinary sodium output.

The changes in sodium excretion caused by angiotensin always could be explained by a concomitant change in filtered load. The present data do not allow to postulate a specific interference of angiotensin with tubular sodium reabsorption in essential hypertension.

Die hier vorgelegten Daten sind im Zusammenhang mit Untersuchungen erhoben worden, deren Gegenstand die Faktoren waren, die eine unterschiedliche Empfindlichkeit gegenüber exogen zugeführtem Angiotensin bei Kranken mit essentieller Hypertonie bewirken.

Eine Infusion isotoner Natriumchloridlösung führt beim Menschen bei leichter Hydrierung zu einer erhöhten Natriumausscheidung. Die Zunahme der Natriumausscheidung ist dabei vom arteriellen Mitteldruck abhängig. Die folgende Tabelle enthält die Mittelwerte von 40 Patienten mit arteriellen Mitteldrucken zwischen 90 und 140 mm Hg. Die Inulinclearance betrug bei diesen Patienten im Mittel 97 ml/min, der niedrigste Einzelwert war 80 ml/min. Die PAH Clearance hatte einen Mittelwert von 498 ml/min, der niedrigste Einzelwert war 395 ml/min. Es handelte sich also um eine weitgehend homogene Gruppe von Patienten mit essentieller Hypertonie, ohne Zeichen einer renalen Erkrankung.

Wie aus der Tabelle zu ersehen ist, wurde die Natriumausscheidung – hier dargestellt als Natriumclearance, wobei die Plasmakonzentrationen von Natrium keine wesentlichen Änderungen und Abweichungen zeigten – unter vier verschiedenen Bedingungen untersucht. Nach einer Periode isotoner Natriumchloridzufuhr in einer Rate von 4 ml/min, erhielten die Untersuchten eine Angiotensininfusion (Hypertensin CIBA), deren Rate so

*) Mit Unterstützung der Deutschen Forschungsgemeinschaft.

eingestellt war, daß eine Blutdrucksteigerung von systolisch 20 mm Hg erreicht wurde. Nach einer weiteren Kontrollperiode wurde Furosemid als Stoßinjektion (Lasix 20 mg) intravenös verabreicht und sodann erneut Angiotensin infundiert.

Arterieller Mitteldruck mm Hg	90	110	130	>140
Natrium-Clearance ml/min · 1,73 m^2				
Isotone NaCl Lsg. Infusion	1.18	1.52	1.65	2.5
Isotone NaCl Lsg. + Angiotensin (äquipressorische Dosis)	—	0.51	0.99	2.2
Isotone NaCl Lsg. + Furosemid (20 mg i. v.)	13.07	14.1	16.2	19.2
Isotone NaCl Lsg. + Angiotensin	6.4	8.9	9.8	15.5

Betrachtet man die Natriumclearance unter den genannten Bedingungen, so bleibt die Abhängigkeit vom arteriellen Mitteldruck grundsätzlich erhalten. Zwar ändern sich erwartungsgemäß die Absolutwerte, die Zunahme mit dem Systemdruck bleibt aber bei Steigerungen der Natriumclearance um das Zehnfache deutlich erkennbar.

Es handelt sich um ein Phänomen, das unabhängig von Basisnatriumausscheidung oder Wasserausscheidung auftritt, ebenso unabhängig von Filtrationsrate oder PAH Clearance, die unter dem Einfluß von Angiotensin eine Reduktion von etwa 50% des Ausgangswertes erfahren.

Mit höherem arteriellen Druck nimmt in den Versuchen die Wasserrückresorption ausgedrückt als $T_C\ H_2O$ ab. Dies trifft auch zu, wenn zusätzlich zur Infusion von Natriumchlorid Angiotensin infundiert wird. Wird dagegen die Diurese um etwa das Zehnfache unter Einwirkung eines Diureticums gesteigert, so bleibt die dabei zu beachtende Clearance osmotisch freien Wassers – wie hier unter Furosemid – unter den gewählten Bedingungen vom Blutdruck unbeeinflußt. Auch die durch Angiotensin herbeigeführte Verminderung von Inulin- und PAH-Clearance ändert die Größe der C_{H_2O} bei den Gruppen mit unterschiedlichem Mitteldruck nur gering.

Eine Zunahme des Blutdruckes geht nach diesen Beobachtungen also mit einer Zunahme der Natriumausscheidung bei Zufuhr isotoner NaCl-Lösung einher. Dieser Zuwachs in Abhängigkeit vom arteriellen Mitteldruck ist mit einer Abnahme der Rückresorption osmotisch freien Wassers gekoppelt. Wird die Natriumausscheidung durch das Diureticum erhöht, so steigen osmolare Clearance und Urinvolumen gleichmäßig mit dem Blutdruck an. Der Anstieg ist hierbei dann jedoch zusätzlich mit der Filtrationsgröße positiv korreliert.

Wir möchten zur Zeit aus diesen Beobachtungen den Schluß ziehen, daß die durch exogen zugeführtes Angiotensin hervorgerufenen Änderungen der Natriumausscheidung Folge der durch Angiotensin bewirkten Änderungen der Hämodynamik der Niere sind und eine spezielle Wirkung von Angiotensin auf die Natriumreabsorption – wenn überhaupt vorhanden – hier von nachgeordneter Bedeutung ist, weil die durchgehende Druckabhängigkeit der Natriumausscheidung zwar absolut, relativ aber nicht geändert wird.

Countercurrent Considerations Relating to Renal Medullary pCO_2 and Bicarbonate Concentrations*)

C. A. BALDAMUS, E. UHLICH

Summary: In micropuncture samples from vasa rectum collecting duct, and the renal artery, pH, pCO_2 and bicarbonate concentrations were determined.

During bicarbonate infusion the CO_2 pressure in vasa recta blood was the same as in animals infused with saline but about 10 mm Hg above that of renal artery samples. Inhibition of carbonic anhydrase with diamox enlarged the CO_2 pressure difference between renal artery and renal papilla to about 40 mm Hg. So it is concluded that increased medullary tissue pressure is mainly due to delayed dehydration. However, the CO_2 pressure in collecting duct samples in both conditions was significantly higher than in vasa recta samples, indicating delayed dehydration in collecting duct urine. When, in contrast, carbonic anhydrase is infused to remove delayed dehydration along the total nephron, the pCO_2 in collecting duct samples and vasa recta samples became equal. The difference between pCO_2 in renal artery and renal medulla under these circumstances was not significant.

The final high pCO_2 of alkaline urine is obtained in part during its passage through the renal papilla. But at the time the urine leaves the papilla the dehydration of urinary carbonic acid is not in its equilibrium state and so the final urinary pCO_2 is only attained in the urinary tract.

In animals infused with saline, there was no difference in bicarbonate concentration in vasa recta and arteria renalis samples. This suggests that bicarbonate is not involved in the general concentrating process of the medulla. The bicarbonate concentration in vasa recta did not rise before the bicarbonate concentration in collecting ducts reached high values. This was interpreted as a diffusion of bicarbonate from collecting duct to vasa recta.

Since the investigations of Strassburg in 1872 (6), it has been appreciated that the partial pressure of CO_2 of urine can exceed that of blood. Pitts and Lotspeich (3) thought that this could be the result of the delayed dehydration of carbonic acid which is instantaneously formed in HCO_3^- containing tubular fluid by hydrogen ion secretion in exchange for reabsorbed sodium. This mechanism is shown graphically in Fig. 1. The rate of the subsequent dehydration of carbonic acid is dependent upon the presence of carbonic anhydrase. When carbonic anhydrase is present carbonic acid is rapidly dehydrated; in its absence the dehydration is delayed. Since carbonic anhydrase is normally not present in distal tubular urine as shown by Rector et al. (4) and seems also not to be available in collecting duct urine, it is possible that the delayed dehydration of carbonic acid will proceed even when urine has left the renal pelvis and thereby results in a rising pCO_2 as the urine travels through the urinary tract.

Another possible factor contributing to a high urinary pCO_2 is the countercurrent system maintaining a high papillary pCO_2 initially generated by delayed dehydration of carbonic acid in distal tubular and collecting duct urine.

*) Methodical details and further results of this investigation are published in Pflügers Arch. ges. Physiol. **303**, 31 (1968).

OCHWADT and PITTS (2) tested the hypothesis of delayed dehydration of carbonic acid as the reason for the high pCO_2 in alkaline urine. They administered an isotonic bicarbonate solution intravenously to dogs and observed the change in urinary pCO_2 after adding carbonic anhydrase to the infusion. As soon as carbonic anhydrase was detectable in the urine the urinary pCO_2 fell to values found in arterial blood.

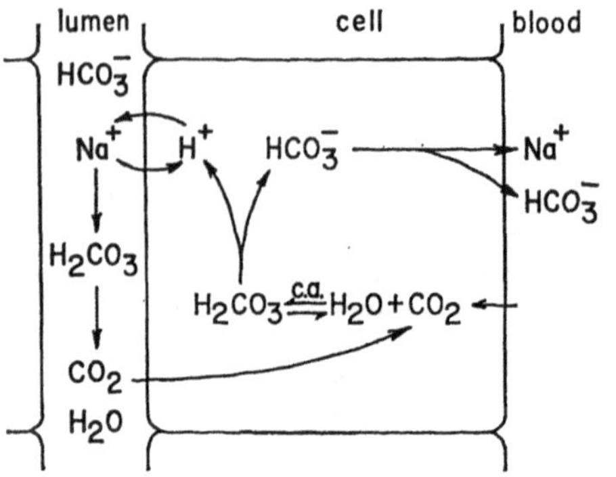

Fig. 1. Renal tubular mechanism of bicarbonate reabsorption.

Although the hypothesis of PITTS and LOTSPEICH (3) was thereby supported it was still unclear whether the pCO_2 rose within the renal medulla or after the urine left the kidney.

The present studies were undertaken with the following questions in mind:

1. Does delayed dehydration of carbonic acid completely account for the high pCO_2 of alkaline urine?
2. What is the effect of delayed dehydration along the whole nephron as produced by administration of diamox on renal medullary and final urine pCO_2?
3. What is the site of origin of the high urinary pCO_2?
4. How is bicarbonate handled in the countercurrent system of the medulla?

To explore these problems micropuncture studies were carried out on rats and CO_2 pressure and bicarbonate concentration were determined in samples of renal artery and vasa recta blood and in collecting duct urine. The pCO_2 values from vasa recta samples were accepted as representative for the pCO_2 of renal medullary tissue because the erythrocytes of vasa recta blood contain sufficient carbonic anhydrase to instantaneously catalyse the dehydration of carbonic acid and the red cell wall is highly permeable for the reactants HCO_3^- and H^+ and the products $CO_2 + H_2O$. Therefore in vasa recta blood carbonic acid and pCO_2 are in equilibrium and no change in pCO_2 occurs during and after sampling. In previous studies we confirmed the validity of this view. In contrast, samples taken from collecting ducts where no carbonic anhydrase seems to be available are not in equilibrium with respect to carbonic acid and pCO_2, resulting in a progressive rise of pCO_2 until equilibrium is reached in the sample pipette.

Since the vasa recta samples were taken immediately adjacent to the collecting duct puncture site and in view of the fact that CO_2 is highly diffusable, it is reasonable to accept vasa recta pCO_2 as being equal to collecting duct pCO_2 at the moment of sampling. Accordingly, the difference between the pCO_2 in the vasa recta and the collecting duct sample after the dehydration reaction came to equilibrium represents the amount of carbonic acid in the urine sample that dehydrates subsequent to the moment of sampling.

For measuring pH in micropuncture samples we constructed a micro-glass-electrode. Following the experience of KHURI et al. (1) who constructed in our laboratory in Berlin a suction type pH electrode, our main innovation was to find pH-sensitive glass and insensitive "inert" glass similar in their melting points and expansion coefficients. These two glasses could be fused together ensuring an absolutely tight junction. In this way, it was possible to get electrodes with a nearly ideal potential response and a stable reading value. In contrast, glass electrodes of KHURI et al. (1) are constructed by using organic resins, wax and other binding materials at the pH glass-inert glass junctions (B and D). In our hands, this method of construction resulted in an unstable mV response and a drifting of the stable reading value, presumably due to minute cracks at the binding sites.

Fig. 2 depicts the main features of the pH microelectrode used in these studies. The pH-sensitive glass capillary (C) (approximate dimensions: inner diameter 20–40 μ, length

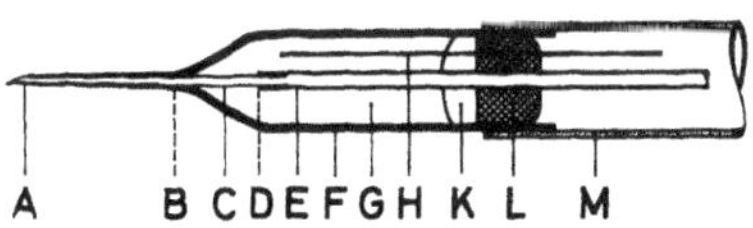

Fig. 2. Details of construction of glass pH electrodes. See text for description.

2–5 mm) is connected by a glass to glass seal at point D with the inner capillary of inert glass (E) and at the point B with the outer capillary of inert glass (F). The chamber between inner and outer glass tubing is filled with reference solution (G) (for example, 0,1 n HCl) and covered with an oil droplet (K). After insertion of a silver-silverchloride wire (H) which serves as reference electrode, the chamber is closed with epoxy cement (L). The whole assembly is then fixed in a thick glass tube (M) for better handling. Samples are sucked in through the tip (A) of the inert glass pipette which can be cut at an outer diameter of 5–10 μ and can be ground to a fine tip. During measuring, the electrode remains immersed in the fluid sample to which electrical contact is established by means of a calomel half cell via saturated KCl-bridge or by means of a Ling-Gerard-microelectrode of low resistance.

The mean potential response at 30° C is 59.4 mV/pH unit and remains constant for several months. During one experiment of 15 hours the base line changed only one mV. The response time depends on the thickness of the wall of the pH glass and is usually about 5–10 seconds. The electrical resistance is about 10^9 Ohm. The pH value can be obtained in sample volumes of 2 nanoliters with a high degree of accuracy and precision.

Micropipettes for collecting samples from vasa recta, collecting ducts, and the renal artery were filled with mercury to prevent loss of CO_2 from the sample. Immediately after sampling the so called "actual pH" was registered, as shown in Fig. 3.

Subsequently, we centrifuged the samples to get rid of the erythrocytes and put the plasma and urine under oil on a slide. Then they were covered with oil in a special chamber at body temperature (38° C) and equilibrated with three known CO_2 pressures. The pH of each sample was measured at each of the three pCO_2's. In this way a CO_2 titration curve was generated for each sample (log pCO_2/pH) by which we could calculate the pCO_2 corresponding to the actual pH. From the known pH and pCO_2 of the sample the bicarbonate concentration was derived according to the HENDERSON-HASSELBALCH equation.

To evaluate the significance of delayed dehydration for high CO_2 pressure in the rat renal medulla and to assess the behaviour of bicarbonate in the countercurrent system we infused an isotonic bicarbonate solution intravenously. In a second group of rats we added a carbonic anhydrase blocker (diamox) to the infusion and in a third series, the enzyme carbonic anhydrase. Finally, a fourth group of rats were studied in the antidiuretic state during slow saline infusion (0.5–1 ml/h).

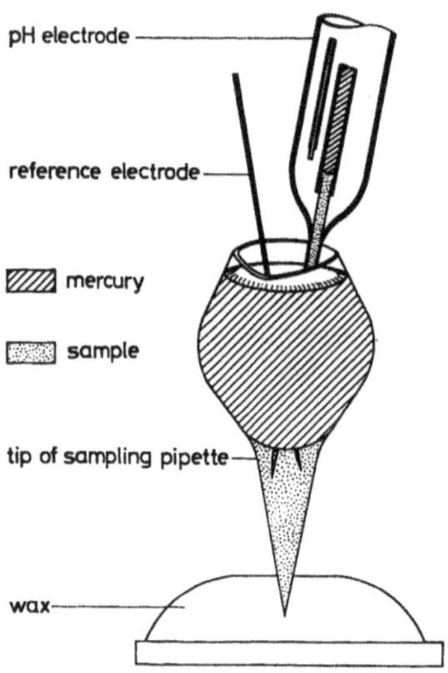

Fig. 3. Details of sample handling during the measurement of the "actual" pH.

These different experimental protocols provided the opportunity for varying factors determining urinary pCO_2 and HCO_3 – concentration. The infusion of HCO_3 – and saline is associated with delayed dehydration of carbonic acid only in distal tubules and collecting ducts. The administration of diamox results in the dehydration being delayed in the proximal tubule as well. In contrast, carbonic anhydrase produces immediate dehydration at all nephron sites when given intravenously.

Our results are shown in Figs. 4 and 5. The pCO_2 of renal artery blood during NaCl infusion (0.5–1 ml/h) is not significantly different when compared to the value obtained during bicarbonate infusion. The values were 45 ± 3 mm Hg and 44 ± 5 mm Hg, respectively. Similarly, no significant change in renal artery pCO_2 was noted with the further addition to the bicarbonate infusion of diamox (51 ± 8 mm Hg) or carbonic anhydrase (48 ± 7 mm Hg).

The pCO_2 of vasa recta blood, and hence of the papilla, was about 11 mm Hg higher than the arterial pCO_2 in the group infused with saline alone. In this group the CO_2 pressure in collecting duct samples could not be measured with our method because the bicarbonate concentration was nearly zero. The difference in pCO_2 between renal papilla and renal artery could be due to delayed dehydration or metabolic CO_2 production. Metabolic CO_2 would be further increased by medullary lactic acid production (5) if this acid is buffered by bicarbonate. On the other hand hydrogen ions mainly secreted in cortical collecting duct cells form, together with bicarbonate ions, carbonic acid. This carbonic acid undergoes delayed dehydration, as expected from the absence of carbonic anhydrase in urine of the distal nephron and forms CO_2. All these mechanisms could be favoured by countercurrent diffusion and could lead to an increase in CO_2 pressure in the papilla.

The group receiving bicarbonate infusions shows the same CO_2 pressure difference between arterial blood (44±5 mm Hg) and vasa rectum (55±9 mm Hg) as the group with saline infusion. The CO_2 of the collecting duct samples (85±20 mm Hg) exceeds the vasa recta CO_2 pressure by about 30 mm Hg. Clearly, delayed dehydration in collecting duct urine did not come to equilibrium until the sample was collected in the sampling pipette.

Extending delayed dehydration to the proximal tubule by adding diamox to the bicarbonate infusion resulted in a CO_2 pressure in the papilla of 92+20 mm Hg as

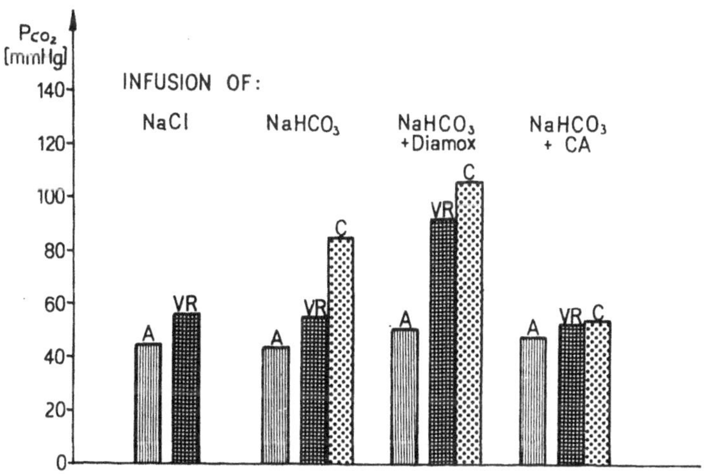

Fig. 4. The response of pCO_2 in samples of renal artery blood (A), vasa recta blood (VR) and collecting duct urine (C) to various experimental conditions.

compared to the arterial value of 51±8 mm Hg. Dehydration of carbonic acid formed in proximal tubules by hydrogen ion secretion is displaced to more distal nephron sites, namely the loops of Henle, because no carbonic anhydrase for immediate dehydration is available. This again leads to a rise in papillary tissue pressure of CO_2 which is accentuated by countercurrent diffusion. The of CO_2 pressure difference between vasa rectum and collecting duct samples in this group is less than that seen during bicarbonate infusions alone, 14 and 40 mm Hg, respectively. This difference can be interpreted according to the following considerations:

After administration of Diamox the flow rate in collecting ducts was much greater than that found in other groups. If one assumes constant hydrogen ion secretion and bicarbonate in excess, this means, per volume of urine less hydrogen ions are available to form carbonic acid. On the other hand, diamox not only delays dehydration of carbonic acid to H_2O and CO_2 by blocking carbonic anhydrase, but also, the hydration of CO_2 to carbonic acid. This process of hydration of CO_2, as shown in Fig. 1, results in the formation of intracellular carbonic acid which will dissociate to H^+ for secretion into tubular lumen and to HCO_3^-. If the intracellular carbonic anhydrase is blocked by Diamox, less hydrogen ions are available for tubular secretion.

When carbonic anhydrase is infused and excreted in the urine, the dehydration of carbonic acid is catalysed along the total nephron. Therefore, if the elevated papillary tissue pressure is due to delayed dehydration, arterial and papillary pCO_2 should be equal under these conditions. Indeed, the vasa recta pCO_2 was 53 ± 12 mm Hg which was not significantly different from that of renal artery blood (48 ± 7 mm Hg) or collecting duct samples (54 ± 12 mm Hg). The absence of a pCO_2 difference between vasa recta and collecting duct samples supports the view that the delayed dehydration was not present in this situation.

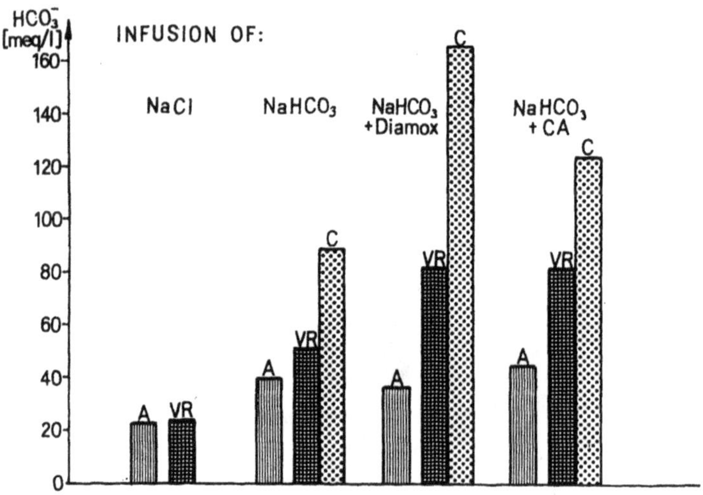

Fig. 5. The response of bicarbonate concentration in renal artery plasma (A), vasa recta plasma (VR) and collecting duct urine (C) to various experimental conditions.

The bicarbonate concentration as shown in Fig. 5 in arterial blood is elevated in the group infused with bicarbonate (40 ± 7 mEq/l) to values nearly twice as high as in the group infused with saline (23 ± 1 mEq/l) alone. Adding diamox or carbonic anhydrase was not followed by gross changes in bicarbonate levels.

In vasa recta plasma (24 ± 5 mEq/l) bicarbonate concentration in the group of saline infusion was the same as in arterial blood. Bicarbonate infusion alone increased the level in vasa recta blood up to 51 mEq/l. Additional diamox or carbonic anhydrase administration was associated with a further rise in vasa recta bicarbonate levels to about 80 mEq/l.

Bicarbonate concentration in collecting ducts increased from values of about zero in saline infused animals to 89 ± 32 mEq/l during bicarbonate infusion. Diamox elevated bicarbonate concentration to 166 ± 31. After addition of carbonic anhydrase to the bicarbonate concentration increased to about 120 mEq/l.

When saline was infused bicarbonate concentration in renal artery plasma and vasa recta plasma was equal, although the osmolality of vasa recta plasma was much higher. Thus, bicarbonate does not seem to be involved in the general process of concentrating in renal medulla. This is in good agreement with the results of ULLRICH et al. (7) who found that both Na^+ and Cl^- concentration in vasa recta plasma in antidiuretic rats equally increased above the values found in arterial plasma. Therefore, they concluded that the bicarbonate concentration in vasa recta and arterial plasma would be the same.

In our experiments where the bicarbonate concentration in collecting ducts exceeded arterial values we found higher bicarbonate concentrations in vasa recta than in arterial plasma. This was the case in all animals which were infused with bicarbonate. The rise in bicarbonate in vasa recta plasma reaches a value which is about one quarter to one half of that of the collecting ducts. A similar phenomenon has been demonstrated for the handling of urea in the countercurrent system (8). A possible interpretation of this finding seems to be diffusion of bicarbonate ions from collecting ducts to vasa recta as soon as the bicarbonate concentration of the collecting ducts exceeds that of vasa recta plasma.

References

1. KHURI, R. N., S. K. AGULIAN, H. OELERT and R. I. HARIK: A single unit pH glass ultramicro electrode. Pflügers Arch. ges. Physiol. **294,** 291 (1967).
2. OCHWADT, B. K. and R. F. PITTS: Effects of intravenous infusion of carbonic anhydrase on carbon dioxide tension of alkaline urine. Amer. J. Physiol. **185,** 426 (1956).
3. PITTS, R. F., W. D. LOTSPEICH: Bicarbonate and the renal regulation of acid base balance. Amer. J. Physiol. **147,** 138 (1946).
4. RECTOR, F. C. jr., N. W. CARTER and D. W. SELDIN: The mechanism of bicarbonate reabsorption in the proximal and distal tubules of the kidney. J. Clin. Invest. **44,** 278 (1965).
5. RUIZ-GUINAZU, A., G. PEHLING, G. RUMRICH und K. J. ULLRICH: Glucose und Milchsäurekonzentration an der Spitze des vaskulären Gegenstromsystems im Nierenmark. Pflügers Arch. ges. Physiol. **274,** 311 (1961).
6. STRASSBURG, G.: Die Topographie der Gasspannung im tierischen Organismus. Pflügers Arch. ges. Physiol. **6,** 65 (1872).
7. ULLRICH, K. J., G. PEHLING und M. ESPINAR-LAFUENTE: Wasser- und Elektrolytfluß im vaskulären Gegenstromsystem des Nierenmarkes. Mit einem theor. Beitrag von R. SCHLÖGL: Salztransport durch ungeladene Porenmembranen. Pflügers. Arch. ges. Physiol. **273,** 562 (1961).
8. ULLRICH, K. J., G. RUMRICH and B. SCHMIDT-NIELSEN: Urea transport in the collecting duct of rats on normal and low protein diet. Pflügers Arch. ges. Physiol. **295,** 147 (1967).

Effects of Diuretics on Active Sodium Transport in Amphibian Membranes

J. EIGLER, J. CRABBÉ

Summary: 1. In isolated amphibian membranes amiloride, when applied to the anatomical outer surface causes a prompt, dose-related and fully reversible decrease of potential difference and short circuit current.

2. Short circuit current remains a quantitative expression of net transport of sodium during exposure of the membrane to amiloride. Short circuit current and Na-influx decrease to the same extent.

3. The effects of vasopressin on the diffusion permeability of water in the absence of osmotic gradients and on the osmotically induced net flow of water are not altered by amiloride.

4. The amiloride-induced decrease of the short circuit current can be reversed by amphotericin B or – if the antibiotic is given first – inhibited.

5. A Na-transport stimulating effect of vasopressin, aldosterone and insulin can also be demonstrated in membranes exposed to small doses of amiloride.

6. The results suggest that amiloride may inhibit the passive entrance of sodium across the dense diffusion barrier of the apical cell membrane.

Introduction

Ever since the fundamental contributions of USSING and his associates regarding the phenomena of transepithelial movement of ions, the so-called short circuit current method – introduced by USSING and ZERAHN (25) – has been used as an experimental tool for the study of transepithelial sodium transport and its modifications by various hormones and drugs.

The principle of the method may be summarized briefly (Fig. 1): The isolated amphibian membrane is mounted between two symmetrical halves of a plexiglass chamber filled with frog RINGER's solution which is oxygenated and stirred by bubbling air. The spontaneous transmembrane potential is recorded on a mV-meter via agar bridges. The potential is the result of active transport of sodium through the epithelial cells from the outside to the inside bathing solution. Chloride follows passively along the electrochemical concentration gradient. An additional pair of electrodes serves to pass a current through the system in reversed direction so as to nullify the spontaneous transmembrane potential. Using ^{22}Na and ^{24}Na for bidirectional sodium flux measurements under these conditions, USSING and ZERAHN (25) have demonstrated that the strength of this current is a quantitative expression of transepithelial net movement of sodium (Na influx minus Na efflux). LEAF et al. (17) have shown this relation (short circuiting current equals net Na transport) to hold true in isolated toad bladder (Bufo marinus) and COFRÉ and CRABBÉ (5) in toad colon as well.

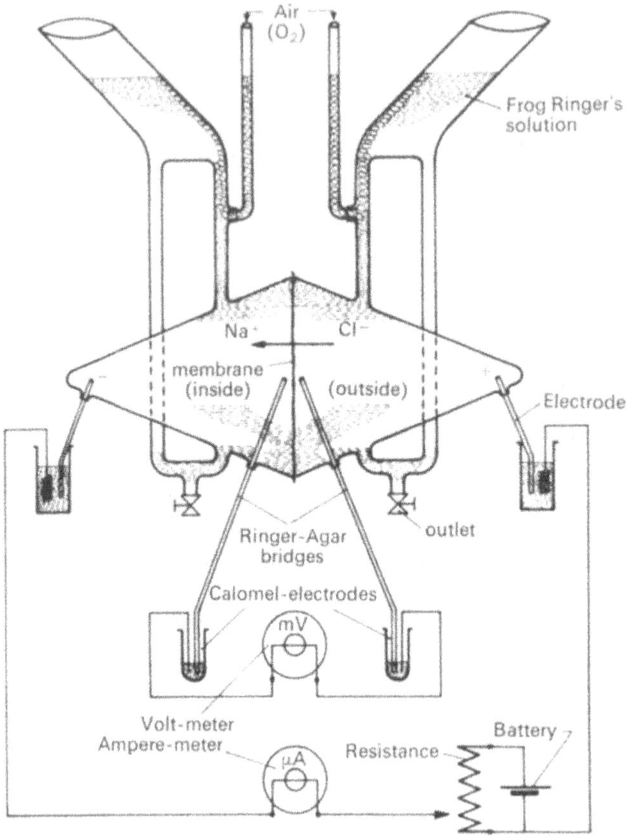

Fig. 1. Schematic representation of the short circuit current method according to USSING and ZERAHN (25).

This method therefore proved to be a rather simple way of measuring transepithelial sodium transport in isolated membranes by continuously or intermittently recording the potential difference (PD) and short circuit current (SCC).

The significance of this "model" with respect to renal physiology stems from the fact that there are many functional similarities between the renal tubule and amphibian membranes.

The use of diuretics in such studies, therefore, appears to be relevant from two different points of view: First, in an attempt to gain further information about the mode of action of the drug in question and second – inasmuchas the mode of action can be defined – to possibly elucidate further the mechanisms involved in active transepithelial ion transport.

During the past years the effects of mercurial diuretics, triamterene, ethacrynic acid and furosemide have been studied in isolated amphibian membranes by various authors (10, 14, 15, 19, 20, 23, 24). Furosemide, which in the kidney presumably inhibits not only transtubular sodium transport but also the passive transfer of anions (4, 6) may serve as a representative example (Fig. 2). Using ventral skin of the European toad (Bufo vulgaris) a marked increase in transmembrane potential relative to the SCC was

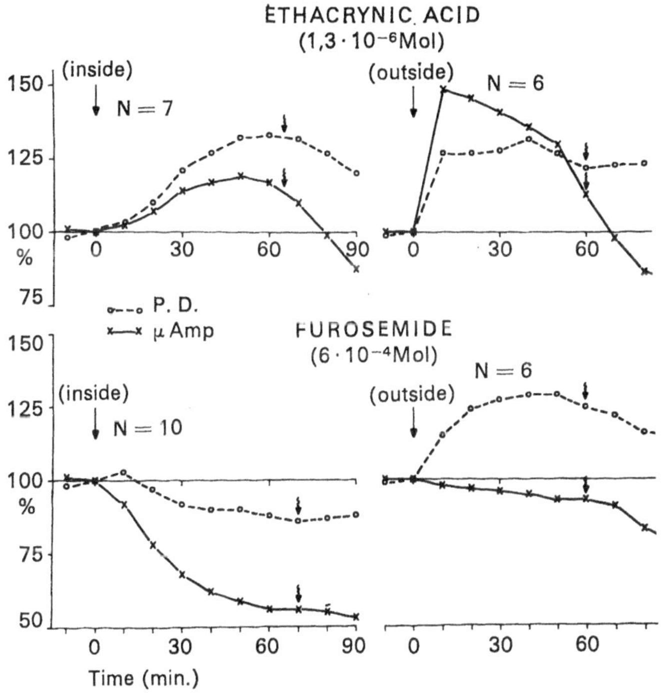

Fig. 2. Effect of ethacrynic acid ($1{,}3 \cdot 10^{-6}$ M) and of furosemide ($6 \cdot 10^{-4}$ M) on potential difference and short circuit current of isolated toad skin (Bufo vulgaris), presented as percent-change of the values at time "zero". Arrows indicate change of bathing solutions and replacement by fresh frog Ringer's. Note difference of response depending on the side of the membrane to which the drug was added. N = number of membranes [Modified from (10)].

observed after addition of furosemide ($6 \cdot 10^{-4}$ M) to the bathing solution, but the SCC – and thus presumably net sodium transport – was depressed only when the drug was added to the solution bathing the inside of the membrane*). This increase in electrical resistance upon addition of the drug probably reflects an inhibition of passive movement of anions across the membrane.

Recently, we have studied in this way amiloride-HCl (MK 870), a new diuretic agent (8, 9, 11, 12). Our results indicate that the drug – beyond its possible use as a therapeutic agent – may prove a valuable tool for the investigation of transcellular sodium transport phenomena. A review of these findings, therefore, will be the subject of this report.

Results

In all isolated membranes examined thus far (frog skin, toad skin, toad bladder, toad colon) amiloride caused a qualitatively similar, almost instantaneous, dose related and

*) The terms "inside" and "outside" refer to anatomical sites: Outside of the skin = apical or mucosal side of the toad bladder = luminal side of the renal tubule. Inside of the skin = basal or serosal side of the toad bladder = interstitial side of the tubular cell.

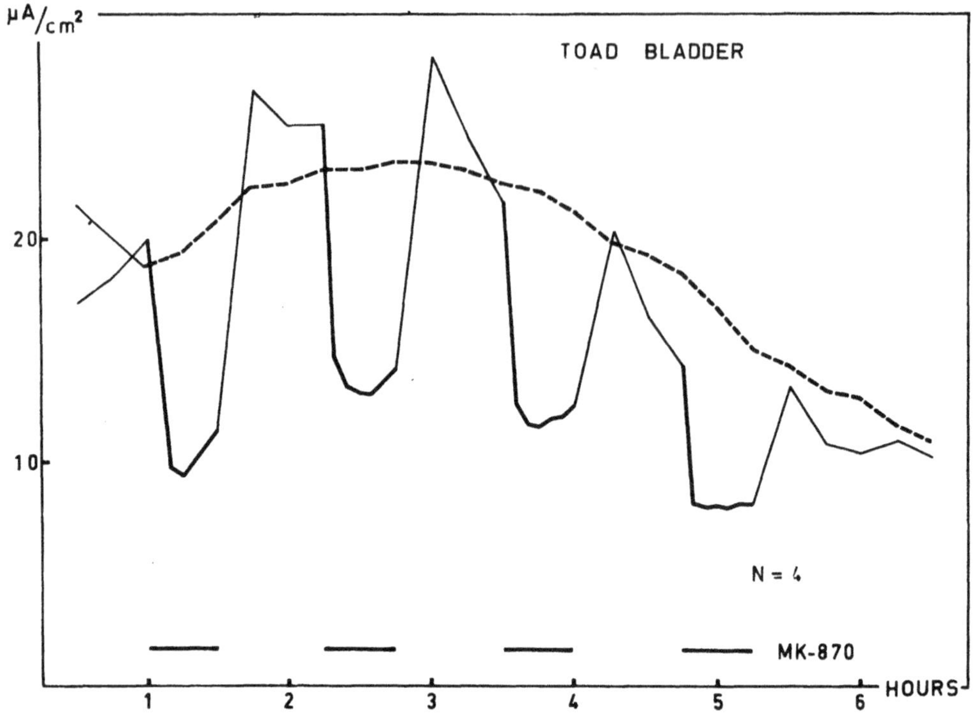

Fig. 3. Effect of amiloride (MK 870) – $4 \cdot 10^{-7}$M – on short circuit current across isolated toad bladder. The drug was added repeatedly to the outside bathing solution for 30 min periods and removed by changing the solution. One half of each bladder served as control (– – – – –) (9).

fully reversible drop of PD and SCC. In the case of the toad bladder such effect could be demonstrated even after application of as little as 10^{-7} M. In our experiments an effect was observed only when the drug was added to the solution bathing the outside of the membrane.

Bentley, however, in a recently published paper (3) has reported a slight decrease in PD and SCC when very high doses (10^{-3} to 10^{-4} M) were added to the inside bathing solution. This effect could not be reversed by replacing the solution with fresh frog Ringer's.

The effect of repeated exposure to $4 \cdot 10^{-7}$ M amiloride on SCC of isolated toad bladder is shown in Fig. 3. It is evident that the drop in electrical activity is fully reversible upon removal of the drug and that the membrane apparently is not permanently damaged during an experimental period of five hours' duration.

PD and SCC were affected to approximately the same extent. This is shown in Fig. 4 for toad skin and toad colon exposed to amiloride, 10^{-6} and $2 \cdot 10^{-5}$ M, respectively, indicating that in all these epithelial structures the response to the drug is qualitatively the same, the differences being of quantitative nature only.

A typical dose-response relation for both toad bladder and skin is given in Fig. 5. The doses used were $4 \cdot 10^{-6}$, 10^{-6} and $4 \cdot 10^{-7}$ M, respectively. Following the replacement of

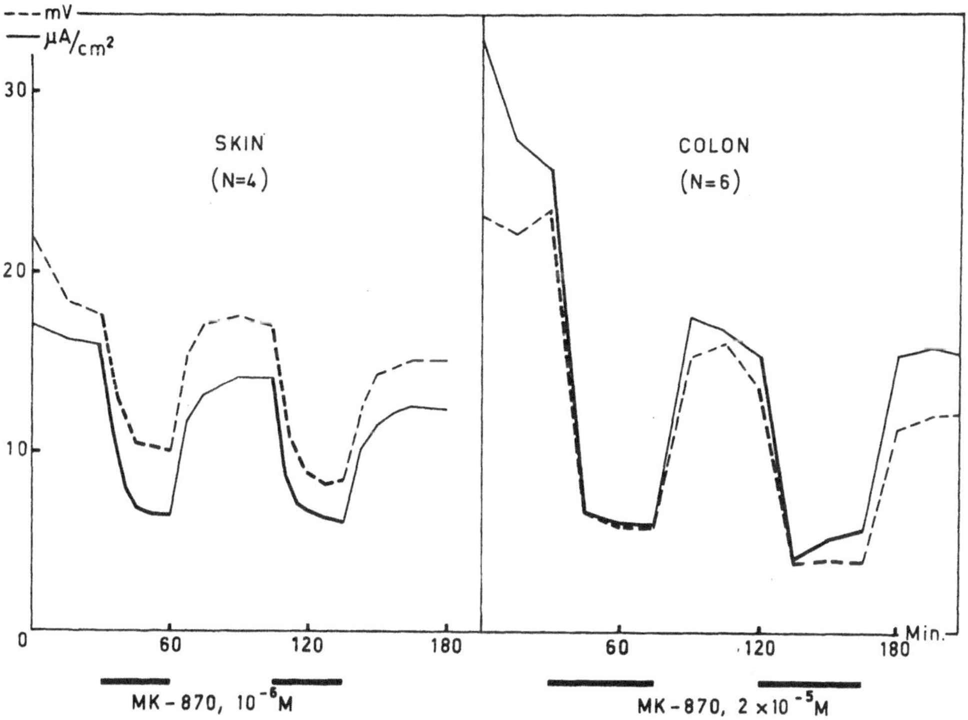

Fig. 4. Effect of amiloride on transmembrane potential (- - - - -) and short circuit current (———) of the isolated skin and colon of the toad Bufo Marinus. Black bars indicate time of exposure. The drug was removed by changing bathing solution (9).

the solution containing the drug by fresh frog Ringer's the increase in electrical activity frequently showed characteristics of a "rebound", a phenomenon which lacks an explanation thus far.

As stated above, addition of the drug to the inside (serosal) bathing solution was without detectable changes of electrical activity. In addition, a normal response to Vasopressin or Insulin was observed after the preparation had been exposed to $2 \cdot 10^{-5}$ M amiloride on the serosal side only (Fig. 6).

In view of the drastic decrease of PD and SCC after exposure of the isolated membrane to amiloride added to the outside bathing solution it seemed advisable to determine whether the SCC under these conditions remained a quantitative expression of transepithelial net flux of sodium. Pertinent data are given in Tables 1 and 2 for frog skin and toad bladder, respectively.

In the case of isolated frog skin (Table 1) sodium influx was measured for three consecutive 60 min periods. Amiloride ($4 \cdot 10^{-5}$ M) was added after the first 60 min control period. The data show that both SCC and influx of sodium were reduced in proportion and to the same extent.

Bidirectional sodium fluxes – using ^{22}Na and ^{24}Na – were measured in isolated toad bladder incubated with $4 \cdot 10^{-7}$ M amiloride (Table 2). The results indicate that SCC

Table 1. Sodium influx (^{22}Na) and mean short circuit current (μval · h^{-1}) across isolated frog skin during three consecutive 60 min periods, one before and two after the addition of 4 · 10^{-5} M amiloride to the outside bathing solution. SCC and Na-influx are reduced to the same extent. [Modified from (12)].

No.	Mean SCC	Na Influx	Mean SCC	Na Influx	Mean SCC	Na Influx
1	4.39	4.32	0.43	0.50	0.43	0.43
2	5.00	4.75	0.47	0.97	0.65	0.65
3	4.12	4.75	0.47	0.94	0.58	1.29
4	5.22	4.68	0.40	0.90	0.40	0.29
5	3.56	4.03	0.11	0.47	0.14	0.25
6	5.22	4.64	0.65	0.94	0.68	1.19
Mean	4.58	4.53	0.42	0.79	0.48	0.68

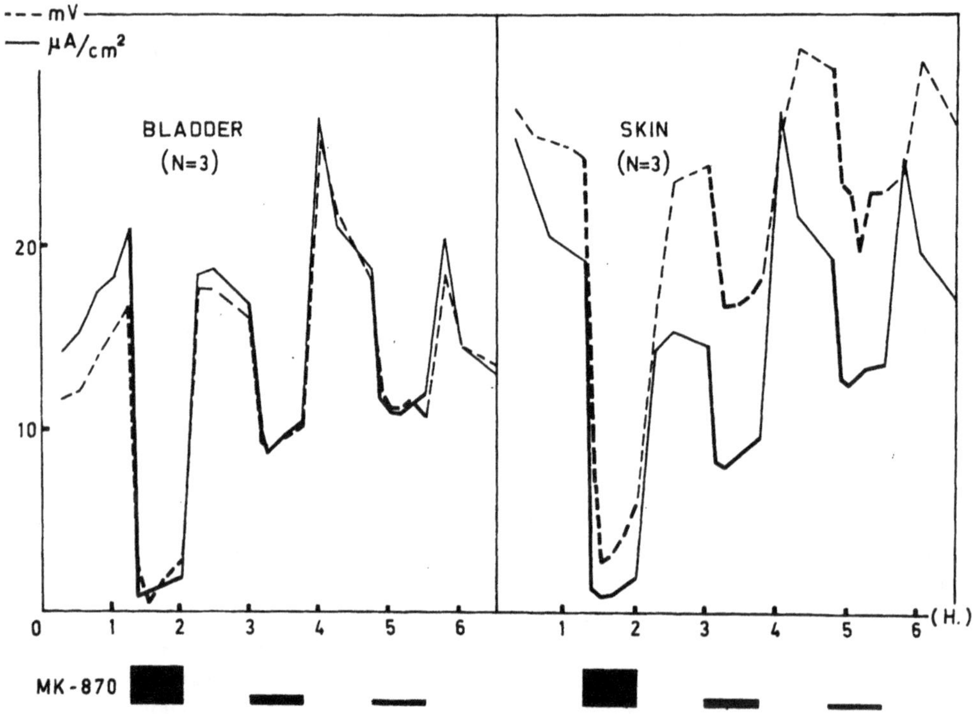

Fig. 5. Effect of decreasing doses (4 · 10^{-6}, 10^{-6}, 4 · 10^{-7} M) of amiloride (MK 870) on transmembrane potential (– – – – –) and short circuit current (———) across isolated bladder and skin of the toad Bufo marinus (9).

remains a reliable quantitative expression of net Na-transport under such circumstances and that amiloride indeed suppresses transepithelial sodium transport.

In contrast to the Na-transport the diffusion permeability and the hydrosmotic flow of water across epithelia remained unaltered after exposure of the membrane to the drug. In frog skin, upon addition of Vasopressin, the diffusion permeability of water in the

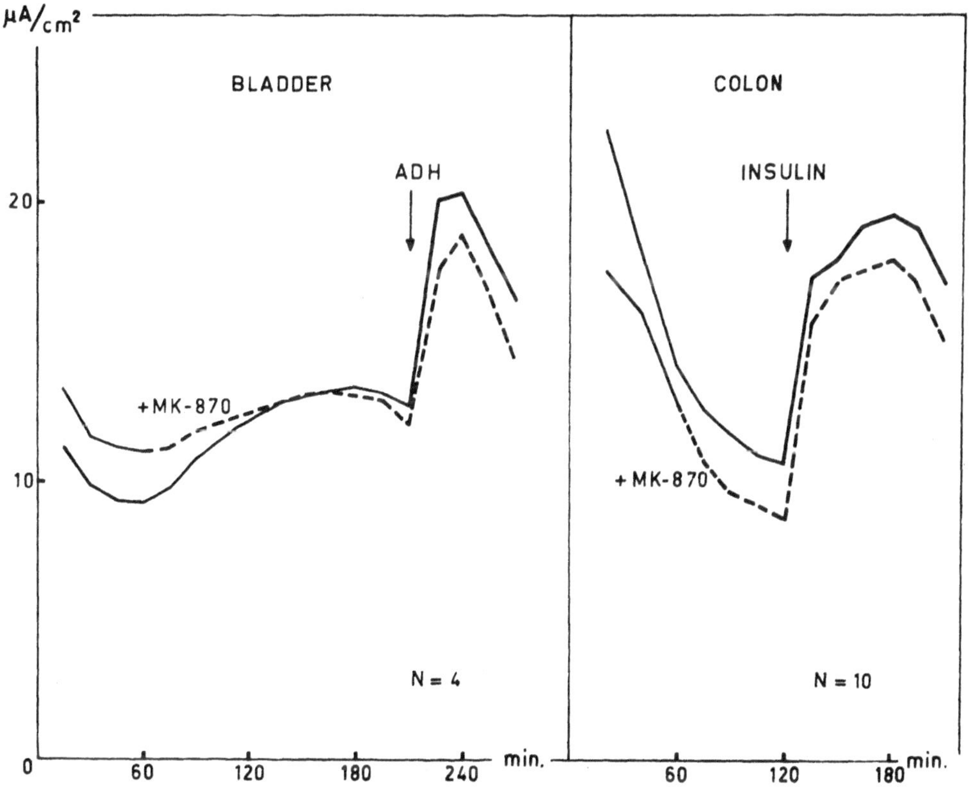

Fig. 6. Paired observations of the short circuit current across isolated bladder and colon of the toad Bufo marinus. One half of each preparation was exposed to $2 \cdot 10^{-5}$ M amiloride at the *serosal* side of the membrane (– – – – –) without detectable changes in electrical activity. Also, subsequent response to Vasopressin (125 mU/ml) or Insulin (125 mU/ml) was normal (9).

Table 2. Bidirectional sodium flux (^{22}Na and ^{24}Na) and mean short circuit current across isolated toad bladder treated with amiloride ($4 \cdot 10^{-7}$ M). Mean ± SEM. N = number of periods (three 30 min periods in four membranes). Note equivalence of short circuit current and net sodium flux. Deviation of the ratio from 100 statistically not significant.

SCC (a)	Na influx M → S (b)	Na efflux S → M (c)	Ratio $\frac{b-c}{a} \cdot 100$
1.992 ± 0.308	3.079 ± 0.484	0.984 ± 0.259	109.1

N = 12 (3 periods in 4 membranes)

absence of an osmotic gradient increases by about 10 per cent (16). In the presence of both Vasopressin and amiloride (200 mU/ml and $4 \cdot 10^{-5}$ M, respectively) the same results were obtained although sodium transport then was greatly reduced (Table 3).

Hydrosmotically induced transepithelial flow across toad skin was studied using a modification of the Ussing chamber (7, 18), which allowed simultaneous measure-

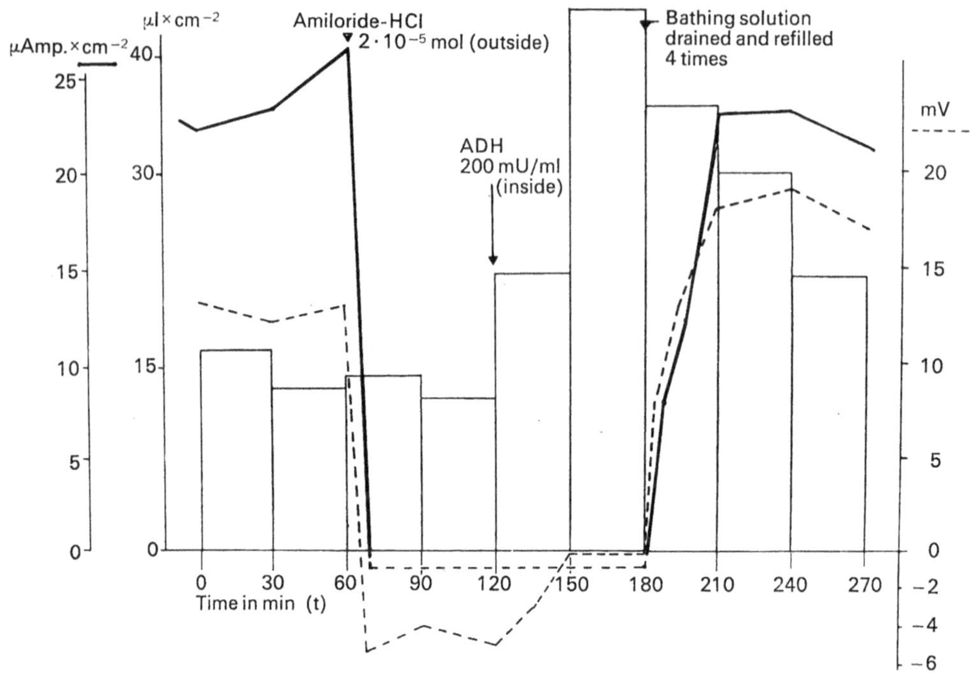

Fig. 7. Effect of amiloride ($2 \cdot 10^{-5}$ M) on transmembrane potential (– – – – –), short circuit current (———) and hydrosmotic water flow across isolated skin of the toad Bufo vulgaris. Osmotic gradient: 190 mOsm/kg H_2O. Note increase in water transfer upon addition of Vasopressin (200 mU/ml) although electrical activity remains close to zero until amiloride is removed by changing bathing solutions several times.

Table 3. Diffusion permeability of water across isolated frog skin during four consecutive 30 min periods; expressed as $\mu l \cdot cm^{-1} \cdot h^{-1}$ (13), Mean ± SEM. After two 30 min control periods Vasopressin (200 mU/ml) was added to four, and Vasopressin in combination with amiloride ($4 \cdot 10^{-5}$ M) to six membranes. Diffusion permeability increased slightly upon addition of Vasopressin irrespective of the presence of amiloride. No osmotic gradient was present. [Modified from (12).]

Group	Substance, Dose	n	1st Period Mean ± SEM ($\mu l \cdot cm^{-2} \cdot h^{-1}$)	2nd Period
A	Control	10	296±12	317±15
B	ADH 200 mU/ml	4	338±16	331±26
C	ADH 200 mU/ml Amiloride-HCl $4 \cdot 10^{-5}$ M	6	356±15	359±16

ments of water flow, potential difference and SCC. An example is illustrated in Fig. 7: In spite of a precipitous drop in electrical activity and a "negative" potential difference – most likely because of a diffusion potential in the reversed direction – following the ap-

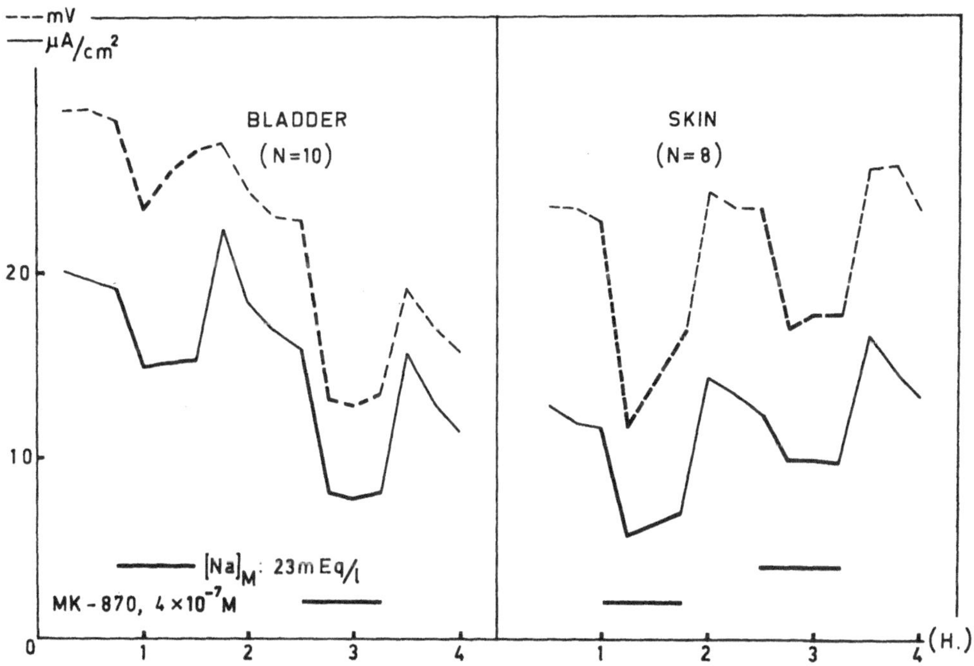

Fig. 8. Effect of lowering Na-concentration of the outside bathing solution in comparison to the effect of amiloride ($4 \cdot 10^{-7}$ M) on transmembrane potential (- - - - -) and short circuit current (———) across isolated bladder or skin of the toad Bufo marinus. Bars indicate time of exposure. Na-concentration: 23 mEq/l. N = number of membranes (9).

Table 4. Hydrosmotic flow ($\mu l \cdot cm^{-2} \cdot h^{-1}$) across isolated toad bladder exposed to $5 \cdot 10^{-6}$ M amiloride before and after addition of small amounts of Vasopressin (25 μU/ml). Osmotic gradient: 180 mOsm/kg H_2O. N = 8 pairs. The difference between controls and amiloride-treated halves was statistically not significant ($p > 0{,}2$) [Modified from (9)].

	Before	ADH	After
Control	3.9 ± 0.8		26.4 ± 5.4
			$P > 0.2$
Amiloride-HCl $5 \cdot 10^{-6}$ M	3.5 ± 0.5		34.7 ± 11.9

plication of $2 \cdot 10^{-5}$ M amiloride, transepithelial water flow along an osmotic gradient of 190 mOsm/kg H_2O was not altered and increased in the typical way when a supramaximal dose of Vasopressin (200 mU/ml bathing solution) was added to the inside bathing solution. After repeated change of bathing solution at both sides of the membrane electrical activity was restored promptly and net water flow decreased gradually.

A more quantitative analysis of these findings was carried out in isolated toad bladder employing the gravimetric method as described by Bentley (2). The results are summarized in Table 4. One portion of the tissue was incubated with $5 \cdot 10^{-6}$ M amiloride

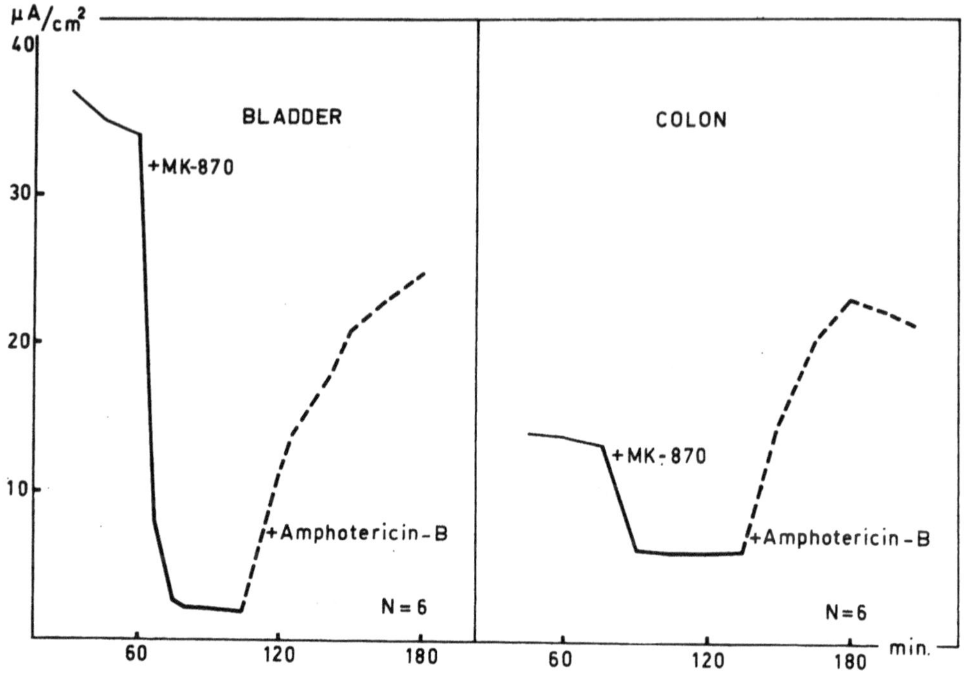

Fig. 9. Effect of amiloride and amphotericin B on short circuit current across isolated toad bladder or colon (Bladder 10^{-6} M and 2,5 µg/ml. Colon: $2 \cdot 10^{-5}$ M and 12,5 µg/ml). N = number of membranes (9).

and later 25 µU/ml Vasopressin were added to both: The increase in transepithelial water flow was the same in control and drug-exposed membranes.

The fact that drug-induced depression of electrical activity occurred only when amiloride was added to the outside of the membrane, the rapidity of its onset of action and the prompt reversibility of its effect upon change of bathing solution – all these findings were taken as suggestive evidence that the drug may cause an inhibition of the presumably passive entrance of sodium across the apical border of the cell. The following data may support this view:

A qualitatively similar response of PD and SCC will be obtained by reducing the Na-concentration of the outside bathing solution (replacing Na by Mg ions). A graphic representation of these measurements in isolated bladder and skin of Bufo marinus is given in Fig. 8.

On the basis of their experiments Lichtenstein and Leaf (18) have postulated that amphotericin B, a polyene antibiotic, causes a change of the permeability characteristics of the dense diffusion barrier at the apical cell membrane, thus facilitating the passive entrance of sodium into the cell. Exposure of the isolated epithelium to both, amphotericin B and amiloride, therefore, seemed of interest.

Isolated toad bladder and colon were incubated in the presence of 10^{-6} and $2 \cdot 10^{-5}$ M amiloride, respectively (Fig. 9). Subsequent addition of amphotericin B (2.5 µg/ml and 12.5 µg/ml, respectively) caused a prompt rise of the SCC.

Results of experiments in reversed sequence are presented in Fig. 10. Here, amphotericin B was given first, causing a marked rise in sodium transport, as had been demonstrated previously (18). In these preparations a decrease in electrical activity did not occur when amiloride was added subsequently, thus supporting the view that amiloride may indeed inhibit the passive entrance of sodium across the apical diffusion barrier of the cell membrane. But even though this assumption may prove to be correct, the chemical nature of the effect remains to be determined.

Finally, the influence of amiloride on the effect of various hormones was studied. When small doses of amiloride are used the stimulatory effect on Na-transport normally initiated by Vasopressin, Aldosterone and Insulin can still be demonstrated. Representative data are presented in Fig. 11. Isolated toad skin was first exposed to $4 \cdot 10^{-7}$ M amiloride and subsequently to 125 mU/ml of Vasopressin or Insulin. In the case of Vasopressin no difference in response between amiloride-incubated and control tissue was noted; the Insulin-induced rise in SCC, however, was less in the amiloride-treated membrane. Assuming an inhibitory effect of amiloride at the site of passive entry of sodium into the cell and of Insulin exerting its effect on sodium transport at the site of the

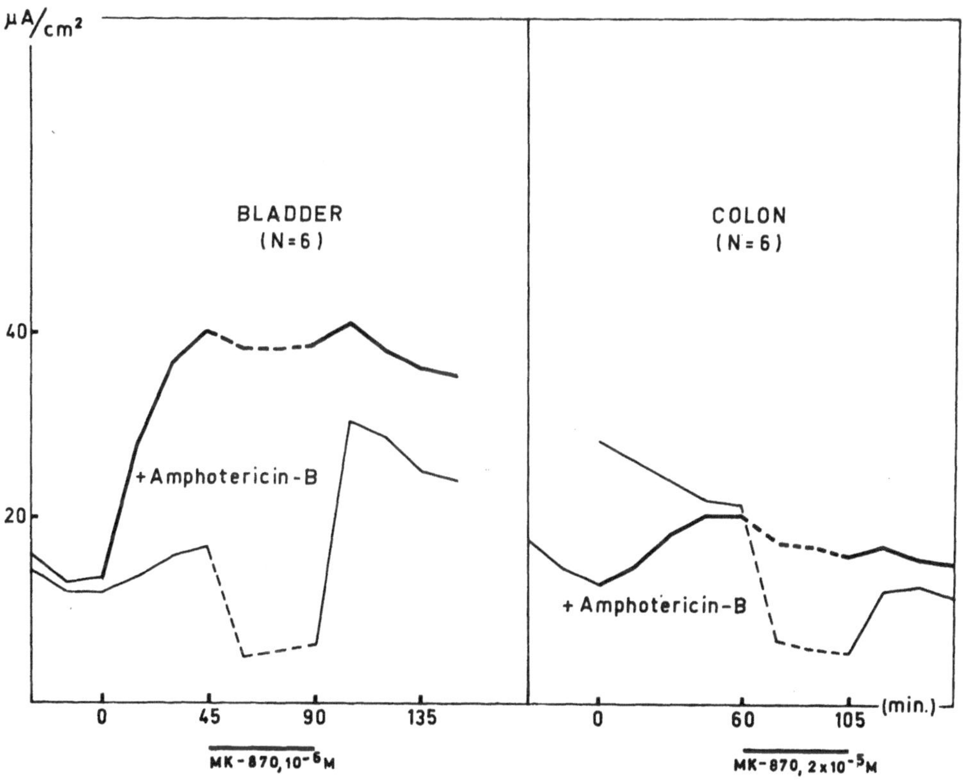

Fig. 10. Effect of amphotericin B and amiloride on short circuit current of isolated toad bladder or colon. Doses as in Fig. 9. N = number of pairs of membranes. Horizontal bars: time exposure to amiloride. Note lack of amiloride-effect in the half first treated with amphotericin B (9).

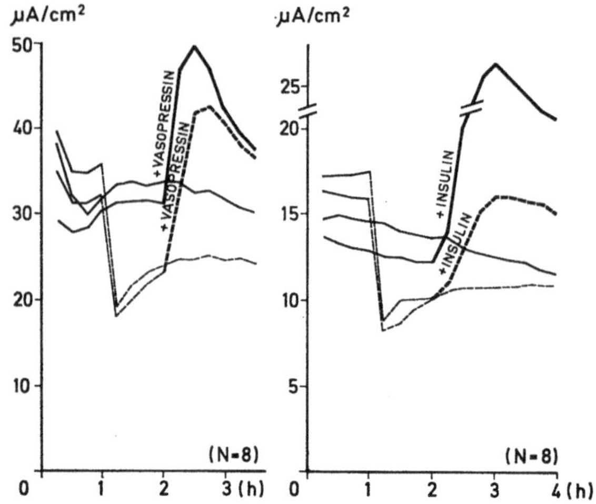

Fig. 11. Effect of amiloride $4 \cdot 10^{-7}$ M (------), and of subsequent exposure to Vasopressin (left) or Insulin (right) on short circuit current across isolated skin of the toad Bufo marinus. Dose of Vasopressin or Insulin: 125 mU/ml. Each skin was cut into four identical pieces. N = number of experiments. Note rather poor response to Insulin in the amiloride-treated membrane (9).

active transport process (Na-"pump") itself, the results could be interpreted in terms of decreased intracellular sodium concentration as a consequence of the action of Amiloride and thus leaving the stimulated Na-pump with less sodium to be transported.

If – in conclusion – an attempt is made to apply these data to the transport mechanisms of the renal tubule, one would have to speak of Amiloride as of a substance which causes its natriuretic effect when added to the luminal side of the tubule. The fact that the distal convolution is regarded as its site of action and that the drug is excreted in the urine – chemically unchanged – at the time of maximal natriuresis (1) would support this hypothesis. The characteristic retention of potassium then could be explained in terms of a decreased transtubular electrical gradient (21, 22). Such interpretation remains speculative at the present time; it seems likely, however, that Amiloride may prove helpful for further analysis of transepithelial electrolyte transport.

References

1. Baer, J. E., C. B. Jones, S. A. Spritzer and H. F. Russo: The potassium-sparing and natriuretic activity of N-amidino-3.5-diamino-6-chloropyrazine-carboxamide hydrochloride dihydrate (amiloride hydrochloride). J. Pharm. exp. Ther. **157,** 472 (1967).
2. Bentley, P. J.: The effects of neurohypophysial extracts on water transfer across the wall of the isolated urinary bladder of the toad, Bufo marinus. J. Endocr. **17,** 201 (1958).
3. Bentley, P. J.: Amiloride: A potent inhibitor of sodium transport across the toad bladder. J. Physiol. **195,** 317 (1968).
4. Buchborn, E. und S. Anastasakis: Angriffspunkt und Wirkungsmechanismus von Furosemid am distalen Nephron des Menschen. Klin. Wschr. **42,** 1127 (1964).
5. Cofré, G. and J. Crabbé: Active sodium transport by the colon of Bufo marinus: Stimulation by aldosterone and antidiuretic hormone. J. Physiol. **188,** 177 (1967).
6. Deetjen, P.: Mikropunktionsuntersuchungen zur Wirkung von Furosemid. Pflügers Arch. ges. Physiol. **284,** 184 (1965).
7. Edelman, I. S., M. J. Petersen and P. F. Gulyassy: Kinetic analysis of the antidiuretic action of vasopressin and adenosine-3',5'-monophosphate. J. Clin. Invest. **43,** 2185 (1964).

8. EHRLICH, E. N., J. EIGLER and J. CRABBÉ: Reversible Inhibition of active Sodium transport by amphibian epithelia upon exposure to Amipramizide. Proc. 2nd Ann. Meet. Europ. Soc. Clin. Invest. Scheveningen 21 (1968).
9. EHRLICH, E. N. and J. CRABBÉ: The mechanism of action of Amipramizide. Pflügers Arch. ges. Physiol. **302**, 79 (1968).
10. EIGLER, J., H. CARL und H. H. EDEL: Zum Wirkungsmechanismus der Ethacrynsäure. – I. Mitteilung: Der Einfluß von Ethacrynsäure und Furosemid auf Membranpotential und Kurzschlußstrom an der Krötenhaut. Klin. Wschr. **44**, 417 (1966).
11. EIGLER, J., J. KELTER und E. RENNER: Wirkungscharakteristica eines neuen Acylguanidins – Amiloride-HCl (MK 870) – an der isolierten Haut von Amphibien. Klin. Wschr. **45**, 737 (1967).
12. EIGLER, J., J. KELTER and E. RENNER: The effect of Amiloride-HCl on sodium and water flux across frog skin. Verh. Ges. f. Nephrol. – Lausanne 1967 (in press.)
13. HAYS, R. M. and A. LEAF: Studies on the movement of water through the isolated toad bladder and its modification by vasopressin. J. gen. Physiol. **45**, 905 (1962).
14. HERMS, W. und K. E. HOFMANN: Untersuchungen an der Froschhaut zur Kenntnis des Wirkungsmechanismus von Diuretika an transportaktiven Membranen. Naunyn-Schmiedebergs Arch. exp. Path. Pharmak. **251**, 355 (1965).
15. JAMISON, R. L.: The action of a mercurial diuretic on active sodium transport, electrical potential and permeability to chloride of the isolated toad bladder. J. Pharm. exp. Ther. **133**, 866 (1961).
16. KOEFOED-JOHNSEN, V. and H. H. USSING: The contributions of diffusion and flow to the passage of D_2O through living membranes. Effect of neurohypophyseal hormone on isolated anuran skin. Acta physiol. scand. **28**, 60 (1953).
17. LEAF, A., J. ANDERSON and L. B. PAGE: Active sodium transport by the isolated toad bladder. J. Gen. Physiol. **41**, 657 (1958).
18. LICHTENSTEIN, N. and A. LEAF: The effect of Amphotericin B on the permeability of the toad bladder. J. Clin. Invest. **44**, 1328 (1965).
19. LINDERHOLM, H.: The frog skin as a model of the kidney tubulus for studies of active transport of ions and the action of diuretics. In: Nierensymposion. Stuttgart, Thieme 1960.
20. LIPSON, S. and R. M. HAYS: The effect of ethacrynic acid and furosemide on sodium transport and ionic permeability in the toad bladder. J. Clin. Invest. **45**, 1042 (1966).
21. MALNIC, G., R. M. KLOSE and G. GIEBISCH: Micropuncture study of renal potassium and sodium excretion in the rat. Amer. J. Physiol. **206**, 674 (1964).
22. MALNIC, G., R. M. KLOSE and G. GIEBISCH: Micropuncture study of distal tubular potassium and sodium transport in rat nephron. Amer. J. Physiol. **211**, 529 (1966).
23. MOLINA, G., J. O. GONZALES und J. G. OROZCO: Einfluß des antidiuretischen Hormons und des Furosemid auf den Natriumtransport. Arzneim.-Forsch. (Drug Res.) **17**, 382 (1967).
24. NAGEL, W. und W. KARGER: Die Wirkung von 4-Chloro-N-(2-sulfamyl-anthranilsäure (Lasix) auf ionenaktive Membranen. Pflügers Arch. ges. Physiol. **281**, 63 (1964).
25. USSING, H. H. and K. ZERAHN: Active transport of sodium as the source of electric current in the short circuited isolated frog skin. Acta physiol. scand. **23**, 110 (1951).

GIEBISCH: I would like to point out that after amiloride the distal transtubular potential difference is significantly reduced. In the experiments which I described before (and in which distal tubular potassium secretion was absent) a mean of -20 mV (lumen negative) was observed.

EDELMAN: I enjoyed Dr. EIGLER's paper very much. I am interested in his analysis of the action of this agent on the permeability of the apical barrier to sodium. One of the controversial areas of work in this field is the analysis of apical versus basal influences in transepithelial sodium transport systems. The experiment which I would like to suggest would be to look at substrate depleted skins or bladders where the degree of substrate-depletion could be determined by the response to exogenous substrate and then see whether this effect (which very likely would be mediated through an effect on the generation on ATP) would influence the degree of inhibition achieved with amiloride.

EIGLER: Thank you very much, Dr. EDELMAN. I hope I have pointed out clearly that this is just a working hypothesis and that none of our experiments really prove that amiloride works at the apical or at the basal border of the cell as far as the transport of sodium is concerned.

CRABBÉ: I might add that it has been possible to reproduce such observations using Triamterene instead of MK 870 (amiloride), and Dr. LEAF reminded me that 4 years ago, FRAZIER had reported in an abstract (J. Clin. Invest. **43**, 1265, **1964**) that guanidinium could also interfere with sodium transport by these preparations. I would like now to have the opinion of organic chemists here about the possible common denominator between these different substances. From the way membranes react to these substances one would be led to assume that both triamterene and amiloride act at about the same site, and might share a common mechanism of action; but would the organic chemists see a clue to this common kind of activity ? Thank you beforehand for the comments.

BAER: Triamterene is a bicyclic pteridine, weakly basic, pK_a 6.2. Amiloride has only one ring, and is a much stronger base, pK 8.7. Although there is a superficial chemical resemblance, one cannot be converted to the other. A number of compounds related to these two have been made in which the pyrimidine ring is opened or closed up, but such compounds do not have the biological properties of triamterene or amiloride.

The Effect of Diuretic Agents and Metabolic Inhibitors on O_2-Consumption and Lactate Production of the Isolated Frog Skin

Sauerstoffverbrauch und Laktatproduktion der isolierten Amphibienhaut von rana temporaria unter Einfluß von Diuretica und Stoffwechselhemmern

W. HERMS

Summary: O_2-consumption (Q_{O_2}) and lactate production of the isolated frog skin (rana temporaria) was measured by Warburg incubation. Several diuretic compounds were added to the incubation medium and changes in respiration as well as lactate production were measured and compared to control skins without the diuretic agent added.

Salyrgan (10^{-4} molar) caused an increase in Q_{O_2} and increase in lactate production. Furosemide and hydrochlorothiazide (5×10^{-4}, 10^{-3} and 2×10^{-4} molar) addition to the incubation medium resulted in a decrease in Q_{O_2}, with no changes in lactate production. With ethacrynic acid there was a slight increase in respiration but no changes in lactate production.

To elucidate further the mechanism of action of diuretic agents with respect to possible metabolic effects, similar experiments were done with metabolic inhibitors known to decrease sodium transport of the frog skin.

NaCN (10^{-3} molar) caused a decrease in Q_{O_2}, but increased lactate production.

2,4 DNP (2×10^{-4} molar) increased oxygen consumption but had no effect on lactate production.

N-ethylmalemide (10^{-5} molar) caused a sharp decrease in respiration and increased lactate production.

p-mercuribenzoate (10^{-3} molar) increased oxygen consumption during the first 60 minutes of incubation. Lactate production was also increased.

The results show:

1. Diuretic agents of different chemical structure do exert different metabolic effects.
2. There is no correlation between the effect of metabolic inhibitors and diuretic agents on respiration and lactate production of the frog skin except for the Hg-compounds salyrgan and p-mercuribenzoate.

Die Untersuchungen verschiedener Autoren (EIGLER, JAMISON, NAGEL und KARGER, HERMS und HOFMANN) über die Beeinflussung des Kurzschlußstroms als Parameter des aktiven Natriumtransportes an der Amphibienhaut haben ergeben, daß Diuretica kein einheitliches Wirkungsmuster zeigen. Um zu klären, ob diese Unterschiede möglicherweise auf einer unterschiedlichen Beeinflussung des Stoffwechsels der Amphibienhaut beruhen, haben wir die Wirkung verschiedener Diuretica auf O_2-Verbrauch und Laktatproduktion an der Haut von *rana temporaria* untersucht. Die Versuche wurden unter Warburg-Bedingungen durchgeführt. Weiterhin wurden vergleichsweise die Effekte verschiedener Stoffwechselhemmer, die sämtlich den aktiven Natriumtransport an der

Amphibienhaut zu hemmen vermögen, in der gleichen Versuchsanordnung hinsichtlich des O_2-Verbrauchs und der Laktatproduktion geprüft.

Abb. 1 zeigt die Wirkung von 10^{-5} Molar Amilorid-HCl (MK 870) sowie Strophanthin (10^{-5} Molar) auf den O_2-Verbrauch. Aufgetragen ist über den zeitlichen Verlauf ein Quotient, gebildet aus der Differenz der mit Pharmakon inkubierten Hauthälfte während der experimentellen Periode gegenüber der Kontrollperiode minus der Differenz der ohne Pharmakon inkubierten Hauthälfte während der experimentellen Periode im Vergleich zur Kontrollperiode, dividiert durch die Mittelwerte der Kontrollperiode. Auf diese Weise sind Spontanschwankungen der Hauthälften mitberücksichtigt, ein Anstieg über Null zeigt eine Zunahme, ein Abfall unter Null eine Abnahme des Sauerstoffverbrauchs an. Beide Pharmaka bewirken einen signifikanten Abfall des O_2-Verbrauchs bereits während der ersten 30 Minuten der Inkubation. Eine Differenzierung, ob der O_2-abhängige Prozeß an der Innen- oder Außenseite der Membran lokalisiert ist, ist mittels der Warburg-Technik nicht möglich. Ebenfalls läßt sich aus dem gleichsinnigen Verhalten der Hemmung des O_2-Verbrauchs nach Inkubation mit Amilorid-HCl und Strophanthin nicht ableiten, daß beide Substanzen an der Membran den gleichen Wirkungsmechanismus haben.

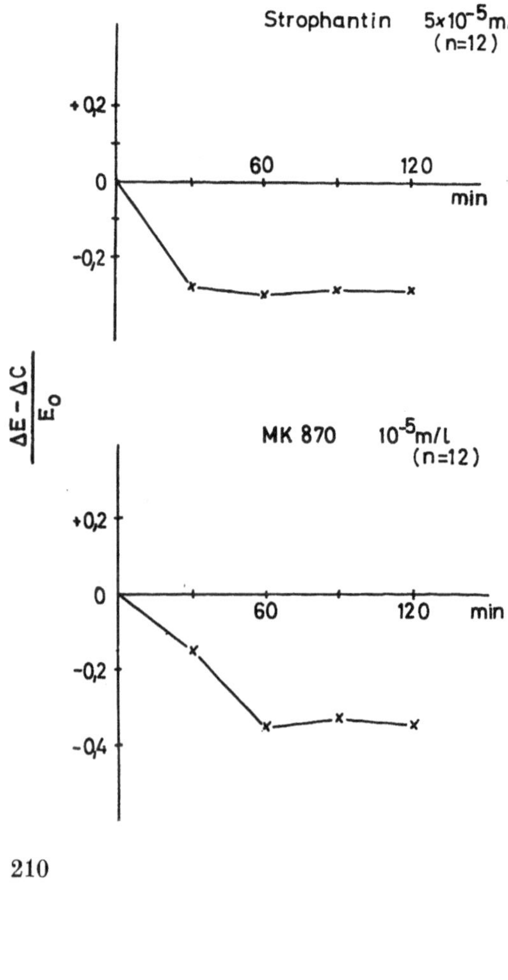

Abb. 1. O_2-Verbrauch der Bauchhaut von rana temporaria unter Einfluß von Amilorid-HCl und Strophanthin.

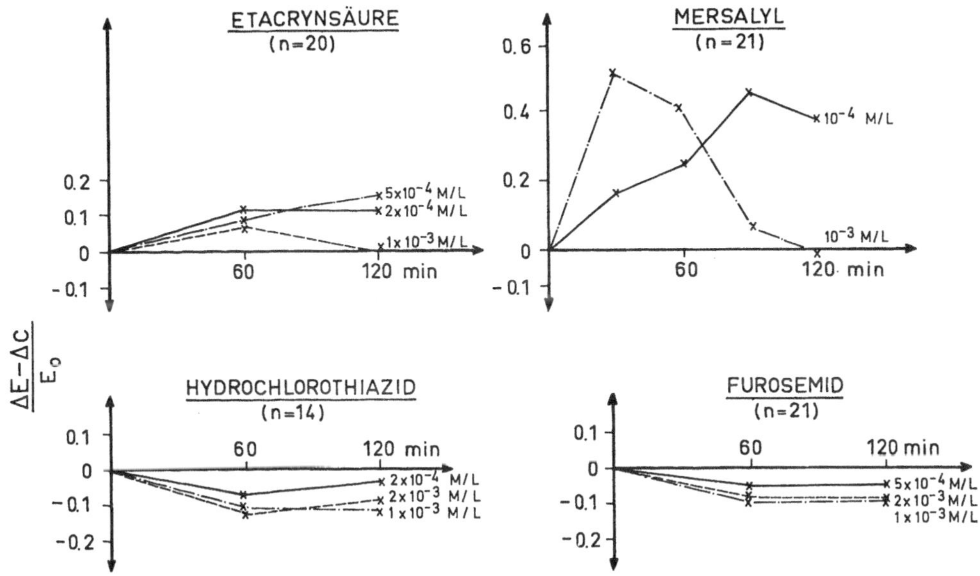

Abb. 2. O_2-Verbrauch der Bauchhaut von rana temporaria bei Inkubation mit verschiedenen Diuretica.

Während Strophanthin und Amilorid-HCl den aktiven Natriumtransport hemmen und entsprechend auch der Sauerstoffverbrauch bei unveränderter Laktatproduktion herabgesetzt ist, zeigen die Diuretica kein einheitliches Verhalten (Abb. 2).

Bei Inkubation mit Etacrynsäure ($2 \cdot 10^{-4}$ Molar, $5 \cdot 10^{-4}$ Molar, $1 \cdot 10^{-3}$ Molar) ist der Sauerstoffverbrauch geringgradig gesteigert.

Bei Inkubation mit Salyrgan in einer Dosierung von 10^{-4} Molar ist der Sauerstoffverbrauch durchgehend gesteigert, bei 10^{-3} Molar ist während der ersten Stunde ein Anstieg, dann ein Abfall zu verzeichnen.

Bei Inkubation mit Furosemid und Hydrochlorothiazid ($5 \cdot 10^{-4}$ Molar, $1 \cdot 10^{-3}$ Molar, $2 \cdot 10^{-3}$ Molar) ist gegenüber den Kontrollhälften eine geringe Abnahme des Sauerstoffverbrauchs festzustellen. Der Abfall ist im Bereich von 10^{-3} und $2 \cdot 10^{-3}$ Molar statistisch signifikant.

Die Beeinflussung der Laktatproduktion (Tabelle 1) zeigt bei Inkubation mit Salyrgan in einer Dosierung von 10^{-4} Molar eine Zunahme auf 112%, bei Inkubation mit 10^{-3} Molar eine Zunahme auf 166% gegenüber den Kontrollansätzen. Die anderen drei Diuretica lassen sämtlich keine signifikanten Änderungen der Laktatproduktion erkennen, mit Ausnahme von Furosemid, das die Laktatproduktion in der Dosierung von 10^{-3} Molar auf 82% gegenüber den Kontrollwerten senkt.

Die Versuche zeigen, daß offenbar die verschiedenen Diuretica unterschiedliche Stoffwechselwirkungen auf die Froschhaut entfalten. Die chemisch verwandten Substanzen wie Hydrochlorothiazid und Furosemid lassen eine gewisse Parallelität erkennen. Bei der Interpretation der Steigerung des Sauerstoffverbrauchs bei Inkubation mit Salyrgan ist zu berücksichtigen, daß das Präparat gleichzeitig Theophyllin in einer Dosierung von

Tabelle 1. Laktatproduktion der Bauchhaut von rana temporaria nach 3stündiger Inkubation mit Diuretica (Salyrgan, Etacrynsäure, Hydrochlorothiazid, Furosemid).

	µg/mg Trockengewicht		%
	Kontr.-Haut	Exper.-Haut	
Mersalyl			
10^{-4} Mol	2,38	2,66	112
10^{-3} Mol	3,00	4,97	166
Etacrynsäure			
2×10^{-4} Mol	1,62	1,65	102
5×10^{-4} Mol	2,00	2,10	105
10^{-3} Mol	2,38	2,30	97
Hydrochlorothiazid			
5×10^{-4} Mol	1,94	1,97	101
10^{-3} Mol	2,20	2,18	108
2×10^{-3} Mol	3,34	3,10	93
Furosemid			
5×10^{-4} Mol	1,86	1,70	91
10^{-3} Mol	3,68	3,76	98
2×10^{-3} Mol	2,43	2,00	82

10^{-5} Molar (bzw. 10^{-4} Molar) enthält. Die alleinige Inkubation der Froschhaut mit Theophyllin läßt indessen erst ab Konzentrationen von $2\cdot10^{-4}$ Molar einen signifikanten Anstieg des O_2-Verbrauchs erkennen, so daß die beschriebenen Änderungen nach Salyrgan nicht auf das Theophyllin bezogen werden können.

Um die Effekte der einzelnen Pharmaka näher zu analysieren, wurden Inkubationsversuche mit Stoffwechselhemmern bekannten Wirkungsmechanismus, die sämtlich den aktiven Natriumtransport an der Amphibienhaut zu hemmen vermögen, durchgeführt. Tabelle 2 zeigt tabellarisch die gemessenen Änderungen:

Tabelle 2. O_2-Verbrauch und Laktatproduktion der Bauchhaut von rana temporaria nach Inkubation mit verschiedenen Stoffwechselhemmern.

	Q_{O_2} µl/h/mg Trockengewicht			P	Laktat µg/mg Trockengewicht		
	Kontr.-Haut	Exper.-Haut	$\frac{\text{Exper.}}{\text{Kontr.}}\times 100$		Kontr.-Haut	Exper.-Haut	$\frac{\text{Exper.}}{\text{Kontr.}}\times 100$
NaCN 10^{-3} Mol n = 6	0,84	0,61	72,6+9,8	0,01	3,10	8,42	271
2,4 DNP 5×10^{-4} Mol n = 6	0,88	1,46	160,5±13,8	0,001	1,64	1,59	97
NEM 4×10^{-4} Mol n = 6	0,88	0,39	47,0±7,2	0,001	2,06	4,70	228
PMB 10^{-3} Mol n = 6	0,86	0,95	110,2±13,5	0,40	2,42	3,16	130

NaCN (10^{-3} Mol) hat eine Abnahme des Sauerstoffverbrauchs bei Steigerung der Laktatproduktion zur Folge.

2,4-Dinitrophenol ($2 \cdot 10^{-4}$ Mol) steigert den Sauerstoffverbrauch bei unbeeinflußter Laktatproduktion.

N-Ethylmalemid (NEM) bewirkt eine Abnahme des Sauerstoffverbrauchs und eine erhebliche Steigerung der Laktatproduktion.

p-Chloromercuribenzoat (PMB) (10^{-3} Mol) läßt während der ersten 60 Minuten eine Steigerung des Sauerstoffverbrauchs erkennen, gefolgt von einem Abfall; im Mittel ist der Sauerstoffverbrauch nicht signifikant vom Kontrollansatz verändert, hingegen ist die Laktatproduktion signifikant gesteigert.

Diese Versuche zeigen:

1. Das Verhalten des Sauerstoffverbrauchs und der Laktatproduktion allein läßt nicht ohne weiteres Rückschlüsse auf die Kopplung von Natriumtransport und Energiestoffwechsel zu. Auch die Kenntnis der ATP-Konzentration allein genügt nicht, da z. B. bei Inkubation mit DNP trotz Hemmung des Natriumtransportes die ATP-Gewebskonzentrationen zwischen 70 bis 80% der Kontrollhäute liegen.
2. Ein Vergleich der durch die Stoffwechselhemmer induzierten Änderungen des Sauerstoffverbrauchs und der Laktatproduktion der Froschhaut und den bei Inkubation mit verschiedenen Diuretica beobachteten Änderungen läßt außer den beiden quecksilberhaltigen Substanzen Salyrgan und PMB keine Parallelität erkennen.

Literatur

1. Eigler, J., H. Carl und H. H. Edel: Klinische Wschr. **44,** 417 (1966).
2. Eigler, J. und J. Crabbé: In: Renal Transport and Diuretics, Spinger, 1969.
3. Herms, W. und K. E. Hofmann: Naunyn-Schmiedebergs Arch. Exp. Path. u. Pharmak. **251,** 355 (1965).
4. Jamison, R. L.: J. of Pharmac. and exper. Therap. **133,** 1 (1961).
5. Nagel, W. und W. Karger: Pflügers Arch. ges. Physiol. **281**, 63 (1964).

Baer: With respect to Dr. Herms' statement, some years ago we reported that 10^{-5} molar chlorothiazide or hydrochlorothiazide will inhibit lactate formation in kidney medulla homogenates (Pharmacologist **4,** 159, 1962). Ethacrynic acid also inhibits this system, as does mercury in almost any form.

The Localization of Transport Processes in the Nephron and their Inhibition by Diuretic Agents as Analyzed by Micropuncture Techniques

P. DEETJEN

Any description of renal transport processes or the mechanism of action of pharmacological agents on the kidney should be predicated upon a knowledge of the nephron site where these processes occur.

For various reasons indirect methods such as clearance techniques and stop flow analysis have fallen from popular use. In the last 10 years micropuncture studies have provided much data concerning transport mechanism in the nephron. Just as the micropuncture technique itself has inherent difficulties, the data that derive from such procedures are at times difficult to interpret. Accordingly, in the following discussion some recent results concerning the localization of action of diuretic agents in the nephron will be presented. In addition, some of the limitations of these micropuncture studies will be delineated.

Micropuncture experiments on kidneys in vivo et situ can be performed on all laboratory animals: on dogs, cats, rats, guinea pigs and golden hamsters. To date, most investigations have been done on rats.

To expose the kidney surface for micropuncture, the rat must be anaestetized. Here, one can make the first mistake. Anaesthetized rats have very poor temperature regulation. At room temperature of 22° C they cool down in 30–50 min from a normal body temperature of 37° – 38° C to 34° C. While the mean arterial pressure stays the same, cardiac output decreases by about 25%. The renal cortical blood flow – in the region where micropunctures are done – decreases by about 50% (Fig. 1) (6). Therefore, the first requirement for a successful micropuncture experiment is sufficient heating of the animal and continuous monitoring of body temperature.

Next, let us consider which tubular measurements are appropriate for the evaluation of diuretic action. An apparently simple and meaningful way of micropuncture analysis of diuretic agents is to measure the inhibition of fractional reabsorption of salt and water at different nephron sites. Unfortunately, here, appearances are deceptive.

To determine fractional reabsorption TF/P_{Inulin} is measured, which is the ratio of the concentration of the (non-reabsorbable) Inulin in tubular fluid and plasma water. In the antidiuretic kidney, one usually finds that TF/P_{In} increases to 2.0–2.5 by the time the filtrate reaches the end of the pars convoluta of the proximal tubule of surface nephrons. By the time the filtrate reaches early and late distal convolutions further increases of TF/P_{In} to 5 and 10, respectively, are usually found.

From the reciprocal value of the TF/P_{In} ratio, fractional reabsorption is calculated. However, a knowledge of endproximal TF/P_{In} itself is not sufficient to determine whether the diuretic has altered the reabsorptive capacity of the tubular epithelium.

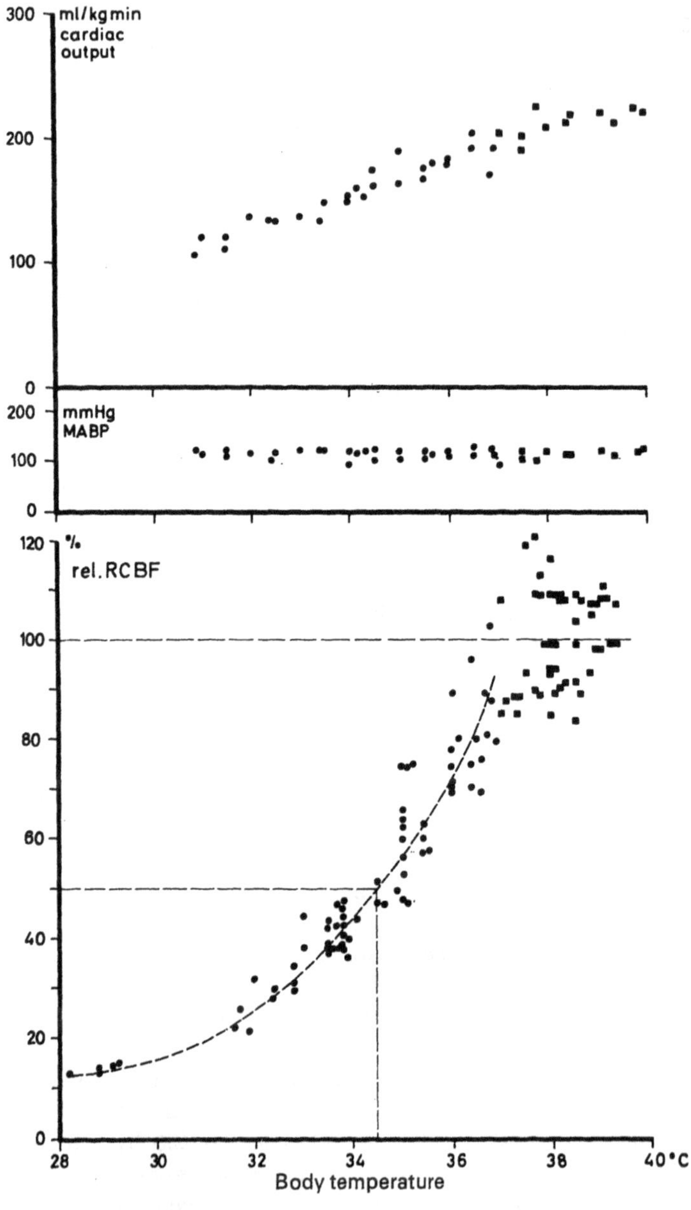

Fig. 1. Cardiac output, mean arterial blood pressure (MABP) and changes in renal cortical blood flow (RCBF) during decrease of body temperature in anesthetized rats.

Table 1. Endproximal TF/P_{Inulin} ratios at GFR in the normal range of 0.95–0.75 ml/g KW · min.

	n	Endproximal TF/P_{Inulin}
Controls	36	2.56 ± 0.49
Furosemide	13	2.42 ± 0.50
Ethacrynic acid	21	2.04 ± 0.61
Amiloride	12	5.29 ± 1.13

If, for instance, endproximal TF/P_{In} quotients of antidiuretic controls are compared with measurements during the action of different diuretics at unchanged GFR (Table 1), it looks, at first sight, as though proximal reabsorption is uninfluenced by furosemide and slightly inhibited by ethacrynic acid, while amiloride increases it. However, such a statement would not be correct.

To explain this apparent discrepancy, let us consider the following. In a wide range of spontaneous or experimental changes of GFR one usually finds, in the antidiuretic kidney, that about 40% of the filtered volume is still present at the end of the proximal convolution. Therefore, not a constant amount but a constant fraction of the filtered volume is reabsorbed. Even though the cause for such behavior was not explained satisfactorily, it was observed (8) that local reabsorption rate (C) and tubular volume ($\pi \cdot r^2 \cdot l$) under many circumstances have a constant proportion

$$K = \frac{C}{\pi \cdot r^2 \cdot l}$$

In spite of the fact that some doubt has been shed on the validity of this relationship (2), a considerable amount of experimental data still warrants its serious consideration. It was observed that dilatation of the tubular lumen is accompanied by proportional increase of C – regardless of whether the dilation was caused by spontaneous increase of intratubular pressure in the course of increased tubular flow rate (9, 24) or by experimental increase of intratubular pressure following ureteral clamping (21, 26).

To express the variables C and r by data more easily to measure during free-flow, several calculations were presented (9, 15, 26). We believe (as explained in the appendix) that the following equation gives a satisfactory description of the behavior of the proximal tubule during free-flow:

$$K = \frac{1}{2t}\left(TF/P_{In} - \frac{1}{TF/P_{In}}\right)$$

From this formula one can derive that the reabsorption capacity (K) can keep a constant value even by arbitrary changes of the TF/P_{In} if these are accompanied by proportional changes of the contact time (t).

Therefore, to prove that a diuretic substance inhibits the reabsorptive capacity the contact time has to be measured in addition to the TF/P_{In} ratio.

It is hardly possible to measure contact times exactly with the common dye injection method. What we measure is a dye passage time where the determination of the beginning and the end of the observation period is subjective and varies from one investigator to the other. That is why most K-values cannot be considered as absolute

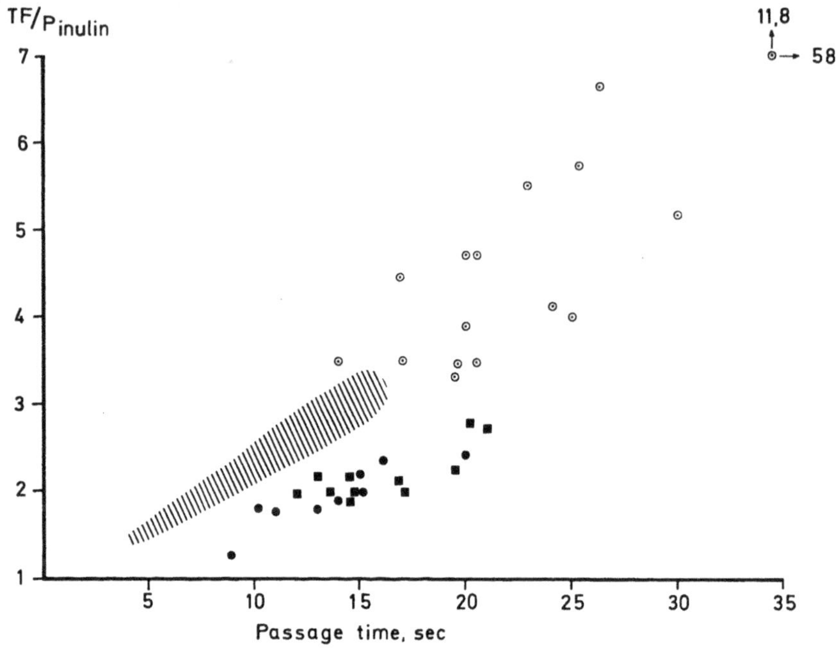

Fig. 2. Relationship between TF/P_{Inulin} and passage time in proximal tubules of rats under the influence of furosemide (●), ethacrynic acid (■) and amiloride (⊙). The shaded area is representative for control values obtained during antidiuresis.

values – but for the same investigator such determination can give comparative results, if it is only neccessary to find out whether the reabsorptive capacity changes or not.

In Fig. 2 you can see the data neccessary for K-determination from experiments with the 3 diuretics mentioned before. From the above formula K was calculated (Table 2). The reabsorptive capacity K of the proximal tubule decreases under furosemide and ethacrynic acid compared to the antidiuretic controls while it stays unchanged during amiloride. The decrease of the reabsorptive capacity under furosemide and ethacrynic acid seems to be essentially unchanged whether the GFR is high or low, the passage time slow or fast, the tubules dilated or nearly collapsed. However, the parameters t and TF/P_{In} are variable. For example, when the glomerular filtrate decreases to less than 50% of the starting level (< 0.4 ml/g · min) during furosemide diuresis, the endproximal TF/P_{In} values are decreased to 1.90 ± 0.45 (3). However, in this case the passage times

Table 2. Reabsorptive capacity K.

	n	K	Difference to Control, P
Controls	28	0.093 ± 0.009	—
Furosemide	9	0.054 ± 0.003	< 0.001
Ethacrynic acid	11	0.054 ± 0.007	< 0.001
Amiloride	16	0.099 ± 0.016	> 0.2

are also reduced and on the average they are not different from those in antidiuretic kidneys. After all, it is apparent that K values calculated from the pertinent mean values of TF/P_{In} and passage times do not differ whether GFR was normal or decreased during furosemide diuresis.

To explain these results we favor the following concept (4, 20): With an unchanged GFR furosemide causes an immense increase of flow rate in the distal nephron. A relatively inflexible section at the end of the tubule, perhaps the so-called Ductus Bellini at the end of the collecting duct, causes an increase of intratubular pressure, which spreads retrogradely to the proximal tubule. The lumen of the proximal tubule then dilatates about 30%. That should lead to an increase of the local reabsorptive rate, C. But, because of diuretic inhibition the increase does not take place, and the ratio $\frac{C}{\pi \cdot r^2 \cdot l}$, the reabsorption constant, decreases. Since the dilatation of the proximal tubule was not caused by an increased filtrate but by this retrograde pressure mechanism, it is understandable that the contact time has to be prolonged. The product of $K \cdot t$ (v. equation 2) can therefore stay in the range of antidiuretic controls as long as the tubular dilatation lasts. With a considerable decrease in GFR, tubular dilatation under Furosemide does not occur. The diuretic still inhibits reabsorptive processes, but the increase of intratubular flow rate in the distal nephron is too small to produce an increase of intratubular pressure. Radius and contact time remain unchanged in the proximal convolution. However, since K is lowered by the diuretic, the TF/P_{In} has to decrease.

Accordingly, at low filtration rate a larger fraction of the filtered volume reaches the end of the proximal tubule, passes distal parts where reabsorption is also mostly inhibited, and is excreted. Indeed, one can see a good relationship between the level of GFR

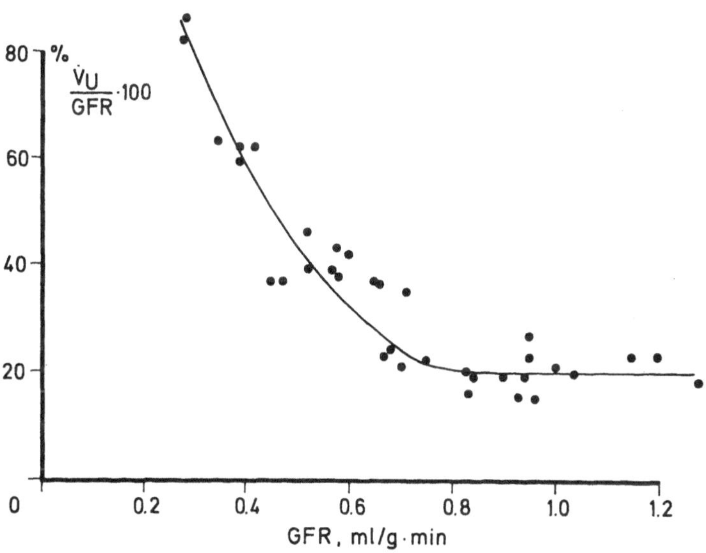

Fig. 3. Relationship between spontaneous variations in GFR and fractional urine excretion during the action of ethacrynic acid.

and the fractional urine excretion under these circumstances. This is demonstrated in Fig. 3 with ethacrynic acid diuresis.

It should be emphasized that this relation between GFR and fractional water reabsorption can only be expected as long as changes in GFR are accompanied by similar changes of flow rate in the tubules. On the other hand, a decrease in GFR under pathological conditions may be due to obliteration of part of the nephrons. Then, also at low GFR diuretic effects on proximal tubules might be compensated as long as the intact nephrons are still normally perfused.

What is the cause for the unexpected increase of endproximal TF/P_{In} values during amiloride diuresis? Since the reabsorption constant K does not show a significant deviation compared to the antidiuretic control (Table 2), the most plausible explanation would be a large increase of resistance in the distal nephron, which leads to retrograde dilatation of the proximal tubule and induces greater reabsorption not hampered by the diuretic.

Our experimental results point to that direction.

If amiloride is injected intravenously into a rat as a single dose of 1.0 mg/kg, a diuresis immediately occurs (Fig. 4). The diuresis is not very distinct compared to ethacrynic acid and furosemide and it ceases after 1 hour. Sodium excretion increases while potassium excretion decreases. Potassium is excreted in the same concentration as plasma – or expressed in another way – the U/P-potassium which is normally between 15–50 (Altromin standard diet) falls to 1.0.

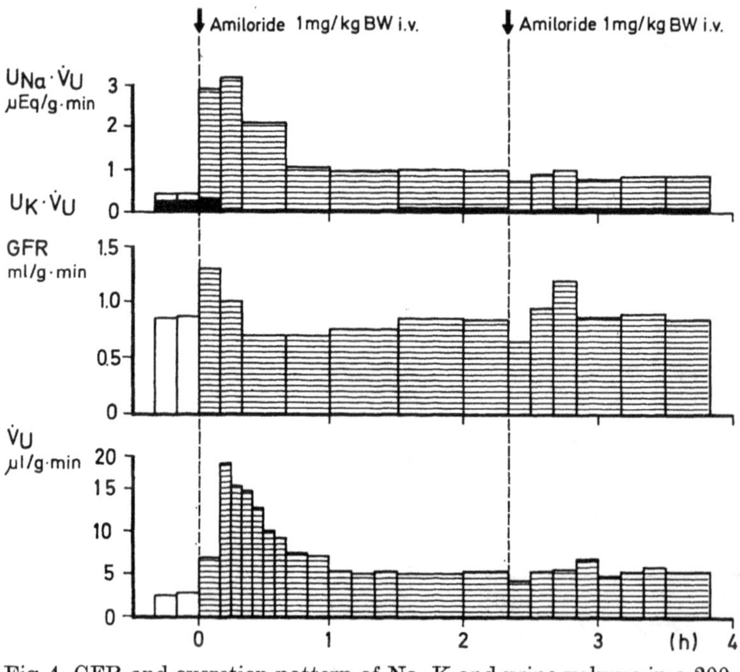

Fig. 4. GFR and excretion pattern of Na, K and urine volume in a 200 g rat. At (↓) 1 mg/kg B. W. amiloride was given intravenously.

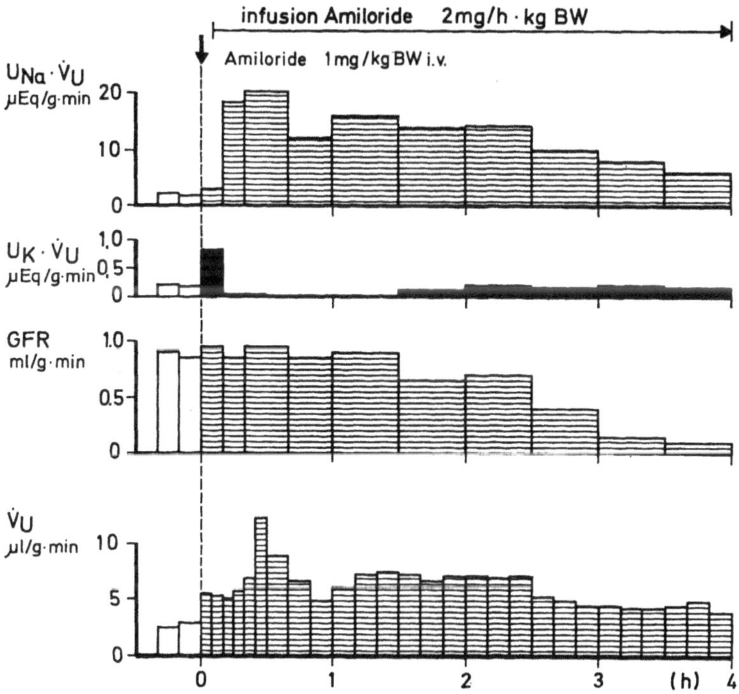

Fig. 5. GFR and excretion pattern of Na, K and urine volume in a 200 g rat. At (↓) 1 mg/kg B. W. amiloride was given intravenously, followed by a constant infusion of 2 mg amiloride/h · kg B. W.

To perform micropuncture experiments, it is of great advantage to have a diuresis as constant and as long-lasting as possible. That is why, after an initial dose of 1.0 mg/kg, we gave a steady infusion of 2.0 mg/kg · h. With this amount, which is per kg body weight more than 10 times higher than effective doses in man, we were able to maintain a diuresis for more than 3 hours. After that, inspite of hyperhydration, neither diuresis nor GFR can be kept from continuous decrease (Fig. 5).

Looking at the kidney surface the proximal tubules appear dilated, their diameter of usually 20 µ is increased to about 24–26 µ. Also the distal convolutions that are visible on the surface are enlarged. Their diameters in antidiuresis are around 9–12 µ, with amiloride they are enlarged to 18–22 µ.

The intratubular pressures in the proximal convolution are increased from 15 ± 2.4 to 37 ± 7.3 mm Hg and in the distal convolution from 9 ± 2.1 to 33 ± 5.4 mm Hg, under these conditions.

The prolongation of the proximal passage time was mentioned already. Also the passage time in Henle's loop of superficial nephrons was also increased from 38.9 ± 10.7 sec to 62 ± 12.7 sec. However, by 50 seconds dye already appears in the kidney pelvis. In sum, this is the picture of partial stopflow. Because the ureter was catheterized or even cut off and widely slit, the drainage block had to be situated intrarenally. We exposed the tip of the kidney papilla which in rats reaches 2 mm into the kidney pelvis. The tissue was swollen, less opaque than normal and tubular structures were difficult to recognize. The papilla was spotted everywhere with little plugs whose number increased toward the tip. When we had previously injected Lissamine green, we could see highly concentrated dye in the tubular section proximal to the plugs, blocking the fluid outflow. The poorly soluble substance was precipitated and had caused an obstruction of the collecting duct drainage system.

This pure mechanical obstruction caused the increase of intratubular pressure in the distal nephron up to the proximal tubule. The consequence is tubular dilatation in a way that never could be provoked by the relatively weak diuretic effect of amiloride and the only small increase in intratubular flow rate.

On the other hand, the tubular dilatation is accompanied by an increase of the fractional reabsorption in the proximal tubule, because under amiloride, unlike furosemide, a compensating inhibition of reabsorption does not occur. This obstruction leads more and more to a decrease of intratubular flow rate and GFR. If care is taken to maintain a higher flow rate in the distal parts of the nephron by a slight mannitol diuresis from the very beginning of the experiment, the precipitation of the substance takes place in extrarenal sites and the obstruction with all its consequences does not occur, even with the high dosage we have used.

Finally, a few comments should be made about the possibilities of recognizing reabsorption inhibition with micropuncture methods in the loop of Henle.

Early distal TF/P_{In} rates in kidneys of similar GFR are, on the average, about 5.8 in antidiuretic controls, about 4.0 during furosemide, and 3.5 during ethacrynic acid (Table 3). However, since the endproximal quotients show differences in all 3 cases, a reabsorption in % of filtered volume can be calculated for Henle's loop of 22% in antidiuretic controls, of 16% under furosemide and even of 21% under ethacrynic acid.

Table 3. Inhibition of reabsorption in the loop of Henle.

	TF/P_{Inulin}		Henle's Loop Reabsorption		
	Early distal	End proximal	% of filtered load	% of loop load	% inhibition
Control	5.8	2.57	22	56	—
Furosemide	4.0	2.42	16	39	30
Ethacrynic acid	3.5	2.04	21	42	25

If volume flow into the loop of Henle is considered, then the reabsorption of this volume will be 56% in antidiuresis, 39% under furosemide, and 42% under ethacrynic acid. Therefore, during the action of these diuretics reabsorption is inhibited by 30 or 25%, respectively.

Little is known about the reabsorptive characteristics in Henle's loop. It was demonstrated (23) that, similar to the proximal convolution, the reabsorption of sodium and water is significantly increased in Henle's loop when intratubular flow rate is experimentally augmented. This response which probably under normal circumstances would contribute to sodium conservation seems to be impeded during the administration of furosemide and ethacrynic acid. The response to these diuretics is characterized by an increase in flow rate which is not accompanied by an increase in reabsorptive rate.

A diuretic cannot be judged by volume excretion only, but also from the excretion fraction of filtered sodium load. In this respect it is of significance that the Na-concentration in the early distal tubular fluid under furosemide and also under ethacrynic acid is higher than under control conditions. In the untouched kidney a Na-concentration of about $^1/_4$ of the plasma-concentration ($TF/P_{Na} = 0.25$) (11) can be found at the early distal site. This low Na-concentration is the result of a continuous Na-reabsorption in the ascending thick limb of Henle's loop without concomittant reabsorption of equivalent amounts of water due to poor water permeability of this tubular section. Under furosemide the early distal TF/P_{Na} increases to 0.7 and nearly 1.0 (14, 17), and under ethacrynic acid to 0.5 and 0.8.

In summary, we should emphasize that micropuncture techniques are particularly prone to artifactural influences and for this reason the data they provide must be meticulously evaluated. Nevertheless, it is only by this type of approach that we can obtain direct information concerning the site and mode of action of diuretic agents. Table 4 summarizes the results from available micropuncture studies on diuretic agents.

Table 4. Localization of diuretic action studied by micropuncture techniques.

	Furosemide	Ethacrynic acid	Hydro-chloro-thiazide	Chlor-thalidone	Mefru-side	Acet-azolamide	Amilo-ride
Proximal convolution	(++)	(+++)		(+)		(+)	—
Henle's loop	+++	++	+		++	+	
Distal convolution	+++	+++	+	+		+	+
References	1*), 3, 4, 12, 13, 14, 17, 18, 20, 22	1*), 7, 16*)	1*), 14, 18	10, 13	19	1*), 12, 18, 25	

*) References No. 1 and No. 16 experiments in dogs, all other in rats.

+++ strong effect
++ moderate effect
+ effect
— no effect
(+) effect can be compensated

Acknowledgements

The author thanks Miss KARIN HARDT for technical assistance in the amiloride experiments and Dipl. phys. WALTER SCHNEIDER for help with the mathematic derivations.

Appendix

The relation between reabsorptive rate C and tubular volume*) ($\pi r^2 l$) which was found to be constant under many experimental conditions is called reabsorptive capacity K

$$K = \frac{C}{\pi r^2 \cdot l}$$

$$C = \dot{V}_o - \dot{V}_l$$

$\dot{V}_o$ means the flow rate at the beginning of the tubule, $\dot{V}_l$ the flow rate at the sampling site.

The tubular volume may also be calculated by the product of contact time t and the flow rate $\tilde{\dot{V}}$, which is determined with the following equation

$$\pi r^2 l = \tilde{\dot{V}} t$$

For determination of $\tilde{\dot{V}}$ and t we use the known and measurable dependency $\dot{V}$ (l):

$$\dot{V}(l) = \frac{\dot{V}_o}{TF/P_{In}(l)}$$

The dependency of TF/P_{In} on the length l we assume to be linearly (5, 26). The slope of the linear function is m. From this follows

$$TF/P_{In}(l) = m \cdot l + 1$$

1. Derivation of contact time:

$$dt = \frac{dl}{v(l)}$$

[v (l) = linear flow velocity in dependence of the tubular length]
t results by integration

$$t = \int_o^l \frac{dl'}{v(l')}$$

or

$$t = \pi r^2 \int_o^l \frac{dl'}{\dot{V}(l')}$$

2. Derivation of $\tilde{\dot{V}}$:

$$\pi \cdot r^2 l = \tilde{\dot{V}} t = \tilde{\dot{V}} \pi r^2 \int_o^l \frac{dl'}{\dot{V}(l')}$$

$$\tilde{\dot{V}} = \frac{l}{\int_o^l \frac{dl'}{\dot{V}(l)}}$$

---

* For the sake of comparison it should be mentioned that by other authors (15, 24) K is defined as reabsorption rate over 2 times the volume.

From equation (1) it results

$$K = \frac{\dot{V}_o - \dot{V}_l}{t \cdot l} \int_o^l \frac{dl'}{\dot{V}(l')}$$

Using equation (3) it is

$$K = \frac{\dot{V}_o - \dot{V}_l}{t \cdot l} \int_o^l \frac{dl'}{\dot{V}_o} \cdot TF/P_{In}$$

Integration and rearrangement finally leads to

$$K = \frac{1}{2t} (TF/P_{In} - \frac{1}{TF/P_{In}}).$$

References

1. Berliner, R. W., J. H. Dirks and W. J. Cirksena: Action of diuretics in dogs studied by micropuncture. In "The Physiology of Diuretic Agents". Conference Monograph N.Y. Academy Sci. p. 424–432 (1966).
2. Brenner, B. M., C. M. Benett and R. W. Berliner: J. Clin. Invest. **47**, 1358–1374 (1968).
3. Deetjen, P.: Pflügers Arch. ges. Physiol. **284**, 184–190 (1965).
4. Deetjen, P.: Micropuncture Studies on Site and Mode of Diuretic Action of Furosemide. In "The Physiology of Diuretic Agents". Conference Monograph N. Y. Academy Sci., p. 408–415 (1966).
5. Deetjen, P. and J. W. Boylan: Pflügers Arch. ges. Physiol. **299**, 19–29 (1968).
6. Deetjen, P. und H. Brechtelsbauer: Pflügers Arch. ges. Physiol. **281**, 26 (1964).
7. Deetjen, P., W. E. Büntig, K. Hardt and Rohde: Diuretic effect of ethacrynic acid in the rat: a micropuncture study about the relationship of site and mode of action. In "Progress in Nephrology", G. Peters (Ed.), Springer, Heidelberg 1969.
8. Gertz, K. H.: Pflügers Arch. ges. Physiol. **276**, 336 (1963).
9. Gertz, K. H., J. A. Mangos, G. Braun and H. D. Pagel: Pflügers Arch. ges. Physiol. **285**, 360–372 (1965).
10. Gertz, K. H. und K. J. Ullrich: Pflügers Arch. ges. Physiol. **274**, 61 (1961).
11. Giebisch, G. and E. E. Windhager: Amer. J. Med. **36**, 643–669 (1964).
12. Holzgreve, H.: this symposion.
13. Holzgreve, H., A. Frick, G. Rumrich, M. Wiederholt und K. J. Ullrich: Wirkungsweise von Diuretica auf den transtubulären Transport von Natriumchlorid in: Normale und Pathologische Funktionen des Nierentubulus. K. J. Ullrich und K. Hierholzer (Ed.) p. 147–154 (Hans Huber, Bern 1965).
14. Horster, M., W. Nagel und K. Thurau: Pflügers Arch. ges. Physiol. **289**, R 68 (1966).
15. Horster, M. and K. Thurau: Pflügers Arch. ges. Physiol. **301**, 162–181 (1968).
16. Levine, D. Z., G. Liebau, H. Fischbach and K. Thurau: Pflügers Arch. ges. Physiol. **304**, 365–375 (1968).
17. Malnic, G., F. L. Vieira and H. Enokibara: Nature (London) **208**, 80–81 (1965).
18. Meng, K.: Arch. Pharmak. exp. Path. **257**, 355–371 (1967).
19. Meng, K. und G. Kroneberg: Arzneim. Forsch. (Drug Res.) **17**, 653–692 (1967).
20. Rector, F. C., F. P. Brunner and D. W. Seldin: Pitfalls in the use of micropuncture for the localization of diuretic action. In "The Physiology of Diuretic Agents". Conference Monograph N. Y. Academy Sci. p. 400–407 (1966).

21. Rector, F. C., F. P. Brunner and D. W. Seldin: J. Clin. Invest. **45**, 590–602 (1966).
22. Rector, F. C., J. C. Sellman, M. Martinez-Maldonado and D. W. Seldin: J. Clin. Invest. **46**, 47–56 (1967).
23. Schnermann, J.: Pflügers Arch. ges. Physiol. **300**, 255–282 (1968).
24. Schnermann, J., M. Wahl, G. Liebau and H. Fischbach: Pflügers Arch. ges. Physiol. **304**, 90–103 (1968).
25. Weinstein, S. W.: Amer. J. Physiol. **214**, 222–227 (1968).
26. Wiederholt, M., K. Hierholzer, E. E. Windhager and G. Giebisch: Amer. J. Physiol. **213**, 809–818 (1967).

Levine: I wonder if I may show two slides concerning the influence of ethacrynic acid on the dog kidney. These studies were done in collaboration with Drs. Thurau, Liebau and Fischbach. In essence, we have confirmed the observations of Dirks et al. that end proximal TF/P Inulin is unchanged during ethacrynic acid administration. However (Fig. 1), we

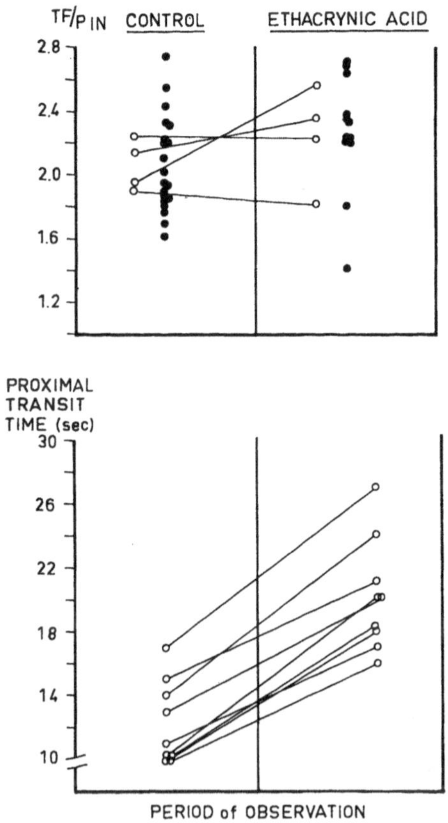

Fig. 1.

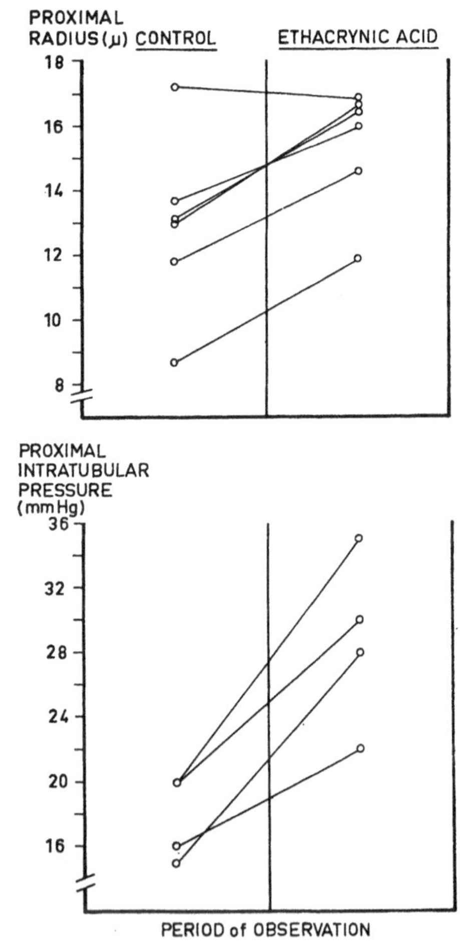

Fig. 2.

can go further and suggest tubular mechanisms which contribute to this constancy. In the top panel you can see that both single observations (black dots) and averages (open circles) for experimental and control periods do not suggest a trend in TF/P Inulin measurements. In the bottom panel we see the passage time uniformly increase in the experimental period. In Fig. 2 you can see that proximal tubular radius and intratubular pressure also increases. In the one case where the radius did not increase, there was a profound fall in GFR. These data then enable us to calculate lateral water flux, and reabsorptive capacity K, during ethacrynic acid administration. The later water flux is slightly reduced and K falls by about 25%. According to the principles Dr. DEETJEN outlined which we agree with entirely, the constancy of fractional reabsorption appears to be made possible by the joint effect of a larger intratubular surface area having a longer exposure time to the filtrate, in spite of a fall in the intrinsic reabsorptive capacity.

HUSMANN: Ich halte Ihre Beobachtung, daß MK 870 in den Tubuli auskristallisieren kann, für besonders wichtig, gerade im Hinblick auf eine Anwendung in der Klinik. Dazu wäre es wertvoll, wenn Sie uns sagen könnten, nach welchen Dosen eine solche Komplikation eintritt.

DEETJEN: Es ist eine oft bestätigte Erfahrung, daß Ratten an Diuretica erst bei sehr viel höheren Dosen pro kg Körpergewicht ansprechen, als Mensch oder Hund. So muß man auch bei Amilorid eine Dosis geben, die etwa 10–15fach über der beim Menschen wirksamen Menge liegt. Eine intrarenale Ausfällung der Substanz haben wir immer dann beobachtet, wenn wir Dauerinfusionen von 2 mg Amilorid/kg BW h gaben, nicht jedoch bei Einzelinjektionen von 1 mg/kg BW.

REUBI: Herr DEETJEN, Sie sagten, daß, wenn das Glomerulumfiltrat abnimmt, die fraktionelle Rückresorption zunimmt. Handelte es sich um eine akute oder um eine chronische Reduktion des Filtrats? Denn, wie Sie sicher wissen, hat vor vielen Jahren die Gruppe von Dr. PITTS gezeigt, daß der diuretische Effekt im akuten Versuch der glomerulären Filtration proportional ist. Demgegenüber konnten wir zeigen, daß bei Menschen mit permanenter Reduktion der glomerulären Filtration der diuretische Effekt bis zu einem kritischen Punkt gleichbleibt. Ich werde das noch morgen zeigen. Eine zweite Frage: Erklären Sie diese Abhängigkeit dadurch, daß der intratubuläre Druck bei guter glomerulärer Filtration so hoch wird, daß es zu einer Dilatation des proximalen Tubulus, zu einer vermehrten proximalen Rückresorption und somit zu einer Abschwächung des diuretischen Effektes kommt?

DEETJEN: Zu Frage 1: Die Variationen im Glomerulumfiltrat waren akute spontane Änderungen, wie man sie bei der Ratte leicht beobachten kann.

Zu der 2. Frage: Daß diese Ergebnisse nicht mit den früheren von Dr. PITTS übereinstimmen, liegt m. M. nach allein in der Tatsache, daß früher Dr. PITTS noch nicht die beiden Substanzen Etacrynsäure und Furosemid in der Hand hatte. Wenn man Hydrochlorothiazid, Chlorothiazid, Chlorthalidon gibt, dann sieht man diese Beziehungen zwischen GFR und Exkretionsfraktion nicht. Das liegt sicher daran, daß nur Furosemid und Etacrynsäure einen signifikanten proximalen Effekt und gleichzeitig einen starken distalen Effekt haben. Nur so kommt es zu der beträchtlichen Erhöhung der distalen Stromstärke.

Es folgt ein Anstieg des intratubulären Druckes, der retrograd zum proximalen Tubulus fortgepflanzt wird und zu dessen Erweiterung führt. Wenn das Filtrat jedoch niedrig ist, dann ist der Zuwachs an intratubulärer Stromstärke im distalen Nephronabschnitt nicht ausreichend, um den Druck so zu erhöhen, daß er retrograd zu einer Dilatation des proximalen Tubulus führt. Dann wird dort die Hemmwirkung der Substanz durch ein Absinken der fraktionellen Resorption offenkundig, weil die Kompensation durch eine Dilatation ausbleibt. Man sieht dann einen Anstieg der fraktionellen Wasserausscheidung bei absinkenden Glomerulumfiltraten.

REUBI: Ganz überzeugt bin ich noch nicht. Man kann von dieser Tubulusgeometrie halten was man will, aber wie bringen Sie Ihre Hypothese in Einklang mit den Beobachtungen von

Herrn Burg an isolierten Tubuli? Wenn wirklich die Stauung am Ende des Tubulussystems dafür verantwortlich ist, müssen Sie entweder eine erhebliche Größenzunahme der Niere beobachten oder eine starke Erhöhung des interstitiellen Druckes. Haben Sie ihn gemessen? Gibt es z. B. bei Tieren mit normaler Filtration eine stärkere Druckzunahme oder eine stärkere Volumenzunahme, als bei Tieren mit reduzierter Filtration?

Deetjen: Die Druckzunahme im proximalen und distalen Konvolut haben wir gemessen. Darüber habe ich berichtet. Wir haben allerdings keine exakten Daten über die Volumenzunahme. Aber es ist ganz zweifelsfrei, daß das Volumen der Niere insgesamt zunimmt. Zur Punktion werden die Nieren in Plexiglasschälchen gelegt, in denen sie mit kleinen Wattebäuschen fixiert werden. Unter einer Diurese mit Furosemid oder Etacrynsäure müssen wir die Watte oft entfernen und dünnere Wattebäusche einlegen, weil die Niere sonst gedrückt würde, so fängt sie an, ihr Volumen zu vergrößern. Die Diskrepanz zu den Befunden von Dr. Burg ist mir durchaus bewußt. Ich weiß auch keine Erklärung dafür, warum bei dem isolierten Tubulus die fraktionelle Resorption im proximalen Tubulus nicht gleichbleibt. Selbst Dr. Burg hat gestern keine Theorie gewagt, um diese Unterschiede zu erklären. Aber wenn z. B. heute morgen bei der Diskussion mit Dr. Hierholzer angeklungen ist, daß sich möglicherweise das Druckvolumendiagramm solcher Tubuli unter Einfluß von Aldosteron ändern kann, dann können auch andere Umstände solche Änderungen des Druckvolumendiagramms zur Folge haben und eine ganz andere Druckvolumencharakteristik des isolierten Tubulus daraus resultieren. Aber das ist eine ganz vage Vorstellung.

Thurau: Ich möchte noch etwas zu den Zweifeln von Herrn Reubi sagen. An der frei fließenden, nicht punktierten Niere läßt sich eine lineare Beziehung zwischen proximalem Tubulusvolumen, d. h. zwischen r^2 und Glomerulumfiltrat nachweisen. Außerdem gibt es kaum einen Zweifel daran, daß bei spontanen Änderungen des Glomerulumfiltrates über einen sehr weiten Bereich die fraktionelle Resorption im proximalen Tubulus konstant bleibt. Aus diesen beiden Beziehungen ergibt sich zwangsläufig der dritte Befund, daß die tubuläre Passagezeit im proximalen Tubulus durch spontane Änderungen des Glomerulumfiltrates nicht variiert wird. – Daß Dr. Burg am isoliert perfundierten Tubulus eine Abhängigkeit der Resorption vom intratubulären Volumen nicht finden konnte, spricht nicht gegen eine solche Beziehung an der intakten Niere.

Heidenreich: Herr Deetjen, ich wollte Sie noch etwas wegen der Ausfällung von Kristallen in den Nephren fragen. Solche Ausfällungen sieht man ja öfters, z. B. auch mit Sulfonamiden. Meist lassen sich diese verhindern, wenn man das pH verändert. Bei einer Substanz wie Amilorid wäre zu erwarten, daß sie im Sauren besser löslich ist. Ich wollte daher fragen, ob Sie das pH gemessen oder variiert haben. – Zweitens möchte ich eine kurze Bemerkung zu Ihrer Betonung der Bedeutung von Mikropunktionsmethoden machen. Diese Bedeutung steht außer Frage, wir benutzen diese Methoden auch, aber andererseits haben Sie z. B. bei Ihren Untersuchungen des Amilorids mit Mikropunktionsmethoden, wenn man von Artefakten absieht, keinerlei Effekte beobachtet. Es ist daher sicher notwendig, mit Clearance- und mit Mikropunktionsmethoden parallel zu arbeiten und darauf zu achten, daß sich die Nierenphysiologie nicht in zwei Richtungen entwickelt, die den Kontakt zueinander verlieren.

Deetjen: Zu Punkt 1: Wir haben beobachtet, daß Amilorid schon im Infusionskatheter ausfällt, wenn wir es in isotoner Kochsalzlösung lösen. Löst man es in Aqua dest., dann unterbleibt diese Ausfällung. Ich kann mir in Analogie vorstellen, daß die Substanz intratubulär in den Endabschnitten leichter ausfallen wird, wenn dort die Kochsalzkonzentrationen erhöht sind. Variationen des pHs haben wir nicht probiert. Dann zu der zweiten Frage: Wenn man einen proximalen Effekt studieren will, dann gibt es m. M. nach keine Alternative zur Mikropunktion. Wenn es sich darum handelt, distale Effekte zu studieren, kann man sicherlich auch aus Stop-flow-Untersuchungen nützliche Hinweise gewinnen.

The Pattern of Inhibition of Proximal Tubular Reabsorption by Diuretics

H. HOLZGREVE

Summary: The mode of action of hydrochlorothiazide, furosemide and acetazolamide was studied in the proximal convoluted tubule of rat kidney by three different micropuncture techniques. The pattern of action of these diuretics was shown to be quantitatively different, but qualitatively similar. Following the administration of these diuretics bicarbonate reabsorption decreased under free flow conditions and the sodium and bicarbonate concentration difference between blood and tubular fluid was reduced during stationary microperfusion with acetazolamide, furosemide and hydrochlorothiazide in decreasing order of effectiveness. Furthermore, following the simultaneous administration of furosemide and acetalozamide an additive effect on the intrinsic reabsorptive capacity of the proximal tubule could not be demonstrated.

Our results can best be explained in terms of inhibition of sodium bicarbonate reabsorption via H^+-ion secretion as first postulated by PITTS and ALEXANDER (11); a mechanism that may be the common pathway in the mode of action of these diuretics in the proximal convoluted tubule of rat kidney.

The analysis of renal action of diuretics is concerned mainly with two questions, namely with the localization within the tubule and the cellular mode of action of these substances. Diuretic action has been demonstrated in both the proximal (1, 2, 3, 7, 9, 12) and distal (7, 9) convoluted tubules accessible to micropuncture. The analysis of the mode of action of diuretics, however, is much more difficult, since underlying cellular and biochemical mechanisms of active transport have not yet fully been clarified. Based on experimentally observed transport phenomena certain models of active transport mechanisms have been worked out. At present, therefore, it is to be shown whether drug induced changes of certain transport characteristics are in correspondence with such models of active transport or not.

Methods

Micropunctures were done in proximal convoluted tubules of male albino rats. Following control periods hydrochlorothiazide (mean doses: 9 mg/kg body weight as a primary dose and 10 mg/kg · h as a sustaining infusion), furosemide (43 mg/kg and 100 mg/kg · h, respectively) or acetazolamide (47 mg/kg and 56 mg/kg · h, respectively) were administered. The fluid loss was exactly replaced. Plasma concentrations of sodium, potassium and chloride were determined after every second micropuncture sample.

Three types of micropuncture techniques were performed:

1. Free flow samples were collected from the last loop of the proximal convoluted tubule accessible to puncture and identified with Lissamine green.

2. Steady state concentrations were measured using the stationary microperfusion method (6, 13). In principle this method consists of the intratubular deposition of an isotonic test solution containing the nonreabsorbable polyethylene glycol between a split oil droplet. This solution remains stationary and has no contact with other tubular fluid. After a few seconds a constant concentration gradient across tubular epithelium is established and then the steady state concentrations of sodium, potassium and chloride in samples of this test solution are measured (11, 14). The steady state concentrations of bicarbonate were calculated according to the formula:

$$TF_{Na} + TF_{K} + (2 \cdot 2{,}66) - TF_{Cl}.$$

TF_{Na}, TF_{K} and TF_{Cl} represent the steady state concentrations in tubular fluid of sodium, potassium and chloride, respectively. The factor $2 \cdot 2.66$ takes into account the calcium steady state concentration in the proximal tubule of the rat (4). A possible change of this value after application of diuretics was disregarded.

3. The reabsorptive half-time was measured using the shrinking drop technique of Gertz (5).

Results and Discussion

During control periods the free flow concentration of chloride in proximal tubular fluid increased from a TF/P-ratio of 1.00 in glomerular filtrate to a mean ratio of 1.24 at the end of the proximal convolution (Fig. 1). After acetazolamide the TF/P-ratio for chloride at the same puncture site reached a value of 1.04 only as a result of decreased bicarbonate reabsorption (1). This effect is to be expected since acetazolamide is a typical inhibitor of

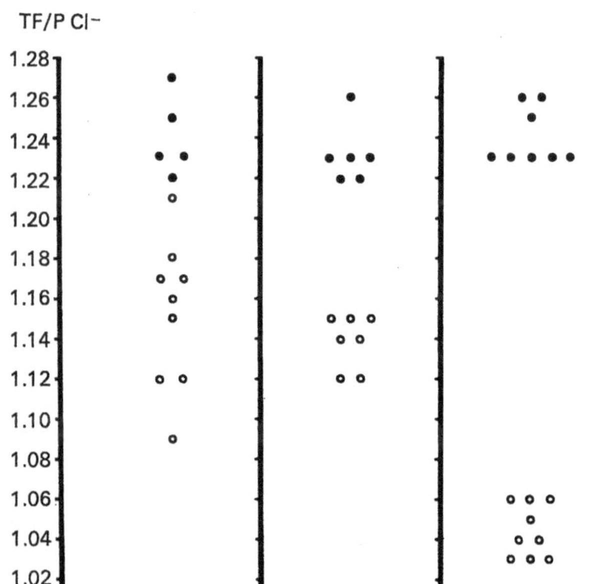

Fig. 1. Tubular fluid (TF) over plasma (P) chloride ratios at the end of the proximal convoluted tubule before (●) and after (○) administration of hydrochlorothiazide, furosemide and acetazolamide. Serum chloride concentrations were corrected for serum water and Gibbs-Donnan equilibrium.

Table 1. Mean sodium, chloride and bicarbonate steady state concentrations before and after administration of hydrochlorothiazide, furosemide and acetazolamide. Bicarbonate concentrations were calculated (for details see methods). n = number of observations.

	Sodium mEq/l			Chloride mEq/l			Bicarbonate mEq/l		
	Before	After	Change	Before	After	Change	Before	After	Change
Hydro-chlorothiazide	105.5 n=10	107 n=12	1.5	107.5 n=11	107 n=15	−0.5	6.5	8.0	1.5
Furosemide	104 n=16	111 n=20	7.0	108.5 n=16	111.5 n=20	3.0	4.5	8.0	3.5
	p < 0.001								
Acetazolamide	108 n=16	118.5 n=18	10.5	109 n=17	111 n=22	2.0	8.5	16.5	8.0
	p < 0.001								

carbonic anhydrase. After administration of hydrochlorothiazide or furosemide, however, the TF/P-ratios for chloride also were found to be diminished at the same puncture site showing mean ratios of 1.15 and 1.14, respectively. This again must be interpreted in terms of decreased reabsorption of bicarbonate.

The contact time of glomerular filtrate with tubular epithelium varies with respect to the diuretic administered (8). By determining the steady state concentrations of sodium, potassium and chloride using the stationary microperfusion method and by calculating the bicarbonate concentration the transport characteristics can be examined independently of changes of contact time. After hydrochlorothiazide the mean steady state concentration of sodium increased by 1.5 mEq/l, after furosemide by 7.0 mEq/l and after acetazolamide by 10.5 mEq/l (Table 1). The sodium concentrations during control periods and following furosemide or acetazolamide were shown to be significantly different ($P < 0.001$). Since serum sodium concentrations remained unchanged these increases of steady state concentrations reflect decreases of the concentration differences between blood and tubular fluid, i. e. the ability of the tubular epithelium to establish a concentration difference between blood and tubular fluid under these experimental conditions is reduced. This was most pronounced after acetazolamide, less after furosemide and insignificantly after hydrochlorothiazide.

The mean steady state concentrations of chloride decreased by 0.5 mEq/l after hydrochlorothiazide and increased after furosemide and acetazolamide by 3.0 and 2.0 mEq/l, respectively.

After administration of hydrochlorothiazide the calculated steady state concentration for bicarbonate increased by 1.5 mEq/l, after furosemide by 3.5 and after acetazolamide by 8.0 mEq/l. Following hydrochlorothiazide and furosemide the serum concentrations of chloride and bicarbonate as derived from the chloride did not change. Following the administration of acetazolamide the serum chloride concentration increased by 3–5 mEq/l. Thus, acetazolamide induced changes characteristic of metabolic acidosis and a decrease of the serum bicarbonate concentration therefore has to be assumed under these conditions. These data indicate that the increase of the steady state concentration of bicarbonate by 1.5 and 3.5 mEq/l after hydrochlorothiazide and furosemide, respectively, reflects a decrease of the concentration difference between blood and tubular fluid (conc. diff. $= P_{HCO_3} - TF_{HCO_3}$) of the same order of magnitude (when P_{HCO_3} constant, increase of TF_{HCO_3} reflects decrease of conc. diff.). Since the serum bicarbonate concentration decreases after acetazolamide, a decrease of the concentration difference between blood and tubular fluid by more than the increase of a steady state concentration of 8 mEq/l must be assumed (decrease of P_{HCO_3} and increase of TF_{HCO_3} are additive with respect to changes of concentration difference).

Thus, the interpretation of transport characteristics given for sodium seems to hold also for bicarbonate: the ability of the tubular epithelium to establish a concentration difference between blood and tubular fluid is reduced, most pronounced following acetazolamide, markedly after furosemide and insignificantly reduced after hydrochlorothiazide. The changes of the values for sodium and bicarbonate are quantitatively correlated, whereas changes of chloride concentrations show no correlation with those of sodium. This is taken as evidence that sodium and bicarbonate steady state concentrations as well as sodium and bicarbonate concentration differences between blood and tubular fluid are consequences of the same active transport mechanism. In view of these data the mechanism of sodium bicarbonate reabsorption via H^+-ion secretion first

Table 2. Reabsorptive half-time (sec) as measured by shrinking drop method (5) before and after administration of hydrochlorothiazide (A), furosemide (B) or acetazolamide (C). When furosemide and acetazolamide were given simultaneously (D), the same doses as in (B) and (C) were used. n = number of tubules studied, each single tubule was studied 2 to 6 times.

	Reabsorptive $t_{1/2}$ (seconds)		
	Before		After
A Hydrochlorothiazide	9.3 n=9	$p < 0.001$	13.8 n=16
			$p < 0.001$
B Furosemide	9.3 n=8	$p < 0.001$	20.4 n=15
			$p < 0.005$
C Acetazolamide	9.0 n=9	$p < 0.001$	24.0 n=15
			$p > 0.1$
D Furosemide and Acetazolamide	9.9 n=13	$p < 0.001$	25.5 n=17

postulated by PITTS and ALEXANDER (10) lends itself as being the transport system which will be inhibited by all the diuretics studied.

The reabsorptive half-time during control periods and after administration of diuretics are given in Table 2. During individual control periods the mean reabsorptive half-times were in the range of 9.0 and 9.9 seconds. Following the administration of diuretics half-times were prolonged: 13.8 seconds after hydrochlorothiazide, 20.4 after furosemide and 24.0 seconds after acetazolamide. If the conclusion based on the above data that these diuretics have a common mode of action proves to be correct, an additive effect would not be expected during simultaneous administration of these drugs. And indeed, following the administration of both furosemide and acetazolamide simultaneously a reabsorptive half-time of 25.5 seconds was measured as compared with 24.0 seconds when acetazolamide alone was given. Therefore, no additive effect on the intrinsic reabsorptive capacity of the proximal tubular epithelium could be demonstrated after simultaneous administration of furosemide and acetazolamide.

References

1. CLAPP, J. R., J. F. WATSON and R. W. BERLINER: Effect of carbonic anhydrase inhibition on proximal tubular bicarbonate reabsorption. Am. J. Physiol., **205,** 693–696 (1963).
2. DEETJEN, P.: Mikropunktionsuntersuchungen zur Wirkung von Furosemid. Pflügers Arch. ges. Physiol. **284,** 184–190 (1965).
3. DIRKS, J. H., W. J. CIRKSENA and R. W. BERLINER: Micropuncture study of the effect of various diuretics on sodium reabsorption by the proximal tubules of the dog. J. clin. Invest., **45,** 1875–1885 (1966).
4. FRICK, A., G. RUMRICH, K. J. ULLRICH and W. E. LASSITER: Microperfusion study of calcium transport in the proximal tubule of the rat kidney. Pflügers Arch. ges. Physiol., **286,** 109–117 (1965).
5. GERTZ, K. H.: Transtubuläre Natriumchloridflüsse und Permeabilität für Nichtelektrolyte im proximalen und distalen Konvolut der Rattenniere. Pflügers Arch. ges. Physiol., **276,** 336–356 (1963).
6. HIERHOLZER, K., M. WIEDERHOLT, H. HOLZGREVE, G. GIEBISCH, R. M. KLOSE and E. E. WINDHAGER: Micropuncture study of renal transtubular concentration gradients of sodium and potassium in adrenalectomized rats. Pflügers Arch. ges. Physiol., **285,** 193–210 (1965).
7. HOLZGREVE, H., A. FRICK, G. RUMRICH, M. WIEDERHOLT and K. J. ULLRICH: Wirkungsweise von Diuretica auf den transtubulären Transport von Natriumchlorid. In: Normale und pathologische Funktionen des Nierentubulus. Ed. by K. J. ULLRICH and K. HIERHOLZER. HUBER, Bern (1965).
8. HOLZGREVE, H.: Hemmung der lokalen und prozentualen Resorption im proximalen Konvolut der Rattenniere nach Gabe von Diuretica. (Abstract). Naunyn-Schmiedebergs Arch. Pharmak. exp. Path., **260,** 146 (1968).
9. MENG, K.: Mikropunktionsuntersuchungen über die saluretische Wirkung von Hydrochlorothiazid, Acetazolamid und Furosemid. Naunyn-Schmiedebergs Arch. Pharmak. exp. Path., **257,** 355–371 (1967).
10. PITTS, R. F. and R. S. ALEXANDER: The nature of the renal tubular mechanism for acidifying the urine. Am. J. Physiol., **144,** 239–254 (1945).
11. RAMSAY, J. A., R. H. J. BROWN and P. C. CROGHAN: Electrometric titration of chloride in small volumes. J. exp. Biol., **32,** 822–829 (1955).
12. RECTOR, F. C. jr., F. P. BRUNNER, J. C. SELLMAN and D. W. SELDIN: Pitfalls in the use of micropuncture for the localization of diuretic action. Ann. N. Y. Acad. Sci., **139,** 400–407 (1966).

13. Shipp, J. C., I. B. Hanenson, E. E. Windhager, H. J. Schatzmann, G. Whittembury, H. Yoshimura and A. K. Solomon: Single proximal tubules of the Necturus kidney. Methods for micropuncture and microperfusion. Am. J. Physiol., **195,** 563–569 (1958).
14. Young, J. A. and E. Schögel: Micropuncture investigation of sodium and potassium excretion in rat submaxillary saliva. Pflügers Arch. ges. Physiol., **291,** 85–98 (1966).

Present Status of Diuretic Therapy

Heutiger Stand der diuretischen Therapie

K. H. BEYER, JR.

The management of edema and of hypertension can be divided in our time into the era B. C. (or before chlorothiazide) and A. D. (or after Diuril, known to most of you as Chlotride). This occurred a decade ago. Most of all, it ushered in an easy capability on the part of the physician to manage many edematous patients effectively with oral therapy that was free of the limitations of prior diuretic agents that were too weak, or that induced self-refractoriness or that required ammonium chloride-induced acidosis and parenteral administration to be most effective.

Since chlorothiazide was introduced to clinical trial new words or expressions have entered our vocabulary, such as saluretic agents, aldosterone antagonists and antikaliuretic or potassium-conserving agents. A whole new constellation of drugs has been brought to the fore, some of which even extend available therapy beyond the promise that the thiazides offered doctor and patient, alike. At first there needed to be the assurance that they worked. Since these drugs were impressive, physician and scientists alike were curious as to how and where they worked. As the capability to salvage patients and to prolong useful life by the support of their homeostasis has become apparent, how to use these agents conjointly has become important. So has the more general need for an insight into electrolyte balance and how this is affected by the interaction of disease and therapy. Thus, the physician may be confronted in his daily practice with clinical problems no more difficult than the assurance that his patient take an adequate but modest dose of a thiazide for a few days at a time. Thus, the patient who has a bothersome premenstrual edema is very likely to respond gratefully to a few days of saluretic-diuretic therapy periodically and without need for concern. At the other extreme might be the hypertensive, digitalized, edematous patient who may, or may not, have a progressive impairment of renal function. Whether the use of modern diuretic therapy is a help or a hazard to such a patient depends on the insight of the physician into the complexity of the problem and his ability to complement adequately with drugs the failing homeostasis.

Today, we have two principal categories of renotropic agents that affect salt and water balance (1):

1. The saluretic drugs;
2. The antikaliuretic agents.

The *saluretic drugs* (omitting organomercurials) include

1. The thiazides and chlorthalidone;
2. Ethacrynic acid;
3. Furosemide.

The Thiazides: In general, the numerous thiazides are represented by chlorothiazide or hydrochlorothiazide and chlorthalidone. Although their dosages vary by almost a thousand-fold, their maximal natriuretic effect is essentially the same and so is their enhancement of potassium excretion. At ordinarily prescribed dosages their chloruretic effect is much the same, but at maximally useful dosages chlorothiazide causes an increased bicarbonate excretion that is less evident for the thiazides that have the least daily dosage. Chlorthalidone has much the same effect on electrolyte excretion, but its duration of action is notably longer than the thiazides, as a group. Actually, any of these drugs can be administered on a once-a-day basis satisfactorily although they are ordinarily administered twice or three times a day. All of them are carbonic anhydrase inhibitors. Whereas this may not be their mode of action, a better explanation still eludes us.

Ethacrynic acid and furosemide are indistinguishable from the thiazides with regard to their clinical effects on electrolyte except that they can produce a greater maximal effect. Thus, these two compounds can be used interchangeably with thiazides, or they may be used to extend therapy for patients who have become refractory to thiazides as the basis for their illness progresses. Ethacrynic acid is a unique compound structurally in that it was designed to bind sulfhydryl groups. Sulfhydryl catalyzed dehydrogenases of the kidney have been thought to be inhibited by organomercurial diuretic agents. Curiously, furosemide, which has the carbonic anhydrase-binding sulfamyl group of the thiazides, more nearly resembles ethacrynic acid in the magnitude of its maximal saluretic effect. Ethacrynic acid is not a carbonic anhydrase inhibitor whereas furosemide is, and to about the same extent as sulfanilamide. The similarity of the magnitude of their saluretic effect, which exceeds that of the thiazides, would seem to relate more to their common sites of action of ethacrynic acid and furosemide along the nephron, including the loop of Henle, rather than to mode of action. Ethacrynic acid is a fairly potent inhibitor of the renal Na-K-Mg-dependent ATPase whereas furosemide is not. Furosemide is a potent diuretic in the rat whereas ethacrynic acid is hardly active in this species.

All of these saluretic agents increase the excretion of sodium, potassium and chloride ions. They are all secreted similarly by the renal tubules, hence they influence uric acid excretion alike. They all cause uric acid retention. Their effect on carbohydrate metabolism is greatest for the thiazides and least, if at all, for ethacrynic acid. Duration of action is least for furosemide and greatest for chlorthalidone.

All of these compounds, administered orally, can cause dehydration. In practice, they can cause hyponatremia, hypokalemia, hypochloremia and metabolic alkalosis. This response is apt to be rendered the more complex by illness and the nature of patient care. I shall have more to say about this after discussing the next general category of compounds.

The antikaliuretic compounds are, in fact, natriuretic by virtue of their ability to inhibit the exchange of potassium for sodium across the distal portion of the nephron. The capacity of the nephron to exchange potassium for sodium is not great as compared to the exchange of hydrogen for sodium, so characteristically these compounds are not nearly so active diuretics as are the saluretic agents. They can be made to induce net potassium retention. Their effect on anion excretion is not remarkable.

The antikaliuretic agents belong to one or the other of two classes. Aldosterone is capable of modulating the exchange of potassium for sodium across the nephron, hence *aldosterone antagonists* increase sodium and decrease potassium excretion. *Spironolactone* is such an agent. It is not active in the absence of aldosterone and it is most effective in conditions wherein excessive aldosterone production is to be found, as in cirrhosis or malignant hypertension. In the laboratory animal its administration is attended by a hyperplasia of the adrenal cortex which is reversible on withdrawal of drug, an adaptive phenomenon characteristic of known antikaliuretic agents.

Triamterene and amiloride inhibit the exchange of potassium for sodium directly and not by blocking the effect of aldosterone. They are active in the adrenalectomized animal. Their chemistry and their collateral pharmacology are quite dissimilar. Amiloride is much the more basic compound. It has the lowest clinical dosage of the antikaliuretic agents. Its duration of action makes it easily adaptable to intermittent therapy as on alternate days. It can be administered conjointly with the customary regimen for saluretic agents, as can the other antikaliuretic compounds mentioned.

The antikaliuretic compounds have been used in practice as diuretic agents but this is not their customary usage. HOLLANDER felt that spironolactone could be used satisfactorily in both edematous and hypertensive therapy if time was sufficient to offset lack of potency. CONWAY considered that when administered on a continuous basis 30 mg of amiloride per day was as effective as was 150 mg of hydrochlorothiazide. On the other hand, neither spironolactone nor triamterene has found favor for use alone and amiloride is not yet generally available.

The reason these agents are seldom used except as adjuncts to saluretic therapy is three-fold:

1. Their diuretic effect is not as great as their natriuretic effect, which, itself, is low compared to thiazides on a peak response basis.
2. The dose-response curves are flat and to obtain maximal natriuresis frank potassium retention may result.
3. Whereas amiloride is the most chloruretic of these compounds, this effect is not commensurate with cation excretion.

From a clinical standpoint, their use alone is rational in those circumstances where the production of aldosterone is sufficient to cause the concomitant excretion of as much or more potassium than sodium by way of this exchange mechanism. Under these conditions the Na/K ratio of excreted cations becomes more favorable to potassium conservation. Indeed, this may be the only practical way to control potassium wasting or to sustain a proper potassium balance in such cases, whether or not a saluretic agent is co-administered. On the other hand, in the presence of substantial impairment of renal function, these compounds may cause hyperkalemia. Thus, they are contra-indicated in severe renal disease or where renal function is believed to be deteriorating.

In preparing for this lecture, I came upon a case report published by MARTIN and FANGER (2) that reads as follows:

> "A 50-year-old male was admitted with dyspnea and chills of two days' duration. He was accustomed to a large wine intake. A fall three days previously caused contusion of the nose and left leg. He was febrile (106.4° F or 41.3° C), dyspneic, and appeared clinically dehydrated with a dry tongue, injected pharynx, and concentrated urine (Sp. Gr. 1.024). Blood pressure was variably elevated from 280/110 to 145/100 mm Hg, and there was cardiac enlargement. The left leg was cold and without peripheral pulses. There was clinical and X-ray evidence of

pneumonia in the right lung. Hematology examination revealed Hb 15.5 gm per cent, white blood count 23,400, neutrophils 80 per cent, band forms 2, lymphocytes 16, monocytes 2. The serum sodium was 125 mEq/l (normal 135–145), potassium 4.1 mEq/l (normal 4–5), chlorides 88 mEq/l (normal 95–105), blood urea nitrogen (BUN) 18 mg per cent (normal 7–25)."

"He was treated with antibiotics and intravenous fluids, receiving 4000 ml of 5 per cent dextrose in normal saline in 7 ½ hours. The fluid administration was predicated on the clinical evidence of dehydration and hyponatremia."

"The patient died on the day of admission, and the autopsy revealed overhydration of the tissues, cardiac hypertrophy, pulmonary congestion and edema, and fatty metamorphosis of the liver."

"A muscle analysis (to be subsequently discussed) obtained from the autopsy revealed overhydration concurring with the autopsy findings. The hyponatremia (125 mEq/l) was a dilution effect resulting from overhydration of the vascular compartment. Hence, the routine electrolyte studies and the clinical impression of dehydration provided misinformation and resulted in incorrected treatment."

This is an interesting case and I would agree that on the basis of the printed information "the clinical impression of dehydration provided misinformation and resulted in incorrect treatment." On the other hand, I see no reason to incriminate the electrolyte studies as being misleading. I should think the low plasma sodium and chloride values would have been helpful in the absence of any history of salt restriction. Certainly, the blood urea nitrogen and potassium values were not indicative of renal impairment or of excessive diuretic therapy.

I can agree with the authors that "Improved understanding and treatment of electrolyte and fluid imbalance will result from determinations of electrolyte and water and acid-base distribution in all compartments of the body." However, this should be interpreted as a general statement. On the whole, experience indicates that substantial changes in the readily assessable plasma values precede alterations in intracellular or total alterations of mass or concentration of electrolytes. For instance, Bergstrom and Hultman (3) have reported data and their interpretation to the effect that 150 mg of hydrochlorothiazide administered daily for a week reduced intramuscular potassium and chloride and increased intracellular sodium, when there has been a 1.9 kg reduction in total body weight and a concomitant induction of both hypokalemia and hypochloremia. When the dosage of furosemide chosen (100 mg) was inadequate to produce comparable reductions in extracellular parameters and body weight loss it did not affect muscle sodium or potassium significantly. Talso and Carbello (4) reported initially that in their experience the thiazides caused a decrease in serum concentration in approximately 85% of patients, but later they reported that these drugs induced no significant change in total exchangeable potassium as measured by the isotope dilution technique (5). Rooth and Furst (6), likewise, noted that polythiazide (1 mg) induced a rather pronounced alkalosis, hypokalemia and reduction in serum chloride in spite of the daily administration of KCL (3 gms). Total exchangeable potassium remained unchanged. On the other hand, it is possible to lower total body potassium as well as plasma potassium concentration with a thiazide, and to reverse that effect with amiloride, as Maronde has shown (7). His data indicate that the plasma potassium concentration returns to normal as the cumulative potassium deficit is replaced by the potassium-sparing agent.

Some 98 per cent of total exchangeable potassium is intracellular and a like percentage of sodium is extracellular. Presently it is believed that a Na-K-Mg-dependent ATPase of the cell membrane is responsible for this potassium gradient across the cell membrane. In a sense, the experiment of MARONDE pits the thiazide-induced exaggerated functional capacity of the Na/K exchange system of the lower nephron against the capability of other cellular Na/K pumps to sustain the total mass of potassium in the body. At low dosages of saluretic agents, body potassium expressed as total mass or as concentration may, or may not, be depressed to the extent of 5% to 10%. However, if the dosage of the drug is sufficient to depress both extracellular potassium and the total exchangeable mass of potassium significantly, its effect can only be reversed by withdrawal or by an antikaliuretic agent which inhibits the renal Na/K exchange to the point that normal equilibrium can be re-established. Such a compound as amiloride can do this alone and, indeed, the co-administration of potassium supplementation with such an agent may precipitate an unwanted hyperkalemia.

From a practical standpoint, these fundamental studies relating extracellular concentration to total body mass or the compartmentalization of ions, such as muscle potassium, lend reassurance to the usefulness of the simple plasma measurements of electrolytes. In other words, plasma potassium or chloride concentrations have to change at least to the point they are recognized to be abnormal before intracellular or pH changes sufficient to influence cellular activity are apt to be present. It is unlikely that we shall know very soon the intracellular potassium concentration of cardiac muscle. Indeed, this would be of uncertain aid unless we knew the balance of ions and the effect of pH thereon. On the other hand, we do know that extreme hyperkalemia or hypokalemia is to be avoided for these changes are reflected in the electrocardiogram and in the response to digitalis.

The physician should understand that, depending on circumstances, the variables of sodium, potassium, chloride, pH and water behave independently of each other. As in the case history cited, the clinical situation can be quite complicated even without restricting sodium, or administering glucose-saline solutions in large volumes, or restricting fluids concomitant with the administration of one or two types of diuretics. Conservative management of the edematous patient who may, or may not, be hypertensive may mean bed rest at first, and certainly means the use of only such a diuretic regimen as may be needed to induce a gradual weight loss and the maintenance of a homeostatic electrolyte balance. Sudden drastic weight loss may impose a greater total hazard to the patient than his prior clinical condition, unless it be for the relief of acute pulmonary edema. Usually a gradual diuresis can be accomplished without substantial reduction of sodium plasma levels. The most satisfactory maintenance of sodium, potassium and chloride plasma levels during diuresis should attend the co-administration of a saluretic agent with a potassium-sparing drug. Their sites of renotropic action combine to emphasize natriuresis, to minimize kaliuresis and to favor a more natural balance of anions. The more severe the condition predisposing to potassium loss the more important the potassium-conserving function of the combined therapy becomes. Sodium, not potassium, is the more physiologic cation to attend the reduction of edema. As indicated previously, the sum of the balanced actions of a saluretic and a potassium-conserving agent does minimize the risk of hypokalemia or hyperkalemia that may attend the vigorous use of either type of agent.

Severe sodium restriction does not seem indicated as an adjunct to saluretic therapy for it is apt to predispose to potassium loss. Diuresis can be a tedious way to remove fluid more directly accessible to paracentesis. However, the precipitous removal of substantial volumes of fluid, as by paracentesis, can have profound effects on the distribution of fluid that depend for their expression on many concurrent circumstances, including plasma protein concentration.

In closing, I should like to reiterate that most clinical conditions that require diuretic therapy, even desperate cases, usually require only effective, not desperate, measures. Moreover, the use of even a "lifesaving" measure should be an informed, not a heroic, procedure. In less dramatic clinical situations, the homeostatic propensities of the patient can save the physician a great deal of needless supplementary therapy if he will give them a chance to respond gradually. Hence, it is of great importance to know well both the clinical situation and the drug and to use moderation in altering either if such remarkable drugs as the modern diuretics are to be used most effectively.

Heutiger Stand der diuretischen Therapie

Die Behandlung von Ödemen und Hypertonie läßt sich zeitlich in eine Ära *vor* Chlorothiazid und eine Ära *nach* Chlorothiazid einteilen (das den meisten von Ihnen als Chlotride oder Diuril bekannt ist), welches vor etwa einem Jahrzehnt eingeführt wurde. In erster Linie versetzte es den Arzt nun in die Lage, auf einfache Weise zahlreiche Ödempatienten einer wirksamen oralen Behandlung zu unterziehen, welche frei von den Einschränkungen früherer Diuretica ist, die zu schwach waren oder zunehmend unwirksam wurden oder die einer Ammoniumchlorid-induzierten Azidose und parenteraler Verabreichung bedurften, um am besten zu wirken.

Seit Chlorothiazid in die klinische Erprobung eingeführt wurde, sind neue Worte oder Begriffe in unser Vokabular eingegangen, wie etwa Saluretica, Aldosteron-Antagonisten und antikaliuretische oder kaliumschonende Mittel. Eine ganze neue Konstellation von Arzneimitteln wurde bereitgestellt, von denen einige sogar noch die Möglichkeiten und Vorteile der Therapie übertrafen, welche bereits die Thiazide dem Arzt wie auch dem Patienten geboten hatten. Zunächst einmal mußte man die Gewißheit haben, daß sie wirksam waren. Da diese Mittel sehr eindrucksvoll in ihrer Wirkung waren, zeigten sich Arzt und Wissenschaftler gleichermaßen neugierig zu erfahren, wie und wo sie wirksam wurden. Da es sich gezeigt hatte, daß man dadurch Patienten retten und mit Unterstützung ihrer Homöostase Leben verlängern kann, ist die Frage, wie diese Medikamente gemeinsam anzuwenden sind, sehr bedeutsam geworden, desgleichen die mehr allgemeine Notwendigkeit für einen Einblick in das Elektrolytgleichgewicht sowie die Frage, wie dieses durch die Wechselwirkung von Krankheit und Therapie beeinflußt wird. So kann sich der Arzt in seiner Alltagspraxis klinischen Problemen gegenübersehen, die nicht weiter schwierig sind; man muß lediglich sicherstellen, daß der Kranke eine mäßige, aber ausreichende Dosis eines Thiazids jeweils einige Tage lang einnimmt. So etwa dürfte eine Patientin mit lästigen prämenstruellen Ödemen sehr wahrscheinlich recht gut auf eine mehrtägige, periodisch verabreichte saluretisch-diuretische Therapie ansprechen, ohne daß Anlaß zur Sorge bestünde. Das andere Extrem könnte der digitalisierte Patient mit

Ödemen und Hypertonie darstellen, bei dem unter Umständen eine fortschreitende Beeinträchtigung der Nierenfunktion besteht. Ob die Anwendung einer modernen Diuretica-Behandlung eine Hilfe oder eine Gefahr für einen solchen Patienten ist, hängt von der Einsicht des Arztes in die Verwickeltheit des Problems und seiner Fähigkeit ab, die versagende Homöostase ausreichend mit Arzneimitteln zu kompensieren.

Wir verfügen heute über zwei Hauptkategorien renotroper Substanzen, welche das Salz- und Wassergleichgewicht beeinflussen (1):

1. Saluretica
2. Antikaliuretica.

Zu den *Saluretica* (ohne organische Quecksilberpräparate) zählen:

1. Thiazide und Chlorthalidon,
2. Etacrynsäure,
3. Furosemid.

Die Thiazide: Allgemein betrachtet werden die zahlreichen Thiazide von Chlorothiazid oder Hydrochlorothiazid und Chlorthalidon repräsentiert. Wenn auch ihre Dosierungen um fast das Tausendfache variieren, so ist doch ihr maximaler natriuretischer Effekt im wesentlichen der gleiche, ebenso die durch sie bedingte Verstärkung der Kaliumausscheidung. In den normalerweise verordneten Dosierungen ist ihre chloruretische Wirkung etwa die gleiche, doch in maximal brauchbaren Dosen führt Chlorothiazid zu einer vermehrten Bikarbonatausscheidung, die bei den Thiaziden, welche die geringste Tagesdosis aufweisen, weniger deutlich ist. Chlorthalidon hat weitgehend den gleichen Effekt auf die Elektrolytexkretion, aber seine Wirkungsdauer ist bemerkenswert länger als die der Thiazidgruppe. Tatsächlich läßt sich jedes dieser Arzneimittel auf einer »Einmal-täglich-Basis« verabreichen; gewöhnlich gibt man sie allerdings zwei- oder dreimal täglich. Sie alle sind Karboanhydrase-Hemmer. Dies mag zwar nicht ihr Wirkungsmodus sein, doch eine bessere Erklärung fehlt uns noch.

Etacrynsäure und Furosemid lassen sich von den Thiaziden in Bezug auf ihre klinischen Wirkungen auf die Elektrolyte nicht unterscheiden, ausgenommen daß sie einen stärkeren Maximaleffekt entfalten können. Demnach kann man diese beiden Mittel abwechselnd mit den Thiaziden benutzen, oder man kann sie dazu verwenden, die Therapie bei Patienten weiterzuführen, die gegenüber den Thiaziden resistent geworden sind mit dadurch bedingtem Fortschreiten ihrer Erkrankung. Etacrynsäure ist strukturell insofern eine einzigartige Substanz, als sie mit der Absicht entwickelt wurde, Sulfhydrylgruppen zu binden. Man hat angenommen, daß Sulfhydryl-katalysierte Dehydrogenasen der Niere durch organische Quecksilberdiuretica inhibiert werden. Seltsamerweise ähnelt Furosemid, welches die Karboanhydrase-bindende Sulfamylgruppe der Thiazide aufweist, noch stärker der Etacrynsäure hinsichtlich des Ausmaßes der maximalen saluretischen Wirkung. Etacrynsäure ist kein Karboanhydrase-Hemmer, wohl aber Furosemid, und zwar in etwa dem gleichen Maße wie Sulfanilamid. Die Ähnlichkeit ihrer saluretischen Wirkungsstärke, die die der Thiazide übertrifft, scheint eher im Zusammenhang mit den gemeinsamen Wirkungsorten von Etacrynsäure und Furosemid am Nephron einschließlich der Henle'schen Schleife zu stehen als mit dem Wirkungsmodus. Etacrynsäure ist im Gegensatz zu Furosemid ein ziemlich starker Hemmer der renalen Na-K-Mg-abhängigen ATPase. Furosemid ist bei der Ratte ein stark wirkendes Diureticum, wogegen Etacrynsäure bei dieser Tierspezies kaum wirksam ist.

Alle diese Saluretica steigern die Ausscheidung von Natrium-, Kalium- und Chloridionen. Sie alle werden in ähnlicher Weise von den Nierentubuli ausgeschieden und beeinflussen folglich die Harnsäureausscheidung gleichermaßen. Sie bewirken sämtlich eine Harnsäureretention. Ihr Effekt auf den Kohlenhydratstoffwechsel ist am stärksten bei den Thiaziden und am geringsten, wenn überhaupt, bei Etacrynsäure. Die Wirkungsdauer ist bei Furosemid am kürzesten und bei Chlorthalidon am längsten.

Alle diese Substanzen können bei oraler Verabreichung eine Wasserverarmung verursachen. In der Praxis können sie zu Hyponatriämie, Hypokaliämie, Hypochlorämie und metabolischer Alkalose führen. Diese Reaktionen können je nach Krankheit und Art der Krankenbetreuung noch verwickeltere Formen annehmen. Hierüber werde ich nach Erörterung der nächsten Hauptkategorie von Substanzen noch mehr zu sagen haben.

Die *antikaliuretischen Mittel* wirken eigentlich natriuretisch dank ihrer Fähigkeit, den Austausch von Kalium gegen Natrium im Bereich des distalen Abschnitts des Nephrons zu hemmen. Das Leistungsvermögen des Nephrons für den Austausch von Kalium gegen Natrium ist im Vergleich zum Austausch von Wasserstoff gegen Natrium nicht groß; folglich sind diese Substanzen charakteristischerweise nicht annähernd so wirksame Diuretica wie die Saluretica. Man kann damit eine ausgeprägte Kaliumretention herbeiführen. Ihre Wirkung auf die Anionen-Ausscheidung ist nicht bemerkenswert.

Die antikaliuretischen Mittel wiederum lassen sich in zwei Klassen einteilen. Aldosteron ist in der Lage, den Austausch von Kalium gegen Natrium im Funktionsablauf des Nephrons zu regulieren; demnach steigern *Aldosteron-Antagonisten* die Natrium- und vermindern die Kalium-Ausscheidung. Ein derartiges Mittel ist *Spironolacton*. Es ist nicht wirksam bei Fehlen von Aldosteron, ist dagegen hochwirksam bei Zuständen, die mit exzessiver Aldosteron-Produktion einhergehen, wie etwa bei Leberzirrhose oder maligner Hypertonie. Bei Versuchstieren ist eine Verabreichung gefolgt von einer Hyperplasie der Nebennierenrinde, die nach Absetzen des Arzneimittels reversibel ist; es handelt sich hier um ein für bekannte antikaliuretische Mittel charakteristisches Anpassungsphänomen.

Triamteren und Amilorid inhibieren den Austausch von Kalium für Natrium direkt und nicht durch Blockierung des Aldosteron-Effektes. Sie sind auch beim adrenalektomierten Tier wirksam. Ihre Chemie und ihre gleichlaufende Pharmakologie sind recht verschieden. Amilorid ist das bei weitem stärker basische Mittel. Es weist die niedrigste klinische Dosierung der Antikaliuretica auf. Auf Grund seiner Wirkungsdauer läßt es sich leicht einer intermittierenden Therapie, etwa an alternierenden Tagen, anpassen. Man kann es gleichzeitig mit dem üblichen Verabreichungsschema für Saluretica geben, ebenso wie die anderen hier genannten antikaliuretischen Substanzen.

Die Antikaliuretica sind in der Praxis als Diuretica angewendet worden, doch dies ist nicht ihr üblicher Verwendungszweck. HOLLANDER war der Ansicht, daß man Spironolacton zur Ödem- wie auch Hypertonie-Behandlung zufriedenstellend benutzen könne, sofern genügend Zeit zur Verfügung stünde, dem Mangel an Wirkungsstärke Rechnung zu tragen. CONWAY hielt 30 mg Amilorid pro Tag bei kontinuierlicher Verabreichung für ebenso wirksam wie 150 mg Hydrochlorothiazid. Andererseits haben sich weder Spironolacton noch Triamteren zur alleinigen Anwendung durchgesetzt, und Amilorid ist zur Zeit noch nicht allgemein erhältlich.

Es gibt drei Gründe dafür, daß diese Mittel fast nur als Adjuvantien zur saluretischen Therapie Verwendung finden:

1. Ihr diuretischer Effekt ist nicht so stark wie ihr natriuretischer Effekt, welcher selbst –nach der Maximalwirkung beurteilt – im Vergleich zu dem der Thiazide gering ist.
2. Die Dosis-Wirkungs-Kurven sind flach, und um eine maximale Natriurese zu erzielen, könnte eine freie Kaliumretention die Folge sein.
3. Amilorid zeigt zwar die stärkste chloruretische Wirkung dieser Substanzen, doch diese Wirkung steht nicht in einem Verhältnis mit der Kationen-Ausscheidung.

Vom klinischen Standpunkt aus ist ihre alleinige Anwendung in solchen Umständen rational, wo die Aldosteron-Produktion ausreicht, die gleichzeitige Ausscheidung von ebenso viel oder mehr Kalium als Natrium auf dem Wege dieses Austauschmechanismus zu verursachen. Unter diesen Bedingungen wird das Na/K-Verhältnis der ausgeschiedenen Kationen günstiger für die Kalium-Konservierung. Dies mag in der Tat der einzige praktische Weg zur Beherrschung von Kaliumverlusten oder zur Aufrechterhaltung einer richtigen Kaliumbilanz in derartigen Fällen sein, gleichgültig ob daneben ein Salureticum verabreicht wird oder nicht. Andererseits können diese Substanzen beim Vorliegen einer erheblichen Beeinträchtigung der Nierenfunktion eine Hyperkaliämie hervorrufen. Sie sind also kontraindiziert bei schweren Nierenkrankheiten oder in Fällen, in denen eine Verschlechterung der Nierenfunktion angenommen wird.

Bei der Vorbereitung dieses Vortrages stieß ich auf einen von Martin und Fanger (2) veröffentlichten Fallbericht, der folgendermaßen lautet:

»Ein 50jähriger Mann wurde mit seit zwei Tagen bestehender Dyspnoe und Schüttelfrösten stationär aufgenommen. Es handelte sich um einen gewohnheitsmäßigen Weintrinker größerer Quanten. Drei Tage zuvor hatte er sich bei einem Sturz eine Prellung der Nase und des linken Beines zugezogen. Er hatte Fieber (41,3 °C), war dyspnoisch und schien klinisch exsikkiert mit trockener Zunge, Rachenrötung und konzentriertem Harn (spez. Gew. 1024). Der Blutdruck war erhöht und variierte zwischen 280/110 und 145/100 mm Hg; es bestand eine Herzvergrößerung. Das linke Bein war kalt und ohne periphere Pulse. Klinisch und röntgenologisch fand sich eine Pneumonie rechts. Die Blutdruckuntersuchungen ergaben folgende Werte: Hb. 15,5 g%, Leukozyten 23400, Neutrophile 80%, Stabkernige 2%, Lymphozyten 16%, Monozyten 2%. Das Serumnatrium betrug 125 mval/l (normal 135–145), Kalium 4,1 mval/l (normal 4–5), Chlorid 88 mval/l (normal 95–105), Blutharnstoff-Stickstoff 18 mg% (normal 7–25).

Er wurde behandelt mit Antibiotica und intravenösen Infusionen von 4000 ml 5%iger Dextrose in physiologischer Kochsalzlösung innerhalb von 7½ Stunden. Die Flüssigkeitsverabreichung erfolgte auf Grund der klinischen Anzeichen von Exsikkose und Hyponatriämie.

Der Patient starb am Aufnahmetag; die Autopsie ergab eine Flüssigkeitsüberfüllung der Gewebe, kardiale Hypertrophie, Lungenstauung und Lungenödem sowie fettige Degeneration der Leber.

Eine mit der Autopsie durchgeführte Muskelanalyse (die später noch zu erörtern ist) ergab übereinstimmend mit den Obduktionsbefunden einen Flüssigkeitsüberschuß. Die Hyponatriämie (125 mval/l) war ein Verdünnungseffekt als Folge der Flüssigkeitsüberladung des Gefäßsystems. Die routinemäßigen Elektrolytuntersuchungen und der klinische Eindruck einer Exsikkose lieferten also falsche Informationen und führten zu einer falschen Behandlung.«

Dies ist ein interessanter Fall, und ich möchte darin zustimmen, daß auf der Basis der veröffentlichten Angaben »der klinische Eindruck einer Exsikkose falsche Informationen lieferte und zu unkorrekter Behandlung führte«. Andererseits sehe ich keinen Grund, die Elektrolytuntersuchungen als irreführend zu beschuldigen. Ich möchte glauben, daß die niedrigen Natrium- und Chloridwerte im Serum aufschlußreich gewesen wären, da ja anamnestisch keine Kochsalzeinschränkung vorlag. Gewiß ließen die Bluthamstoff-Stickstoff- und Kaliumwerte eine Beeinträchtigung der Nierentätigkeit oder eine exzessive diuretische Therapie nicht erkennen.

Ich kann den Autoren darin zustimmen, daß »Bestimmungen der Elektrolyt-, Wasser- und Säure-Basen-Verteilung in allen Systemen des Körpers auch zu besserem Verständnis und besserer Behandlung von Elektrolyt- und Flüssigkeitsgleichgewichtsstörungen führen werden.« Dies sollte man jedoch als eine allgemeine Aussage auslegen. Insgesamt gesehen zeigt die Erfahrung, daß es vor den intrazellulären oder Gesamtänderungen der Elektrolytmenge oder -konzentration zu wesentlichen Veränderungen in den leicht zu ermittelnden Plasmawerten kommt. Zum Beispiel haben BERGSTRÖM und HULTMAN (3) Befunde dazu mitgeteilt und Stellung genommen zu der von ihnen beobachteten Wirkung, daß 150 mg Hydrochlorothiazid – eine Woche lang täglich verabreicht – den intramuskulären Kalium- und Chloridgehalt verminderten und den intrazellulären Natriumgehalt steigerten in Fällen, in denen das Gesamtkörpergewicht um 1,9 kg abnahm und gleichzeitig eine Hypokaliämie wie auch Hypochorlämie herbeigeführt wurde. In Fällen, wo die gewählte Dosierung von Furosemid (100 mg) nicht ausreichte, um vergleichbare Verminderungen in den extrazellulären Parametern und einen Gewichtsverlust zu erzeugen, wurde auch der Natrium- und Kaliumgehalt im Muskel nicht signifikant beeinflußt. TALSO und CARBELLO (4) berichteten zunächst, daß nach ihrer Erfahrung die Thiazide bei etwa 85% der Patienten eine Abnahme in der Serumkonzentration verursachten, teilten aber später mit, daß diese Arzneimittel keine signifikanten Änderungen des gesamten austauschbaren Kaliums herbeiführten, wie Messungen mittels der Isotopenverdünnungstechnik ergaben (5). ROOTH und FURST (6) stellten gleichfalls fest, daß Polythiazid (1 mg) eine ziemlich ausgeprägte Alkalose, Hypokaliämie und Abnahme des Serumchlorids auslöste trotz täglicher Verabreichung von KCl (3 g). Das gesamte austauschbare Kalium blieb unverändert. Andererseits ist es möglich, den Gesamtkaliumgehalt des Körpers wie auch die Plasma-Kalium-Konzentration mit einem Thiazid zu senken und mit Amilorid diesen Effekt wieder umzukehren, wie MARONDE gezeigt hat (7). Seine Befunde lassen erkennen, daß die Plasma-Kalium-Konzentration zu Normwerten zurückkehrt, wenn man das kumulative Kaliumdefizit mit Hilfe des kaliumeinsparenden Mittels ausgleicht.

Etwa 98 Prozent des gesamten austauschbaren Kaliums befinden sich intrazellulär und ein ähnlicher Prozentsatz an Natrium extrazellulär. Heute glaubt man, daß eine Na-K-Mg-abhängige ATPase der Zellmembran verantwortlich ist für dieses Kaliumgefälle durch die Zellmembran hindurch. In gewissem Sinne stellt das Experiment von MARONDE die Thiazid-induzierte gesteigerte funktionelle Kapazität des Na/K-Austauschsystems des unteren Nephrons und die Fähigkeit anderer zellulärer Na/K-Pumpen, die Gesamtmenge an Kalium im Körper zu erhalten, einander konträr gegenüber. Bei niedrigen Saluretica-Dosen kann das Körper-Kalium – ausgedrückt in Gesamtmenge oder in Konzentration – unter Umständen bis zu 5% oder 10% erniedrigt sein. Wenn jedoch die

Dosierung des Arzneimittels ausreicht, sowohl den extrazellulären Kaliumgehalt als auch die austauschbare Gesamtmenge an Kalium signifikant herabzusetzen, so läßt sich dieser Effekt nur durch Absetzen des Mittels oder durch Verabreichung einer antikaliuretischen Substanz umkehren, welche den renalen Na/K-Austausch so weit inhibiert, daß ein normales Gleichgewicht wiederhergestellt werden kann. Eine derartige Substanz wie Amilorid kann dies allein bewirken, und die gleichzeitige Verabreichung von Kaliumzusätzen mit einem solchen Mittel könnte tatsächlich eine unerwünschte Hyperkaliämie auslösen.

Aus praktischer Sicht liefern diese grundlegenden Untersuchungen über die Beziehungen der extrazellulären Konzentration zur Gesamtmenge im Körper oder zum örtlich abgeteilten Ionengehalt, wie etwa Muskel-Kalium, eine erneute Bestätigung für die Nützlichkeit einfacher Serumelektrolytbestimmungen. Anders ausgedrückt müssen sich die Serum-Kalium- oder -Chloridkonzentrationen zumindest so weit ändern, daß man sie als abnorm erkennen kann, noch bevor intrazelluläre oder pH-Änderungen, die zur Beeinflussung der zellulären Aktivität ausreichen, vorhanden sein dürften. Es ist unwahrscheinlich, daß wir schon sehr bald über die intrazelluläre Kaliumkonzentration des Herzmuskels Bescheid wissen werden. Dies wäre freilich nur eine unsichere Hilfe, sofern wir nicht auch das Ionengleichgewicht und den Effekt des pH darauf kennen würden. Andererseits ist uns bekannt, daß man eine extreme Hyperkaliämie oder Hypokaliämie vermeiden muß, denn diese Veränderungen spiegeln sich im Elektrokardiogramm und im Ansprechen auf Digitalis wider.

Der Arzt sollte verstehen, daß sich je nach den Umständen die veränderlichen Werte für Natrium, Kalium, Chlorid, pH und Wasser unabhängig voneinander verhalten. Wie in der zitierten Kasuistik kann die klinische Situation recht kompliziert sein, auch ohne Natriumeinschränkung oder Verabreichung von Glukose-Kochsalz-Lösungen in großen Mengen oder Flüssigkeitsbeschränkungen gleichzeitig mit der Anwendung einer oder zweier Diuretica-Arten. Die konservative Behandlung des Ödempatienten, der möglicherweise auch an Hypertonie leidet, dürfte zunächst einmal Bettruhe bedeuten, und sicherlich bedeutet sie auch die Anwendung nur eines solchen Diuretica-Therapieschemas, wie es gerade notwendig sein mag, um einen allmählichen Gewichtsverlust herbeizuführen und ein homöostatisches Elektrolytgleichgewicht aufrechtzuerhalten. Ein plötzlicher, drastischer Gewichtsverlust kann für den Patienten eine größere Gesamtgefahr bilden als sein vorheriger klinischer Zustand, es sei denn, es ginge um die Beseitigung eines akuten Lungenödems. Gewöhnlich kann man eine allmähliche Diurese erzielen ohne erhebliches Absinken der Serumnatriumspiegel. Die befriedigendste Aufrechterhaltung der Natrium-, Kalium- und Chloridspiegel im Serum während der Diurese dürfte man durch die gleichzeitige Verabreichung eines Salureticums mit einem kaliumeinsparenden Mittel erreichen. Durch die jeweiligen Angriffspunkte ihrer renotropen Wirkung bewirken sie vereint eine Verstärkung der Natriurese, eine starke Verminderung der Kaliurese und die Förderung eines natürlicheren Anionengleichgewichtes. Je schwerer der Krankheitszustand ist, der zum Kaliumverlust prädisponiert, umso wichtiger wird die kaliumeinsparende Funktion der kombinierten Therapie. Natrium, nicht Kalium, ist das physiologischere Kation, das mit der Reduzierung von Ödemen einhergeht. Wie schon vorher angedeutet, senken die ausgewogenen Wirkungen eines Salureticums und eines kaliumsparenden Mittels gemeinsam das Risiko einer Hypokaliämie oder Hyperkaliämie, welches die energische Anwendung der einen oder der anderen Arzneimittelart begleiten kann, auf ein Minimum.

Eine starke Natriumeinschränkung scheint nicht indiziert zu sein als Unterstützung zur saluretischen Therapie, da sie doch zu Kaliumverlusten prädisponieren kann. Eine Diurese kann eine langwierigere Art der Ausschwemmung von Flüssigkeit sein, die man besser und direkter durch Bauchpunktion entfernen könnte. Die plötzliche Beseitigung erheblicher Flüssigkeitsmengen, etwa durch Bauchpunktion, kann allerdings tiefgreifende Wirkungen auf die Flüssigkeitsverteilung haben, deren Ausdruckswerte von zahlreichen nebeneinander bestehenden Umständen einschließlich der Serum-Eiweiß-Konzentration abhängt.

Abschließend möchte ich nochmals darauf hinweisen, daß die meisten klinischen Zustände, die einer diuretischen Therapie bedürfen, selbst verzweifelte Fälle, gewöhnlich nur wirksame, aber nicht verzweifelte Maßnahmen erfordern. Darüber hinaus sollte die Anwendung selbst eines »lebensrettenden« Verfahrens eine wohlbedachte, nicht eine heroische Maßnahme sein. In weniger dramatischen klinischen Situationen können die körpereigenen Homöostase-Regulationsmechanismen des Patienten dem Arzt einen großen Teil unnötiger Substitutionstherapie ersparen, wenn er ihnen Gelegenheit gibt, allmählich zu reagieren. Folglich ist es von großer Bedeutung, sowohl über den klinischen Zustand als auch über das Arzneimittel gut Bescheid zu wissen und nur maßvoll den Zustand oder die Therapie zu verändern, wenn man solch bemerkenswerte Medikamente wie die modernen Diuretica auf die wirksamste Weise einsetzen will.

Literatur / References

1a. Beyer, K. H. and J. E. Baer: Pharmacological Reviews **13,** 517 (1961).
1b. Beyer, K. H. and J. E. Baer: Newer Diuretics. Fortschritte der Arzneimittelforschung **2,** 9 (1960).
1c. Baer, J. E. and K. H. Beyer: Renal Pharmacology. Annual Review of Pharmacol. **6,** 261 (1966).
2. Martin, H. F. and H. Fanger: Rhode Island Med. J. **49,** 303 (1966).
3. Bergstrom, J. and E. Hultman: Acta Med. Scand. **180,** 363 (1966).
4. Talso, P. J. and A. J. Carballo: N. Y. Acad. Sci. Ann. **88,** 822 (1960).
5. Talso, P. J., C. E. Miller, A. J. Carballo and I. Vasquez: Metab. Clin. Exper. **9,** 456 (1960).
6. Rooth, G. and C. Furst: Acta Med. Scand. **176,** 51 (1964).
7. Maronde, R. F.: Personal communication to W. H. Wilkinson. See article by Dr. Wilkinson in this monograph.

Pharmacology of Antikaliuretic Substances

Pharmakologie antikaliuretischer Substanzen

J. E. BAER

There is good evidence that excreted K^+ is derived from the distal segment of the nephron, and that its rate of excretion may be importantly dependent on the Na^+ load at this site. The K^+-losing action of potent diuretics has been attributed to an increase in unreabsorbed Na^+ available for exchange with K^+. Acute experiments show that the relative Na/K excreted is not identical for all diuretics, and that H^+ as well as K^+ may contribute to ionic balance of the excreted urine.

The ability of cortical steroids, notably aldosterone, to decrease the Na^+/K^+ ratio, and of spironolactone to reverse this effect, defines one Na-K exchange mechanism. The organomercurials have only limited K-sparing action; the effect is not observed unless K excretion is initially high. In dogs, the K-sparing action is very evident in the presence of alkaline urine caused by pretreatment with acetazolamide (1, 2), although the natriuretic action of organomercurials is often less effective when urine is alkaline.

Chlorazanil, a triazine ("Orpidan"), is a weak natriuretic agent that does not cause K^+ loss. SHIDEMAN (3) found it to have weak K^+-sparing properties in rats over a limited dose range. Chlorazanil blocked the kaliuretic response to KCl or acetazolamide. The K-sparing action is not generally characteristic of the triazine, pyrimidine, or pteridine structures, however.

The effects of triamterene and amiloride (Fig. 1) on Na^+ and K^+ excretion are qualitatively different from those of the primary aldosterone antagonists such as spironolactone. Thus, in adrenalectomized rats the latter will exactly reverse the tendency of a mineralocorticoid to block Na^+ excretion and to enhance K^+ excretion, thus restoring the ratio of Na^+/K^+ excreted to that obtained in the absence of deoxycorticosterone (DOC) (Table 1). Triamterene will increase Na^+ excretion to a greater extent, and also sub-

Table 1. Cation excretion in adrenalectomized rats.

	Dose µg/rat p. o.	µEq/rat/7 hours			
		0 Doca		12γ Doca	
		Na^+	K^+	Na^+	K^+
Control	–	73±7	16±2	40	22
Spironolactone	800	74	20	62	22
Triamterene	200	87	12	51	19
Amiloride	100	90	9	114	10

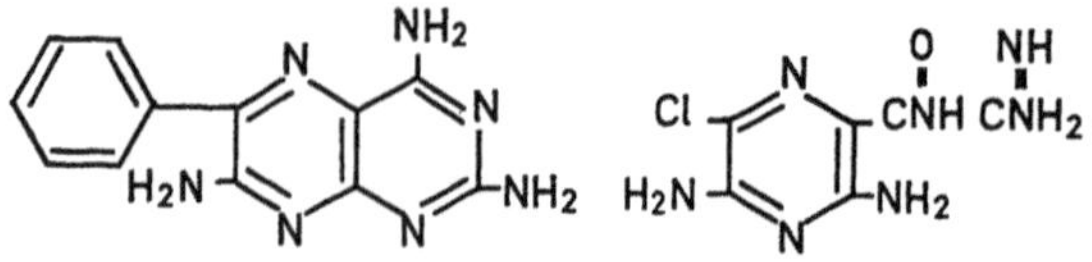

Triamterene
pKa = 6,19

Amiloride (MK-870)
pKa = 8,67

Fig. 1 – Abb. 1

stantially decrease K^+ excretion, so that the effect of the salt-retaining steroid is more than reversed. Amiloride, which is unique in that it is a relatively strong base, has a similar effect at a much lower dose (4, 5). Furthermore, both compounds are active in adrenalectomized rats given no DOC, indicating that antagonism of mineralocorticoid action is not the basis for their activity.

In normal rats treated with acetazolamide or a thiazide, amiloride will increase Na^+ and decrease K^+ excretion to a greater extent than would be expected on the basis of the action of the drugs given separately (Table 2). The organomercurial diuretic meralluride

Table 2. Cation excretion in normal fasted rats.

	Dose mg/kg p. o.	μEq/rat/5 hours	
		Na^+	K^+
Control	–	25	35
Amiloride	.625	203	57
HCTZ	.625	230	183
Amiloride +	.625	560	90
HCTZ	.625		
Acetazolamide	25.	600	250
Amiloride +	.4	900	110
Acetazolamide	25.		

has weak natriuretic action in rats. We have been unable in numerous experiments to show any K^+ retaining action of Hg^{++} in rats receiving acetazolamide, nor does the meralluride act synergistically to increase Na^+ excretion (Table 3 and 4). Whether this

Table 3. Electrolyte excretion in normal fasted rats.

	Dose mg/kg	μEq/rat/5 hours		
		Na^+	K^+	Cl^-
Control		58	97	73
Acetazolamide	25 p. o.	610	373	87
Acetazolamide	25 p. o.	528	363	77
+ Meralluride	2 mg Hg i. m.			
Acetazolamide	25 p. o.	698	440	128
+ Meralluride	4 mg Hg i. m.			
Acetazolamide	25 p. o.	1257	110	352
+ Amiloride	0.5 i. m.			

Table 4. Effect of Hg diuretic on K^+ excretion in rats (μEq/rat).

	Control	Meralluride 4 mg Hg/kg	Acetazolamide	Acetazolamide + 2 mg Hg/kg	Acetazolamide + 4 mg Hg/kg
A	97		373	363	440
B			250	280	310
C			480	637	623
D	21	34	393	343	370
E	17		413	437	417
F	15	13	270		307
				366	411

is a species difference, or whether it relates to inherent mechanisms of action, the Hg^{++} diuretic is very different from amiloride in the rat with respect to K^+-sparing activity.

The pharmacology of amiloride has been reported previously in some detail (6, 7). In clearance experiments in dogs, amiloride increases Na^+ excretion modestly, but decreases K^+ excretion (6). The K^+-sparing effect of amiloride is seen in clearance experiments with dogs pretreated with NH_4Cl or $NaHCO_3$ (Fig. 2 and 3). Amiloride is at least as effective as meralluride in such experiments. In NH_4Cl-treated dogs, meralluride had no consistent effect on K^+ secretion (Fig. 2). Acetazolamide increases the excretion of Na^+ and K^+; Pitts and others (1, 2) have shown that meralluride will inhibit K^+ excretion induced by the carbonic anhydrase inhibitor. Amiloride effectively inhibits the kaliuretic action of acetazolamide in dogs. In $NaHCO_3$-treated dogs, both amiloride and meralluride depressed K^+ excretion (Fig. 3).

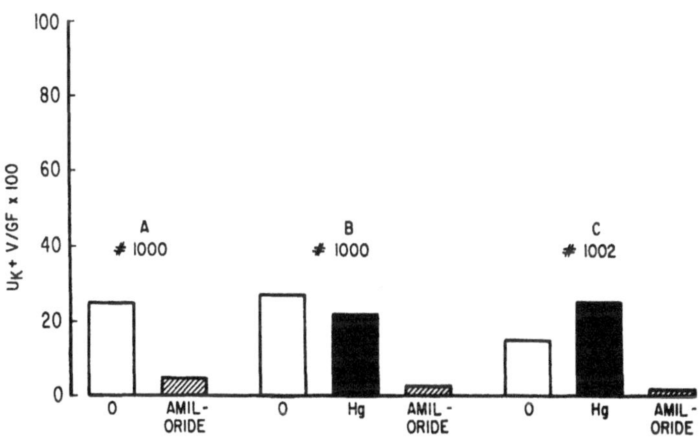

Fig. 2. Clearances in NH_4Cl treated dogs (15 ml/min NaCl).
Amiloride: 0.5 mg/kg Prime, 0.6 mg/kg/hr
Meralluride: 2 mg Hg/kg Prime, 2 mg Hg/kg/hr

Abb. 2. Clearance-Untersuchungen bei NH_4Cl-behandelten Hunden (15 ml/min NaCl).
Amilorid: 0,5 mg/kg Anfangsdosis, 0,6 mg/kg/h
Merallurid: 2 mg Hg/kg Anfangsdosis, 2 mg Hg/kg/h

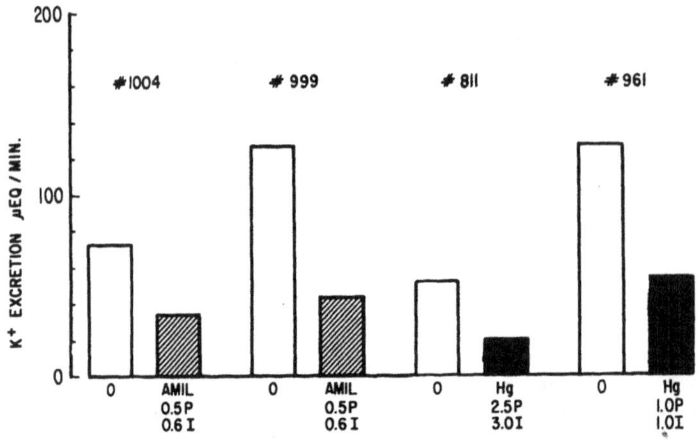

Fig. 3. Clearances in $NaHCO_3$ treated dogs (PO_4 buffer 3 ml/min).

Abb. 3. Clearance-Untersuchungen bei $NaHCO_3$-behandelten Hunden (PO_4-Puffer 3 ml/min).

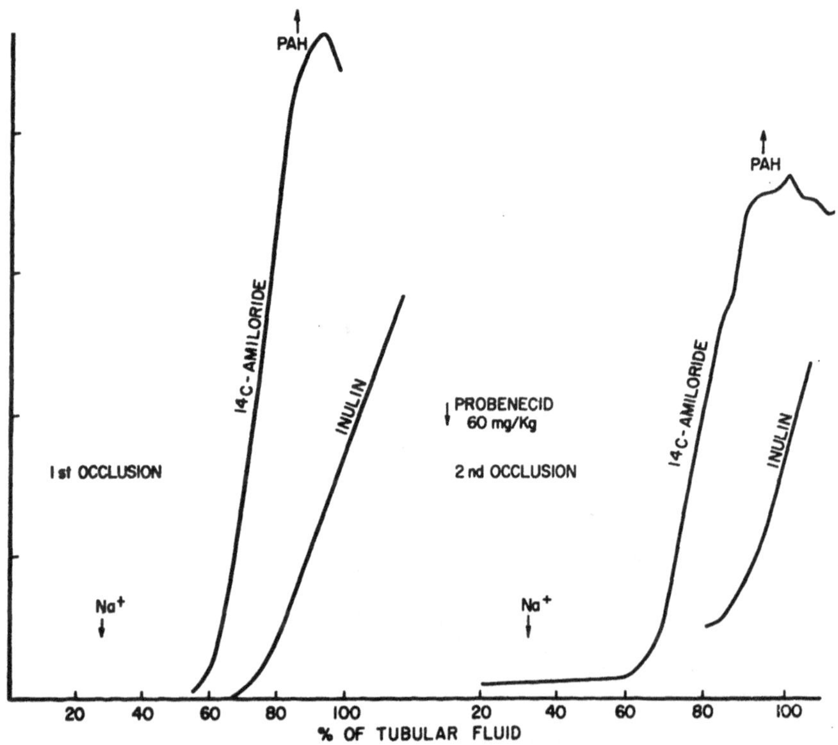

Fig. 4. Modified stop-flow in dog ureter occluded for 3 min, then amiloride + Inulin i. v.

Abb. 4. Modifizierter Stop-flow beim Hunde-Ureter, Verschluß für 3 min, dann Amilorid und Inulin i. v.

A distal site for the K^+-sparing action of amiloride is indicated in stop-flow studies in dogs (6). Concurrent with the depression in K^+ concentration, there is an elevation in the Na^+ content of distal samples, suggesting that amiloride inhibits distal reabsorption of Na^+. In stop-flow studies, the pH of distal samples was elevated by 1 to 2 pH units by amiloride; chloride concentration was unchanged. The relative importance of proximal vs. distal effects on H^+ excretion (and on HCO_3-reabsorption) remains to be established.

Amiloride is slowly but completely excreted in the urine following parenteral administration to rats, mice, and dogs (6). In modified stop-flow studies, amiloride and inulin were injected shortly before deocclusion of the ureter (Fig. 4). The appearance of amiloride preceded that of inulin, confirming the impression from conventional stop-flow studies that amiloride is secreted in the proximal portion of the nephron. The pattern was not modified by pre-treatment with probenecid, indicating that the transport of amiloride is not blocked by probenecid.

The availability of effective K^+-sparing agents provides the clinician with a tool for the selective modification of this parameter. The effect on renal Na-K and Na-H exchange processes provides a rationale for the use of combinations of amiloride with thiazides as well as with the more potent saluretic agents.

Pharmakologie antikaliuretischer Substanzen

Es liegen eindeutige Befunde dafür vor, daß ausgeschiedenes K^+ aus dem distalen Abschnitt des Nephrons stammt und daß seine Ausscheidungsrate sehr wesentlich vom Na^+-Gehalt an dieser Stelle abhängig sein kann. Die K^+-ausscheidende Wirkung starker Diuretica hat man einer Zunahme an nichtrückresorbiertem Na^+ zugeschrieben, das zum Austausch mit K^+ zur Verfügung steht. Akute Experimente zeigen, daß das relative Exkretionsverhältnis von Na/K nicht gleich ist für alle Diuretica und daß H^+ wie auch K^+ zum Ionengleichgewicht des ausgeschiedenen Urins beitragen kann.

Die Fähigkeit von Nebennierenrindensteroiden, vornehmlich Aldosteron, den Na^+/K^+-Quotienten zu vermindern, und von Spironolactone, diesen Effekt umzukehren, kennzeichnet einen Na-K-Austauschmechanismus. Die organischen Quecksilberpräparate haben nur eine begrenzte K-einsparende Wirkung; der Effekt wird nicht beobachtet, sofern nicht die K-Ausscheidung anfänglich hoch ist. Bei Hunden ist die K-einsparende Wirkung sehr deutlich bei Vorliegen von alkalischem Urin, herbeigeführt durch Vorbehandlung mit Acetazolamid (1,2), wogegen die natriuretische Wirkung von organischen Quecksilberpräparaten oft weniger ausgeprägt ist, wenn der Urin alkalisch ist.

Chlorazanil, ein Triazin (»Orpidan«), ist eine schwache natriuretische Substanz, welche keinen K^+-Verlust herbeiführt. SHIDEMAN (3) stellte fest, daß es bei Ratten schwache K^+-einsparende Eigenschaften innerhalb eines begrenzten Dosierungsbereiches besitzt. Chlorazanil blockiert die kaliuretische Reaktion auf KCl oder Acetazolamid. Die K-einsparende Wirkung ist jedoch nicht allgemein charakteristisch für Triazin, Pyrimidin oder Pteridin-Strukturen.

Die Wirkungen von Triamteren und Amilorid (Abb. 1) auf die Na^+- und K^+-Ausscheidung sind qualitativ verschieden von denjenigen der primären Aldosteron-Antagonisten wie Spironolacton. So etwa kehrt die letztgenannte Substanz bei adrenalektomierten Ratten die Tendenz eines Mineralokortikoids, die Na^+-Ausscheidung zu blockieren und die K^+-Ausscheidung zu verstärken, genau um und führt so das Ausscheidungsverhältnis von Na^+/K^+ wieder zu dem zurück, welches man bei Fehlen von Desoxycorticosteron (DOC) erhält (Tab. 1). Triamteren steigert in größerem Maße die

Tab. 1. Kationenausscheidung bei adrenalektomierten Ratten.

	Dosis γ/Ratte p. o.	µval/Ratte/7 Stunden 0 DOCA		12γ DOCA	
		Na^+	K^+	Na^+	K^+
Kontrolle	—	73±7	16±2	40	22
Spironolacton	800	74	20	62	22
Triamteren	200	87	12	51	19
Amilorid	100	90	9	114	10

Na^+-Ausscheidung und vermindert auch die K^+-Ausscheidung beträchtlich, so daß die Wirkung des salzretinierenden Steroids mehr als nur aufgehoben wird. Amilorid, das insofern einzigartig ist, als es eine verhältnismäßig starke Base ist, hat eine ähnliche Wirkung in viel niedrigerer Dosis (4, 5). Darüber hinaus sind beide Substanzen wirksam bei adrenalektomierten Ratten, die kein DOC erhalten haben, was erkennen läßt, daß ein Antagonismus der Mineralocorticoidwirkung nicht ihre Wirksamkeitsgrundlage ist.

Bei normalen Ratten unter Verabreichung von Acetazolamid oder einem Thiazid steigert Amilorid die Na^+- und vermindert die K^+-Ausscheidung in stärkerem Maße, als man entsprechend der Wirkung der getrennt verabreichten Arzneimittel erwarten würde (Tab. 2). Das organische Quecksilberdiureticum Merallurid zeigt bei Ratten eine

Tab. 2. Kationenausscheidung bei normalen Ratten – Nüchternwerte.

	Dosis mg/kg p. o.	µval/Ratte/5 Stunden Na^+	K^+
Kontrolle	—	25	35
Amilorid	0,625	203	57
Hydrochlorothiazid	0,625	230	183
Amilorid + Hydrochlorothiazid je	0,625	560	90
Acetazolamid	25,0	600	250
Amilorid + Acetazolamid	0,4+25,0	900	110

schwache natriuretische Wirkung. Es ist uns in zahlreichen Experimenten nicht gelungen, irgendeine K^+-retinierende Wirkung von Hg^{++} bei Ratten nachzuweisen, die Acetazolamid erhalten haben, und ebensowenig wirkt das Merallurid synergistisch zur Steigerung der Na^+-Ausscheidung (Tab. 3 und 4). Ob dies nun auf einem Spezies-Unterschied beruht oder ob es in Beziehung steht zu inhärenten Wirkungsmechanismen, das Hg^{++}-Diureticum unterscheidet sich jedenfalls erheblich vom Amilorid bei der Ratte in Bezug auf die K^+-einsparende Aktivität.

Tab. 3. Elektrolytexkretion bei normalen Ratten – Nüchternwerte.

	Dosis mg/kg	µval/Ratte/5 Stunden		
		Na^+	K^+	Cl^-
Kontrolle		58	97	73
Acetazolamid	25 p. o.	610	373	87
Acetazolamid + Merallurid	25 p. o. 2 mg Hg i. m.	528	363	77
Acetazolamid + Merallurid	25 p. o. 4 mg Hg i. m.	698	440	128
Acetazolamid + Amilorid	25 p. o. 0,5 i. m.	1257	110	352

Tab. 4. Effekt des Hg-Diureticums auf die K^+-Exkretion bei Ratten (µval/Ratte).

	Kontrolle	Merallurid 4 mg Hg/kg	Acetazolamid	Acetazolamid 2 mg Hg/kg	Acetazolamid 4 mg Hg/kg
A	97		373	363	440
B			250	280	310
C			480	637	623
D	21	34	393	343	370
E	17		413	437	417
F	15	13	270		307
				366	411

Über die Pharmakologie von Amilorid ist bereits früher im einzelnen berichtet worden (6, 7). Bei Clearance-Versuchen bei Hunden steigert Amilorid die Na^+-Ausscheidung mäßig, vermindert jedoch die K^+-Ausscheidung (6). Der K^+-einsparende Effekt von Amilorid wird bei Clearance-Experimenten mit Hunden beobachtet, die mit NH_4Cl oder $NaHCO_3$ vorbehandelt wurden (Abb. 2 und 3). Amilorid ist mindestens so wirksam wie Merallurid in derartigen Experimenten. Bei NH_4Cl-behandelten Hunden zeigt Merallurid keinen übereinstimmenden Effekt auf die K^+-Sekretion (Abb. 2). Acetazolamid steigert die Ausscheidung von Na^+ und K^+; Pitts und andere (1, 2) haben gezeigt, daß Merallurid die durch den Karboanhydrasehemmer induzierte K^+-Ausscheidung hemmt. Amilorid hemmt wirksam die kaliuretische Wirkung von Acetalozamid bei Hunden. Bei $NaHCO_3$-behandelten Hunden unterdrückte Amilorid wie auch Merallurid die K^+-Exkretion (Abb. 3).

Daß die K^+-einsparende Wirkung von Amilorid distal erfolgt, geht aus Stop-flow-Untersuchungen bei Hunden hervor (6). Gleichzeitig mit der Senkung der K^+-Konzentration kommt es zu einer Erhöhung des Na^+-Gehaltes distal entnommener Proben, was vermuten läßt, daß Amilorid die distale Rückresorption von Na^+ hemmt. In Stop-flow-Untersuchungen wurde der pH-Wert distal entnommener Proben durch Amilorid um 1 bis 2 pH-Einheiten erhöht; die Chloridkonzentration war unverändert. Die relative Bedeutung der proximalen im Vergleich zu den distalen Effekten auf die H^+-Ausscheidung (und auf die HCO_3-Rückresorption) müßte noch ermittelt werden.

Amilorid wird langsam, aber vollständig im Urin ausgeschieden nach parenteraler Verabreichung an Ratten, Mäuse und Hunde (6). In modifizierten Stop-flow-Untersuchungen wurde Amilorid und Inulin kurz vor Beseitigung des Ureterverschlusses injiziert (Abb. 4). Das Erscheinen von Amilorid ging dem von Inulin voraus, was den Eindruck aus konventionellen Stop-flow-Untersuchungen verstärkt, daß Amilorid im proximalen Anteil des Nephrons sezerniert wird. Das Erscheinungsbild wurde nicht durch Vorbehandlung mit Probenecid verändert, ein Zeichen dafür, daß der Transport von Amilorid nicht durch Probenecid blockiert wird.

Die Verfügbarkeit wirksamer K^+-einsparender Substanzen gibt dem Kliniker ein Hilfsmittel für die selektive Modifizierung dieses Parameters in die Hand. Der Effekt auf die renalen Na-K- und Na-H-Austauschprozesse bietet einen Maßstab für die Anwendung von Kombinationen von Amilorid mit Thiaziden wie auch mit den stärker wirkenden Saluretica.

Literatur / References

1. Berliner, R. W.: Harvey Lectures **55**, 141 (1960).
2. Pitts, R. F. et al.: J. Pharmacol. Exper. Therap. **123**, 89 (1958).
3. Skulan, T. W. and F. E. Shideman: J. Pharmacol. Exper. Therap. **148**, 356 (1965).
4. Glitzer, M. S. and S. L. Steelman: Nature (Lond.) **212**, 191 (1966).
5. Bicking, J. B. et al.: J. Med. Pharm. Chem. **8**, 683 (1965).
6. Baer, J. E. et al.: J. Pharmacol. Exper. Therap. **157**, 472 (1967).
7. Baer, J. E. and K. H. Beyer: An. Rev. Pharmacol. **6**, 261 (1966).

Oelert: Wie rasch ist der Wirkungseintritt von Amilorid?

Baer: There is no delay in the onset of action of amiloride. When given intravenously to dogs, sodium excretion increases a little more slowly than with intravenous ethacrynic acid.

The Clinical Assessment of Diuretic Agents

Die klinische Erprobung von Diuretica

W. H. WILKINSON

Summary: The clinical evaluation of a new diuretic agent is the comprehensive assessment of its clinical utility and safety. The mode of action, comparative effectiveness in relation to other drugs and areas of practical application are defined by well planned and executed pharmacologic studies. A definition of risk is achieved through routine safety assessment and by special studies of organ function in all patients receiving the compound.

The transition of a chemical from the laboratory to the clinic and human trial is justified if the compound has attributes that have not been achieved or equalled by previous diuretic agents. Studies in man are devised that parallel toxicologic and pharmacologic evaluations in animals. While never completely separable, clinical studies divide themselves into evaluations of effectiveness and comparisons with other diuretic agents, and studies that are primarily concerned with safe use of the drug in conditions where its application is anticipated. Some recent studies conducted with a new diuretic agent, amiloride (MK-870), illustrate some of the steps that are essential today for the adequate evaluation of a new drug of this class. Since these drugs augment and, in some ways, complement other diuretics, their administration to patients receiving natriuretic, saluretic agents has been more frequent.

Classes of Diuretics

The various classes of diuretics that are presently employed differ in their sites of action upon the nephron. Through their differing potencies, patterns of electrolyte elimination and effects on free water clearance, they have diverse areas of utility and effectiveness.

1. Potent Natriuretic Agents

It is appropriate to consider mercurial diuretics, ethacrynic acid, and furosemide together since they share the capability of providing diuresis in resistant edema states.

Mercurials have the disadvantage of being pH dependent and requiring injection, but have advantages of effectiveness, and in some cases they reduce potassium excretion. Their favorable action on free water clearance may be useful with other measures in the treatment of chronically ill, hyponatremic patients with edema (1).

Ethacrynic acid and furosemide are thought to act chiefly to inhibit salt transport in the ascending limb of the loop of Henle. Both drugs are effective orally and parenterally, and both agents cause a prompt natriuresis and diuresis. Neither drug potentiates the maximal action of the other. There is suggestive evidence that both furosemide and ethacrynic acid induce a shift in the pattern of blood flow through the kidney that may account for their greater diuretic effectiveness. While single dose studies have shown that these agents have a favorable sodium-to-potassium urinary excretion ratio, their potent natriuretic and chloruretic effects in edematous patients have often led to the development of metabolic alkalosis and secondary aldosteronism, and with the resulting increase in potassium excretion, this advantage is nullified.

2. Moderately Effective Natriuretic-Antihypertensive Agents

A second group of drugs that include the thiazides and phthalimidines are less potent but still highly effective clinically. While these drugs may cause metabolic alkalosis, the tendency is usually less than that observed with ethacrynic acid or furosemide, probably because these more potent diuretics also produce hydrogen ion depletion. The thiazides are also distinguished from the more potent agents by their inability to interfere with the urinary concentrating mechanism. Other possible differences are a relatively greater depression of glomerular filtration and renal plasma flow. The effects of thiazides on carbohydrate metabolism have been documented with greater certainty than for furosemide or ethacrynic acid, where studies are continuing. Both groups of drugs may cause hyperuricemia.

Perhaps the greatest advantages of this class of drugs are their extremely low toxicity at any dose, and their broad utility alone or as adjunctive agents in the treatment of edema or hypertension. When it is possible to employ them on an intermittent basis, these drugs, as well as the more potent compounds, are much less apt to induce excessive potassium and chloride loss and metabolic alkalosis.

3. Potassium-Conserving Mild Natriuretic Agents

A third category of drugs act to conserve potassium, as well as being mildly diuretic. Spironolactone is recognized to be a true aldosterone antagonist, since its activity can be titrated against that of a mineralo-corticoid. The other agents in this general class, triamterene and amiloride, inhibit the exchange of sodium for potassium and hydrogen in the distal tubules and are active in adrenalectomized animals and the human counterpart. The definition and measurement of effectiveness in the case of a potassium-retaining agent requires assessment of natriuretic as well as antikaliuretic potency.

Clinical studies with spironolactone have shown that prediction of the optimal effective dose is far from a simple matter. If the dose of spironolactone could be calculated only on a basis of the amount of circulating aldosterone, its antikaliuretic activity in hypertension should be achieved at doses lower than those needed in cirrhosis or the nephrotic syndrome. In fact, however, non-edematous hypertensive patients require about the same amount of spironolactone to prevent hypokalemia as do nephrotic or cirrhotic patients (9).

Triamterene and amiloride HCl (MK-870) appear to have certain quantitative differences, but are similar qualitatively. Both drugs produce natriuresis while causing a lowering of potassium and hydrogen ion secretion and a reduction in blood pH. Comparative studies indicate that amiloride is more potent than triamterene on a dosage basis, and may be more effective. Some of the studies employed in the recent evaluation of amiloride are illustrative of techniques available, and utilized in the clinical investigation of all types of diuretic agents at present.

Studies on Blood and Urinary Electrolytes

The evaluation of the natriuretic effectiveness of diuretic agents usually begins with single dose studies, utilizing increasing doses of the drug beginning at subeffective levels.

The effects on urinary and serum electrolytes following administration of increasing doses of amiloride were determined, and the doses required to produce natriuresis and potassium retention were found to be from 4 to 15 mg (11).

A more elaborate dose range study is then planned. Such studies are usually undertaken in normal volunteers selected to form a homogeneous population. They receive rigidly fixed diets and are rotated sequentially through the drug or drugs at the doses selected. Suitable drug free intervals between trials are employed to avoid residual effects.

Such a study was recently performed by Foltz (2) to determine the effects of MK-870 and ethacrynic acid on urinary potassium excretion. Ethacrynic acid in doses of 50 mg to 150 mg increased potassium excretion over control. While there was a reduction in kaliuresis with administration of amiloride alone, this was not clearly evident except in the 24 hr collection. The combination of ethacrynic acid plus amiloride cancelled the ethacrynic acid-induced kaliuresis over a 24-hr collection. Ethacrynic acid is a drug that acts chiefly within 10–12 hrs, while amiloride's activity extends over about 24 hrs. The later period of sodium retention and preferential potassium excretion that is induced by volume depletion, however, may actually augment the effectiveness of the second diuretic.

The comparative effectiveness of amiloride and triamterene was examined by Wilson et al. (3), who utilized a standardized assay procedure in which the therapeutic efficacy of these drugs at ceiling dosages were compared. Each agent was administered in a sequence that attempted to eliminate the effects of external factors. The urinary excretions of sodium and chloride were greater and potassium less, following amiloride at the doses employed, regardless of the sequence of drug administration.

Traditionally, evaluations of diuretic potency are based on single dose tests. Patients, however, are treated sometimes for prolonged periods with the continuous administration of fixed doses. Therefore, a dose response study of a drug over prolonged periods to determine the net gain or loss of electrolytes under standardized conditions is a logical approach to the problem of responsiveness of patients under chronic conditions of use.

Conway (4) has studied diuretic responses in two groups of five non-edematous patients who received amiloride 30 mg and hydrochlorothiazide 100 mg/day. After a four-day control period, patients were started on amiloride or hydrochlorothiazide with the dietary intake of electrolytes kept constant. While the maximal excretion of sodium and chloride was far greater with hydrochlorothiazide on the first day, the total excretion of sodium with amiloride was actually slightly greater in the five-day period.

Evaluations of this type, while not commonly employed, should be applicable especially to diuretics and other therapy where daily continuous treatment might be anticipated.

Effects on Body Electrolytes

Studies of blood levels of sodium or potassium are useful insofar as experience allows one to be certain that any changes are reflective of alterations in the total body composition; however, they may be misleading. For this reason, great effort has been exerted in recent years to find suitable methods for estimating intracellular levels of electrolytes under various clinical states, and with the use of diuretics. Some of the techniques that have been available for several years are just beginning to find practical application in clinical studies of new drugs. Methods for the determination of intracellular electrolytes include the metabolic balance study, which utilizes measurements of total intake and output of electrolytes, radio-isotopic dilution methods, and total body counting. Biopsy techniques have been employed less frequently, but the development of ultramicromethods offer promise for wider clinical application in the future (7, 10).

The utilization of whole body radio-activity counters in clinical studies began about 10 years ago. The technique applied to potassium balance is based on the detection of gamma radiation from the ^{40}K isotope which is present in a constant proportion of 0.0118% of all natural potassium.

A special, sensitive large volume scintillator detector is employed for accurate determinations of whole-body potassium in patients. The equipment consists of a thalium activated sodium iodide crystal spectrometer with four sodium iodide crystals about the patient who is in a steel-walled room. After calibration, these crystals move up and down, scanning the gamma radiation spectrum of ^{40}K during one hour. The total body potassium method offers the advantages of rapid measurement and the possibility of repeated studies without significant radiation hazard. LAWRENCE (5) and his associates estimated total body potassium before therapy, after one week of treatment with ethacrynic acid or furosemide, and after a second week, with amiloride added to the baseline diuretic therapy. There was evidence of potassium depletion after the first week even though serum levels remained constant. After the second week serum levels tended to increase while the total body content of potassium was restored to pre-therapy levels. These same investigators demonstrated a lack of correlation between the serum potassium level and total body potassium content.

Isotope dilution studies utilizing ^{42}K to determine total exchangeable potassium has a serious disadvantage; it requires about 30 to 40 hours for the isotope to achieve equilibrium, and the method underestimates total body potassium.

Most recent determinations utilizing exchangeable potassium, total body potassium, and metabolic balance studies, show that the total loss in body potassium is as great as ten percent following continuous thiazide therapy for two or more weeks.

The metabolic study was utilized in studies by MARONDE (6) to determine the effects of amiloride on intracellular potassium. Patients with mild to moderate essential hypertension, without edema or any evidence of cardiac failure or significant renal disease, received a constant measured diet which contained approximately 90 mEq potassium/24 hrs. Twenty-four-hour urine and weekly stool collections were made, and uneaten food was taken into account for balance calculations. After a period of stable sodium and potassium balance, hydrochlorothiazide 150 mg was given in divided doses for varying periods, averaging over 30 days. At the end of this period amiloride HCl was added, and sodium and potassium balance under the influence of the two drugs was measured.

The first patient accumulated a total net loss of over 700 mEq K^+ in two months on hydrochlorothiazide. With the addition of 10 mg, and then 20 mg, of amiloride there was a cumulative gain of over 200 mEq K^+ within 10 days. The serum potassium levels increased only by 0.5 mEq/l during this same period, while the patient's weight remained constant at 62 kg. Most of the increase in potassium content, therefore, must necessarily have occurred within the intracellular compartment.

The balance study may serve also to discriminate fine differences in responsiveness to dose. The following patient was given various doses of amiloride plus hydrochlorothiazide 150 mg. There was an initial significant loss of both sodium and potassium with hydrochlorothiazide alone; with the addition of amiloride 10 mg, potassium losses were reversed, while sodium excretion showed a further increase.

These trends were accentuated when the dose was increased to 20 mg. At a dosage of 5 mg/day, however, the patient once again went into negative potassium balance and positive sodium balance. These data, plus data derived from other studies, suggest that 10 mg/day or more is the most effective dose of amiloride in reversing a thiazide-induced kaliuresis.

In a third study, the response to the administration of 60 mEq potassium chloride daily was compared to that of amiloride 20 mg/day. In this patient, the negative potassium balance caused by continuous hydrochlorothiazide administration was reversed with both potassium chloride and amiloride. As might be anticipated, sodium losses increased significantly when the two diuretic agents were utilized together. It is interesting to note that there was no significant alteration in the urinary excretion of aldosterone with potassium chloride, but in all studies with amiloride, there was an increase. The mechanism of this increase is not clear, but it may represent a mechanism for control of the antikaliuretic action of the drug.

Sodium loss with thiazides was greatest in the first several days of drug therapy and then rapidly decreased. The loss of potassium, however, continued beyond the first week to 10 days, with the cumulative excretion forming a curve that leveled off usually at 300 to 600 mEq. The net loss in potassium in these studies was about 10% of the estimated total body content of potassium. These findings are in close agreement with studies performed by Bergstrom (7) et al., utilizing whole body counting and tissue analyses, and by Remenchick (8) et al., utilizing both whole body counting and estimates based on total exchangeable potassium. Studies have not been completed as yet on patients receiving diuretic therapy on an intermittent basis, but it is reasonable to assume that the kaliuretic activity could be mitigated or even prevented by use of the drugs intermittently.

Safety Evaluations

The routine performance of hepatic function tests in normal subjects and in patients receiving diuretic therapy for prolonged periods is part of every evaluation. The sensitivity and lack of specificity of enzymatic tests of hepatic function is well known, and a pattern of elevations in numbers of patients is more significant than any single slight increase over normal values. If a significant elevation does occur, however, and the condition of the patient warrants such a trial, repeated enzyme studies following discontinuance of the drug, and then a third test following reinstitution of therapy should be useful in assigning the responsibility for a liver function test abnormality. This so-called "rechallenging" of the patient is an extremely useful tool for clarifying problems related to laboratory values, just as the liver biopsy, in the presence of a possible drug-related jaundice, may be valuable.

Routine hematologic testing for safety is in a somewhat less satisfactory state in the study of new drugs. The clinician, justifiably, is less willing to re-expose a patient with the occurrence of a neutropenia of questionable etiology.

Also, bone marrow biopsy specimens and sections are obtained less frequently in the evaluation of new drugs than are liver biopsies; this is partly reflective of the greater utility of the liver biopsy. Routinely, as part of a chronic safety evaluation, tests of all the coagulation factors are obtained, as well as the routine blood counts. These studies, however, were originally developed for purposes other than drug evaluations, and it is questionable whether coagulation studies in a limited number of subjects have great utility.

The effects of a diuretic agent on renal function are exhaustively examined and become part of the pharmacologic as well as safety assessment of the compound. Almost always, any comparative evaluations that may be initiated include routine, periodic tests of the serum uric acid and the blood urea or creatinine. Studies of carbohydrate metabolism have become exceedingly complex in recent years. Whereas a few years ago studies included only the two hour post-prandial or fasting glucose test, blood insulin assays and tests of peripheral glucose handling, as well as the routine blood glucose, are included as special studies in the examination of new agents.

Part of the conventional evaluation of diuretics and other drugs today includes efforts by isotope studies to trace as precisely as possible the metabolic and excretory pathways of the compound. Often such studies parallel prior investigations performed in animals, but occasionally there may be surprises with studies in man providing useful, new information.

Die klinische Erprobung von Diuretica

Zusammenfassung: Die klinische Auswertung eines neuen Diureticums besteht in der umfassenden Beurteilung des klinischen Nutzens und der Sicherheit. Die Wirkungsweise, die Wirksamkeit im Vergleich zu anderen Medikamenten und praktische Anwendungsgebiete werden durch gut geplante und ausgeführte pharmakologische Untersuchungen bestimmt. Eine Definition des Risikos wird durch spezielle Untersuchungen der Organfunktion und durch routinemäßige Tests der Organfunktion bei allen Patienten erreicht, die das Medikament erhalten.

Bei einem chemischen Präparat ist der Übergang vom Laboratorium in die Klinik und in die Erprobung am Menschen gerechtfertigt, wenn das Mittel Eigenschaften hat, die von früheren Diuretica nicht erreicht wurden. Es wurden Untersuchungen am Menschen entwickelt, die den toxikologischen und pharmakologischen Auswertungen bei Tieren entsprechen. Wenn man sie auch niemals vollkommen voneinander trennen kann, so kann man doch klinische Untersuchungen aufteilen in Beurteilungen der Wirksamkeit und Vergleiche mit anderen Diuretica und in Untersuchungen, die sich primär mit der gefahrlosen Anwendung des Mittels bei Erkrankungen beschäftigen, bei denen es vermutlich zur Anwendung kommen wird. Einige neuere Untersuchungen, die mit dem neuen Diureticum Amilorid (MK-870) durchgeführt wurden, zeigen einige der Schritte, die heute für eine ausreichende Auswertung eines neuen Mittels dieser Klasse erforderlich sind. Da diese Mittel andere Diuretica in ihrer Wirkung verstärken und in gewisser Weise ergänzen, werden sie häufiger bei Patienten gegeben, die natriuretische oder saluretische Mittel erhalten.

Einteilung der Diuretica

Die verschiedenen Klassen von Diuretica, die gegenwärtig verwendet werden, unterscheiden sich in ihrem Angriffspunkt am Nephron. Durch ihre unterschiedliche Wirksamkeit, die verschiedenartigen Elektrolytausscheidungen und Wirkungen auf die Wasserausscheidung haben sie unterschiedliche Anwendungs- und Wirkungsbereiche.

1. Stark natriuretisch wirksame Substanzen

Man kann Quecksilberdiuretica, Etacrynsäure und Furosemid zusammen betrachten, da alle diese Mittel die Fähigkeit haben, bei therapieresistenten Ödemzuständen eine Diurese hervorzurufen.

Quecksilberdiuretica haben den Nachteil, daß sie pH-abhängig sind und injiziert werden müssen, ihre Vorteile sind die hohe Wirksamkeit und die in manchen Fällen verminderte Kaliumausscheidung. Ihre günstige Wirkung auf die Wasserausscheidung kann zusammen mit anderen Maßnahmen bei der Behandlung chronisch kranker hyponatriämischer Patienten mit Ödemen nützlich sein (1).

Man nimmt an, daß die Wirkung von Etacrynsäure und Furosemid hauptsächlich darin besteht, daß sie den Salztransport in dem aszendierenden Schenkel der Henle'schen Schleife hemmen. Beide Mittel wirken oral und parenteral und beide führen zu einer prompten Natriurese und Diurese. Keines der Mittel potenziert die maximale Wirkung des anderen. Es gibt Anzeichen dafür, daß sowohl Furosemid als auch Etacrynsäure eine Änderung des Durchblutungsschemas der Niere hervorrufen, die vielleicht für die stärkere diuretische Wirksamkeit verantwortlich ist. Während Untersuchungen mit Einzeldosen gezeigt haben, daß diese Mittel einen günstigen Na/K-Ausscheidungsquotienten haben, führt doch ihre sehr starke natriuretische und chloruretische Wirkung bei ödematösen Patienten oft zur Entwicklung einer metabolischen Alkalose und sekundärem Aldosteronismus. Durch die resultierende Steigerung der Kaliumausscheidung wird dieser Vorteil wieder aufgehoben.

2. Mäßig starke natriuretisch wirkende Antihypertonica

Eine zweite Gruppe von Pharmaka, zu denen Thiazide und Phthalimidine gehören, ist weniger stark aber klinisch doch noch hoch wirksam. Diese Mittel können zwar eine metabolische Alkalose verursachen, die Tendenz dazu ist aber gewöhnlich geringer als die von Etacrynsäure oder Furosemid, wahrscheinlich weil diese stärkeren Diuretica auch zu einem Mangel an Wasserstoffionen führen. Die Thiazide unterscheiden sich auch dadurch von den stärkeren Mitteln, daß sie den Mechanismus der Harnkonzentration nicht beeinflussen können. Andere mögliche Unterschiede sind die relativ stärkere Einschränkung der glomerulären Filtration und des Plasmaflusses durch die Nieren. Die Wirkungen der Thiazide auf den Kohlehydratstoffwechsel sind besser bekannt als die von Furosemid oder Etacrynsäure; die Untersuchungen mit diesen letzten Mitteln sind noch im Gange. Beide Gruppen von Medikamenten können zu einem erhöhten Harnsäurespiegel im Blut führen.

Der vielleicht größte Vorteil dieser Klasse von Medikamenten ist ihre extrem niedrige Toxizität bei jeder Dosierung und ihr weites Anwendungsspektrum allein oder mit anderen Medikamenten zusammenn bei der Behandlung von Ödemen oder Hypertonie. Wenn eine intermittierende Anwendung möglich ist, führen diese Mittel wie auch die noch stärkeren sehr viel weniger leicht zu exzessivem Kalium- und Chloridverlust und zu metabolischer Alkalose.

3. Schwach natriuretisch und antikaliuretisch wirksame Substanzen

Eine dritte Kategorie von Mitteln wirkt mild diuretisch, führt aber nicht zum Kaliumverlust. Spironolacton ist anerkanntermaßen ein echter Aldosteronantagonist, da seine Aktivität gegen die von Mineralcorticoiden titriert werden kann. Die anderen Mittel dieser allgemeinen Klasse, Triamteren und Amilorid, hemmen den Austausch von Natrium gegen Kalium und Wasserstoff in den distalen Tubuli und wirken auch bei adrenalektomierten Tieren und entsprechenden Menschen. Die Definition und Messung der Wirksamkeit im Falle Kalium-konservierender Mittel erfordert die Bestimmung sowohl der natriuretischen als auch der antikaliuretischen Wirksamkeit.

Klinische Untersuchungen mit Spironolacton haben gezeigt, daß eine Voraussage über die optimal wirksame Dosis ganz und gar nicht leicht ist. Wenn die Dosis von Spironolacton nur auf der Basis der Menge des zirkulierenden Aldosterons berechnet werden könnte, sollte man erwarten, daß deren antikaliuretische Aktivität bei der Hypertonie bei Dosen erreicht wird, die niedriger sind als die bei Zirrhose oder beim nephrotischen Syndrom erforderlichen. In Wirklichkeit sind die zur Verhinderung von Hypokaliämie erforderlichen Mengen von Spironolactone bei nicht ödematösen Hochdruckkranken und bei nephrotischen oder zirrhotischen Patienten ungefähr gleich (9).

Triamteren und Amilorid-HCl (MK 870) haben anscheinend gewisse quantitative Unterschiede, sind aber qualitativ ähnlich. Beide Pharmaka führen zu einer Natriurese bei erniedrigter Kalium- und Wasserstoffionenausscheidung sowie einer Herabsetzung des Blut-pH. Vergleichende Untersuchungen zeigen, daß Amilorid bei gleicher Dosierung stärker und vielleicht wirksamer ist als Triamteren. Einige der Untersuchungen, die bei der kürzlich erfolgten Erprobung des Amilorid vorgenommen wurden, zeigen sehr anschaulich die zur Zeit bei der klinischen Erprobung aller Arten von diuretischen Mitteln verfügbaren und angewendeten Methoden.

Untersuchung von Blut- und Urinelektrolyten

Die Untersuchung der natriuretischen Wirksamkeit diuretischer Mittel beginnt gewöhnlich mit der Untersuchung der Wirkung von Einzeldosen, wobei man ansteigende Dosen des Medikamentes verwendet, beginnend unterhalb des Wirkspiegels.

Die Wirkungen auf Urin- und Serumelektrolyte nach Gabe ansteigender Dosen von Amilorid wurden bestimmt, und es wurde gefunden, daß die zur Erzielung einer Natriurese und einer Kaliumretention erforderlichen Dosen zwischen 4 und 15 mg lagen (11).

Dann wird eine sorgfältigere Untersuchung der Variationsbreite der Dosis angelegt. Solche Untersuchungen werden gewöhnlich an gesunden Freiwilligen vorgenommen, die so ausgewählt sind, daß sie eine homogene Gruppe bilden. Sie bekommen eine fest vorbestimmte Ernährung und erhalten nacheinander das oder die Mittel in der ausgewählten Dosierung. Ausreichend lange Intervalle ohne Gabe von Medikamenten dienen der Vermeidung von Restwirkungen.

Eine solche Untersuchung wurde kürzlich von FOLTZ (2) durchgeführt, um die Wirkungen von MK-870 und Etacrynsäure auf die Kaliumausscheidung im Urin zu bestimmen. Dosen von 50 bis 150 mg Etacrynsäure steigerten die Kaliumausscheidung gegenüber den Kontrollen. Es bestand zwar eine Einschränkung der Kaliurese bei Gabe von Amilorid allein, diese war aber erst im 24-Stunden Sammelurin deutlich nachweisbar. Die Kombination von Etacrynsäure mit Amilorid hob die durch die Etacrynsäure bewirkte Kaliurese, gemessen am 24-Stunden Sammelurin, auf. Etacrynsäure ist ein Medikament, das hauptsächlich innerhalb von 10–12 Stunden wirkt, während sich die Wirkung von Amilorid über 24 Stunden erstreckt. Die spätere Periode der Natriumretention und die bevorzugte Kaliumausscheidung, die durch den Volumenmangel entsteht, kann die Wirksamkeit des zweiten Diureticums sogar erhöhen.

Von WILSON (3) wurde die Wirkung von Amilorid und Triamteren verglichen. Er benutzte ein standardisiertes Auswertungsverfahren, bei dem die therapeutische Wirksamkeit dieser Mittel bei Höchstdosen verglichen wurde. Die Aufeinanderfolge der Mittel wurde so gewählt, daß äußere Faktoren nach Möglichkeit ausgeschaltet waren. Nach Amilorid war bei den verwendeten Dosen die Ausscheidung von Natrium und Chloriden höher und die von Kalium geringer, unabhängig von der gewählten Aufeinanderfolge der Mittel.

Traditionsgemäß basieren die Erprobungen der diuretischen Wirksamkeit auf Tests mit Einzeldosen. Patienten werden jedoch manchmal über längere Zeiträume hin mit kontinuierlicher Gabe bestimmter Dosen behandelt. Die Untersuchung der Reaktion auf eine über längere Zeiträume hin gegebene Dosis eines Mittels zur Bestimmung des echten Gewinns oder Verlustes von Elektrolyten unter genormten Bedingungen ist deshalb eine logische Methode zur Lösung des Problems der Reaktionsweise von Patienten bei chronischer Anwendung des Medikaments.

CONWAY (4) untersuchte die diuretischen Reaktionen bei zwei Gruppen von fünf nichtödematösen Patienten, die 30 mg Amilorid und 100 mg Hydrochlorthiazid pro Tag erhalten hatten. Nach einer Kontrollperiode von vier Tagen erhielten die Patienten Amilorid oder Hydrochlorothiazid, wobei die Zufuhr von Elektrolyten mit der Nahrung konstant gehalten wurde. Während die maximale Ausscheidung von Natrium und Chlorid am ersten Tag bei Hydrochlorothiazid weit größer war, war innerhalb der ganzen 5-Tages-Periode die Gesamtausscheidung von Natrium doch leicht höher bei Amilorid.

Auswertungen dieser Art werden zwar im allgemeinen nicht angewendet, sie erscheinen aber zweckmäßig besonders bei Diuretica und anderen Therapeutica, bei denen eine fortlaufende tägliche Anwendung erwartet werden kann.

Wirkungen auf den Elektrolythaushalt

Untersuchungen des Blutspiegels von Natrium oder Kalium sind insoweit nützlich, als man nach Erfahrung sicher sein kann, daß Veränderungen dieser Werte Veränderungen der Gesamt-Körperelektrolyte widerspiegeln; sie können aber auch irreführend sein. Aus diesem Grunde hat man in den letzten Jahren große Anstrengungen unternommen, geeignete Methoden zur Bestimmung der intrazellulären Elektrolytspiegel bei verschiedenen klinischen Zuständen zu finden, auch bei Anwendung von Diuretica. Einige der Methoden, die schon seit mehreren Jahren zur Verfügung stehen, beginnen erst jetzt bei klinischen Untersuchungen neuer Medikamente praktische Anwendung zu finden. Methoden für die Bestimmung der intrazellulären Elektrolyte sind zum Beispiel Stoffwechsel-Bilanzuntersuchungen, wobei Messungen der Gesamt-Aufnahme und -Ausscheidung von Elektrolyten verwendet werden, sowie Radioisotopen-Verdünnungsmethoden. Probeexzisions-Techniken sind weniger häufig verwendet worden, die Entwicklung von Ultra-Mikromethoden eröffnet aber Aussicht auf eine breitere klinische Anwendung in der Zukunft (7, 10).

Die Verwendung von Ganzkörper-Radioaktivitätsbestimmungen bei klinischen Untersuchungen begann ungefähr vor 10 Jahren. Die für die Kalium-Bilanz angewendete Technik basiert auf der Entdeckung der Gammastrahlung des Isotops K^{40}, das in einem konstanten Verhältnis von 0,0118% in allem natürlichen Kalium enthalten ist. Für genaue Bestimmungen des Gesamt-Körperkaliums bei Patienten wird ein spezieller, empfindlicher Scintillationszähler mit großem Volumen verwendet. Die Ausrüstung besteht aus einem Thallium-aktivierten Natriumjodid-Kristallspektrometer, wobei vier Natriumjodidkristalle um den Patienten herum angeordnet sind und dieser sich in einem Raum mit Stahlwänden befindet. Nach der Kalibrierung bewegen sich diese Kristalle auf und ab und zeichnen das Gammastrahlungsspektrum von K^{40} über eine Stunde hin auf. Die Methode der Bestimmung des Gesamt-Körperkaliums hat die Vorteile einer schnellen Messung und die Möglichkeit wiederholter Untersuchungen ohne wesentliche Strahlengefährdung. Lawrence (5) und Mitarbeiter bestimmten das Gesamt-Körperkalium vor der Behandlung, nach einwöchiger Behandlung mit Etacrynsäure oder Furosemid und nach einer zweiten Woche, während der außer der diuretischen Basistherapie noch Amilorid gegeben wurde. Nach der ersten Woche bestanden Zeichen für Kaliummangel, obwohl die Serumspiegel konstant blieben. Nach der zweiten Woche zeigten die Serumwerte eine Tendenz zum Anstieg, während der Gesamtkaliumgehalt des Körpers zu der Höhe vor der Behandlung zurückkehrte. Diese gleichen Untersucher wiesen eine fehlende Korrelation zwischen Serumkaliumspiegel und Gesamtkaliumgehalt des Körpers nach.

Isotopen-Verdünnungsmethoden mit K^{42} zur Bestimmung des gesamten austauschbaren Kaliums haben einen schwerwiegenden Nachteil; das Isotop braucht etwa 30 bis 40 Stunden zur Erreichung des Gleichgewichts und die Methode unterschätzt den Gesamtgehalt des Körpers an Kalium.

Ganz neue Bestimmungen unter Verwendung von austauschbarem Kalium, Gesamt-Körperkalium und Stoffwechsel-Bilanzuntersuchungen zeigen, daß der Gesamtverlust an Körperkalium nach einer fortlaufenden Thiazidbehandlung von zwei oder mehr Wochen ungefähr 10 Prozent beträgt.

Die metabolische Methode wurde bei den Untersuchungen von Maronde (6) benutzt, um die Auswirkungen von Amilorid auf das intrazelluläre Kalium zu bestimmen. Patienten mit geringer bis mäßiger essentieller Hypertonie ohne Ödeme oder irgendwelche Hinweise auf Herzinsuffizienz oder signifikanter Nierenerkrankung erhielten eine konstante genau bestimmte Diät, die ungefähr 90 mval Kalium/24 Stunden enthielt.

Der 24-Stunden-Urin und der Stuhl wurden gesammelt und nicht gegessene Nahrung wurde bei Bilanzberechnungen berücksichtigt. Nach einer Periode stabiler Natrium- und Kaliumbilanz wurden 150 mg Hydrochlorothiazid über verschiedene Zeiträume in geteilten Dosen gegeben, im Durchschnitt 30 Tage lang. Am Ende dieser Periode wurde Amilorid-HCl noch zusätzlich gegeben und die Natrium- und Kaliumbilanz wurde unter dem Einfluß der beiden Mittel gemessen.

Der erste Patient hatte nach zweimonatiger Behandlung mit Hydrochlorothiazid schließlich einen Gesamtverlust von über 700 mval K. Nach Zugabe von 10 mg und dann 20 mg Amilorid kam es zu einem kumulativen Gewinn von über 200 mval K^+ innerhalb von 10 Tagen. Die Serum-Kaliumspiegel nahmen während der gleichen Periode nur um 0,5 mval/l zu, während das Gewicht des Patienten konstant bei 62 kg blieb. Der größte Teil der Zunahme des Kaliumgehalts muß sich daher notwendigerweise im intrazellulären Raum abgespielt haben.

Die Bilanzuntersuchung kann auch dazu dienen, feine Differenzen der Reaktion auf verschiedene Dosen zu unterscheiden. Der folgende Patient erhielt verschiedene Dosen von Amilorid plus 150 mg Hydrochlorothiazid. Bei Hydrochlorothiazid allein kam es anfänglich zu einem signifikanten Verlust sowohl von Natrium als auch von Kalium; nach Zugabe von 10 mg Amilorid wurde der Kaliumverlust ausgeglichen, während die Natriumausscheidung eine weitere Zunahme zeigte.

Diese Tendenzen wurden verstärkt, wenn die Dosis auf 20 mg erhöht wurde. Unter einer Dosis von 5 mg/Tag zeigte der Patient jedoch wieder eine negative Kaliumbilanz und eine positive Natriumbilanz. Diese Daten sowie die von anderen Untersuchungen lassen vermuten, daß 10 mg/Tag oder mehr beim Amilorid die wirksamste Dosis zur Aufhebung der Thiazid-induzierten Kaliurese ist.

In einer dritten Untersuchung wurde die Reaktion auf eine Gabe von 60 mval Kaliumchlorid täglich mit der von 20 mg Amilorid pro Tag verglichen. Bei diesem Patienten wurde die durch die fortlaufende Hydrochlorothiazidgabe verursachte negative Kaliumbilanz sowohl mit Kaliumchlorid als auch mit Amilorid ausgeglichen. Wie zu erwarten, nahmen die Natriumverluste signifikant zu, wenn die beiden Diuretica zusammen gegeben wurden. Interessant ist, daß mit Kaliumchlorid keine signifikante Veränderung der Ausscheidung von Aldosteron im Urin eintrat, daß es aber bei allen Untersuchungen mit Amilorid zu einem solchen Anstieg kam. Der Mechanismus dieses Anstiegs ist nicht klar, es handelt sich aber möglicherweise um einen Mechanismus der Kontrolle der antikaliuretischen Wirkung des Mittels.

Der Natriumverlust war bei Thiaziden in den ersten Tagen der medikamentösen Behandlung am größten und nahm dann sehr schnell ab. Der Kaliumverlust setzte sich jedoch über die erste Woche bis zu 10 Tagen fort, wobei die kumulative Ausscheidung eine Kurve darstellte, die gewöhnlich bei 300 bis 600 mval abfiel. Der Kaliumverlust betrug bei diesen Untersuchungen ungefähr 10% des geschätzten Gesamt-Körpergehalts von Kalium. Diese Befunde stimmen gut mit Untersuchungen überein, die von BERGSTROM (7) und Mitarb. durchgeführt wurden, die Ganzkörperzählungen und Gewebsanalysen verwendeten und von REMENCHICK (8) und Mitarb., die Ganzkörperzählungen verwendeten sowie Schätzungen, die sich auf das gesamte austauschbare Kalium gründen. Die Untersuchungen an Patienten unter intermittierender diuretischer Therapie sind zur Zeit noch nicht abgeschlossen, man kann aber wohl annehmen, daß die kaliuretische Aktivität durch die intermittierende Anwendung der Mittel gemildert oder sogar unterdrückt wird.

Prüfungen der Gefahrlosigkeit

Die routinemäßige Durchführung von Leberfunktionsproben bei normalen Personen und bei Patienten, die für längere Zeit unter diuretischer Therapie stehen, ist Teil jeder Prüfung. Die Empfindlichkeit und der Mangel an Spezifität enzymatischer Tests der Leberfunktion ist sehr wohl bekannt und eine schematische Erhöhung bei einer großen Anzahl von Patienten ist von größerer Bedeutung als irgendein einzelner leichter Anstieg über Normalwerte. Wenn es jedoch zu einer signifikanten Erhöhung kommt und der Zustand des Patienten einen solchen Versuch rechtfertigt, müßten zur Feststellung der Ursache des pathologischen Ausfalls des Leberfunktionstests wiederholte Enzymuntersuchungen nach Absetzen des Medikaments und ein dritter Test nach Wiederbeginn der Therapie nützlich sein. Dieses sogenannte »rechallenging« des Patienten ist ein extrem nützliches Verfahren zur Klärung von Problemen bezüglich Laborwerten, genau so wie die Leberbiopsie bei einer möglicherweise durch ein Medikament bedingten Gelbsucht wertvoll sein kann.

Die routinemäßige hämatologische Testung auf Gefahrlosigkeit ist bei der Untersuchung neuer Arzneimittel etwas weniger befriedigend. Der Kliniker ist verständlicherweise beim Auftreten einer Neutropenie fraglicher Ätiologie weniger gewillt, einen Patienten der Noxe nochmals auszusetzen.

Auch Knochenmarksbiopsien- und Schnitte werden bei der Erprobung neuer Medikamente weniger häufig angewendet als Leberbiopsien; das spiegelt teilweise den größeren Wert der Leberbiopsie wieder. Routinemäßig werden als Teil chronischer Sicherheitsprüfungen Bestimmungen aller Gerinnungsfaktoren durchgeführt sowie in jedem Falle Blutbilder. Diese Untersuchungen wurden jedoch ursprünglich für andere Zwecke als Arzneimittelprüfungen entwickelt und es ist fraglich, ob Gerinnungsuntersuchungen bei einer begrenzten Zahl von Patienten einen großen Wert haben. Die Auswirkungen der Diuretica auf die Nierenfunktion sind erschöpfend untersucht worden und sind fester Bestandteil sowohl der pharmakologischen Prüfungen als auch der Prüfungen auf Gefahrlosigkeit geworden. Fast immer gehören zu jeglicher vergleichender Prüfung, die eingeleitet wird, routinemäßige wiederholte Bestimmungen der Serum-Harnsäure und des Blut-Harnstoffs oder Kreatinins. Untersuchungen des Kohlehydratstoffwechsels sind in den letzten Jahren äußerst komplex geworden. Während vor wenigen Jahren die Untersuchung nur aus einer Bestimmung des Blutzuckers 2 Stunden nach einer Mahlzeit oder im Nüchternzustand bestand, werden jetzt bei der Prüfung eines neuen Mittels außerdem Blutinsulin-Analysen und Tests der peripheren Glukoseverwertung neben den routinemäßigen Blutzuckeruntersuchungen durchgeführt.

Als Teil einer konventionellen Auswertung von Diuretica und anderer Medikamente versucht man heute, so genau wie möglich durch Isotopenuntersuchungen den Weg des Präparates im Stoffwechsel und die Ausscheidungsweise zu verfolgen. Oft stimmen solche Untersuchungen mit früheren Erforschungen am Tier überein, gelegentlich kann es aber auch Überraschungen geben bei Untersuchungen am Menschen mit nützlichen, neuen Informationen.

Literatur / References

1. EPSTEIN, F. H.: Regulation of major body electrolytes; M. H. MAXWELL, C. R. KLEEMAN: Clinical disorders of fluid and electrolyte metabolism, McGraw-Hill Co., New York, 1962.
2. FOLTZ, E. L.: To be published.
3. LANT, A. F., J. J. SMITH and G. M. WILSON: Clinical evaluation of amiloride (MK-870), a potassium-sparing diuretic. Clin. Pharmacol. and Therap. 10 (1) Jan.-Feb. 1969.
4. HITZENBERGER, G., H. KAMPFFMEYER and J. CONWAY: The diuretic effect of desmethylpipazuroyl-guanidine (MK-870) in man, Clin. Pharm. & Therap. **9**, 71–79, Jan.-Feb. (1968).
5. JOHNY, K. V., J. R. LAWRENCE, A. R. CLARKSON and B. W. WORTHLEY: Total body potassium studies in patients on diuretics using whole body monitor – International Nephrology Society, Oct. 1967.
6. MARONDE, R. F.: To be published.
7. BERGSTROM, J., E. HULTMAN: The effect of thiazides, chlorthalidone and furosemide on muscle electrolytes and muscle glycogen in normal subjects, Acta. Med. Scand. **180**, 363–376 (1966).
8. REMENCHIK, A. P., L. C. JOHNSTON: Potassium depletion produced by administration of chlorthalidone to nonedematous patients with arterial hypertension, Amer. J. Med. Sci. **250**, 171–176 (1966).
9. GANTT, C.: Personal communication.
10. LUND, P. K., J. C. MATHIES: X-ray spectroscopy in biology and medicine. VII. Ultramicro determination of potassium in human tissue and blood serum, Amer. J. Clin. Path. **44**, (4) 398–404, Oct. 1965.
11. BULL, M. B., J. H. LARAGH: Amiloride. A potassium-sparing natriuretic agent, Circulation **37**, 45–53, Jan. 1968.

GROSS: In some of your cases, hydrochlorothiazide was given in a dose of 150 mg per day for months. Is this to be considered a normal dosage?

WILKINSON: The usual dose is 100 mg per day, preferrably on an intermittent basis.

JAHRMÄRKER: The continuous longterm application of the diuretic serves mainly as a toxicity-study. But due to induced hyper-aldosteronism or other adaptive mechanisms, the effect on the mineral metabolism changes, which is in itself an interesting problem. Information on the direct pharmacological action of the diuretic will be achieved better by alternating short term trials. The preference of normal volunteers in such trials is generally accepted in view of uniformity of the results.

WILKINSON: We are talking about the clinical trial versus the controlled comparative study. We certainly would not make final conclusions without a clinical trial. I tried to select some of the techniques employed by us.

LEPPLA: In some of your trials, you found a cumulative potassium loss amounting up to 700 mval. This will cause the serious danger of potassium deficiency with all its hazards including nephropathy.

WILKINSON: This particular patient was an extreme example. As a rule, when the patient approaches a loss of 10% from his calculated body potassium, intervening therapy is started. These studies are performed in a metabolic ward and within a program investigating potassium substitution therapy.

LEPPLA: Let us assume that the subject suffering the 700 mval potassium loss has a total body potassium of 3,500 mval, which is a normal figure for a person weighing 70 kg. This loss would amount to 20% of the body potassium and could not be considered as without risk. If there were no signs of potassium deficiency one could question whether the balance study led to correct results. The safer way would be to measure body potassium by total body gamma counting of the natural ^{40}K radioactivity.

Effects of Combined Application of Antikaliuretic Agents and Diuretics

Kombinierte Anwendung antikaliuretischer Substanzen mit konventionellen Diuretica*) **)

Kh. R. KOCZOREK, H. JAHRMÄRKER, H. HOFMANN, W. VOGT, P. SCHMIEDEK, B. SIMON, E. BALDE

Summary: The potassium-sparing natriuretic agents constitute an important advance in present diuretic therapy. Today, the application of a strong acting saluretic compound alone belonging to the group of conventional diuretics (thiazides, furosemide, ethacrynic acid) as a rule should be avoided in the management of edema of various origin. The combined diuretic therapy with antikaliuretic agents together with conventional diuretics should be given preference and more attention. Clinical-pharmacological studies during recent years have taught us clearly that this combined diuretic therapy provides the better results at less incidence and reduction of unwanted side effects in the homoiostasis of electrolytes and water. The pattern of diuresis as a result of the combined application of antikaliuretic agents and conventional diuretics seems to be more of the physiological type, that means especially a better sodium/chloride-ratio in the daily voided urine without potassium loss. Fixed combinations of diuretic agents, however, are not desirable as during any combined therapy over a longer period of time there will be phases requiring a change of dose-relation of the individual components, demanded by alterations occurring in the electrolyte-water balance resp. in the acid-base balance sooner or later during the course of this type of therapy. Even in a nearly recompensated patient, we face different regulatory situations than we do in the same patient under conditions of severe decompensation.

Progesterone fulfills all of the criteria of specific aldosterone-antagonism as the steroidal spirolactones do. With progesterone, especially when combined with a conventional diuretic we could achieve diuresis of sodium and chloride with loss of edema also. Progesterone nowadays is known as the biological prototype of aldosterone antagonists.

Triamterene and amiloride possess special mechanisms of renal handling of electrolytes and water. These two synthetic substances with anti-aldosterone effects only on the renal level exert their action through mechanisms totally different from that of aldosterone antagonists. But in common with progesterone and the spirolactones, triamterene and amiloride are potassium-sparing natriuretic agents. The simultaneous antichloruretic effects of these antikaliuretic diuretics as shown in our diagrams are important for the management and prevention of hypochloremic alkalosis. In patients with such a disturbance a disproportion may be existent between the quantity of sodium demanding reabsorption and the amount of reabsorbable anion available for this purpose. This fact necessarily maintains an accelerated rate of sodium-hydrogen and sodium-potassium exchange with the consequence that metabolic alkalosis will persist until chloride is provided in sufficient amounts for normalization of the sodium-cation exchange.

The advantages of the combined diuretic therapy are discussed, including the intermittent treatment of outpatients over long periods, presenting multiple examples for the application

*) Mit Unterstützung durch die Deutsche Forschungsgemeinschaft.

**) Technische Assistenz: Frau HANNA GROHMANN und Frl. BARBARA RÖSING.

of antikaliuretic agents of the above mentioned types alone and together with conventional diuretics in the management of patients with congestive heart failure, liver cirrhosis with ascites and nephrotic syndrome.

From our data presented in this paper it is obvious, that an understanding of the characteristic mechanisms of the different diuretics is essential for the proper and safe use of such powerful agents.

Die (patho)physiologischen Mechanismen, die der Niere zur Konservierung und Elimination von Elektrolyten unter differenten Bedingungen zur Verfügung stehen, sind so vielschichtiger Natur, daß unsere Kenntnisse der einzelnen Funktionsabläufe und ihrer endokrinen als auch nicht-endokrinen Steuerungsmöglichkeiten sich in gewissen Zeitabständen immer wieder als ergänzungsbedürftig erweisen. Es ist daher verständlich, wenn es den Pharmazeuten noch nicht gelungen ist, ein Diureticum mit derart gekoppelten Eigenschaften zu entwickeln, daß nacheinander oder gleichzeitig die verschiedenen Ionenresorptions- und Austauschmechanismen in optimaler Weise beeinflußt würden, deren Aufgabe in den proximalen und distalen Nephronabschnitten die Modifizierung der Elektrolytausscheidung im Endharn ist. Von einem solchen Diureticum müßte man erwarten, daß es bei oraler Wirksamkeit die renale Elimination von Elektrolyten und Wasser in einem Verhältnis fördert, das weitgehend der Zusammensetzung des extrazellulären Flüssigkeitsraumes entspricht. Es müßte diese Wirkung auch bei Daueranwendung behalten und dürfte keine toxischen Nebenwirkungen zeigen.

Diesen Anforderungen, die der Therapeut stellen muß, wird heute noch keines der bekannten Diuretica gerecht. Alle bisher synthetisierten diuretischen Substanzen führen bei alleiniger Anwendung über kürzere oder längere Zeit in mehr oder minder ausgeprägtem Maße zu Störungen der Ionengleichgewichte des Organismus. Es ist aber dennoch möglich, diese therapeutischen Forderungen annähernd zu erfüllen, wenn man den Weg über die kombinierte Anwendung der sog. konventionellen Diuretica mit einem Aldosteron-Antagonisten oder einer anderen antikaliuretischen Substanz in der Behandlung von pathologischen Wasseransammlungen verschiedener Genese beschreitet.

Eine erfolgreiche diuretische Kombinationsbehandlung setzt allerdings genaue Kenntnisse der Wirkungsbilder der einzelnen Substanzen und der ihnen zugrundeliegenden Wirkungsprinzipien voraus. Dabei ist das Problem zu berücksichtigen, daß der Organismus im Verlauf der Krankheit eine durchaus wechselnde Natriumretention aufweisen kann.

Kochsalzrestriktion

Schon vor der Erkenntnis der Bedeutung des Aldosterons für die normale und pathologische Regulation des Elektrolyt- und Wasserhaushaltes galt im therapeutischen Bemühen des Arztes die Erfahrung, daß ohne Kochsalz eine Ödembildung nicht möglich ist. Und auch heute noch ist der *Kochsalz- und damit Natriumentzug in der Nahrung eine der wirksamsten Maßnahmen* in der Therapie der mit Ödemen einhergehenden Erkrankungen. Beispielsweise werden bei einer wirklich streng kochsalzarmen Ernährung ca. 90% der Herzkranken praktisch ödemfrei und bleiben es auch. Meistens jedoch – besonders bei ambulanten Patienten – kann eine ausreichende Einschränkung der Kochsalzzufuhr nicht so straff durchgeführt werden wie es erforderlich wäre. Einen

Ausweg aus dieser Situation stellt die Anwendung der Saluretica dar, die wir heute als sog. konventionelle Diuretica den Aldosteron-Antagonisten und den anderen Anti-Aldosteron-Substanzen gegenüberstellen.

Konventionelle Diuretica

Zu diesen diuretisch wirksamen Pharmaca gehören neben den Quecksilberpräparaten und Carboanhydrasehemmern – auf die wir heute in der Klinik meist verzichten können – vor allem die Sulfonamid-Diuretica vom Typ des Chlorothiazids und seine Derivate, sowie das Chlorthalidon. In jüngster Zeit sind als besonders stark und sehr rasch wirkende Saluretica das Furosemid und die Etacrynsäure hinzugekommen. Mit Hilfe dieser Substanzen gelingt es, die renale Kochsalz- d. h. Natriumausscheidung und sekundär hierzu auch die Wasserausscheidung zu steigern. Jedoch stellte sich jeweils bald heraus, daß ein Teil der Patienten mit hydropischen Erkrankungen aus hepatischer, cardialer oder renaler Ursache gegenüber diesen modernen Diuretica refraktär wurde. Als weiterer Nachteil dieser an sich potenten Diuretica wirkte es sich aus, daß vielfach die im proximalen Tubulus erzeugte Natriurese anschließend im distalen Tubulus teilweise in eine Kaliurese umgewandelt werden kann, und zwar dann, wenn im distalen Abschnitt des Nephron unter einer erhöhten Aldosteronaktivität ein gesteigerter Ionenaustausch von Natrium gegen Kalium stattfindet. Daher werden durch die Anwendung der Saluretica vor allem diejenigen Ödemkranken von Kaliumverlusten mit ihren unerwünschten Komplikationen bedroht, deren Natriumretention hauptsächlich durch einen sekundären Aldosteronismus unterhalten wird. Es ist deshalb eine geläufige Erfahrung, daß die Anwendung solcher potentiell kaliopenisch wirkenden Diuretica gerade bei Patienten mit einer Leberzirrhose mit Ascites oder einem nephrotischen Syndrom, aber auch bei vielen Fällen von Herzinsuffizienz nicht selten zu bedrohlichen Kaliummangelzuständen führen kann.

Aldosteron-Antagonisten

Nachdem man nach den Ergebnissen zahlreicher experimenteller und klinischer Untersuchungen über die Pathogenese der Ödeme der verschiedenen Krankheitsgruppen sowohl für die Refrakterität gegen die konventionellen Diuretica als auch für deren – therapeutisch absolut unerwünschte – Kaliummehrausscheidung eine gesteigerte Aldosteronaktivität im distalen Abschnitt des Nephrons verantwortlich machen konnte, war es naheliegend, nach Möglichkeiten zu forschen, die es erlaubten, speziell den Aldosteroneinfluß auf diesen Anteil der Natriumrückresorption im renalen Tubulussystem auszuschalten. Hierfür boten sich drei Wege an:

1. Man konnte versuchen, die Stimuli und/oder tropen Faktoren auszuschalten, die eine pathologische Aldosteronaktivität auslösen bzw. vermitteln können. Dies Vorhaben erwies sich jedoch insofern als schwierig, als viele Auslösungsmechanismen des Aldosteronismus diskutiert wurden, und man ist sich wohl auch heute noch nicht einig, ob hämodynamische, reflektorische, humorale, intrazelluläre oder pH-abhängige Mechanismen im Vordergrund stehen. Man bemüht sich daher, an der zugrundeliegenden Störung anzugreifen, indem man z. B. bei der hydropischen Herzinsuffizienz mit denjenigen

Maßnahmen eine Diurese vorzubereiten und einzuleiten versucht, die die Herzfunktion bessern (Bettruhe, Glykosidgaben, evtl. Sauerstoff, venendrucksenkende Maßnahmen, Frequenztherapie etc.).

2. Man konnte versuchen, die Aldosteronbiosynthese in der Nebennierenrinde durch chemische Substanzen wie Amphenon B, Metopiron (SU-4885) oder Triparanol zu hemmen. Diese Versuche haben letzten Endes zu keinen befriedigenden Resultaten geführt, da die verwendeten Stoffe, abgesehen von manchen unerwünschten Nebenwirkungen, nicht nur die Aldosteronsynthese, sondern auch die Biosynthese der anderen Nebennierenrindensteroide blockieren. Sie fallen damit (in der vorliegenden Form) für die Routinebehandlung aus. Nicht zuletzt gilt dies für die 11-beta-Hydroxylasehemmer auch darum, weil durch sie eine Kette von Kompensationsmechanismen einschließlich einer gesteigerten ACTH-Freisetzung ausgelöst wird und sie u. a. so eine gesteigerte Sekretion von mineralotropen Corticosteroiden wie 11-Desoxycortisol und Cortexon zur Folge haben. Diese beiden letztgenannten Substanzen können dabei in solchen Mengen auftreten, daß sie die Hemmung der Aldosteronsynthese wieder zunichtemachen und weiterhin eine gesteigerte Natriumretention begünstigen. Man hat allerdings versucht, die Natriurese doch zu erzwingen, indem man zusätzlich zu den 11-beta-Hydroxylasehemmern einen ACTH-Hemmer (z. B. Prednison) verabreichte und auf diese Weise auch die gesteigerte Sekretion von 11-Desoxycortisol und Cortexon verhinderte. Möglicherweise sind aber Substanzen wie Amphenon B und Metopiron als Prototypen neuer Pharmaca anzusehen, die vielleicht eines Tages eine spezifische Hemmung nur der Aldosteronsynthese ohne Aufstau anderer mineralotroper Substanzen erlauben. Über die Effekte von Substanzen wie Aminoglutethimide auf die Nebennierenfunktion des Menschen (Fishman et al. 1967) liegen noch keine ausreichenden Erfahrungen vor, um ihre künftige Bedeutung im täglichen Therapieplan sicher abschätzen zu können. Zunehmendes Interesse erfahren derzeit wieder, im Zusammenhang mit dem Renin-Angiotensin-System, die *Anti-Aldosteron-Eigenschaften des Heparins*, die erstmals von Majoor et al. (1957) näher untersucht worden sind, und auch gewisser Heparinoide (wie z. B. des Versuchspräparates Ro I – 8307). Neben einer Reihe anderer Autoren können wir auf Grund eigener Beobachtungen und bisher unveröffentlichter Untersuchungsergebnisse (Koczorek 1959 und 1960) die Anti-Aldosteron-Effekte des Heparins und des Heparinoids Ro I–8307 (Koczorek 1964) bei hydropischen Patienten mit sekundärem Aldosteronismus bestätigen. Bei diesen Untersuchungen überraschte uns auch der erhebliche diuretische (und natriuretische) Effekt der gleichzeitigen Anwendung von Heparin und Spironolactone (Abb. 21), insbesondere beim cardialen Hydrops.

3. Man konnte versuchen, die Aldosteronaktivität direkt am Erfolgsorgan auszuschalten, also besonders am Tubulusapparat der Nieren. Solche Substanzen mit den gewünschten aldosteronantagonistischen Eigenschaften hat man schließlich in der Gruppe der Steroid-Spirolactone auch gefunden. Den konventionellen Diuretica gegenüber haben diese Aldosteronantagonisten zwei sehr wesentliche Vorzüge. Sie haben einmal einen anderen Angriffspunkt am Nephron und vor allem einen von den konventionellen Diuretica völlig verschiedenen Wirkungsmechanismus. Obwohl selbst von meist schwächerer diuretischer Wirkung, machen sie wegen dieser besonderen Eigenschaften einen weiteren Anteil von sog. therapierefraktären Patienten der Ausschwemmung überschüssigen Kochsalzes und Wassers zugänglich. Zum anderen Mal führt ihr Einsatz nicht zu Kaliumverlusten,

sondern im Gegenteil oft sogar zu einer Kaliumretention mit Normalisierung des unter der Einwirkung von Mineralocorticoiden und der diuretischen Therapie verminderten Kaliumbestandes des Organismus.

Unsere Kenntnisse über Aldosteronantagonisten sind also eng verknüpft mit dem patho-physiologischen Verständnis der Aldosteronwirkung in der Pathogenese hydropischer Krankheitsbilder. Wir konnten 1957 an mehr als 100 Fällen von sekundärem Aldosteronismus verschiedener Genese zeigen, daß äquivalente Aldosteronmengen im Harn mit einer quantitativ unterschiedlichen Natriumausscheidung einhergehen (BUCHBORN, KOCZOREK und WOLFF, 1957). Als Ursachen dieser wechselnden Beziehung zwischen Aldosteronausscheidung und Natriurese wurde in der Folgezeit von verschiedenen Arbeitsgruppen eine Reihe von modifizierenden Faktoren aufgeklärt, die sich nur z. T. als krankheitsspezifisch erwiesen und unter denen Veränderungen der Natriumzufuhr, der Körperlage, der intrarenalen Hämodynamik, der tubulären Aldosteronempfindlichkeit und des hepatischen Aldosteronmetabolismus (vgl. Beitrag MULLER, S. 421) neben anderen zu nennen sind.

Progesteron - Biologischer Prototyp der Aldosteronantagonisten

Besonders wichtig im Hinblick auf die Aldosteronantagonisten ist die Gruppe der normalen und pathologischen Graviditäten. Hier fanden sich in unseren Untersuchungen (KOCZOREK, WOLFF und BEER, 1957) bei normalen Schwangerschaften sehr hohe Aldosteronaktivitäten im Harn bei regelrechten Elektrolytverhältnissen, insbesondere also ohne eine Beeinflussung der renalen Natriumausscheidung, so daß quasi das Bild einer tubulären Aldosteron-»Refraktärität« vorlag, oder nach heutiger Nomenklatur: Ein renales Escape-Phänomen. Da sich parallel zu dieser erhöhten Aldosteronausscheidung, zumal im letzten Trimenon der Normalgravidität, regelmäßig auch eine erhöhte Progesteronproduktion findet, lag die Vermutung nahe, daß die natriumretinierende Wirkung solch hoher Aldosteronmengen im Harn Gravider durch eine gleichzeitig erhöhte, natriumeliminierende Progesteronaktivität neutralisiert werden könnte.

Wir hatten bei normalen Schwangerschaften Aldosteronausscheidungen im Urin von 16 µg bis 108 µg pro Tag gemessen, progressiv ansteigend vom 4. bis 9. Monat. Die Werte normaler, nichtgravider Frauen hatten wir zwischen 0,6 µg und 7,0 µg Aldosteron/24 Stunden-Urin liegend gefunden. Bei Spätgestosen war die Aldosteronausscheidung mit Werten zwischen 15 µg und 72 µg Aldosteron/Tag gegenüber den gesunden Graviden im letzten Schwangerschaftsmonat um ca. 30% vermindert. Bei beiden Gruppen waren die Werte post partum innerhalb weniger Tage zur Norm zurückgekehrt. Unter dem Eindruck dieser Befunde war die Ursache des Aldosteronismus dieser beiden untersuchten Gruppen in den Bedingungen der Gravidität selbst zu suchen.

Aus den Untersuchungen von LANDAU u. Mitarb. (1955) und auch aus eigenen Beobachtungen an Normalpersonen und Ödemkranken (KOCZOREK 1957) wußten wir, daß Progesteron in Mengen von 50–300 mg/d einen starken natriuretischen Effekt besitzt. Wir haben seinerzeit darum einen Antagonismus zwischen natriumbewahrenden und natriumeliminierenden Faktoren angenommen und den *Hyperaldosteronismus der Gravidität als Anpassungsvorgang an die durch die Bedingungen der Schwangerschaft gesteigerte Produktion des natriuretisch wirkenden Progesterons* gedeutet.

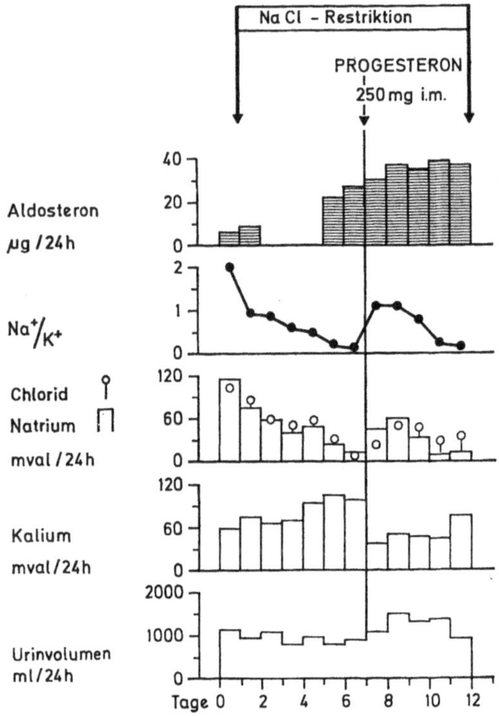

Abb. 1. Nachweis des aldosteronantagonistischen Effektes einer einmaligen, intramuskulären Progesterongabe bei einem gesunden Mann (B.L., 35 Jahre) mit einer durch diätetischen Salzentzug gesteigerten Aldosteronproduktion. – Der steile Anstieg des Na/K-Quotienten im Urin trotz der erhöhten Aldosteronaktivität spiegelt die vermehrte Natriurese und verminderte Kaliurese unter dem Progesteroneinfluß deutlich wider. Die nach Progesteroninjektion weiterhin zunehmende Aldosteronurie läßt erkennen, daß dieser Effekt nicht über eine Hemmung der adrenalen Aldosteronbiosynthese zustande kommt. Die renale Chloridausscheidung unter Progesteron nimmt im Verhältnis zur Natriumelimination weniger stark zu, als man es bei den herkömmlichen Diuretica z. B. aus der Thiazidreihe beobachten kann. Aldosteron wurde nach der Methode von NEHER und WETTSTEIN (J. Clin. Invest.: **35,** 800; 1956) bestimmt. (Nach KOCZOREK 1960).

Ein solcher Antagonismus konnte schließlich auch zwischen exogen zugeführtem Aldosteron und Progesteron an Addison-Patienten (LANDAU u. Mitarb. 1958, KOCZOREK 1961) und an adrenalektomierten Ratten (KAGAWA 1958) im sog. Kagawa-Test nachgewiesen werden. Wir fanden auch bei Normalpersonen unter Salzentzug, d. h. mit hoher endogener Aldosteronproduktion eine Zunahme der Natriumausscheidung ohne gleichzeitige Steigerung der Kaliumausscheidung nach parenteralen Gaben von 60–250 mg Progesteron. Die Aldosteronproduktion erfuhr dabei keine Hemmung; es wurde im Gegenteil sogar eine weitere Steigerung der Aldosteronurie beobachtet (KOCZOREK 1957; KOCZOREK und WOLFF 1960; KOCZOREK 1960), wie das Beispiel in Abb. 1 zeigt. Schließlich führt Progesteron auch zu einer Umkehr der Aldosteronwirkung auf die Wasserstoff-Ionenausscheidung im Urin, während das Gestagen bei Abwesenheit von Mineralocorticoiden im Organismus solche Effekte (ebenso wie die Spirolactone) nicht erkennen läßt (= Abb. 3). Seither konnte die natriuretische Wirksamkeit des Progesterons auch an Fällen von sekundärem Aldosteronismus bei dekompensierter Leberzirrhose (Abb. 5) und Herzinsuffizienz und auch beim nephrotischen Syndrom (Abb. 6) mehrfach bestätigt werden (KOCZOREK 1957; KOCZOREK und WOLFF 1960; DUCOMMUN und ENGEL 1960; JØRGENSEN und EILERSEN 1960; JENKINS 1961; KOCZOREK 1962). Nachdem neueste Untersuchungen die Korrelation zwischen Aldosteron und Progesteron bei Graviditäten und Spätgestosen auch anhand ihrer Sekretionsraten (Lit. bei KOCZOREK 1962) zeigen konnten und Progesteron nach allen vorliegenden Untersuchungen den Kriterien eines spezifischen Aldosteronantagonisten durchaus entspricht, muß man im Progesteron den ersten überhaupt beschriebenen und bisher einzigen, näher bekannten körpereigenen Aldosteronantagonisten sehen.

Wenn auch somit während der letzten Jahre von einigen Arbeitsgruppen mehrfach gezeigt worden ist, daß die aldosteronantagonistischen Wirkungen des Progesterons in gleicher Weise wie die Spirolacton-Effekte zur erfolgreichen Therapie (vor allem in Kombination mit konventionellen Diuretica) von verschiedenen Ödemkrankheiten ausgenutzt werden können, wird Progesteron als Aldosteronantagonist in Zukunft doch nur für klinisch-experimentelle Fragestellungen seine Bedeutung behalten.

Früher von uns erhobene Befunde über extrarenale Effekte der Spirolactone und von Progesteron hatten wir (Koczorek, von Bubnoff und Riecker 1962) dahingehend interpretiert, daß die Aldosteronantagonisten neben ihren bekannten renalen Auswirkungen auch die Ionenverteilung an anderen Körperzellen beeinflussen können, »sei es über eine Auswirkung der renal erzeugten Bilanzstörung oder sei es durch direkten Angriff an den zellulären Substraten«. Neuere Untersuchungen über den Einfluß von Aldosteron und Aldosteronantagonisten (Baethmann et al. 1968; Koczorek et al. 1968) auf den Elektrolyttransport beim experimentellen Hirnödem und beim chronischen Hirnödem

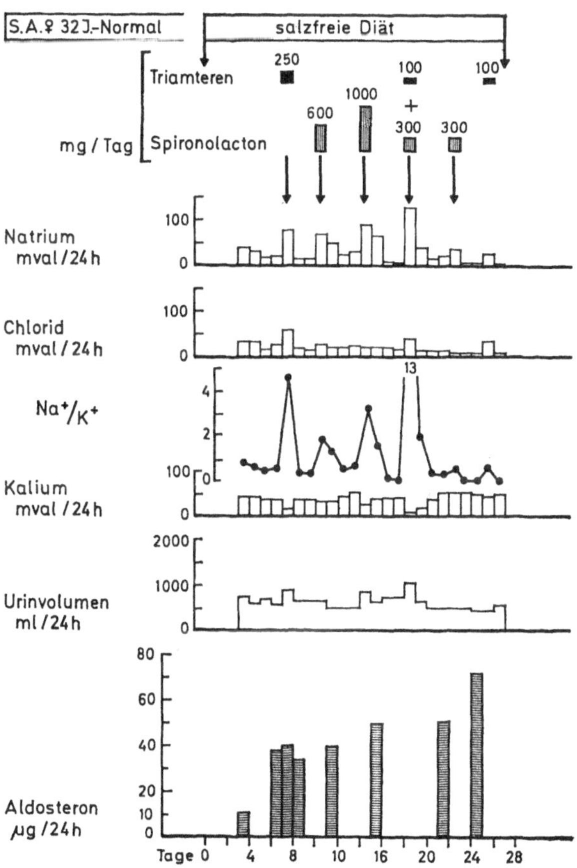

Abb. 2. Vergleich der Wirkung einmaliger und kombinierter Gaben von Spironolacton und Triamteren in verschiedener Dosierung auf die renale Elektrolyt-, Wasser- und Aldosteronausscheidung einer gesunden Frau (S.A., 32 Jahre) mit einem durch Natriumrestriktion hervorgerufenen Hyperaldosteronismus. – Die ersten Messungen der verschiedenen Parameter im Urin wurden am vierten Tag nach Beginn des diätetischen Salzentzugs vorgenommen. Die kombinierte Anwendung von Triamteren und Spironolacton führt zu einer stärkeren Beeinflussung der Elektrolytzusammensetzung des Endharnes als die jeweiligen Substanzen allein. Diese Abbildung zusammen mit Abb. 1 zeigen auch deutlich die Ähnlichkeit der Effekte von Progesteron, Spironolacton und Triamteren in qualitativer Hinsicht, auch wenn das quantitative Ausmaß der renalen Auswirkungen unterschiedlich ist (Nach Koczorek 1960).

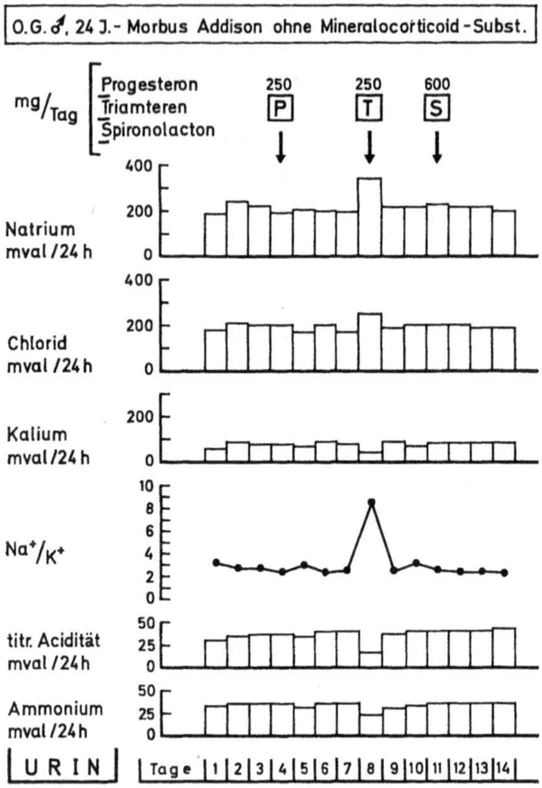

Abb. 3. Vergleich der Wirkung von Progesteron, Triamteren und Spironolacton auf die renale Ausscheidung von Natrium, Chlorid, Kalium, Wasser, titrierbare Azidität und Ammonium bei einem 24jährigen Patienten (O.G.) mit einem M. Addison während einer Phase ohne Mineralocorticoidsubstitution. Progesteron und Spironolacton bleiben als Aldosteronantagonisten ohne erkennbare Wirkung, während Triamteren seine typischen Effekte auf die renale Elektrolytausscheidung behält (Nach Koczorek 1961).

des Menschen, weisen ebenfalls auf extrarenale Effekte der Aldosteronantagonisten hin, lassen jedoch gleichzeitig vermuten, daß eine Steigerung des Elektrolyttransportes unter Aldosteronantagonisten zwischen intra- und extrazellulären Räumen nur dann möglich ist, wenn der Organismus die Fähigkeit behält, auf den Einfluß der Aldosteronantagonisten mit einem reaktiven Aldosteronismus zu antworten (siehe auch Beitrag Reulen et al., S. 469). Extrarenale Effekte an elektrolytaustauschenden Zellen ließen sich für die Spirolactone (Moll und Koczorek 1961) und für Progesteron (Koczorek und Moll 1961) auch am Rattendarm nachweisen. Auf die Steigerung des Elektrolyttransportes durch Aldosteron an verschiedenen Zellmembranen bei der adrenalektomierten Ratte haben Senft und Mitarb. ausdrücklich hingewiesen (Senft und Losert 1963; Losert, Senft und Senft 1964).

Kriterien des Aldosteronantagonismus

Die Kriterien eines spezifischen Aldosteronantagonismus einer diuretischen Substanz lassen sich scharf umreißen. Sie sollen hier noch einmal zusammengefaßt werden. Von einer aldosteronantagonistisch wirksamen Substanz muß man erwarten, daß sie

1. an den mineralaustauschenden Zellgrenzflächen alle Aldosteronwirkungen verhindert, d. h. an der Niere a) zu einer Steigerung der Natriurese, b) zu einer Verminderung der

Kaliurese, und c) zu einer Verminderung der Wasserstoff-Ionenausscheidung (gemessen an titrierbarer Azidität und Ammoniumausscheidung) führt;

2. die aldosteronantagonistischen Effekte auch außerhalb der Niere an anderen elektrolytaustauschenden Körperzellen entfaltet, wenn diese unter einem Aldosteroneinfluß stehen;

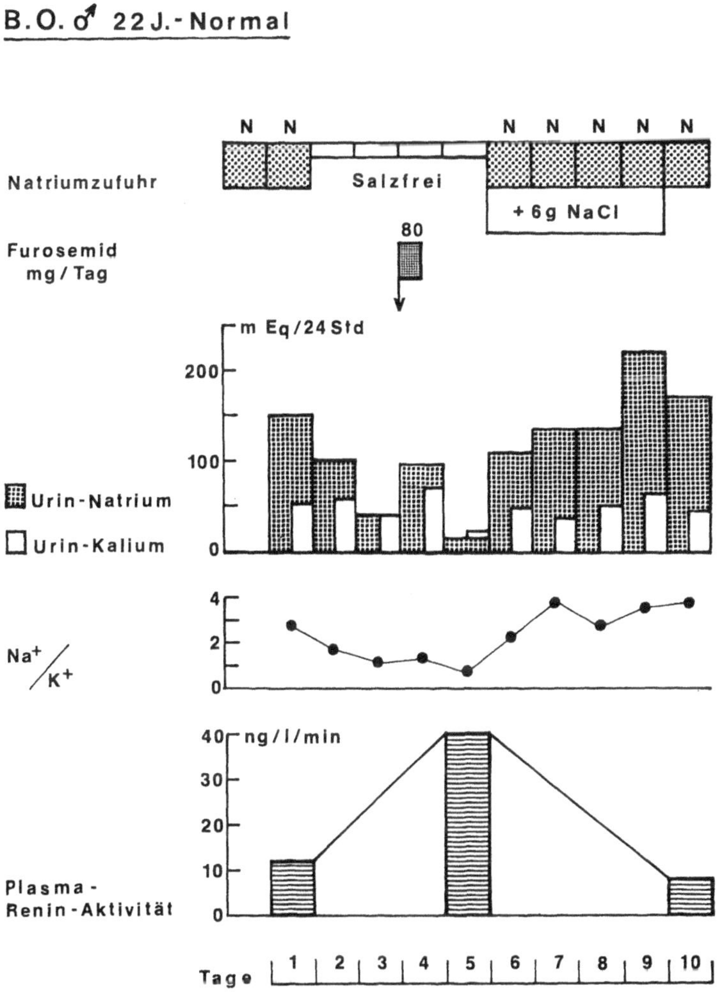

Abb. 4. Verhalten der Plasma-Renin-Aktivität bei einem gesunden, männlichen Probanden (B.O., 22 Jahre) unter normaler (freigewählter) Natriumzufuhr, Salzentzug (salzfreie Diät und zusätzlich 80 mg Furosemid am dritten Tag der salzfreien Untersuchungsperiode) und anschließender erhöhter Natriumzufuhr (täglich zusätzlich 6 g Kochsalz zur normalen Kost). – Die Änderung der Plasma-Renin-Aktivität unter diesen Bedingungen weist auf die Verknüpfung des Renin-Angiotensin-Systems mit der adrenalen Aldosteronproduktion hin (nach Koczorek und Mitarbeitern 1967). Die Plasma-Renin-Aktivität wurde nach der Methode von Boucher et al. [Canad. Med. Assoc. J. 90, 194 (1964) bestimmt].

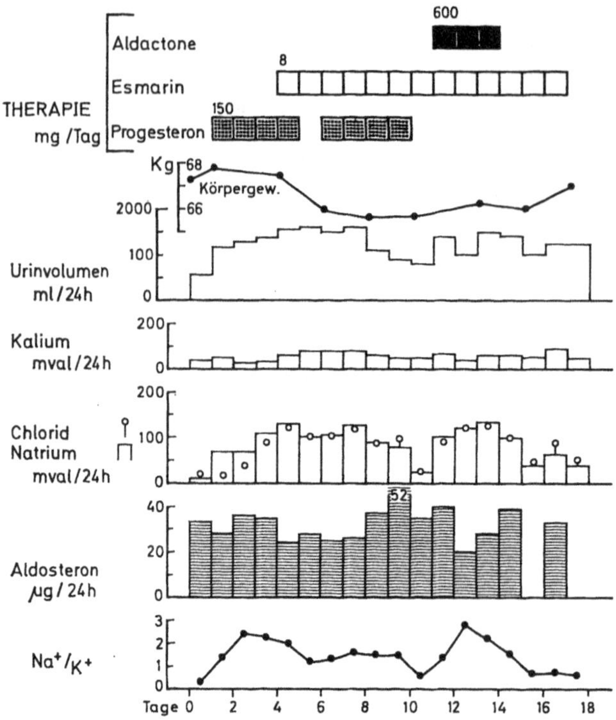

Abb. 5. Diuretische Behandlung einer 69jährigen Patientin (J.A.) mit einer posthepatitischen, dekompensierten Leberzirrhose (und Herzinsuffizienz bei Hypertonie) mit Progesteron bzw. der Kombination Progesteron/Esmarin und Aldactone/Esmarin. – Beginn der Behandlung am 4. 7. 1961 (= Tag 0 in der Abb.). Serum-Kalium-Konzentration am 5. 7. 1961 = 3,55 mval/l; am 18. 7. 1961 = 4,15 mval/l. Sonstige (in der Abbildung nicht verzeichnete) Therapie: salzfreie Leberschonkost, Vitamine, Verdauungsfermente, Laevoral-Trinkkuren, Glykoside und täglich 5 mg Prednisolon. Unter Progesteron allein war entsprechend den aldosteronantagonistischen Eigenschaften des Gestagenes ein Anstieg der Natriumausscheidung mit einem Anstieg des Na/K-Quotienten und einem, im Verhältnis zur Natriurese, geringeren Anstieg der Chloridausscheidung zu beobachten. Die Wasserbilanz wurde negativ. Unter der kombinierten Anwendung Progesteron/Esmarin (= Trichlormethiazid) fand sich eine ähnliche Elektrolytzusammensetzung im Endurin wie unter der nachfolgenden kombinierten Anwendung von Aldactone/Esmarin. – Einen wesentlich stärkeren diuretischen Effekt hatte etwa 1½ Jahre später der kombinierte Einsatz von Aldactone/Esmarin/Heparin bei der Patientin, der innerhalb von 21 Tagen zu einem Verlust von 9 kg Ödemflüssigkeit geführt hat. Vergl. hierzu auch die Wirkung von Heparin auf die Elektrolytausscheidung des Patienten J. K. in Abb. 21.

3. die antagonistischen Wirkungen nur in Anwesenheit von Aldosteron (oder einem aldosteronähnlichen Corticoid) erkennen läßt;
4. die Wirkungen an den gleichen Lokalisationen ausübt wie der Mineralocorticoid-Agonist, also insbesondere keine Hemmung der adrenocorticalen Aldosteronproduktion bzw. -sekretion hervorruft, wie man es von den 11-beta-Hydroxylasehemmern, dem Triparanol und den Heparinoiden kennt;
5. die Nierendurchblutung und die Glomerulumfiltration nicht unmittelbar beeinflußt; und daß
6. die aldosteronantagonistischen Effekte durch eine Steigerung der Aldosteronmenge wieder durchbrochen werden können.

Allen diesen Forderungen werden bisher nur Progesteron und die synthetischen Spirolactone gerecht. Aus dieser Gruppe ist das Spironolacton (= Aldactone oder Aldactone A) am bekanntesten geworden. *Von Triamteren und von Amilorid* (= MK 870 = Amipramidine = Amipramizide in der Literatur), einem Guanidin-Derivat mit triamterenähnlicher Wirkung, die wir in den letzten Jahren ebenfalls klinisch überprüften, *werden diese Kriterien nicht in allen Punkten erfüllt.*

Erwähnenswert in diesem Zusammenhang erscheint uns, daß die durch Butazolidin bewirkte Natriumretention durch die Spirolactone nicht beeinflußt werden kann. Hingegen ist noch zu überprüfen, ob Triamteren und Amilorid in dieser Situation wirksam sind.

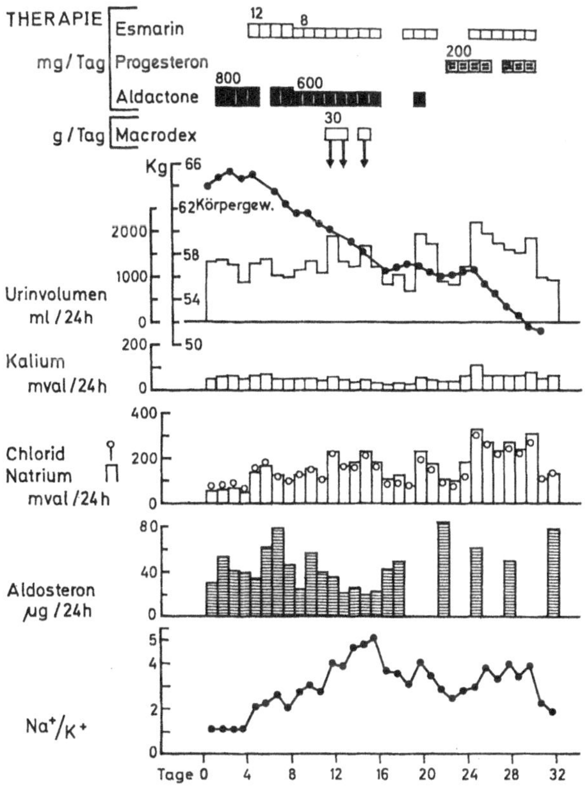

Abb. 6. Kombinierte diuretische Behandlung einer 21jährigen Patientin mit einem nephrotischen Syndrom bei Lupus Erythematodes (K. W.) – Diese Patientin hatte vor Beginn des in dieser Abbildung dargestellten Behandlungsabschnitts unter ACTH, Masoten (Na-bindender Kationenaustauscher), salzarmer Diät und gelegentlichen Diureticagaben (Navidrex, Esidrix) innerhalb von 20 Tagen rund 10 kg Wasser eingelagert. Bereits bei der Klinikaufnahme hatten massive Ödeme bestanden, bei einer Erniedrigung des Gesamteiweißes auf 4,2% und einer nephrotischen Dysproteinämie im Elektrophoresediagramm. Die Ursache der Hypoproteinämie war in einer Proteinurie mit Eiweißverlusten von 8–10 g Eiweiß/24 Std. zu sehen. Als Ausdruck der vorwiegenden Nierenbeteiligung des Erythematodes visceralis disseminatus im Sinne der Erythematodes – Nephritis bestand eine Hypertonie mit Blutdruckwerten von 180/110 mm Hg. Die Funktionsdiagnostik der Niere hatte eine hochgradige Verminderung des Glomerulumfiltrates auf etwa ¼ der Norm bei relativ geringerer Einschränkung der Nierendurchblutung ergeben, wie dies für die Nierenmanifestation des Erythematodes charakteristisch ist. Die diuretische Kombinationsbehandlung mit Aldactone/Esmarin und Progesteron/Esmarin, sowie Makrodexinfusionen als Plasmaexpander führte zu einer kontinuierlichen Ausschwemmung der Ödeme mit einer Abnahme des Körpergewichts von 62,2 kg auf 51,4 kg. Bei der Entlassung aus der Klinik bestanden nur noch geringe prätibiale Ödeme. Sonstige (in der Abbildung nicht verzeichnete) Therapie: Penicillin, Propoquin und Dianabol, sowie salzfreie Diät. Serumelektrolyte am Beginn der kombinierten Behandlung: Natrium = 137 mval/l, Kalium = 3,95 mval/l, Standardbikarbonat = 23 mval/l, pH = 7,36. Serumelektrolyte am Ende der kombinierten Behandlung: Natrium = 144 mval/l, Kalium = 4,72 mval/l, Standardbikarbonat = 22,8 mval/l. Der Rest-N-Wert war unter der Diuresetherapie von 88 mg% vor Beginn der Medikation auf 27 mg% abgesunken. Auffällig ist hier, daß die Kombination Progesteron/Trichlormethiazid eine stärkere Natrium-Diurese herbeigeführt hat, als die Kombination Aldactone/Trichlormethiazid (Nach Koczorek und Edel 1961).

Substanzen, die in ihren peripheren Auswirkungen auf den Elektrolyt-Wasser-Haushalt dem Wirkungsbild der Aldosteronantagonisten gleichen, ihre Effekte aber über einen Eingriff in die Aldosteronbiosynthese mit Verminderung der adrenalen Aldosteronsekretion erreichen, sollten unter dem Begriff der Aldosteron-Synthese-Hemmer zusammengefaßt und beschrieben werden. Eine solche Einteilung würde es erlauben, den Begriff der Anti-Aldosteron-Substanzen für Pharmaka wie das Triamteren und das Amilorid zu reservieren; Pharmaka, die in ihrer diuretischen Charakteristik das Wirkungsbild der Aldosteronantagonisten simulieren, ihre Effekte aber weder über einen spezifischen Aldosteronantagonismus noch über einen Einfluß auf die Aldosteronbiosynthese erreichen, sondern einen eigenen, noch nicht sicher abgeklärten Wirkungsmechanismus haben (s. auch Beitrag EIGLER und CRABBÉ, S. 195).

Triamteren und Amilorid = Synthetische Anti-Aldosteron-Substanzen mit eigenem Wirkungsmechanismus

Die strukturelle Ähnlichkeit der Aldosteronantagonisten Progesteron und der Spirolactone mit ihren Mineralocorticoid-Agonisten Aldosteron, Cortexon und verschiedenen synthetischen Cortisol-Derivaten ist augenscheinlich. Ihnen allen ist die Steroid-Konfiguration gemeinsam. Aufgrund erster Beobachtungen wurden früher auch dem nichtsteroidalen 2,4,7-Triamino-6-Phenylpteridin (= Triamteren) aldosteronantagonistische Eigenschaften zugeschrieben, da die Substanz alle Effekte des Aldosterons auf die renale Elektrolytausscheidung aufzuheben vermochte.

Eine Ähnlichkeit von *Triamteren* mit den Aldosteronantagonisten ergibt sich jedoch nur insofern, als die Elektrolytzusammensetzung des Endharnes sich im Hinblick auf die Verminderung der Kalium- und Wasserstoff-Ionenelimination bei Steigerung der Natriurese qualitativ gleichen. Aber schon das quantitative Ausmaß der renalen Auswirkungen scheint bei beiden Substanzgruppen unterschiedlich zu sein. Bei etwa vergleichbarer Natriurese durch Triamteren und Spironolacton ist die Verminderung der Kaliumausscheidung oft unter Triamteren stärker ausgeprägt. Wesentlich für die Charakterisierung ist vor allem jedoch, daß Triamteren seinen Einfluß auf den renalen Elektrolytumsatz nicht nur bei einem Aldosteronismus (vgl. Abb. 2) zeigt, sondern ihn auch dann noch beibehält, wenn der Organismus nicht unter dem Einfluß von Aldosteron (oder anderen Mineralocorticoiden) steht (Abb. 3). In diesem Zusammenhang ist weiterhin wichtig, daß Triamteren den Natrium/Kalium-Quotienten des Speichels nicht zu ändern vermag, wie es von den Spirolactonen bekannt ist. Darüber hinaus spricht gegen einen Aldosteronantagonismus von Triamteren, daß kombinierte Gaben von Spirolactonen und Triamteren eine Natriurese verursachen, die bei weitem die Effekte einer maximal wirksamen Dosis von Triamteren übertrifft. Würde Triamteren spirolactonähnliche Eigenschaften haben, müßte der maximal mögliche Triamtereneffekt dem Effekt einer Kombination Spirolacton/Triamteren gleich sein. Diese Tatsache spricht ebenso gegen eine teilweise aldosteronantagonistische Triamterenwirkung. Auch die Annahme eines dissoziierten aldosteronantagonistischen Triamtereneffektes, der nur auf die Beeinflussung des Natrium-Ions gerichtet wäre, ist als unrichtig abzulehnen. Solche Annahmen stiften nur unnötige Verwirrung bei der Charakterisierung der Triamterenwirkungen.

Das triamterenähnliche *Amilorid* ist in seiner antikaliuretischen Wirkung ebenfalls unabhängig von der Anwesenheit von Mineralocorticoiden im Organismus. Die bisher vorliegenden eigenen Ergebnisse weisen uns Amilorid als eine Substanz mit der stärksten von uns beobachteten Hemmwirkung auf die Kaliurese aus. Näheres über die pharmakologischen Eigenschaften des Amilorid findet sich im Beitrag K. H. BEYER (S. 235) und im Beitrag J. E. BAER (S. 247).

Synthetische Aldosteronantagonisten

Die größten Erfahrungen über die klinische Anwendung von synthetischen Aldosteronantagonisten wurden mit der Gruppe der Spirolacton-Diuretica gesammelt. Bei der Suche nach synthetischen Aldosteronantagonisten waren die amerikanischen Forscher CELLA und KAGAWA (1957) auf zwei neue Steroide gestoßen, denen bald weitere Derivate folgten.

Es handelt sich bei diesen Stoffen um 17-Spirolacton-Steroide, d. h. um Substanzen, die wie das Desoxy-Corticosteron 11-Desoxyverbindungen sind, sich aber von den genuinen Nebennierenrindensteroiden dadurch unterscheiden, daß sie anstelle der alpha-Ketol-Seitenkette und der Hydroxylgruppe an C-17 einen Propionsäure-gamma-Lactonring tragen. Die peroral wirksame Substanz SC-9420 hat unter den Namen Spironolacton und Aldacton weite klinische Verbreiterung und Beachtung gefunden. In der Grundlagenforschung wurde sie ebenfalls erfolgreich angewendet. Das Aldacton ragt unter diesen neuen Substanzen besonders hervor, weil es seinen diuretischen Effekt bei peroraler Wirksamkeit und guter Verträglichkeit entfaltet. Einzelheiten über die pharmakologischen Eigenschaften und die klinische Wirksamkeit der Spirolactone finden sich in den Übersichten zu diesem Thema (BARTTER 1960; KOCZOREK 1961; BUCHBORN und KOCZOREK 1962; KRÜCK, KOCZOREK und BETZIEN 1962).

Antikaliuretische Diuretica als Gruppenbezeichnung

Den Aldosteronantagonisten, dem Triamteren und dem Amilorid ist *gemeinsam*, daß sie als Diuretica einen vorwiegend distalen Angriffspunkt am Nierentubulus haben, unabhängig von ihrer Struktur, und daß sie die Kaliumausscheidung nicht steigern und bei Kaliumverlust-Situationen sogar zur Kaliumretention führen. Diese Eigenschaften lassen es als zweckmäßig erscheinen, sie unter dem *Begriff der antikaliuretischen Substanzen bzw. Diuretica* zusammenzufassen und so den konventionellen Diuretica, zu denen wir auch Furosemid und die Etacrynsäure zählen, mit mehr proximal im Tubulus gelegenen Angriffspunkt und Tendenz zu Kaliumverlusten gegenüberzustellen. Innerhalb dieser Gruppen ist die Stärke der Wirkung auf die Ionenbewegungen bei den verschiedenen Substanzen verschieden groß. Allen diesen antikaliuretischen Substanzen ist aber außerdem gemeinsam, daß sie zu einer Verminderung der Wasserstoffionenausscheidung führen und ferner auch *antichloruretisch* wirken, *in dem Sinne, daß die Chloridausscheidung hinter der gesteigerten Natriurese zurückbleibt.* Dabei laufen nach unseren Ergebnissen antikaliuretische und antichloruretische Wirksamkeit in ihrer Stärke weitgehend parallel, und zwar anscheinend zunehmend in der Reihenfolge Progesteron – Spirolactone – Triamteren – Amilorid. Somit hat diese Diuretica-Gruppe auch für die Behandlung von Störungen des Säure-Basen-Haushalts große Bedeutung.

Abb. 7. Verhalten der renalen Elektrolyt- und Wasserausscheidung bei einem 49jährigen Patienten (L.F.) mit einer hydropischen Herzinsuffizienz (Ödeme und Aszites) nach altem Hinterwandinfarkt und fraglichem frischen Vorderwandinfarkt unter der Behandlung mit der diuretischen Dreierkombination Salureticum-Aldosteronantagonist-antikaliuretische Substanz Triamteren. Die Abbildung zeigt zunächst den Anstieg des Körpergewichts, dem unter der kombinierten diuretischen Therapie dann eine Ausschwemmung folgt. Es ist auch erkennbar, wie unter Anwendung der antikaliuretischen Substanzen die Chlorid- hinter der Natriumausscheidung zurückbleibt. – Die Basistherapie mit Bettruhe, Salzrestriktion und Glykosiden ist in der Abbildung weggelassen worden. Der größere Effekt der Dreierkombination auf die Natriurese gegenüber den Tagen, an denen das Salureticum entweder nur mit Aldactone oder Triamteren kombiniert worden war, ist eindeutig zu erkennen. Der Anstieg der Serum-Kalium-Konzentration von 4,10 mval/l auf 5,54 mval/l entspricht der verminderten renalen Kaliumausscheidung durch die antikaliuretischen Substanzen.

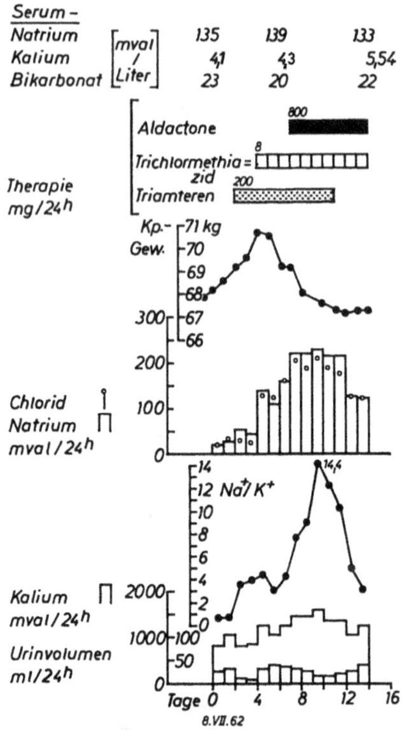

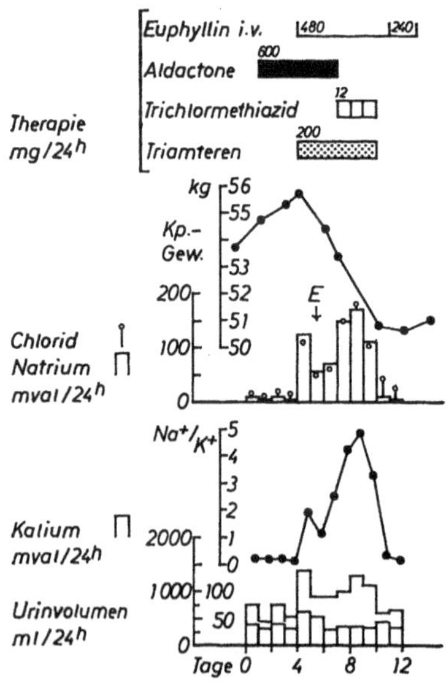

Abb. 8. Kombinierte diuretische Behandlung einer 54jährigen Patientin (K. K.) mit hydropischer Herzinsuffizienz bei kombiniertem Mitralvitium. – In voraufgegangenen Behandlungsperioden hatten weder das Thiazid-Derivat (Esmarin) allein noch Triamteren allein zu einer Senkung des Körpergewichts geführt. Unter gleichzeitigem Einsatz beider Substanzen war das Körpergewicht von 55,5 kg auf 53,7 kg innerhalb von sechs Tagen gesunken. Danach war es unter Triamteren allein einige Tage lang stationär geblieben und war dann wieder angestiegen. – Die anschließende alleinige Aldactone-Medikation in der hier verzeichneten Dosierung erwies sich als wirkungslos. Die Kombination Aldactone/Triamteren leitete jedoch einen steilen Gewichtssturz von 55,7 kg auf 50,7 kg ein. In der Aldactone-Nachphase war die kombinierte Triamteren/Thiazid-Auswirkung auf die Urinelektrolyte stärker ausgeprägt als in den früheren Behandlungsperioden, möglicherweise wegen der oft zu beobachtenden Nachwirkung des Aldosteronantagonisten, die auch aus den klinisch-pharmakologischen Untersuchungsergebnissen der Abb. 2 zu erkennen ist. Die Serumelektrolyte blieben während dieser Behandlung unverändert im Normbereich. Ein Anstieg des Rest-N wurde nicht beobachtet. Sonstige therapeutische Maßnahmen: Bettruhe, salzfreie Diät, Glykoside und Antibiotica (der klinische Verlauf war durch eine interkurrente Pneumonie kompliziert). E = Erbrechen.

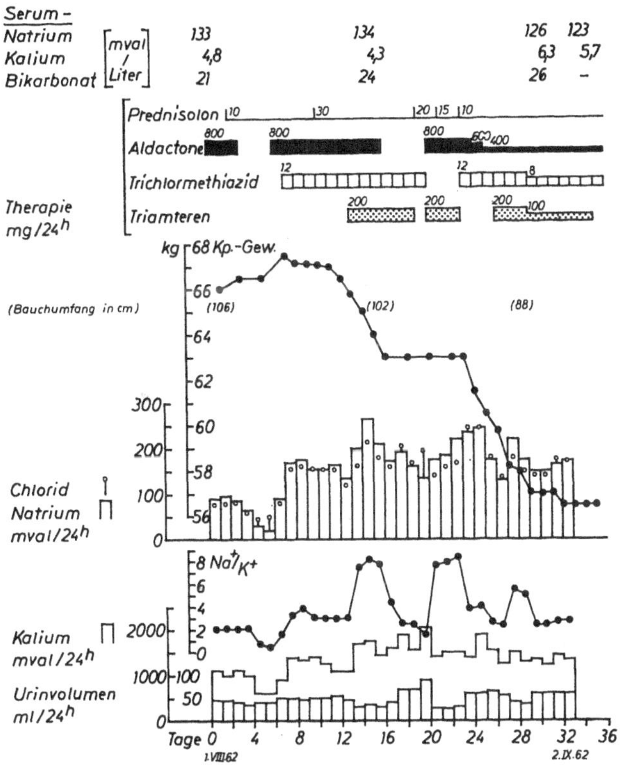

Abb. 9. Auswirkungen kombinierter diuretischer Medikationen auf den Elektrolyt-Wasserhaushalt eines 50jährigen Patienten (S. A.) mit einer atrophischen, postdystrophischen Leberzirrhose mit Aszites, bei dem außerdem eine (mäßig schwere) chronische diffuse Glomerulonephritis mit nephrotischem Einschlag vorlag. Unter der diuretischen Kombinationsbehandlung kam es zur weitgehenden Ausschwemmung des Aszites und der peripheren Ödeme, nachdem der Patient auf Aldactone allein nicht mehr angesprochen hatte. Die Gewichtsabnahme in der hier dargestellten Behandlungsphase betrug 11,0 kg in 25 Tagen. Sie wurde ohne wesentliche Störungen im Elektrolytmetabolismus erzielt. Der Anstieg des Serumkaliums am 30. Tag auf 6,3 mval/l war passager; am 11.9.1962 wurde eine Serumkaliumkonzentration von 5,1 mval/l gemessen (Serumnatrium = 130 mval/l; Bikarbonat 20 mval/l). Am gleichen Tag war der vorübergehend bis auf 68 mg% (am 16.8. 1962) erhöht gefundene Rest-N-Wert wieder auf 51 mg% abgefallen. Vor der Entwicklung der Refrakterität gegen den Aldosteronantagonisten konnte das Körpergewicht des Patienten innerhalb von 29 Tagen allein mit täglich 800 mg Aldactone (nur an drei aufeinanderfolgenden Tagen waren zusätzlich 10 mg eines Hydrochlorothiazidpräparates gegeben worden) von 76,5 kg (am 1.7.1962) bis auf 65,5 kg gesenkt werden. Insgesamt wurden also in dem geschilderten Fall durch diuretische Maßnahmen mit Spironolacton allein und in Kombination mit Triamteren und einem Thiazid-Diureticum im Zeitraum vom 29.6.–2.9.1962 rund 20 kg überschüssig als Aszites und periphere Ödeme eingelagertes Wasser wieder entfernt. Die Diät wurde salzarm gehalten. Die gleichen Diuretica-Kombinationen sind bei diesem Patienten in wechselnder Anordnung bei ambulanter und stationärer Behandlung bis jetzt (= 6 Jahre) wirksam geblieben; Elektrolytstörungen traten nicht auf.

Diuretische Kombinationsbehandlung

Alle ihre Eigenschaften zusammen machen die Aldosteronantagonisten und die anderen antikaliuretischen Substanzen zu idealen Kombinationspartnern für die verschiedenen Thiazid-Derivate, das Furosemid und vor allem auch die Etacrynsäure, da die potenten natriuretischen Eigenschaften der konventionellen Diuretica meist mit ebenso potenten, meist dosisabhängigen kaliumverlierenden Eigenschaften verknüpft sind.

Bei der Kombinationsbehandlung (und auch beim alleinigen Einsatz) von kaliumverlierenden Ödemkranken sind Triamteren und Amilorid den Spirolactonen in einem wichtigen Punkt überlegen, nämlich der Geschwindigkeit des Wirkungsbeginns. Ihr Effekt setzt noch am Tage der Anwendung ein – dies ist gut an den Beispielen in den Abb. 10–12 für Amilorid und in den Abb. 7 und 9 für Triamteren zu erkennen – und nach

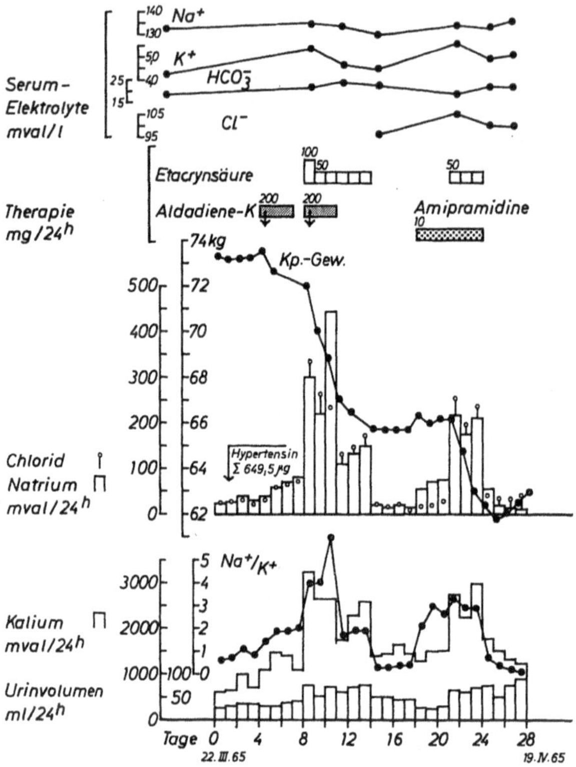

Abb. 10. Kombinierte diuretische Behandlung eines 61jährigen Patienten mit einer dekompensierten Leberzirrhose und (leichtem) Diabetes mellitus mit Aldadiene-Kalium, einem intravenös applizierbaren Spirolactonderivat, und Etacrynsäure. – Es handelt sich um den gleichen Patienten wie in Abb. 11. Dort findet sich auch die eingehende Darstellung der Wirkung der kombinierten Anwendung von Amilorid (= Amipramidine) und Etacrynsäure auf seinen Elektrolyt-Wasser-Haushalt. Hier ist diese Behandlungsphase nur zum Vergleich mit den Effekten der Kombination Aldadiene-Kalium/Etacrynsäure wiedergegeben. Bei diesem Vergleich ist vielleicht zu berücksichtigen, daß am ersten Tag der Kombination Aldadiene-Kalium/Etacrynsäure die doppelte Dosis Etacrynsäure (= 100 mg) gegeben worden ist. Denn es ist auffallend, daß hier die Kombination von Aldadiene-Kalium mit Etacrynsäure zu einem stärkeren Natrium- und Körpergewichtsverlust geführt hat als die Kombination Amilorid/Etacrynsäure, obwohl die alleinigen Anwendungen von 10 mg Amilorid und 200 mg Aldadiene-Kalium (jeweils drei Tage lang) sich als äquinatriuretisch erwiesen hatten. Andererseits ist zu erkennen, daß bei diesen äquinatriuretischen Dosen Amilorid entschieden stärker antikaliuretisch und antichloruretisch wirkte als das Spirolacton-Derivat. Die antikaliuretischen (und für Amilorid auch der antichloruretische Effekt) Wirkungen haben auch sofortige Auswirkungen auf die entsprechenden Ionenkonzentrationen im Serum. – Die Bemerkung »Hypertensin« in der Abbildung weist auf einen Angiotensin-Infusions-Test hin, dessen Auswirkungen hier nicht diskutiert werden sollen.

24 Stunden ist eine Wirkung nicht mehr nachweisbar. Dieser rasche Wirkungseintritt ermöglicht ein Abfangen von Kaliumverlusten schon am ersten Tag der Behandlung. Die etwas stärkere Beeinflussung der Kalium- und Wasserstoffionenelimination durch Triamteren und der noch stärkere Effekt von Amilorid im Vergleich zu Spironolacton bei annähernd gleicher Wirksamkeit auf die Natriurese ist ebenfalls beachtenswert. Diesen

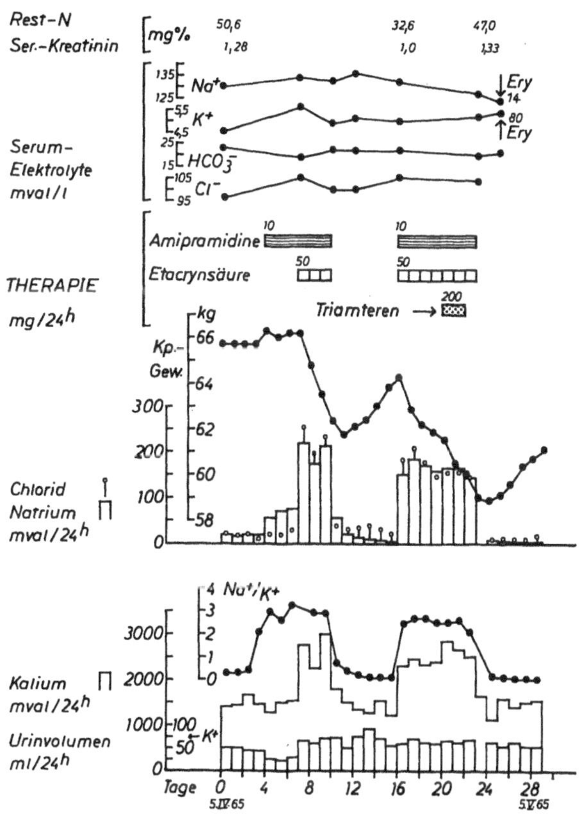

Abb. 11. Kombinierte diuretische Behandlung eines 61jährigen Patienten (S. K.) mit dekompensierter Leberzirrhose und (leichtem) Diabetes mellitus mit Amilorid (= Amipramidine = MK 870) als antikaliuretischer Substanz. – Das in seiner Wirkungscharakteristik triamterenähnliche Guanidinderivat führt zu einem sofortigen Rückgang der Kaliurese mit Anstieg der Natriurese. Die Chloridausscheidung blieb dabei weit hinter der Natriurese zurück. Die Wirkung auf die Elektrolytzusammensetzung im Urin spiegelte sich in gegensätzlichen Bewegungen der Serumelektrolyte wider, insbesondere des Chlorids und des Kaliums. Der leichte Abfall der Serumbikarbonatkonzentration reflektierte eine unter alleiniger Amilorid-Gabe einsetzende vermehrte Bikarbonat-Diurese bzw. Wasserstoffionenretention. Eine Steigerung der Wasserausscheidung trat unter der hier verwendeten Amilorid-Menge nicht auf. Andererseits blieb aber auch ein weiterer Gewichtsanstieg aus. Der Zusatz von täglich 50 mg Etacrynsäure führte unter Steigerung der Natrium-Chlorid-Wasserdiurese sofort zu einem steilen Abfall des Körpergewichts. Nach einem Rückgang der Natriurese und Wiederanstieg des Körpergewichts in einem medikationsfreien Intervall konnten gleich gute Effekte mit der Diuretica-Kombination in der folgenden zweiten Behandlungsphase beobachtet werden. Bei relativ stabilem Verhalten der anderen gemessenen Ionenkonzentrationen im Serum fand sich allerdings zunehmend eine Tendenz zur Hyponatriämie. Dabei war der Natriumgehalt der Erythrozyten mit 14 mval/l niedrig, was für eine vorwiegende Mangel-Hyponatriämie spricht (Jahrmärker, von Bubnoff und Riecker 1960), während das Erythrozytenkalium mit einer Konzentration von 80 mval/l an der unteren Normgrenze lag. Hierbei ist zu berücksichtigen, daß eine Behandlungsperiode mit der Kombination Aldadiene-Kalium/Etacrynsäure vorausgegangen war, die bereits zu einer Mobilisierung des Aszites mit einer Gewichtsabnahme von 73,6 kg bis auf 65,7 kg innerhalb von 10 Tagen geführt hatte (s. hierzu Abb. 10). – Aus der Abb. 11 ist auch zu erkennen, daß die zusätzliche Gabe von Triamteren zur Amilorid/Etacrynsäure-Kombination keinen additiven oder potenzierenden Effekt auf die Elektrolytausscheidung hatte, wie wir ihn von einer Kombination Spironolactone/Etacrynsäure/Triamteren kennen. Dies Verhalten erlaubt u. a. die Annahme, daß Amilorid und Triamteren den distal-tubulären Kationenaustausch in der Niere auf eine einander ähnliche Weise beeinflussen.

Effekt kann man mit Vorteil zur raschen Behebung von Kaliummangelzuständen ausnutzen. Er kann sich aber auch nachteilig durch zu rasche Entwicklung einer Hyperkaliämie erweisen. Im Einzelfall ist die richtige Wahl des saluretischen Kombinationspart-

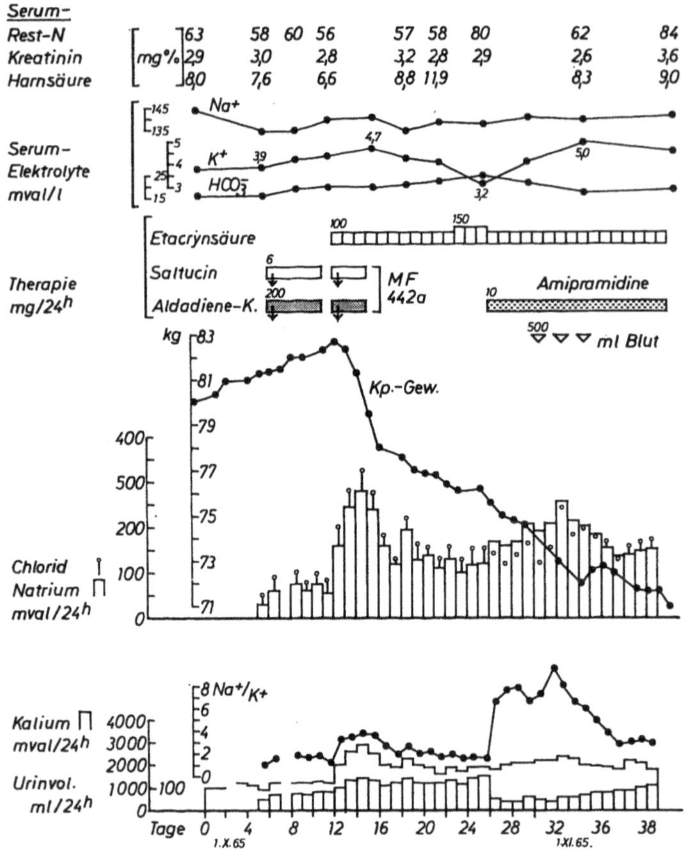

Abb. 12. Kombinierte diuretische Behandlung eines 59jährigen Patienten mit dekompensierter Leberzirrhose und chronischer Glomerulonephritis. – Die Ergebnisse der Untersuchung des Elektrolyt-Wasserhaushaltes zeigen erstens die Möglichkeit der erfolgreichen Kombination eines Aldosteronantagonisten (Aldadiene-Kalium) mit zwei saluretischen Substanzen, die verschiedene Angriffspunkte am Nephron haben, der Etacrynsäure und einem Derivat der Thiazidreihe (= Thiabutazid = Saltucin). Saltucin und Aldadiene-Kalium standen bei diesen Untersuchungen als intravenös anwendbares Versuchspräparat MF 442a (Boehringer/Mannheim) zur Verfügung. Zweitens zeigen die Ergebnisse, daß Amilorid (= Amipramidine in der Abbildung) bei längerer kombinierter Anwendung mit Etacrynsäure in fixer Dosisrelation seine antikaliuretischen und antichloruretischen Eigenschaften allmählich verlieren kann, wobei in diesem Fall der Wirkungsverlust nach sechs Tagen einsetzte. Etwa zu diesem Zeitpunkt begann auch der Kombinationseffekt von Amilorid/Etacrynsäure auf die Natriurese nachzulassen und der Verlauf der vorher stetig fallenden Körpergewichtskurve flachte ab bzw. wurde (in engem Bereich) schwankend. Einen nahezu gleichen Körpergewichtsabfall über die Ausschwemmung pathologischer Wasseransammlungen konnte man bei diesem Patienten während eines früheren stationären Aufenthaltes unter der diuretischen Kombinationstherapie mit Aldactone (tägl. 400 mg) / Saltucin (täglich 10 mg) / Triamteren (täglich 200 mg) beobachten. Unter dieser »Dreierkombination« war das Körpergewicht in der Zeit vom 19.12.1964–5.1.1965 von 82,1 kg auf 71,3 kg abgesunken. Das Glomerulumfiltrat war am 15.12.1964 mit Hilfe der endogenen Kreatinin-Clearance auf 31,6 ml/min/1,73 m² vermindert gefunden worden. Die Serum-Kalium-Konzentration hatte damals vor Beginn der diuretischen Therapie 3,75 mval/l und am Ende 6,45 mval/l betragen. Unter der anschließenden alleinigen Behandlung mit intermittierenden Gaben von Saltucin fiel dieser erhöhte Serum-Kalium-Spiegel innerhalb von 3 Tagen wieder auf 4,1 mval/l zurück. – Sonstige Therapie während der Untersuchungen: Salzfreie, eiweißreiche Leberschonkost, Antibiotica, Laevoral, Verdauungsfermente, Vitamine.

ners entscheidend, das heißt, kaliuretische und antikaliuretische Wirksamkeit müssen bei der diuretischen Kombination sorgfältig aufeinander abgestimmt werden. Ist die günstigste Kombination einmal ermittelt, so kann sie mit Erfolg oft als intermittierende Dauertherapie auch ambulant über längere Zeiträume (unter wöchentlicher oder 14tägiger Elektrolytkontrolle) weitergeführt werden (Abb. 18 und Abb. 19).

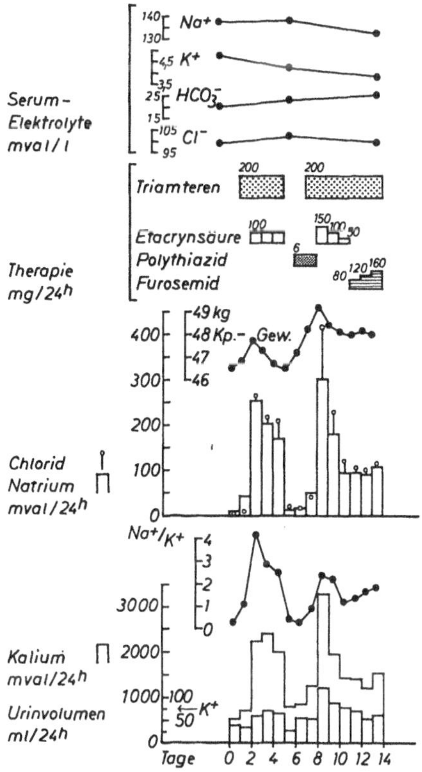

Abb. 13. Untersuchungsergebnisse bei einer 68-jährigen Patientin (P. M.) mit dekompensierter atrophischer Leberzirrhose in einer diuretischen Behandlungsphase, in der sich die Kombination Etacrynsäure/Triamteren als eindeutig wirksamer erwiesen hat, als die Kombination Furosemid (= Lasix)/Triamteren. Unter Etacrynsäure fand sich hier eine dosisabhängige Steigerung der Natrium-Chlorid- und Wasserausscheidung, allerdings auch der Kaliurese. 200 mg Triamteren konnten bei 150 mg Etacrynsäure eine stark überwiegende Chlorurese nicht verhindern. Unter Furosemid war ein solcher dosisabhängiger Effekt auf die Elektrolyt- und Wasserausscheidung nicht vorhanden, obwohl der Effekt der Kombination Furosemid/Triamteren etwas stärker ausgeprägt war als unter Triamteren allein. Auch in früheren Behandlungsperioden war bei dieser Patientin eine Dosissteigerung von Furosemid, ob es nun allein gegeben wurde oder zusammen mit einer antikaliuretischen Substanz (außer Triamteren waren Aldactone-A, Aldadiene-Kalium oder Amilorid als Kombinationspartner eingesetzt worden). Der Effekt der Dosissteigerung war übrigens auch mit intravenös appliziertem Furosemid nicht zu erreichen. Die Kombination Triamteren/Etacrynsäure behielt ihre diuretische Wirksamkeit bei dieser Patientin nach ihrer Entlassung aus der stationären Behandlung auch als intermittierende Langzeittherapie, ohne gröbere Schwankungen der über einen Zeitraum von mehreren Monaten wiederholt kontrollierten Serum-Elektrolyt-Konzentrationen zu zeigen. Die Patientin richtete dabei die Einnahme der Diuretica-Kombination nach dem Ergebnis ihrer täglichen Körpergewichtskontrolle selbst aus. Während dieser Zeit hatte sie auch ihre alte Tätigkeit als Putzfrau in einem Bürobetrieb für einige Stunden täglich freiwillig wiederaufgenommen, »um etwas gegen die Langeweile zu Hause zu tun«. Sonstige Therapie: Salzfreie bzw. salzarme Leberschonkost, Vitamine, Verdauungsfermente, Laevoral.

Der Nachteil eines verzögerten vollen Wirkungseintritts von Spironolacton haftet dem neuen, intravenös applizierbaren Aldosteronantagonisten Aldadiene-Kalium, ebenfalls ein Spirolacton-Derivat (= SC 14266), nicht mehr an. Aldadiene-Kalium besitzt die ungefähr gleichen zeitlichen Wirkungscharakteristica wie Triamteren und Amilorid hinsichtlich des Beginns der Wirkung. Hingegen kann die Wirkung wie bei allen anderen Spirolactonderivaten den Zeitraum von 24 Stunden überdauern.

Während man sich heute über die günstigen Auswirkungen einer kombinierten Anwendung von antikaliuretischen Substanzen und konventionellen Diuretica auf den Ionenhaushalt von *hydropischen Lebererkrankungen* weithin einig ist (vgl. Beitrag Sherlock, S. 365) und den kombinierten Einsatz von Diuretica auch beim *nephrotischen Syndrom* (vgl. Beitrag Reubi, S, 381) akzeptiert, möchten viele Therapeuten ein solches Vorgehen bei der hydropischen Herzinsuffizienz nur für die schweren Zustände gelten lassen. Man hört dann nicht selten den Einwand, bei der kardialen Insuffizienz spiele der sekundäre

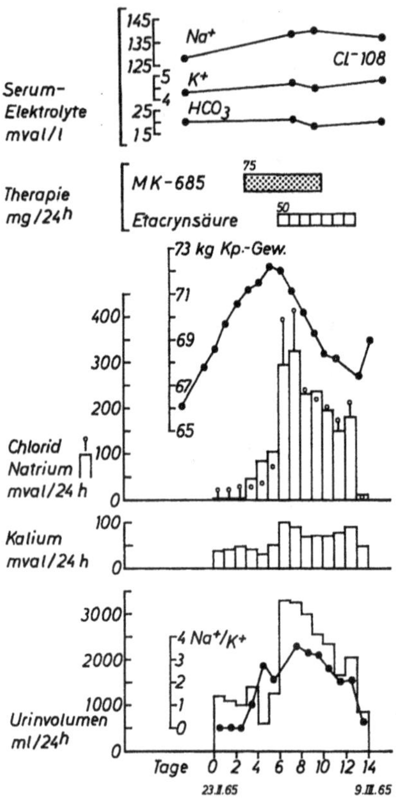

Abb. 14. Behandlung einer 58jährigen Patientin (M.F.) mit einem chemischen Vorläufer von Amilorid, dem Versuchspräparat MK 685, und Etacrynsäure. Es handelte sich um eine schwere hydropische Herzinsuffizienz mit Cirrhose cardiaque (ausgeprägter Aszites und periphere Ödeme) bei einem Mitralvitium und Hypertonie sowie chronischer Pyelonephritis mit kompensierter Retention. Bei Vergleichsuntersuchungen hat sich MK 685 schließlich als weniger wirksam und mit mehr Nebenwirkungen behaftet als MK 870 = Amilorid erwiesen und wurde zugunsten von Amilorid aufgegeben. Die Abbildung zeigt jedoch deutlich die qualitative Ähnlichkeit im Wirkungsbild, die MK 685 im Vergleich zu Amilorid aufweist. – Sonstige Therapie: Salzfreie Leberschonkost, Laevulose-Glucose-Infusionen, Vitamine, Bettruhe und Glykoside.

Aldosteronismus nicht die große Rolle, die man ihm für die Wasseransammlung von Lebererkrankungen zugestehen müsse. Dem lassen sich wesentliche Argumente entgegenhalten (vgl. Beitrag Muller, S. 421). Doch selbst wenn die Diskussion über den Pathomechanismus der renalen Salz-Wasser-Retention bei der Herzinsuffizienz noch um verschiedene Hypothesen kreisen, auf die hier nicht näher eingegangen werden kann, sollte man sich in diesem Zusammenhang der Ausführungen von Ch. K. Friedberg auf dem, 1959 in Herrenchiemsee abgehaltenen Symposion über Diurese und Diuretica erinnern, der mahnte, daß ein *Kaliummangel wahrscheinlich die am häufigsten übersehene Elektro-*

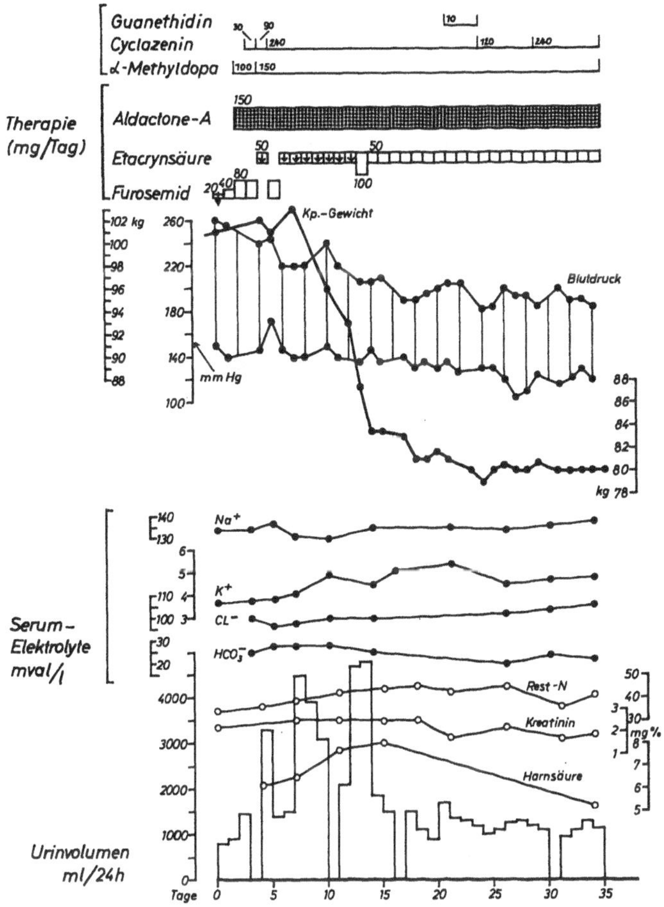

Abb. 15. Kombinierte diuretische Behandlung eines 46jährigen Patienten (K. H.) mit einem Aldosteron-Antagonisten (= Aldactone-A) und Etacrynsäure, bei dem eine schwere hydropische Herzinsuffizienz bei Hypertonie bestand. Neben der antihypertensiven und diuretischen Medikation waren als Basistherapie (in der Abbildung nicht vermerkt) Bettruhe, salzfreie Diät, Glykoside (täglich 0,375 mg Lanicor oral) und Antikoagulantien (täglich 1,5 mg Marcumar) verordnet worden. In der Abbildung bedeuten die in der Therapierubrik angegebenen Kästchen mit eingezeichnetem Pfeil, daß an diesen Tagen Etacrynsäure bzw. Furosemid intravenös appliziert worden ist. An allen anderen Tagen wurden die Medikamente oral gegeben. Die diuretischen und blutdrucksenkenden Maßnahmen waren in den letzten Wochen vor der stationären Aufnahme ohne Erfolg geblieben. Ein Versuch zu Beginn der stationären Behandlung, eine Diurese mit Gewichtsabnahme durch die kombinierte Gabe von Aldactone-A und Furosemid zu erzwingen, hatte keinen merkbaren Erfolg. Unter Etacrynsäure plus Aldactone A setzte dagegen sofort eine starke Diurese ein, und ohne Nachlassen der diuretischen Wirkung wurden innerhalb von 17 Tagen rund 23 kg Ödemflüssigkeit ausgeschwemmt. Unerwünschte Änderungen der Serumelektrolyte traten dabei nicht auf. Es ist bemerkenswert, daß der vorübergehende Anstieg des Harnsäurespiegels sich trotz weiterer Gabe von Etacrynsäure/Aldactone wieder normalisierte. Auch die vorübergehenden Anstiege des Kreatinins und Reststickstoffs waren schließlich reversibel, eine Beobachtung, die fast regelmäßig anzutreffen ist. Unter der diuretischen Therapie kam es hier mit der Gewichtsabnahme zu einer Wiederansprechbarkeit auf antihypertensive Substanzen. Der Patient konnte in wesentlich besserem Allgemeinzustand mit intermittierender diuretischer Therapie wieder nach Hause entlassen werden.

lytstörung bei Herzkranken sei und der Kaliummangel auch dann bereits vorliegen könne, wenn das Plasmakalium noch normal gemessen würde. Die Herzinsuffizienz an sich hat ja als Ausdruck der Störung des Zellstoffwechsels, insbesondere der Beeinträchtigung der Aufrechterhaltung des normalen intra-zellulären Ionengefälles, eine vielfach nachgewiesene Tendenz zu einer Verminderung des Kaliumbestandes. Die Verminderung des Gesamtkaliumbestandes muß mehr als 100 mval betragen, um überhaupt am Serumkaliumspiegel erkennbar zu werden. Man muß auch daran denken, daß diese Kaliummangeltendenz der Herzinsuffizienz verstärkt wird durch Appetitlosigkeit, einseitige Diätformen, Diarrhöen u. a., abgesehen von den Auswirkungen der diuretischen Maßnahmen.

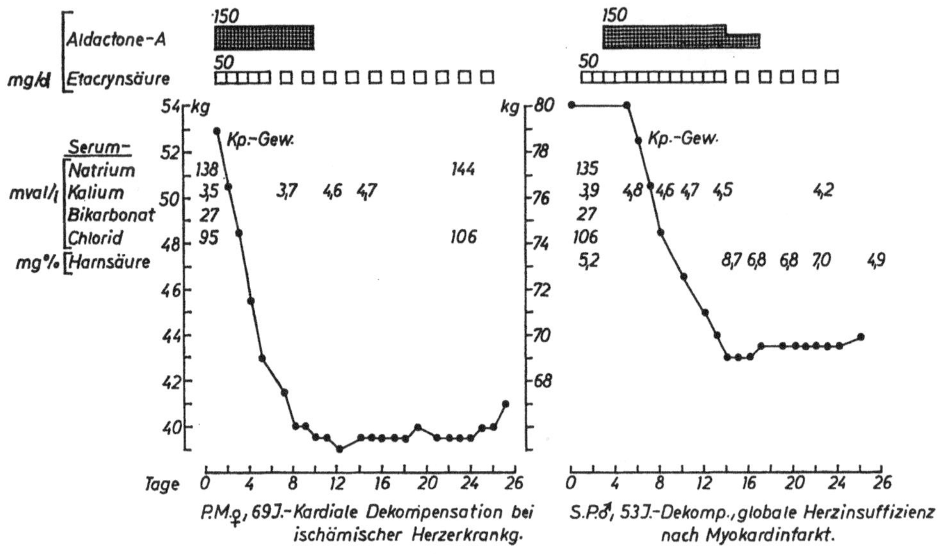

Abb. 16. Ödemausschwemmung mit der diuretischen Kombination Aldactone-A/Etacrynsäure bei einer 69jährigen Patientin (P. M.) und einem 53jährigen Patienten (S. P.) mit schwerer Dekompensation im Elektrolyt-Wasserhaushalt bei Herzinsuffizienz. Sonstige Therapie bei beiden Kranken: Salzfreie Diät, Glykoside und Antikoagulantien. In beiden Fällen konnten die Patienten, die vorher als therapierefraktär galten, anschließend weitgehend ödemfrei und in gebessertem Allgemeinzustand aus der stationären Beobachtung entlassen werden.

Bei unseren Untersuchungen, die wir seit Mitte 1964 mit der salidiuretisch sehr wirksamen Etacrynsäure bei bisher 80 Patienten über kürzere und längere Beobachtungsperioden durchgeführt haben, (Koczorek und Hofmann 1966) fanden wir, daß bei der Behandlung von 61 Patienten mit *hydropischer Herzinsuffizienz verschiedener Ätiologie* (arteriosklerotische und hypertensive Herzerkrankungen, erworbene und angeborene Vitien, Myokardiopathien, primäre und sekundäre pulmonale Hypertonien) die Kombination der Etacrynsäure mit einer antikaliuretischen Substanz der alleinigen Anwendung der Etacrynsäure überlegen und vorzuziehen war. Durch die Kombinationsbehandlung konnte die beim Einsatz größerer Etacrynsäuremengen zu beobachtende rasche Neigung zur Ausbildung einer hypochlorämischen und/bzw. hypokaliämischen Alkalose praktisch völlig ausgeglichen werden, und zwar unter additiver bis überadditiver diuretischer Wirkung. Dabei betrug die maximale kumulative Gewichtsabnahme in der Patientengruppe, die Etacrynsäure allein erhalten hatte, niemals mehr als rund 8,0 kg. Dagegen erreichte die maximale kumulative Gewichtsabnahme in der mit Etacrynsäure plus antikaliuretischer Substanz behandelten Patientengruppe Werte bis zu 23,0 kg. Als antikaliuretische Substanz wurde bei der Kombination mit Etacrynsäure meistens Aldactone-A gewählt (Abb. 15, 16 und 21). Doch wir konnten ähnlich günstige therapeutische Ergebnisse verzeichnen, wenn wir statt des Aldosteronantagonisten eine andere antikaliuretische Substanz wie Amilorid (Abb. 14, 17 und 20) oder auch Triamteren (Abb. 13) zusammen mit der Etacrynsäure verordneten (Koczorek, Engelhardt und Hofmann 1968).

Dreier-Kombinationen von Diuretica

Hervorzuheben ist noch die Möglichkeit der Kombination von antikaliuretischen Substanzen vom Triamterentyp mit den Spirolactonen, allein (Abb. 8) und zusammen mit den konventionellen Diuretica.

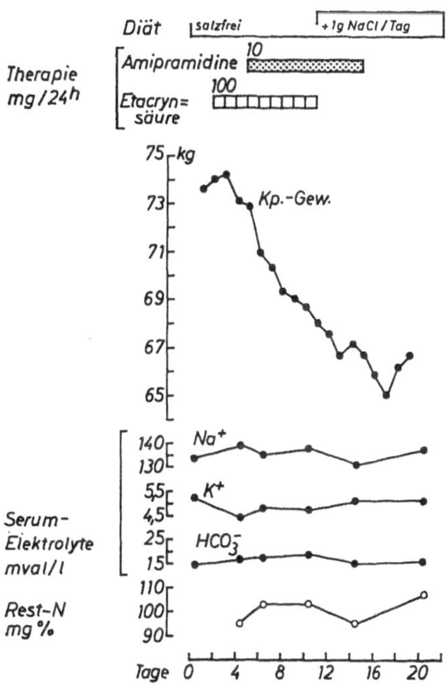

Abb. 17. Diuretische Kombinationstherapie mit Amilorid/Etacrynsäure eines 62jährigen Patienten (U. H.), der bei einer globalen Herzinsuffizienz mit Cirrhose cardiaque nach Myokardinfarkt und bei polycystischer Nierendegeneration einen erheblichen allgemeinen Hydrops und ausgeprägten Aszites entwickelt hatte. Die Glomerulumfiltration (endogene Kreatinin-Clearance) war auf 10,8 ml/min/1,73 m^2 eingeschränkt. Es handelte sich somit um einen Hydrops, bei dem kardiale, hepatische und renale Komponenten pathogenetisch beteiligt waren. Mit Hygroton, Lasix und Aldactone-A hatten sich in voraufgegangenen Behandlungsperioden wirklich effektive Diuresen nicht mehr erzielen lassen. Bessere Diuresen wurden schließlich mit Etacrynsäure und intravenös appliziertem Aldadiene-Kalium und vor allem, wie die Abbildung zeigt, mit der Kombination Etacrynsäure/Amipramidine = Amilorid bei streng salzfreier bzw. salzarmer (1 g NaCl-Zulagen pro Tag) Diät erreicht. Unter Weiterführung dieser Behandlungsweise wurden die Ödeme dieses Patienten fast vollständig ausgeschwemmt. Insgesamt nahm sein Körpergewicht vom 25. 8. 1965 (= Tag 3 in der Abbildung) bis zum 29. 9. 1965 von 74,2 kg bis auf 59,8 kg ab und er konnte wieder nach Hause entlassen werden. Seine kardialen Symptome (Dyspnoe, Einflußstauung) hatten sich zu diesem Zeitpunkt entscheidend gebessert und auch subjektiv hatte sich der Patient deutlich leistungsfähiger gefühlt. Die Konzentration der harnpflichtigen Substanzen im Serum (Rest-Werte um 100 mg% und Serum-Kreatinin um 5 mg% schwankend) hatten durch die diuretische Therapie keine wesentliche Änderung erfahren und entsprachen seiner reduzierten endogenen Kreatinin-Clearance.

Es gibt z. B. Patienten, bei denen weder die Kombination Triamteren plus konventionelles Diuretikum noch die Kombination Aldactone bzw. Aldactone-A plus konventionelles Diuretikum eine Ödemausschwemmung herbeiführt, die sog. *Dreier-Kombination* Triamteren-Aldosteronantagonist-konventionelles Diuretikum aber den gewünschten Erfolg bringt (Abb. 7 und 9). Analoges gilt für die Kombination Amiloride/Aldosteronantagonist/Saluretikum. An diese Möglichkeit der Dreier-Kombination *bei diuretisch scheinbar refraktären Patienten* sollte daher öfters gedacht werden.

Interessant genug, können anscheinend Amilorid und Triamteren nicht mit dem gleichen additiven oder potenzierenden Effekt in einer Dreierkombination mit einem der konventionellen Diuretica genutzt werden, wie aus der Abb. 11 zu erkennen ist. Dieses Verhalten kann als Hinweis auf die Ähnlichkeit der Wirkungsprinzipien von Amilorid und Triamteren gewertet werden.

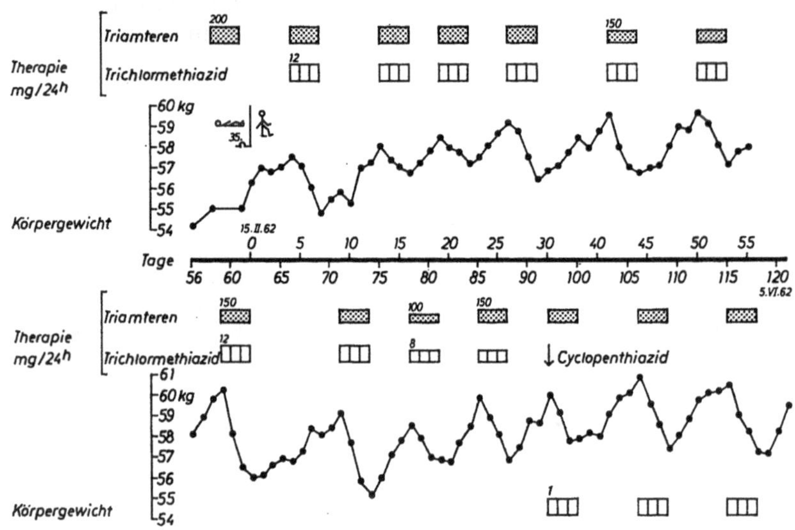

Abb. 18. Ergebnis des Versuchs einer ambulanten intermittierenden diuretischen Langzeitbehandlung einer 20jährigen Patientin (F. G.) mit einem nephrotischen Syndrom mit der Kombination Triamteren/Trichlormethiazid bzw. Triamteren/Cyclopenthiazid, wobei die Patientin die Einnahme der Medikamente unter täglicher Kontrolle ihres Körpergewichtes selbst steuerte. Diese ambulante Behandlung hatte begonnen, nachdem während eines 35tägigen stationären Aufenthaltes die Reaktion der Patientin auf die Diuretica durch tägliche Elektrolytkontrollen im Harn geprüft worden war. In der Abbildung wird diese intermittierende kombinierte Langzeittherapie bis zum 120. Tag nach der Entlassung aus der stationären Beobachtung (5. 6. 1962) dargestellt; sie wurde jedoch in gleicher Weise noch einen Monat lang weitergeführt. In der Regel sollten in solchen Fällen die Gewichtsschwankungen kleiner gehalten werden durch häufigere einmalige Diuretica-Dosen. Die Kontrolluntersuchung der Serum-Elektrolytkonzentration am 6. 7. 1962 brachte die folgenden Werte: Natrium = 130 mval/l; Kalium = 3,93 mval/l und Standardbikarbonat = 26,0 mval/l. Der Rest-N wurde mit 26,0 mg% gemessen. Auch bei zwischenzeitlichen Kontrollbestimmungen waren unter diesen therapeutischen Maßnahmen niemals hyper- oder hypokaliämische Werte beobachtet worden. Das Allgemeinbefinden der Patientin, die wieder ihren Beruf als Stenotypistin aufgenommen hatte, war relativ gut. Die Diät wurde salzarm gehalten.

Es sind auch diuretische Dreier-Kombinationen möglich, bei denen man versucht, die unterschiedlichen Angriffspunkte zweier konventioneller Diuretica im Nephron zusammen mit einem Aldosteronantagonisten (oder einer anderen antikaliuretischen Substanz) auszunutzen. Ein Beispiel eines solchen Behandlungsversuchs ist in Abb. 12 dargestellt.

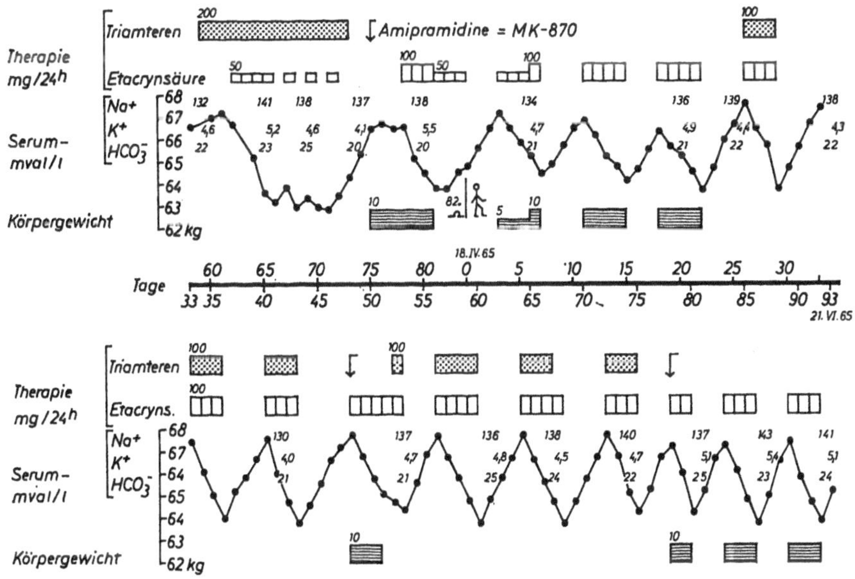

Abb. 19. Intermittierende diuretische Langzeitbehandlung eines 42jährigen Patienten (R. R.) mit einem nephrotischen Syndrom bei chronischer membranöser Glomerulonephritis. Nach einem stationären Aufenthalt von 82 Tagen (maximales Körpergewicht während dieser Zeit = 78,0 kg; minimales Gewicht unter Kombinationstherapie mit Etacrynsäure und einem Guanidin-Derivat = 62,7 kg) wurde der Patient mit den Kombinationen Triamteren/Etacrynsäure oder Amilorid/Etacrynsäure ambulant weiterbehandelt (Amilorid als quergestreifte Blöcke dargestellt.) Amilorid ist heute der systematische Name für MK 870, das bisher auch als Amipramidine bezeichnet worden ist. Der Patient kontrollierte sein Körpergewicht täglich selbst und nahm eine der beiden (während seines stationären Aufenthaltes unter klinisch-pharmakologischen Kontrollen erprobten) Kombinationen dann ein, wenn sein Gewicht von einer Minimalbasis von weniger als 64 kg auf einen Wert von etwa 68 kg zugenommen hatte. In ungefähr 14tägigen Abständen (meistens) wurden Kontrolluntersuchungen, vor allem der Serumelektrolyte durchgeführt. Die Ergebnisse zeigten niemals wesentliche Abweichungen von den Normbereichen. Es ist zu erwähnen, daß der Patient immer nur zu einer mäßigen Einschränkung der Kochsalzaufnahme bereit war. Immerhin konnte er auf die vorgezeichnete Weise seine Ödembildung vom Tag der Entlassung aus der stationären Behandlung (18.4.1965) bis Oktober 1965 selbst unter Kontrolle halten und seiner beruflichen Tätigkeit als Elektrokaufmann nahezu voll nachgehen. Auch hier wären kleinere Gewichtsschwankungen (vgl. Abb. 18) wünschenswert gewesen. Sonstige Therapie in diesem Zeitraum: Cortisonderivate, Antibiotica. Der nach unten gerichtete Pfeil in der Abbildung weist auf den Wechsel von Triamteren auf Amilorid hin, das dann in gestreiften Blöcken unterhalb der Gewichtskurven eingezeichnet ist.

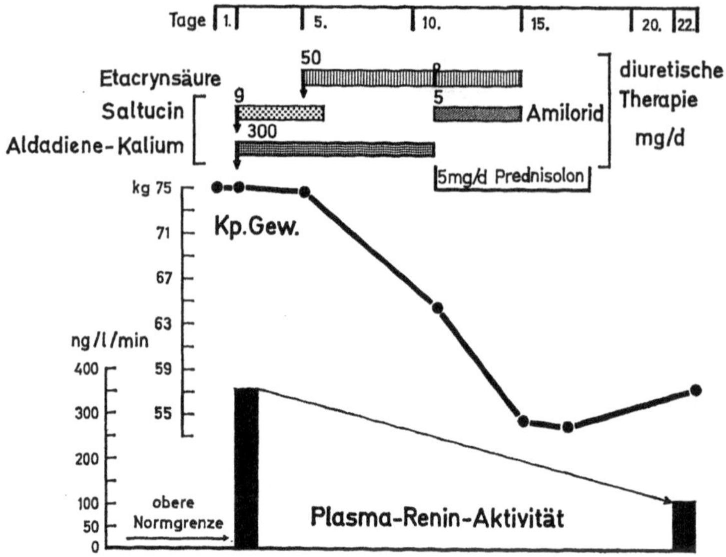

Abb. 20. Verhalten der Plasma-Renin-Aktivität bei einer 64jährigen Patientin (R. K.) mit schwerer hydropischer Herzinsuffizienz bei Aortenklappenstenose (und rel. Mitralinsuffizienz) unter kombinierter diuretischer Therapie, die zur Ödemausschwemmung mit einer Abnahme des Körpergewichts von rund 20 kg geführt hatte. Saltucin = Thiabutazide. In der Abbildung nicht vermerkte sonstige Therapie: Salzfreie Diät, Glykoside, Antikoagulantien (= Sintrom) und Bettruhe. Die Serum-Elektrolytkonzentrationen am 17. Untersuchungstag betrugen: Natrium = 133 mval/l; Kalium = 5,1 mval/l; Standardbikarbonat = 20 mval/l und Chlorid = 106 mval/l. Die Blutdruckwerte lagen zwischen 110–120 mm Hg systolisch und 70–80 mm Hg diastolisch.

Abb. 21. Detaillierte Darstellung der Auswirkungen einer kombinierten diuretischen Therapie auf den Elektrolyt-Wasser-Haushalt (Urin-Elektrolyte, Serum-Elektrolyte, Erythrozyten-Natrium, Erythrozyten-Kalium) und die Plasma-Renin-Aktivität bei einem 44jährigen Patienten (J. K.) mit schwerer hydropischer Herzinsuffizienz bei Aortenklappenstenose. – Wie in Abb. 20 gingen auch hier die Abnahme des Körpergewichts (14 kg) und Ödemausschwemmung mit einer Abnahme der Plasma-Renin-Aktivität einher. Der Blutdruck des Patienten vor Beginn der diuretischen Therapie lag bei 115/80 mm Hg. Natrium und Kalium im Erythrozyten sind als Konzentrationsänderungen gegenüber dem Mittelwert der Norm angegeben, der für das Erythrozyten-Natrium in unserem Labor nach Riecker und von Bubnoff (1959) mit 16,4 mval/l und für das Erythrozyten-Kalium mit 81,1 mval angesetzt wird. Sonstige Therapie: Salzfreie Diät und Glykoside. Am 22. Behandlungstag wurde wegen einer Lungenembolie für einige Tage Heparin (= Liquemin) eingesetzt. Die Antikoagulantientherapie wurde später mit Sintrom weitergeführt. – Es ist beachtenswert, daß es unter der Heparinwirkung zu einer Steigerung der Natriurese und einem Sturz des Körpergewichts kam, die den diuretischen Kombinationseffekt von Aldactone-A und Etacrynsäure wesentlich übertrafen. Die am 3. Tag der Heparingabe sehr verstärkt einsetzende Diurese mit Abnahme des Körpergewichts von 56,5 auf 53,4 kg erschien so bedrohlich, daß am Folgetag für 4 Tage täglich 2 g NaCl zur salzfreien Diät zugesetzt und außerdem im gleichen Zeitraum insgesamt 1250 ml Plasma infundiert wurden. Gleichzeitig wurde die Aldactone-A-Medikation reduziert bzw. gestoppt. Unter diesen Maßnahmen flachte die Körpergewichtskurve unter Rückgang der Natriurese wieder ab. Die exogene Zufuhr von Aldosteron (Aldocorten CIBA) und der Übergang der Heparin- auf die Sintrom-Medikation führten schließlich zu einem weiteren drastischen Rückgang der Natriurese, Abfall des Natrium/Kalium-Quotienten im

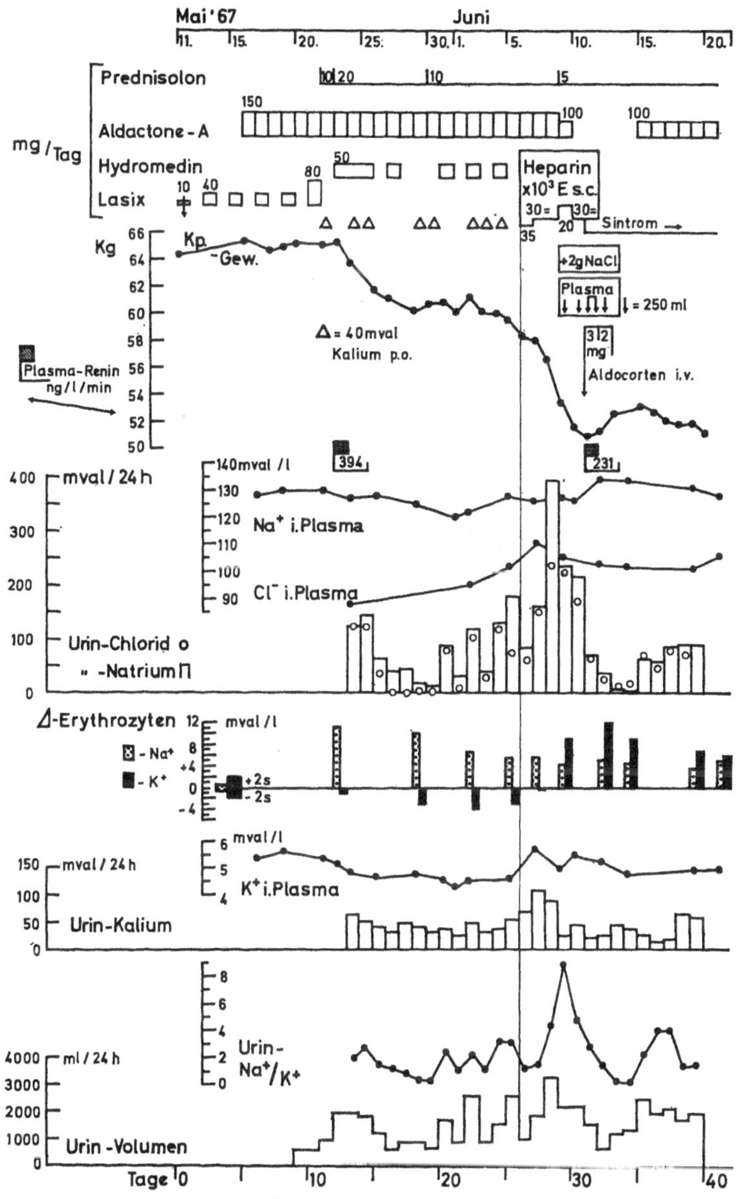

Urin unter 1 und allmählichem Wiederanstieg des Körpergewichts. Einige Tage später führte dann Aldactone-A wieder zur Abnahme des Körpergewichts unter Zunahme der Natrium-Chlorid-Diurese und Abnahme der Kaliurese. Insgesamt wurde so die Ausschwemmung der Ödeme des Patienten ohne anhaltende Störungen des Elektrolyt-Wasserhaushaltes erreicht und er wurde alsbald operationsfähig (Implantation eines Starr-Edwards-Ventils in der Chirurgischen Universitätsklinik München). Der Patient ist jetzt ambulant unter Glykosidgaben voll kompensiert.

Auf die Anwendung von *Glucorticoiden* als unterstützende Maßnahme bei der diuretischen Therapie wird im Beitrag von JAHRMÄRKER, KOCZOREK, AVENHAUS u. GROHMANN (S. 433) eingegangen.

Abschließend kann man also feststellen, daß man heute bei der Behandlung von Ödemkrankheiten einer kombinierten diuretischen Therapie fast immer den Vorzug vor der alleinigen Anwendung eines stark wirksamen Saluretikums geben sollte. Diese Feststellung muß man auch für die Behandlung des cardialen Hydrops gelten lassen, da uns detaillierte klinisch-pharmakologische Untersuchungen der letzten Jahre zunehmend gelehrt haben, daß die kombinierte Therapie mit antikaliuretischen Substanzen plus einem konventionellen Diureticum eindeutig bessere Ergebnisse bringen kann, und zwar insofern, als sich einerseits die Effekte der einzelnen Substanzen auf die renale Eliminierung von Kochsalz (mit einem wesentlich günstigeren Verhältnis von Natrium zu Chlorid im Endharn) und Wasser addieren oder gar potenzieren, und, als sich andererseits ihre unerwünschten Auswirkungen auf den Elektrolyt- (bzw. Säure-Basen-) Haushalt ausgleichen oder gar nicht erst in Erscheinung treten. Oder kürzer formuliert: Die kombinierte diuretische Therapie von Ödemkrankheiten liefert bessere erwünschte Resultate bei Reduktion der unerwünschten Nebenwirkungen. Starre Diuretica-Kombinationen (= multiple Substanzen in einem einzigen Präparat) sind jedoch abzulehnen, denn es wird während einer Kombinationstherapie immer Phasen geben, in denen man die Dosis-Relation der Pharmaka zueinander wird ändern müssen, da sich während einer solchen Behandlung früher oder später zwangsläufig neue Gleichgewichte im Elektrolyt-Wasser- bzw. Säure-Basen-Haushalt des Organismus einstellen werden. Schon bei einem auch nur annähernd rekompensierten Patienten stehen wir anderen regulatorischen Situationen gegenüber als bei dem gleichen Patienten während eines schwer dekompensierten Zustands.

Literatur / References

BAETHMANN, A., KH. R. KOCZOREK, H. J. REULEN, W. WESEMANN, H. F. HOFMANN, A. ANGSTWURM und W. BRENDEL: Die Beeinflussung des traumatischen Hirnödems durch Aldosteron, Aldosteronantagonisten und Dexamethason im Tierexperiment. In: Postoperative Störungen des Elektrolyt- und Wasserhaushalts. Pathophysiologie und Therapie. F. K. Schattauer Verlag, Stuttgart – New York, 1968, S. 163.

BARTTER, F. C.: The Clinical Use of Aldosterone Antagonists. Charles C. Thomas, Publisher; Springfield, Illinois, USA, 1960.

BUCHBORN, E. und KH. R. KOCZOREK und H. P. WOLFF: Aldosteronausscheidung und tubuläre Nierenfunktion. Klin. Wschr. **35**, 452 (1957).

BUCHBORN, E. und KH. R. KOCZOREK: Aldosteronantagonisten und ihre klinische Anwendung. Verh. dtsch. Ges. inn. Med. **68**, 649 (1962).

CELLA, J. A. and C. M. KAGAWA: Steroidal lactons. J. Am. Chem. Soc. **79**, 4808 (1957).

DUCOMMUN, P. et E. ENGEL: Déclenchement de la diurèse par l'association de progestérone et d'un dérivé de l'iso-indoline dans un cas d'oedèmes réfractaires. Schweiz. med. Wschr. **90**, 561 (1960).

FISHMAN, L. M., G. W. LIDDLE, D. P. ISLAND, N. FLEISCHER and O. KÜCHEL: Effects of aminoglutethimide on adrenal function in man. J. Clin. Endocrinol. & Metab. **27**, 481 (1967).

FRIEDBERG, CH. K.: The use of diuretics in heart disease. In: Diurese und Diuretica. Springer-Verlag. Berlin – Göttingen – Heidelberg, 1959, S. 221.

HEMPEL-JØRGENSEN, P. and P. EILERSEN: Antagonism of aldosterone by progesterone. Effects of progesterone in two cases. Acta Med. Scand. **168**, 55 (1960).

JAHRMÄRKER, H., M. v. BUBNOFF u. G. RIECKER: Über Hyponatriämiesyndrome und ihre Analyse durch Elektrolytbestimmung in Erythrocyten. Klin. Wschr. **39,** 317 (1960).
JENKINS, J. S.: Progesterone and norethisterone in cyclical oedema and ascites. Brit. Med. J. **5256,** 861 (1961).
KAGAWA, C. W.: Blocking urinary electrolyte effects of desoxycorticosterone with progesterone in rats. Proc. Soc. Experim. Biol. Med. 99, 705 (1958).
KOCZOREK, KH. R., H. P. WOLFF und M. L. BEER: Über die Aldosteronausscheidung bei Schwangerschaften und bei Schwangerschaftstoxikosen. Klin. Wschr. **35,** 497 (1957).
KOCZOREK, KH. R.: Untersuchungen über natriuretische, aldosteronantagonistische Effekte des Progesterons bei Gesunden und Ödemkranken. Unveröffentlichte Befunde 1957-1959.
KOCZOREK, KH. R.: Diskussionsbemerkung: Über den natriuretischen Effekt von exogenem Progesteron bei Normalpersonen (eigene Beobachtungen).
a) Internationales Symposion über Diurese und Diuretica. Herrenchiemsee, 17.-20. Juni 1959.
b) In: Diurese und Diuretica. Herausg. E. Buchborn und K. D. Bock. Springer-Verlag. Berlin – Göttingen – Heidelberg, 1959, S. 343.
KOCZOREK, KH. R.: Natriuretische Progesteroneffekte beim sekundären Aldosteronismus. In: SCHWIEGK, H. und H. JAHRMÄRKER: Therapie der Herzinsuffizienz. Handbuch der inneren Medizin, IX. Band, S. 551. Springer-Verlag, Berlin – Göttingen – Heidelberg 1960.
KOCZOREK, KH. R.: Über aldosteronantagonistische Eigenschaften des Progesterons. Klin. Wschr. **38,** 826 (1960).
KOCZOREK, KH. R. und H. P. WOLFF: Über Erfahrungen mit Aldosteron-Antagonisten. Simposio sull'aldosterone. Siena, März 1960. Referat: Folia endocrinol. **13,** 290 (1960).
KOCZOREK, KH. R.: Untersuchungen über die Auswirkungen von Spironolactone-, Triamteren-, oder Progesterongaben auf den Elektrolyt-Wasser-Haushalt beim M. ADDISON. Bisher unveröffentlichte Befunde 1961.
KOCZOREK, KH. R. und H. H. EDEL: Zur Ödembehandlung des nephrotischen Syndroms mit Spironolactone und Progesteron. Bisher unveröffentlichte Befunde 1961.
KOCZOREK, KH. R.: Physiologie und Pathophysiologie der Aldosteroninkretion. In: KRÜCK, KOCZOREK und BETZIEN: Klinische Anwendung der Aldosteron-Antagonisten. Georg Thieme Verlag, Stuttgart 1962, S. 2.
KOCZOREK, KH. R.: Pharmakologie der Spirolactone. In: KRÜCK, KOCZOREK und BETZIEN: Klinische Anwendung der Aldosteron-Antagonisten. Georg Thieme Verlag, Stuttgart 1962, S. 29.
KOCZOREK, KH. R., M. v. BUBNOFF und G. RIECKER: Über extrarenale Wirkungen von aldosteron-antagonistischen Substanzen. Untersuchungen an Erythrozyten. In: KRÜCK, KOCZOREK und BETZIEN: Klinische Anwendung der Aldosteron-Antagonisten. Georg Thieme Verlag, Stuttgart 1962, Seite 111.
KOCZOREK, KH. R. und H. CH. MOLL: Über den Einfluß von Progesteron auf die Resorption von Natrium aus dem Magen-Darmtrakt von Ratten. Unveröffentlichte Befunde 1962.
a) Diskussionsbemerkung auf dem Symposion über Transport und Funktion intrazellulärer Elektrolyte, Schüren, Juni 1967.
b) In: Transport und Funktion intrazellulärer Elektrolyte. Herausgeber: F. Krück. Urban & Schwarzenberg, München – Berlin – Wien, 1967, S. 151.
KOCZOREK, KH. R.: Die aldosteronantagonistischen Spirolactone. Grundlagen ihrer Indikation und Anwendung. Internist **2,** 640 (1964).
KOCZOREK, KH. R.: Clinical experience with MK 870 – a new, antikaluric agent in diuretic therapy. Symposion on MK 870 (= Amipramidine = Amiloride). New York, December 1965.
KOCZOREK, KH. R.: Neue Diuretika im klinischen Vergleich. Diuretika-Symposion der Fa. C. F. Boehringer & Söhne GmbH, Mannheim, Februar 1966.
KOCZOREK, KH. R. und H. HOFMANN: Zur Behandlung der hydropischen Herzinsuffizienz mit Etacrynsäure, einem neuartigen Salidiuretikum. Verh. dtsch. Ges. inn. Med. **72,** 910 (1966).
KOCZOREK, KH. R., D. ENGELHARDT und H. HOFMANN: Effects of ethacrynic acid in combination with antikaluric agents (spironolactone or SC-14266, triamterene, amipramidine

= MK 870) in patients with pathological fluid retention. Abstr. Intern. Congr. Nephrology, Washington, D. C. 1966, p. 224.

KOCZOREK, KH. R.: Differentialtherapeutische Überlegungen beim Einsatz von Triamteren. In: Therapie mit Triamteren. Georg Thieme Verlag, Stuttgart 1967, S. 49.

KOCZOREK, KH. R., B. SIMON, P. SCHMIEDEK, W. VOGT und B. LÜDERITZ: Funktionsstörungen des Renin-Angiotensin-Systems bei Leberkrankheiten. V. Lebertagung der Sozialmediziner, Bad Mergentheim, 13.–15. 10. 67.

KOCZOREK, KH. R., W. VOGT, P. SCHMIEDEK und H. JOST: Die Auswirkungen von Störungen der Leberfunktion auf das Renin-Angiotension-System. Dtsch. Ges. Kreislaufforsch., 33. Jahrestagung, Bad Nauheim 1967; Referat: Klin. Wschr. **45,** 896 (1967).

KOCZOREK, KH. R., H. ANGSTWURM, A. BAETHMANN, D. ENGELHARDT, H. J. REULEN, P. SCHMIEDEK, W. VOGT, B. SIMON, E. FRICK und W. BRENDEL: Aldosteronausscheidung beim Pseudotumor cerebri – einer klinischen Form des Hirnödems unbekannter Ursache. In: Postoperative Störungen des Elektrolyt- und Wasserhaushaltes. Pathophysiologie und Therapie. F. K. Schattauer Verlag, Stuttgart – New York 1968, S. 177.

KRÜCK, F., KH. R. KOCZOREK und G. BETZIEN: Klinische Anwendung der Aldosteron-Antagonisten. Georg Thieme Verlag, Stuttgart 1962.

LANDAU, R. L., D. M. BERGENSTAL, K. LUGIBIHL and M. E. KASCHT: The metabolic effects of progesterone in man. J. Clin. Endocrinol. & Metab. **15,** 1194 (1955).

LANDAU, R. L. und K. LUGIBIHL: Inhibition of the sodium-retaining influence of aldosterone by progesterone. J. Clin. Endocrinol. Metabol. **18,** 1237 (1958).

LOSERT, W., C. SENFT und G. SENFT: Extrarenale Wirkungen des Aldosterons und der Spirolactone. Naunyn-Schmiedebergs Arch. exp. Path. Pharmak. **248,** 450 (1964).

MAJOOR, C. L. H., H. PRENEN, P. J. J. VAN MUNSTER und R. J. A. F. M. SCHLATMANN: Het diuretische effect van heparine, in het bijzonder bij patiënten met het nefrotische syndroom. Ned. Tijdschr. Geneesk. **101,** 1301 (1957).

MOLL, H. CH. und KH. R. KOCZOREK: Über den Einfluß eines Aldosteron-Antagonisten (SC-8109) auf die Resorption von Natrium aus dem Magen – Darmtrakt von Ratten. Klin. Wschr. **40,** 825 (1962).

SENFT, G. und W. LOSERT: Der Einfluß von Aldosteron und Aldosteron-Antagonisten auf die Verteilung von Elektrolyten zwischen dem intra- und extrazellulären Raum. Naunyn-Schmiedeberg's Arch. exp. Path. Pharmak. **245,** 113 (1963).

MULLER: Ich glaube auch, daß wir früher den Hyper-Aldosteronismus bei der Herzinsuffizienz unterschätzt haben, da das Problem der Metabolic-Clearance-Rate noch nicht bekannt war. Wir wissen heute, daß die Leberdurchblutung beim Herzpatienten vermindert ist und daher eine normale oder nur leicht erhöhte Aldosteron-Ausscheidung im Urin einem höheren aktiven Aldosteronspiegel im Blut entsprechen kann. Trotzdem bin ich mit der Anwendung von Spironolactonen bei Herzpatienten zurückhaltend, da man viel eher eine Hyperkaliämie mit Werten von 6 mval/l erreichen kann, als bei der Lebercirrhose, wo diese Gefahr praktisch nicht besteht.

KOCZOREK: Ich danke Herrn MULLER und darf vielleicht entgegnen, daß wir bei der Behandlung der vorhin vorgestellten größeren Patientengruppe mit hydropischer Herzinsuffizienz Aldactone-A mit dem auch hinsichtlich der renalen Kaliumausscheidung recht wirksamen Diureticum Etacrynsäure kombiniert haben. Nach unseren Erfahrungen kann man die Dosen der einzelnen Substanzen bei der kombinierten diuretischen Therapie so aufeinander abstimmen, daß man auch bei der Herzinsuffizienz nicht in bedrohliche Hyperkaliämie-Bereiche gerät. Meist war der Kaliumhaushalt der Patienten mit 50 mg Etacrynsäure und 150 mg Aldactone-A/Tag auch über längere Zeit ausgeglichen.

HEINZ: Sie haben eine große Zahl von Einzelverläufen gezeigt. Haben Sie unter diesen Bedingungen, bei Patienten unterschiedlicher Art, bei wechselnden Kombinationen verschiedener Diuretica und variablen Dosierungen einen Versuch einer statistischen Auswertung gemacht, oder kennen Sie ein Verfahren, das die Untersuchung derart vieler Variablen überhaupt zuläßt? Weiterhin: Haben Sie Chlorverluste bei der Kombination von Etacrynsäure und Amilorid gesehen?

KOCZOREK: Die Frage nach der statistischen Auswertung unserer Ergebnisse ist dahingehend zu beantworten, daß es möglicherweise lohnend sein würde, dies nachzuholen, da wir über ein recht großes Befundmaterial verfügen. Andererseits glaube ich aber doch, daß sorgfältig über längere Zeit dokumentierte Einzelverläufe hinsichtlich der Wirkungscharakteristik und der Wirksamkeit neuer Substanzen mehr (oder zumindest nicht weniger) aussagen können, als eine Statistik der Reaktionen einer ganzen Gruppe von Patienten; die wegen der ausgeprägten biochemischen Individualität des einzelnen Patienten für echte statistische Aussagen doch zu heterogen zusammengesetzt wäre. Wir wissen ja alle, daß selbst der Einzelpatient in verschiedenen Stadien seiner Erkrankung auf gleiche Medikationen recht unterschiedliche Reaktionen zeigen kann. – Nun noch die Frage nach den Chloridverlusten unter der Kombination Amilorid/Etacrynsäure: Ich habe in meinem Vortrag darauf hingewiesen, daß alle klinisch bisher eingesetzten antikaliuretischen Substanzen gleichzeitig auch zu einer Chloridretention führen, und zwar zunehmend in der Reihenfolge Progesteron, Spironolacton, Triamteren und am stärksten Amilorid. Diese Chloridretention ist bei der einzelnen Substanz, ebenso wie die antikaliuretische Wirkung, von der angewandten Dosis abhängig. Chloridverluste bei Kombination mit einem konventionellen Diureticum können daher wie die Kaliumverluste durch Änderungen des Mengenverhältnisses der einzelnen Substanzen zueinander vermieden werden.

KRÜCK: Diuretica und antikaliurische Substanzen wirken additiv auf die Natriumausscheidung. Wie groß schätzen Sie die Gefahr einer dadurch induzierten Hyponatriämie?

KOCZOREK: Ich habe keine extreme Hyponatriämie beobachtet. Manchmal sahen wir dagegen bei erfolgreicher diuretischer Therapie sogar einen Anstieg von Werten, die bei Behandlungsbeginn im unteren Grenzbereich gelegen hatten.

JAHRMÄRKER: Von terminalen Zuständen abgesehen ist dies eine Frage der vorsichtigen und intermittierenden Dosierung. Ein plötzlicher großer Gewichtsverlust soll jedenfalls vermieden werden.

REUBI: Wenn Sie sagen, man sollte ganz allgemein die Diuretica mit antikaliurischen Substanzen kombinieren, bin ich nicht einverstanden. Bei der Behandlung einer Hypertonie ist dies oft nicht nötig, oder eine Kaliumsubstitution ausreichend. In anderen Fällen sind sie trotzdem nicht davon dispensiert, regelmäßig das Kalium zu bestimmen, um eine Hyperkaliämie zu vermeiden. Eine Kombination ist aber sicher ratsam, wenn der Patient auf ein Diureticum allein nicht genügend reagiert, z. B. beim nephrotischen Syndrom. Unter Umständen gibt es Kontraindikationen, etwa durch eine Niereninsuffizienz. Wenn bei kombinierter Anwendung beispielsweise von Etacrynsäure und Spironolacton eine Hyponatriämie entsteht, kann man immer noch Prednison geben, um die Wasserausscheidung zu fördern und die Natriumkonzentration zu normalisieren. Insgesamt scheint mir eine kombinierte Behandlung nicht generell indiziert, ggf. aber eine genaue Definition erforderlich, welche Kombination gemeint ist.

KOCZOREK: Ich glaube, unsere Ansichten liegen nicht so weit auseinander, wie Ihre Ausführungen auf den ersten Blick vermuten lassen könnten. Erstens habe ich mich in meinem Beitrag nicht auf die Behandlung von Hypertonikern bezogen, sondern nur auf Patienten mit Ödemen aus renalen, cardialen oder hepatischen Ursachen. Zweitens wissen wir übrigens aus Doppelblindversuchen, daß die Aldosteronantagonisten – ich rede jetzt nicht von der antikaliuretischen Substanz Triamteren oder Amilorid – einen günstigen Effekt in der Langzeitbehandlung der Hypertonie haben, und zwar in geringen Dosen, bei denen selbst über lange Zeiträume hinweg keine Hyperkaliämie verzeichnet wurde. – Die von uns beobachteten Fälle wurden übrigens hinsichtlich des Elektrolythaushaltes regelmäßig überwacht, so daß die Therapie veränderten Situationen leicht angepaßt werden konnte. Und noch etwas zu einem letzten unerledigten Punkt: Ich habe nur betont, daß man bei der Behandlung der hydropischen Herzinsuffizienz die Ansicht, es genügten bei diesen Patienten Diuretica allein vielleicht doch revidieren und korrigieren sollte, denn die Effekte der kombinierten diuretischen Therapie sind auch bei dieser Gruppe von Ödemkranken nach unseren Untersuchungen eindeutig günstiger, nicht nur hinsichtlich der Elimination von überschüssigem Wasser, sondern auch besonders hinsichtlich der Nebenwirkungen im Elektrolythaushalt. Allerdings muß die kombinierte diuretische Therapie bei schweren Fällen elastisch gehandhabt werden unter Vermeidung von starren Schemata.

MULLER: Was haben Sie eigentlich gegen die salzlose Diät? Wenn ein Patient, wie in Ihren Versuchen, in einigen Tagen 3–4 kg an Gewicht zunimmt, muß eine wesentliche Salzzufuhr stattgefunden haben.

KOCZOREK: Bei der intermittierenden Langzeittherapie handelte es sich um ambulante Patienten, die noch ihrem Beruf nachgingen und unter keinen Umständen auf einer salzfreien Diät zu halten waren. Im übrigen behandeln wir unsere Patienten grundsätzlich (abgesehen von der Bettruhe und den selbstverständlichen Glykosidgaben bei Herzkranken) mit einer Reduktion der Salzzufuhr; doch ist es auch in der Klinik auf den offenen Allgemeinstationen sehr schwierig, eine strenge Natriumrestriktion durchzuführen. Das ist wohl eher eine Frage streng überwachter Stoffwechselstationen. Praktisch sind meistens salzarme Diäten mit einem Natriumgehalt von 30–40 mval/Tag zu erreichen.

On the Urinary Excretion of a New Antikaliuretic Agent

Über die Harnausscheidung einer neuen antikaliuretischen Substanz

E. SCHMID, G. FRICKE

Neben dem Nachweis der pharmakologischen Wirkungen sind Untersuchungen über Resorption, Verteilung, Metabolismus und Ausscheidung bei neu eingeführten Arzneimitteln von besonderem Interesse.

Eine intensive Fluoreszenz ermöglicht die Bestimmung des K-retinierenden Diureticum Amilorid im Harn noch bei Konzentrationen im Nanogramm-Bereich. Wir ent-

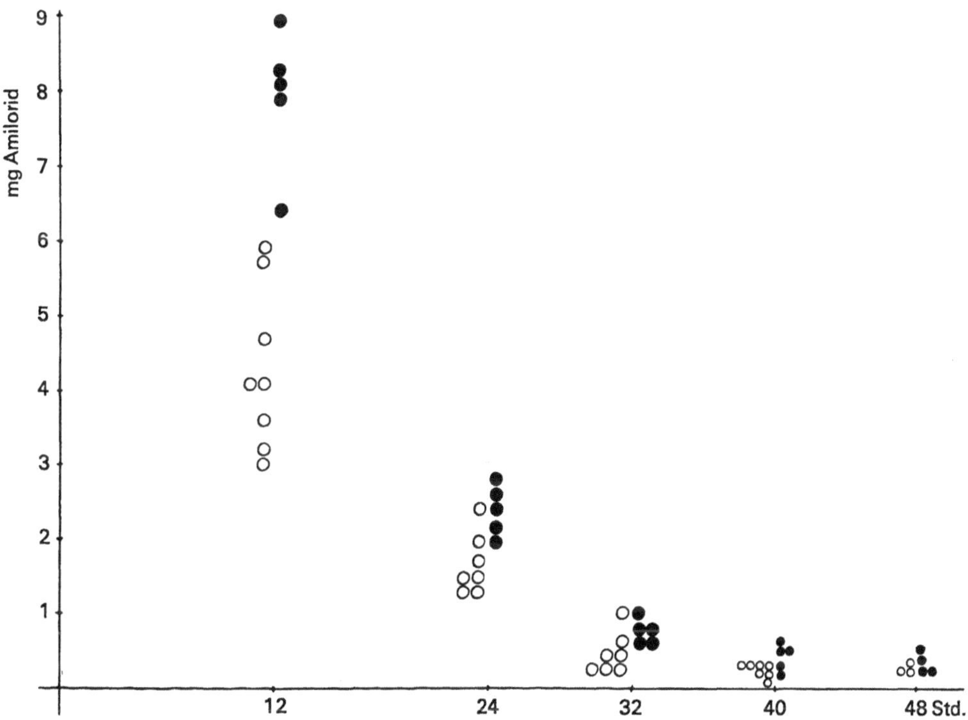

Abb. 1 a. Ausscheidung von Amilorid im Harn nach 20 mg per os als Einzeldosis bei gesunden Probanden. ○ = Einnahme zum Frühstück, ● = bei 4 Std. Nahrungskarenz.

Fig. 1 a. Excretion of amiloride in urine after oral administration of a single dose of 20 mg to healthy experimental subjects. ○ = drug taken at breakfast, ● = after abstention from food for 4 hours.

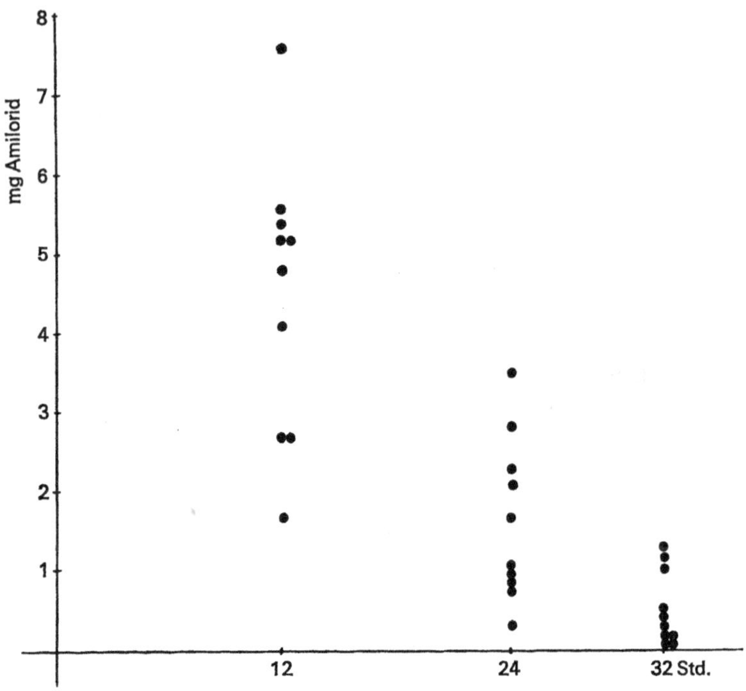

Abb. 1b. Harnausscheidung von Amilorid bei Kranken mit dekompensierter Leberzirrhose.

Fig. 1b. Urinary excretion of amiloride by patients with decompensated cirrhosis of the liver.

wickelten folgende Methode: Isolierung von Amilorid durch Dünnschicht-Bandchromatographie des Nativharns auf Kieselgel-G mit dem Fließmittelsystem Isopropanol: Ammoniak 85:15, Zweitentwicklung im System Isopropanol: Äthylazetat: Ammoniak 47:47:6.

Extraktion der Amilorid-haltigen Zone mit n/10 NaOH, Fluoreszenzmessung mit dem Aminco-Bowman-Spektrophotofluorometer ($\lambda_A = 366$ nm, $\lambda_F = 422$ nm).

Die Untersuchung von 184 Sammelharnen von 39 Probanden führte zu folgenden Ergebnissen:

1. Nach Zufuhr von 10 bzw. 20 mg Amilorid, als Einzeldosis zum Frühstück oder kurz darauf eingenommen, wurden innerhalb von 24 Stunden 28% im Mittel wiedergefunden. Über den Verbleib des Rests waren zunächst keine Aussagen möglich. Insbesondere ergaben die Versuche keinen Hinweis auf eine Harnausscheidung fluoreszierender Metaboliten. Dies steht im Gegensatz zu früheren Untersuchungen mit Spironolacton, bei denen wir neben dem Hauptmetaboliten Aldadiene 7 weitere Abbauprodukte fanden. Bei 4stündiger Nahrungskarenz lag die Wiederfindung von Amilorid bei den gleichen Probanden mit 55% der applizierten Dosis doppelt so hoch wie nach Einnahme zum Frühstück. Dies spricht dafür, daß die Harnausscheidung des Pharmakons wesentlich von der enteralen Resorption bestimmt wird, deren Beeinflussung durch Nahrungsbestandteile noch nicht geklärt wurde.

2. Von besonderem Interesse erschien uns die Frage, welche Pharmakon-Mengen bei gesicherter Leberzirrhose und portalem Hochdruck wiedergefunden werden. 10 Patienten, davon 6 mit ausgeprägtem Ascites, nahmen 20 mg Amilorid zum Frühstück ein. Die Ausscheidungsgeschwindigkeit und die Wiederfindung unterschied sich bei dieser Gruppe nicht von den Befunden bei Kontrollpersonen.

3. Hinsichtlich des zeitlichen Verlaufs der Amilorid-Ausscheidung fanden wir ein Maximum zwischen der 4. und 8. Stunde nach Applikation. Nach 10 mg ließen sich ab der 12. Stunde meist nur noch Spuren nachweisen, während nach einer Einzeldosis von 20 mg die Ausscheidung erst nach 40–48 Std. abgeschlossen war (Abb. 1). Diese Ergebnisse sind mit Angaben über Eintritt und Dauer des klinischen Effekts auf Wasser- und Elektrolyt-Ausscheidung zu vereinbaren. Beziehungen zwischen der Wiederfindung von Amilorid und der Diurese bestehen nicht. Wird Amilorid zusammen mit dem Salureticum Etacrynsäure verabreicht, so kommt es zu einer erheblichen Zunahme des Harnvolumens ohne gleichzeitige Erhöhung der Amilorid-Ausscheidung.

4. Im klinischen Versuch wurde dieser Effekt bei 9 von 10 Patienten mit zuvor therapieresistentem Ödem oder Ascites bestätigt. Als Nebenwirkungen trat ein kurzfristiger Stupor bei einer Kranken mit Leberzirrhose auf, bei der der Ascites zu rasch ausgeschwemmt wurde.

Die Laborproben verhielten sich bis auf den Anstieg des Serum-Harnsäure-Spiegels in einem Falle unauffällig.

On the Urinary Excretion of a New Antikaliuretic Agent

Investigations of the absorption, distribution, metabolism, and excretion of newly introduced drugs, in addition to studies of their pharmacological actions, are of particular interest.

It is possible to determine the K-retaining diuretic compound amiloride in urine at concentrations within the nanogram range due to its intense fluorescence. We have developed the following method: Isolation of amiloride by thin layer chromatography of urine on Kieselgel-G with the fluid system isopropanol: ammonia 85:15, second partition with the system isopropanol: ethylacetate: ammonia 47:47:6.

Extraction of the amiloride-containing zone with n/10 NaOH, measurement of fluorescence with the Aminco-Bowman-spectrophotofluorometer ($\lambda_A = 366$ nm, $\lambda_F = 422$ nm).

Examination of 184 urines from 39 experimental subjects gave the following results:

1. After administration of 10 or 20 mg amiloride, taken as single dose at breakfast or shortly afterwards, an average amount of 28% was recovered within 24 hours. It was not possible at first to elucidate the fate of the residue. The experiments gave no indication in particular about urinary excretion of fluorescent metabolites. This was in contrast to earlier studies with spironolactone, in which we had found 7 further dissociation products in addition to the chief metabolite aldadiene. After the same subjects had abstained from food for 4 hours 55% of the administered dose of amiloride were recovered, this being twice as much as the amount recovered after administration at breakfast. This indicates that the urinary excretion of the drug is largely determined by enteral absorption. The influence of components of food on this has not been clarified.

2. We were particularly interested in the question what amount of drug would be recovered in confirmed cirrhosis of the liver with portal hypertension.

10 patients, 6 of whom had pronounced ascites, received 20 mg amiloride at breakfast. There was no difference between this group and a control group in the velocities of excretion and recovery.

3. As regards the course of time of amiloride excretion we observed a maximum between the 4th and 8th hour after administration. After a dose of 10 mg only traces were shown after 12 hours, whilst after a single dose of 20 mg excretion continued for 40–48 hours afterwards (Fig. 1). These results are compatible with known statements about the beginning and duration of the clinical effects of water and electrolyte excretion. There is no relationship between recovery of amiloride and diuresis. If amiloride is administered together with the saluretic ethacrynic acid, urinary volume increases greatly, but there is no simultaneous increase of excreted amiloride.

4. Clinical trials confirmed these effects in 9 out of 10 patients who had treatment-resistant edema or ascites. One patient with cirrhosis of the liver, whose ascites was too quickly removed, had a short-lasting stupor as side-effect.

Laboratory tests gave results within the normal range, with the exception of a rise of serum uric acid levels in one case.

Serum Electrolytes During Combined Administration of Ethacrynic Acid and Amiloride

Das Verhalten der Serum-Elektrolyte unter der Verabreichung einer Etacrynsäure-Amilorid-Kombination

F. HUSMANN, P. SUCHAN

In der Literatur finden sich mehrere Hinweise auf die kaliumretinierende Eigenschaft des Amilorid (N-Amidino-3,5-diamino-6-chlor-pyrazinamid-hydrochlorid) (1–4). Wir haben nachzuprüfen versucht, ob diese Eigenschaft erhalten bleibt, wenn Amilorid gemeinsam mit einem Diureticum verabfolgt wird.

Als Diureticum wählten wir für unsere Untersuchungen Etacrynsäure und verabreichten Dosen von 50 bis 150 mg Etacrynsäure mit 5,0 bis 15,0 mg Amilorid über einen Zeitraum von 12 Wochen. Als Versuchspersonen dienten 10 Patienten mit vorwiegend cardial bedingten Ödemen. Die Behandlung erfolgte ausschließlich stationär. In einer Vorbeobachtungsperiode von jeweils 8 Tagen wurden lediglich Cardiaca, Coronardilatatoren o. ä. verabreicht. Während der gesamten Versuchsdauer wurde einheitlich eine kochsalz- und flüssigkeitsarme Diät gegeben.

Kontrolliert wurde die Einwirkung des Kombinationspräparates auf den Serum-Kalium, -Natrium-, -Calcium- und -Chlorid-Spiegel. Die Bestimmung der genannten Kationen erfolgte flammenphotometrisch; das Anion wurde mit einem Chlorocounter erfaßt. – Die statistische Auswertung der Ergebnisse nahmen wir nach dem Student-Test vor. Eine Signifikanz wurde angenommen, wenn die Irrtumswahrscheinlichkeit unter 5% lag, d. h. wenn $p < 0{,}05$ war.

Unsere Untersuchungen ergaben, daß unter der Behandlung mit der Etacrynsäure-Amilorid-Kombination in der von uns gewählten Dosierung der Serum-Kalium-Wert leicht ansteigt (von 4,67 auf 4,84 mval/l). Dieser Anstieg ist nicht signifikant. Er findet sich fast ausschließlich bei Patienten mit normo- oder hypokaliämischen Ausgangswerten. In anderen Fällen ist unter der Therapie ein Absinken zu beobachten, das besonders ausgeprägt war bei einem Patienten mit einem Ausgangswert von 6,6 mval/l Kalium. Dieser Wert ging unter der Applikation des Kombinationspräparates auf 5,5 mval/l zurück. Bleiben diese Werte bei der statistischen Auswertung unberücksichtigt, so findet sich ein Anstieg des Serum-Kalium-Wertes von durchschnittlich 4,44 auf 4,76 mval/l, ein Ergebnis, das an der Signifikanzgrenze liegt.

Diese Befunde deuten auf eine gewisse Abhängigkeit des Verhaltens des Serum-Kalium-Spiegels von der Höhe des Ausgangswertes hin, wobei hohe Ausgangswerte unter der Therapie eher einen Rückgang erkennen lassen, niedrige mehr einen Anstieg zeigen. Ein analoges Verhalten läßt der Serum-Natrium-Spiegel erkennen. In den Fällen, in denen der Ausgangswert über 130 mval pro Liter lag, fand sich unter der Behandlung eine Abnahme des Natrium-Spiegels. Werte unterhalb von 130 mval/l wiesen einen Anstieg auf, der am stärksten ausgeprägt war bei einem Patienten mit einem Ausgangswert von 121,8 mval/l, der unter der Therapie auf 147,0 mval/l anstieg. Dieses Verhalten dürfte verantwortlich sein für die Tatsache, daß sich unter der Behandlung keine Signifikanz bei der Änderung des Serum-Natrium-Spiegels nachweisen läßt, wenn alle Patienten gemeinsam berücksichtigt werden (Rückgang von 138,59 auf durchschnittlich 133,11 mval/l). Die gesonderte Betrachtung der beiden genannten Gruppen läßt einen deutlichen Rückgang des Serum-Natrium-Spiegels in der einen, einen ebensolchen Anstieg in der anderen Gruppe erkennen. Für eine Signifikanzberechnung ist allerdings die Fallzahl zu klein.

Der Serum-Calcium-Spiegel sinkt unter der Therapie von durchschnittlich 5,29 signifikant auf 4,95 mval/l ab. Niedrige Ausgangswerte ändern sich dabei kaum, während der Rückgang um so größer ist, je höher der Ausgangswert liegt. Im Extremfall fanden wir einen Rückgang um 0,65 mval/l, nämlich von 5,65 auf 5,0 mval/l.

Der Chloridgehalt des Serums läßt, abgesehen von einer Ausnahme, einen Rückgang erkennen (von durchschnittlich 95,92 auf 92,50 mval/l), der aber nicht signifikant ist wegen der starken Schwankung der Ausgangswerte (zwischen 87,9 und 110,5 mval/l).

Unsere an einem relativ kleinen Patientengut gewonnenen Ergebnisse deuten darauf hin, daß unter der Therapie mit einer Kombination von Etacrynsäure und Amilorid in der von uns gewählten Dosierung die Serumelektrolyte sich in Abhängigkeit von der Höhe der Ausgangswerte ändern. Wir möchten mit diesem kurzen Beitrag eine Überprüfung an einem größeren Krankengut anregen, wobei auch die Relation Amilorid zu Etacrynsäure variiert werden sollte.

Serum Electrolytes During Combined Administration of Ethacrynic Acid and Amiloride

The literature contains several references to the potassium-retaining properties of amiloride hydrochloride (N-amidino-3,5-diamino-6-chloro-pyrazinamide-hydrochloride), (1–4). We have attempted to investigate whether this property is preserved if amiloride hydrochloride is administered jointly with another diuretic agent.

For studies we selected ethacrynic acid as a diuretic agent and we administered it in doses of 50 to 150 mg with 5.0 to 15.0 mg of amiloride hydrochloride for a period of 12 weeks. 10 patients with predominantly cardiac edema served as experimental subjects. Treatment was only carried out while the patients were hospitalized. During a pre-observation period of 8 days the patients only received cardiac drugs, coronary-dilating agents, etc. During the entire duration of the test the patients received a uniform low-salt and low-fluid diet.

The action of the combination drug on the serum-potassium, serum-sodium, serum-calcium and serum-chloride level was determined. The stated cations were determined with the flame-photometer and the anion was determined with a chlorocounter. The statistical analysis of the results was performed according to the Student-test. The results were assumed to be significant if the probability of error was less than 5%, i. e., if p was <0.05.

Our studies showed that during treatment with the combination of ethacrynic acid and amiloride in the dosage selected by us the serum-potassium-level shows a mild increase from 4.67 to 4.84 mEq/l. This increase is not significant. It is found almost exclusively in patients with normokalemic or hypokalemic starting values. In other cases a decrease can be observed during treatment and this was particularly pronounced in one patient with a starting value of 6.6 mEq/l of potassium. During the administration of the combination drug this value decreased to 5.5 mEq/l. If these values are not considered in the statistical analysis, one finds a mean increase of the serum-potassium-level from 4.44 to 4.76 mEq/l, a result which is close to the border of significance. These findings indicate a certain dependency of the reactions of the serum-potassium-level on the magnitude of the starting value and in this context higher starting values had a tendency to show a decrease during treatment, whereas low starting values had a tendency to show an increase. The serum-sodium-level shows a similar reaction. Cases in which the starting value was above 130 mEq/l showed a decrease of the sodium-level during treatment. Values below 130 mEq/l showed an increase which was most pronounced in one patient with a starting value of 121.8 mEq/l which during treatment increased to 147.0 mEq/l. These reactions are probably responsible for the fact that during treatment it is not possible to demonstrate significance in the changes of the serum-sodium-level if one considers all patients jointly (a decrease from 138.59 to a mean of 133.11mEq/l). A separate evaluation of the two stated groups shows a definite decrease of the serum-sodium-level in one group and a corresponding increase in the other group. However, the number of cases is too small to determine the significance.

During treatment the serum-calcium-level decreases from a mean of 5.29 to 4.95mEq/l, and this is significant. In this context low starting values hardly change, whereas the decrease is the more pronounced the higher the starting value. In one extreme case we found a decrease by 0.65 mEq/l, i. e., from 5.65 to 5.0 mEq/l.

With one exception the chloride level of the serum shows a decrease (from a mean of 95.92 to 92.50 mEq/l) which, however, is not significant on account of the strong fluctuation of the starting values (from 87.9 to 110.5 mEq/l).

Our results, which were obtained in a relatively small patient group, indicate that during treatment with a combination of ethacrynic acid and amiloride hydrochloride with the dosage level selected by us the serum electrolytes change with a dependency on the magnitude of the starting values. With this brief contribution we would like to stimulate re-examination on a larger patient group during which the ratio of amiloride hydrochloride to ethacrynic acid should also be varied.

Literatur / References

1. Baer, J. E., C. M. Mucha, S. A. Spitzer and H. W. Yee: Federation Proc. **25**, 197 (1966).
2. Hitzenberger, G. H., Kampffmeyer and J. Conway: Clin. Pharm. Therap. **9**, 71 (1968).
3. Reynolds, T. B. and H. C. Pelle: Clin. Research **14**, 184 (1966).
4. Singh, B. N., D. E. Richmond, J. D. Wilson, H. A. Simmonds and J. D. K. North: British Med. J. **1967**, I, 143.

Clinical Results with Ethacrynic Acid in Combination with MK 870*)

Klinische Ergebnisse mit Etacrynsäure in Kombination mit MK 870*)

K. W. FRITZ, R. RICHTER

Bei insgesamt 30 Ödemkranken, 13 Patienten mit kardialen, 11 mit renalen und 6 mit hepatischen Ödemen, wurde die Wirkung von Etacrynsäure allein und in Kombination mit MK 870 untersucht. Die Dosis betrug 100 mg Etacrynsäure täglich über 2 Wochen, denen nach 7 Tagen 20 mg MK 870 täglich zugesetzt wurden. Am ersten Therapietag kam es unter Etacrynsäure zu einem Anstieg der Diurese von 1050 ml als Durchschnittswert zweier Vortage auf 1850 ml, also um 76%. Die Ausscheidung von Natrium stieg von vorher 80 mval/die auf 195 mval/die an, damit um 144%. Die Ausscheidung von Chlor nahm von 85 mval/die um 141% auf 205 mval/die zu, die Ausscheidung von Kalium von 35 mval/die um 57% auf 55 mval/die. Die Konzentration der drei Elektrolyte im Urin änderte sich für Natrium um +38% von 76 auf 105 mval/l, für Chlor um +37% von 81 auf 111 mval/l und für Kalium um −9% von 33 auf 30 mval/l.

Verglichen mit Furosemid ergibt sich damit ein wesentlich höherer Elektrolytverlust relativ zur diuretischen Wirkung. Frühere Untersuchungen mit dieser Substanz in Dosierungen von 40 und 80 mg täglich zeigten bei einem Diuresezuwachs um 125% nur geringe Zunahmen der Natriumkonzentration von 86 mval/l auf 96 mval/l (+12%), und der Chlorkonzentration von 99 auf 105 mval/l (+6%), für Kalium eine deutliche Abnahme der Konzentration von 42 auf 28 mval/l (−33%).

Der Natrium/Kalium-Quotient stieg unter Hydromedin von 2,5 auf 3,6 am ersten Therapietag, fiel dann aber innerhalb von 7 Tagen auf den Ausgangswert ab. In dieser Zeit ließ sich eine durchschnittliche Gewichtsabnahme von 1,3 kg erreichen. Die Serumkonzentrationen von Natrium und Kalium blieben dabei unverändert, während das Serum-Chlor eine fallende und das Serumbikarbonat eine steigende Tendenz zeigte, in Einzelfällen mit deutlich alkalotischen Werten.

Die Zugabe von MK 870 in der zweiten Therapiewoche hatte eine Verstärkung des diuretischen Effektes zur Folge. Die Gewichtskurve, die in den letzten Tagen der ersten Woche horizontal verlaufen war, zeigte wieder eine fallende Tendenz, und es kam nochmals zu einer Gewichtsabnahme von durchschnittlich 1,5 kg in der zweiten Woche. Die Tagesharnmengen nahmen entsprechend leicht zu. Während die renale Chlorausscheidung dabei unverändert blieb, stieg die Natriumausscheidung deutlich an. Damit kam es zu einer Umkehrung des Natrium/Chlor-Quotienten von 0,93 in der ersten Therapiewoche auf 1,13 in der zweiten Therapiewoche. Die Kaliumausscheidung fiel gleichzeitig

*) Amilorid

deutlich ab, so daß auf Grund dieses Verhaltens beider Elektrolyte der Natrium/Kalium-Quotient einen erheblichen Anstieg auf 6,2 am ersten Tag mit MK 870 erkennen ließ. In den folgenden Tagen fiel dieser wieder ab, lag aber auch noch am letzten Tag der zweiten Woche mit 3,2 über dem Ausgangswert. Entsprechend sank jetzt die Serum-Natriumkonzentration auf 138,5 mval/l, während das Serum-Kalium auf 4,9 mval/l anstieg. Die Serum-Chlorkonzentration wurde nicht beeinflußt, dafür zeigte die Serum-Bikarbonatkonzentration eine fallende Tendenz.

Das Verhalten der renalen Ausscheidung wie auch der Serumkonzentrationen war in den drei Patientengruppen nicht einheitlich. Der beste diuretische Effekt ließ sich mit einer Gewichtsabnahme von durchschnittlich 5 kg in den 2 Therapiewochen bei den cardialen Ödemen erzielen. Bei den renalen Ödemen kam es am ehesten zu Azidosen, während die Patienten mit hepatischen Ödemen keinen Anstieg des Serum-Kaliums, dafür aber eine Neigung zur Hyponatriämie erkennen ließen.

Aus diesen Werten ergibt sich, daß die Kombination von Etacrynsäure mit MK 870 einen günstigen therapeutischen Effekt aufweist, da die diuretische Wirkung der Etacrynsäure verstärkt, der renale Kaliumverlust vermieden und die Neigung zur metabolischen Alkalose ausgeglichen werden kann. Bei gleicher Dosierung der Etacrynsäure ist aber der Effekt von MK 870 auf die Serum-Kaliumkonzentration und den Bikarbonatspiegel unterschiedlich. Abgesehen von den Unterschieden bei verschiedener Ödemgenese nahm die Tendenz zur Hyperkaliämie zu, wenn bei gleicher Relation höhere Dosen von Etacrynsäure zur Ausschwemmung benötigt wurden. Entsprechend sahen wir einen Patienten, der unter nur 50 mg Etacrynsäure gut ausschwemmte und trotz täglich 20 mg MK 870 plus Zulage von 26 mval Kalium täglich mit seiner Serumkonzentration im unteren Normbereich blieb. Wurde die Kombination von 100:20 mg beider Substanzen als Langzeittherapie nur zwei- oder dreimal pro Woche gegeben, zeigten Kontrollen bei 10 Patienten über 6 Wochen allerdings keine Abweichungen der Serumkonzentrationen aus dem Normbereich. Ähnlich wie bei der Kombination von Diuretica mit Spironolacton erscheint jedoch eine fixe Kombination der Etacrynsäure mit der kaliumretinierenden Substanz nicht vorteilhaft. Eine optimale Einstellung wird sich nur durch eine individuell variierbare Kombination erreichen lassen.

An Nebenwirkungen ergab sich vor allem eine Neigung zum Anstieg des Harnsäurespiegels, der bei einem Patienten von einem Normalwert von 7 mg% ausgehend 18 mg% erreichte. Sonstige Nebenwirkungen waren einmal ein Verwirrtheitszustand und nach langer Gabe von Etacrynsäure (insgesamt 23,3 g) Drehschwindel und Schwerhörigkeit, die sich nach Umsetzen auf Furosemid als teilweise reversibel erwiesen. Gelegentlich kam es zur Verstärkung einer vorbestehenden metabolischen Azidose, die bei einem Patienten mit beginnender renaler Insuffizienz innerhalb von 14 Therapietagen mit der Kombination zu einem Abfall des venösen pH von 7,25 auf 7,09 führte.

Clinical Results with Ethacrynic Acid in Combination with MK 870 (Amiloride)

The effect of ethacrynic acid alone and in combination with MK 870 was studied in a total of 30 patients with edema; 13 patients with cardiac edema, 11 with renal edema, and 6 with hepatic edema. The daily dose was 100 mg ethacrynic acid for 2 weeks to which, after 7 days, 20 mg MK 870 were added per day. On the first day of treatment with ethacrynic acid an increase of diuresis from 1050 ml as the mean value from two previous days to 1850 ml occurred, i. e., an increase of 76%. The excretion of sodium increased from a previous value of 80 mEq/day to 195 mEq/day, i. e., by 144%. The excretion of chloride increased from 85 mEq/day by 141% to 205 mEq/day, the excretion of potassium increased from 35 mEq/day by 57% to 55 mEq/day. The urinary concentration of these three electrolytes changed by +38% from 76 to 105 mEq/l in the case of sodium, for chloride it changed by 37% from 81 to 111 mEq/l, and for potassium it changed by −9% from 33 to 30 mEq/l.

Thus, in comparison to furosemide a considerably higher loss of electrolytes is found as compared with the diuretic effect. Previous studies with this substance with dosage levels of 40 and 80 mg per day, associated with an increase of the diuresis by 125%, showed only minimal increases of the sodium concentration from 86 mEq/l to 96 mEq/l (+12%), and of the chloride concentration from 99 to 105 mEq/l (+6%), and in the case of potassium they showed a definite decrease of the concentration from 42 to 28 mEq/l (−33%).

During treatment with ethacrynic acid the sodium-potassium ratio increased from 2.5 to 3.6 on the first day of treatment, but it subsequently decreased within 7 days to the starting value. During this period it was possible to achieve a mean weight loss of 1.3 kg. However, the serum levels of sodium and potassium remained unchanged, whereas the serum-chloride showed a decreasing and the serum-bicarbonate an increasing tendency. In individual cases this was associated with definitely alkalotic values.

The addition of MK 870 during the second week of treatment resulted in an increase of the diuretic effect. The weight curves which had pursued a horizontal course during the last few days of the first week, once again showed a downward tendency and a mean weight loss of 1.5 kg occurred again during the second week. The daily urine output showed a corresponding mild increase. The sodium excretion increased definitely, whereas the renal chloride excretion remained unchanged. Thus a reversal of the sodium-chloride ratio occurred from 0.93 during the first week of treatment to 1.13 during the second week of treatment. At the same time the potassium excretion decreased markedly and thus, on the basis of these reactions of the two electrolytes, the sodium-potassium ratio showed a considerable increase to 6.2 on the first day with MK 870. During the subsequent days it once again decreased, but even on the last day of the second week it still was 3.2 and thus it was above the starting value. Correspondingly, the serum-sodium concentration now decreased to 138.5 mEq/l, whereas the serum potassium increased to 4.9 mEq/l. The serum chloride concentration was not affected, but the serum-bicarbonate level showed a downward tendency.

The reactions of renal excretion as well as of the serum levels were not uniform in the three patient groups. The best diuretic effect – with a mean weight loss of 5 kg during the two week treatment period – could be achieved in patients with cardiac edema. In patients with renal edema acidosis occurred most readily, whereas patients with hepatic edema did not demonstrate an increase of the serum-potassium but instead of this they showed a tendency to hyponatremia.

These results indicate that combination of ethacrynic acid with MK 870 has a favourable therapeutic effect since the diuretic effect of ethacrynic acid is intensified, renal potassium loss is avoided and the tendency to metabolic alkalosis can be compensated. However, with an identical dosage level of ethacrynic acid, the effect of MK 870 on the serum-potassium level and on the bicarbonate level is diverse. Apart from the different etiologies of the edema, an increased tendency towards hyperkalemia was noted with higher doses of ethacrynic acid needed for better elimination of edema, the relation remaining the same. In agreement with this, we observed one patient who – while only receiving 50 mg ethacrynic acid – showed a good diuretic effect and whose serum potassium concentration remained in the lower range of normal despite daily administration of 20 mg MK 870 plus addition of 26 mEq of potassium per day. However, if the combination of 100 mg ethacrynic acid and 20 mg MK 870 was administered as longterm treatment, only 2 or 3 times per week, controls in 10 patients over 6 weeks failed to show deviations of the serum concentrations from the normal range. However, similar to a combination of diuretics with spironolactone, a fixed combination of ethacrynic acid with the potassium retaining substance does not appear to be advantageous. Optimal dosage can only be achieved by an individual, variable combination.

As far as side effects are concerned we usually observed a tendency towards an increase in the uric acid level which in one patient reached 18 mg%, starting from a normal value of 7 mg%. Other side effects which were observed were one case with mental confusion and, after prolonged administration of ethacrynic acid (total 23.3 g) a case with vertigo and decreased auditory acuity which, after the patient was switched to furosemide, were found to be partially reversible. Occasionally, potentiation of a pre-existing metabolic acidosis occurred which in one patient with beginning renal failure produced a decrease of the venous pH from 7.25 to 7.09 within 14 days of treatment with this combination.

Amiloride in Edematous Patients

Amilorid-Anwendung bei der Ödemausschwemmung

N. HEINZ

Im Folgenden wird über Ergebnisse mit Amilorid in Kombination mit Etacrynsäure bei insgesamt 38 Patienten berichtet. Unser Krankengut ist nicht homogen, ganz überwiegend ist aber eine Herzinsuffizienz Ursache der Salz- und Wasserretention gewesen. Alle Patienten haben eine Diät mit einer Kochsalzbeschränkung auf höchstens 3 g in 24 Std. erhalten.

Da in den kleinen Gruppen, über die ich berichten kann, das bisher vorliegende Zahlenmaterial nicht normal verteilt ist, wurde von einer weiteren statistischen Bearbeitung abgesehen.

Die bei uns und anderweitig festgestellten besonderen Charakteristika der Wirkung, nämlich Kaliumretention und Begünstigung einer hyperchlorämischen Azidose, lassen eine Kombination des allein nur relativ schwachen Diureticums Amilorid mit Etacrynsäure sehr erfolgversprechend erscheinen.

Wir haben überwiegend die Kombination 5 mg Amilorid + 25 mg Etacrynsäure eingesetzt. Die Ergebnisse sind in Tab. 1 zusammengestellt.

Tab. 1. Diurese mit 5 mg Amilorid + 25 mg Etacrynsäure. (N = 15)

	Vortage			Behandlungstage		
	3	2	1	1	2	3
Urin ml/24 h	722	836	839	1 095	1 261	1 207
Na mval/24 h	44	48	42	101	110	102
K mval/24 h	42	43	42	42	36	40
Na/K Quotient	1,1	1,1	1,0	2,5	3,1	2,6
Chlorid mval/24 h	73	75	75	103	122	122

Diurese mit 10 mg Amilorid + 50 mg Etacrynsäure (N = 11)

	Vortage			Behandlungstage		
	3	2	1	1	2	3
Urin ml/24 h	780	760	780	1 550	1 540	1 630
Na mval/24 h	51	49	42	155	156	148
K mval/24 h	40	43	38	36	48	54
Na/K Quotient	1,3	1,1	1,1	4,3	3,3	2,7
Chlorid mval/24 h	73	66	57	150	141	106

Die Größe der Diurese, die wir mit der Kombination erreicht haben, hängt vom Umfang der Kochsalz- und Wasserretention ab, maximal wurden in 24 Std. bei 5 + 25 mg 5300 (!) ml Urin ausgeschieden. Resistenz trotz Flüssigkeitsretention haben wir zweimal bei ätiologisch völlig anders geartetem Ödem, nämlich bei Ascites infolge Peritonealcarcinose gesehen, bei allen cardial oder infolge Leberzirrhose Dekompensierten war mit höchstens 10 + 50 mg bei der erwähnten NaCl-Restriktion eine befriedigende Diurese möglich.

Eine Mittelwertsbildung über die ersten drei Behandlungstage hinaus erschien mir sinnlos – bei der hier gewählten Dosis erlischt die Diurese trotz Fortführung der Therapie nach Eintritt der Gewichtskonstanz. Der Urin-Na/K-Quotient ging auf Werte um 1,0 oder sogar darunter zurück, schon für die Behandlungstage 5.–7. streut demnach der Urin Na/K-Quotient zwischen 1,0 und 10,0, je nach dem Umfang der dann noch laufenden Diurese.

Kein Patient erhielt eine Kaliumsubstitution, trotzdem stieg der Kaliumspiegel im Serum an, Schwierigkeiten mit einer Hypokaliämie hatten wir bei keinem Patienten (Tab. 2).

Tab. 2. Serumelektrolyte während der Amilorid-Etacrynsäure-Diurese.

1.	5 + 25 mg Vorperiode	Behandlungsperiode (3. Tag) (N = 15)
Na	134,9	134,5
K	4,33	4,86
Cl	100,7	99,6
2	10 + 50 mg Vorperiode	Behandlungsperiode (3. Tag) (N = 11)
Na	134,4	134,1
K	4,47	4,74
Cl	102,9	96,9

Gegenstand besonderer Aufmerksamkeit müssen, damit das Präparat nicht in Mißkredit gerät, bedrohliche Hyperkaliämien sein. Wir haben drei Beobachtungen gemacht, die alle Patienten mit leichter Azotämie (Kreatininspiegel 2–3 mg%) betreffen. Die Hyperkaliämien (7,1–7,5 mval/l) treten unter Umständen sehr schnell, z. B. binnen 2 Tagen, auf. Sie waren aber mit Natrium-Polystyrolsulfonat gut zu beherrschen.

Ich halte eine Therapie mit Amilorid – auch in der Form einer Kombination mit Etacrynsäure – ab einem Serumkreatininspiegel von 1,5 mg% für nicht indiziert und gefährlich. Da bei geriatrischen Patienten häufig – z. B. infolge renaler Arteriosklerose oder chronischer Pyelonephritiden latente Niereninsuffizienten vorliegen, scheint mir das Präparat generell für ältere Patienten weniger geeignet zu sein. Für die Behandlung der Herzinsuffizienz- und Leberzirrhose-Salz- und Wasserretention ist es hervorragend geeignet.

Addendum: Inzwischen wurden insgesamt 64 Patienten mit variablen Amilorid-Etacrynsäure-Kombinationen und unterschiedlicher Kochsalzrestriktion behandelt. Für die oben genannten Dosiskombinationen und eine Kochsalzrestriktion auf 3 g/die hat die statistische Auswertung mit dem Wilcoxon-Test bei ungefähr gleichen Mittelwerten folgendes ergeben: Bei 5 mg Amilorid + 25 mg Etacrynsäure (N = 24) und der doppelten Dosis (N = 13) nehmen das Urinvolumen, die Natriumausscheidung und die Chloridausscheidung zu, der Serumchloridspiegel nimmt ab ($p < 0{,}01$), der Serumkaliumspiegel steigt an ($p < 0{,}05$), für den Serumnatriumspiegel und für die Kaliurese lassen sich keine gerichteten Bewegungen gegenüber der Vorperiode sichern.

Amiloride in Edematous Patients

This is a report on the results obtained with amiloride in combination with ethacrynic acid in a total of 38 patients. Our patient material is not homogenous, but in the large majority of cases, heart failure was the cause of the salt and water retention. All patients received a diet, the salt content of which was limited to a maximum of 3 g per 24 hours.

Statistical analysis was precluded by the fact that the small number of samples reported here were not normally distributed. The particular characteristics of the effect which was observed in this study and by other investigators, i. e. potassium retention and enhancement of hyperchloremic acidosis, make a combination of the diuretic agent amiloride (which by itself has only a relatively weak action) in connection with ethacrynic acid, appear to be very promising.

Usually, a combination of 5 mg of amiloride with 25 mg ethacrynic acid was used. The following table indicates the responses obtained.

Table 1. Diuresis with 5 mg Amiloride + 25 mg Ethacrynic Acid. (N = 15)

	pre-treatment days			treatment days		
	3	2	1	1	2	3
Urine ml/24 h	722	836	839	1 095	1 261	1 207
Na mEq/24 h	44	48	42	101	110	102
K mEq/24 h	42	43	42	42	36	40
Na/K ratio	1.1	1.1	1.0	2.5	3.1	2.6
Chloride mEq/24 h	73	75	75	103	122	122

Diuresis with 10 mg of Amiloride + 50 mg of Ethacrynic Acid. (N = 11)

	pre-treatment days			treatment days		
	3	2	1	1	2	3
Urine ml/24 h	780	760	780	1 550	1 540	1 630
Na mEq/24 h	51	49	42	155	156	148
K mEq/24 h	40	43	38	36	48	54
Na/K ratio	1.3	1.1	1.1	4.3	3.3	2.7
Chloride mEq/24 h	73	66	57	150	141	106

The intensity of the diuresis which we achieved with this combination depends on the extent of the salt and water retention. The maximum urine excretion per 24 hours with 5 mg amiloride and 25 mg ethacrynic acid was 5300 (!) ml of urine. In two cases with edema of an entirely different etiology, i. e. ascites due to cancer of the peritoneum, we observed resistance despite fluid retention. In all other patients with decompensation due to cardiac factors or due to cirrhosis of the liver, a satisfactory diuresis was possible with NaCl restriction and combined therapy with 10 mg amiloride and 50 mg ethacrynic acid. In my opinion, it is useless to determine the mean values after the first three days of treatment – with the dosage level which was selected for this study, diuresis ceases after a constant weight has been achieved despite the continuation of treatment. The urinary Na/K-ratio decreased to values around 1.0 or even lower, and by the 5th to 7th day of treatment, the urinary Na/K-ratio scatters from 1.0 to 10.0 depending on the extent of the diuresis which is still taking place.

No patient received potassium substitution, nevertheless, the serum-potassium level increased. In no patient did we have difficulties with hypokalemia.

Table 2. Serum Electrolytes During Diuresis with Amiloride and Ethacrynic Acid.

1.	5 + 25 mg preceding period	treatment period (3rd day) (N = 15)
Na	134.9	134.5
K	4.33	4.86
Cl	100.7	99.6
2.	10 + 50 mg preceding period	treatment period (3rd day) (N = 11)
Na	134.4	134.1
K	4.47	4.74
Cl	102.9	96.9

In order to avoid adverse reactions to this drug, one must pay particular attention to dangerous hyperkalemia which we observed in three patients (serum potassium level 7.1–7.5 mEq/l), all of whom had mild azotemia (serum creatinine level 2–3 mg%). Under certain circumstances, hyperkalemia may occur very rapidly, i. e. within two days. However, they were well controlled with sodium polystyrolsulfonate.

In my opinion, treatment with amiloride – even in combination with ethacrynic acid – is not indicated and dangerous in the face of a serum-creatinine level of 1.5 mg% or higher. Since geriatric patients frequently e. g. due to renal arteriosclerosis or chronic pyelonephritis have latent renal failure, it appears to me that this drug is generally less suitable for elderly patients. It is excellently suited for the treatment of cardiac insufficiency, cirrhosis of the liver as well as salt- and water retention.

Addendum: In the meantime we have observed and studied a total of 64 edematous patients with the various fixed ethacrynic acid-amiloride-combinations under varying degrees of NaCl-restriction. For the above-mentioned fixed combination and a sodium restriction of 3 g/die, the statistical evaluation with the Wilcoxon-test showed the following results:

Under 5 mg amiloride and 25 mg ethacrynic acid, respectively under the double dose, there was an increase in urine volume and in sodium and chloride secretion while the serum chloride level decreased significantly ($p < 0.01$) and the serum potassium level rose ($p < 0.05$); serum sodium and potassium secretion did not show any significant changes compared with the control period.

The Action of Amiloride on the Sodium Transport at the Erythrocyte Membrane

Die Wirkung von Amilorid auf den Natrium-Transport an der Erythrozytenmembran

F. WESSELS

Bereits in früheren Untersuchungen hatten wir bei essentiellen Hypertonikern eine Erhöhung des Natriumgehalts der Erythrozyten festgestellt, die nach unseren Untersuchungen wahrscheinlich durch eine Steigerung der Natriumpermeabilität bedingt ist (6). Unter einer Behandlung mit Saluretica nahm die Natriumkonzentration der Erythrozyten parallel zur Blutdrucksenkung ab (4).

Wir prüften daher in vitro mit ^{22}Na den Einfluß verschiedener Saluretica sowie des Diazoxides auf den aktiven und passiven Natriumtransport der Erythrozyten mit folgenden Ergebnissen:

Hydrochlorothiazid sowie Mefrusid lassen den Natriumstoffwechsel der Erythrozyten unbeeinflußt. Das war auch zu erwarten, da diese Substanzen bekanntlich nur in metabolisierter Form wirken (1, 3).

Etacrynsäure, Furosemid und Diazoxid verlangsamen dosisabhängig einmal den Natriumeinstrom als den Parameter der Natriumpermeabilität sowie auch den aktiven Natriumtransport der Erythrozyten. Die Hemmung des Natriumeinstroms trat bei allen Substanzen bereits bei einer wesentlich niedrigeren Dosierung ein als die des Natriumausstromes. Dadurch kam es bei Wirkstoffkonzentrationen, wie sie wahrscheinlich auch im Serum nach Gabe von Furosemid (5) und Diazoxid in akut blutdrucksenkenden Dosen vorliegen, zu einer Abnahme des Natriumgehaltes der Erythrozyten. Dieser Befund könnte bei Übertragung auf die Gefäßmuskulatur und unter Berücksichtigung der Untersuchungen FRIEDMANS (2) evtl. den blutdrucksenkenden Effekt dieser Substanzen erklären.

In Fortführung dieser Untersuchungen testeten wir jetzt auch das neue kaliumsparende Saluretieum MK 870 (Amilorid).

Wie die Abbildung zeigt, hemmt MK 870 (Amilorid) ebenfalls dosisabhängig den aktiven Natriumtransport der Erythrozyten. Auf eine Hemmung der Natriumpumpe in den distalen Tubuli wird auch der saluretische Effekt dieses Pharmakons zurückgeführt. Der Wirkungsmechanismus, über den Amilorid den aktiven Natriumtransport hemmt, ist noch weitgehend ungeklärt. Die Membran-ATPase bleibt jedenfalls von Amilorid unbeeinflußt (Forschungslabor MSD).

Auf den Natriumeinstrom der Erythrozyten als dem Gradmesser der Natriumpermeabilität hat Amilorid dagegen keinen Einfluß. Das führt dazu, daß Amilorid in vitro den Natriumgehalt der Erythrozyten erhöht.

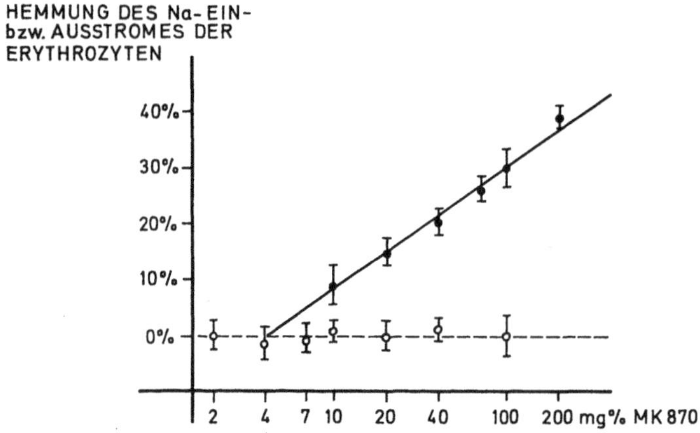

Einfluß von MK 870 auf den Natriumein- und -ausstrom der Erythrozyten
Influence of MK 870 on the sodium influx and outflow of erythrocytes

——— Efflux- / .... Influx- } Hemmung   = $\bar{x} \pm 2S$ n = 8   Inhibition of { outflow ——— / influx ....

Hinsichtlich des kaliumsparenden Effektes von MK 870 fällt auf, daß Triamteren, das ja auch kaliumsparend wirkt, ebenfalls nur den aktiven Natriumtransport und nicht die Natriumpermeabilität der Erythrozyten herabsetzt, während die zu einem Kaliumverlust führenden Saluretica Furosemid und Etacrynsäure zusätzlich die Natriumpermeabilität der Erythrozyten vermindern.

The Action of Amiloride on the Sodium Transport at the Erythrocyte Membrane

In earlier investigations on patients suffering from essential hypertension I had found an increased sodium content of the erythrocytes, which I thought to be due to an increase of permeability for sodium (6). On treatment with saluretics the concentration of sodium in erythrocytes fell in parallel with the fall of blood pressure (4).

I examined, therefore, in vitro with ^{22}Na the influence of various saluretics and of diazoxide on active and passive sodium transport of erythrocytes and found:

Hydrochlorothiazide and mefruside do not influence the sodium metabolism of erythrocytes. This was to be expected, as these compounds only act when metabolized (1, 3).

Ethacrynic acid, furosemide and diazoxide retard both the influx of sodium as parameter of sodium permeability and the active sodium transport of erythrocytes. This is dose-dependent. All compounds inhibited sodium influx at a much lower dosage than sodium outflow. In consequence, a decrease in the sodium content of the erythrocytes was analogue the serum blood levels of furosemide- (5) and diazoxide-doses sufficient for an acute lowering of blood pressure. These findings may possibly explain the blood pressure lowering effect of these compounds as being due to transmission to the muscular layers of blood-vessels, taking into account FRIEDMAN's studies (2).

I continued these investigations by testing the new potassium saving saluretic MK 870 (amiloride).

As shown in the illustration, MK 870 also inhibits dose-dependently the active sodium transport of erythrocytes. The saluretic action of this drug is also thought to be due to inhibition of the sodium pump in the distal tubules. The mechanism of action by which MK 870 inhibits active sodium transport is as yetlargely unexplained. Membrane ATPase is uninfluenced by MK 870 (Research Laboratories MSD).

Amiloride has no influence on the sodium influx into erythrocytes as a parameter of sodium permeability. Amiloride, therefore, increases the sodium content of erythrocytes in vitro.

So far as the potassium-saving effect of MK 870 is concerned, it is remarkable that triamterene, which is also potassium-saving, also only lowers the active sodium transport and does not lower the sodium permeability of erythrocytes, whilst the saluretics furosemide and ethacrynic acid, which both cause a loss of potassium, in addition reduce the sodium permeability of erythrocytes.

Literatur / References

1. Baumung, H. und K. Formanek: Med. Pharmacol. exp. **14,** 317 (1966).
2. Friedman, S. M., J. D. Jamieson and C. Friedman: Circulation Res. **7,** 44 (1959).
3. Kroneberg, G., K. Meng, L. Heilmeyer, E. S. Mazzei, H. J. Holtmeier und F. Marong in: Diureseforschung, IV. Symposion in Freiburg i. Br., Thieme, Stuttgart 1967.
4. Losse, H., H. Zumkley und H. Wehmeyer: z. Kreislaufforschung **51,** 43 (1962).
5. Muschaweck, R. und P. Hajdu: Arzneim.-Forsch. **14,** 44 (1964).
6. Wessels, F., G. Junge-Hülsing und H. Losse: z. Kreislaufforschung **56,** 374 (1967).

Diuretics in the Treatment of Hypertension

Bedeutung der Diuretica für die Hypertoniebehandlung

E. WOLLHEIM

Summary: 1. Concerning the pathogenesis of essential (primary) hypertension, the following factors have been established:

a) The inheritance factor of the disease

b) The importance of environmental influences for the manifestation of this inheritance in the progress of life

c) The characteristic behaviour of the hemodynamics: In the stage of cardio-vascular and renal compensation, the active blood volume is decreased by 10 to 15%. In more than 90% of these patients, the cardiac output is normal, or more often, slightly decreased. In a special group of 8%, an increase of cardiac output is found. Total peripheral resistance is elevated in every patient in correlation to his cardiac output. The smaller arteries and arterioles of patients with essential hypertension reveal a special sensitivity against all different irritations.

2. In patients with malignant hypertension, a definite life-prolonging effect of hypotensive therapy could be shown.

3. At present, only symptomatic treatment is possible in most types of arterial hypertension. For this purpose, drugs with different central or peripheral sites of action are available, for instance saluretic substances as thiazides, furosemide, mefroside and ethacrynic acid.

4. All these drugs decrease active blood volume and cardiac output in acute experiments. But this reaction alone is not responsible for the hypotensive effect. During chronic application of these substances the hemodynamic factors return to the values before treatment.

5. The effect of these substances is to be understood by a decrease of the total peripheral resistance connected with the increase in sodium excretion. This could be shown by investigations of the renal functions under the influence of these substances.

6. A combination of different drugs will increase the therapeutic effect while side effects decrease.

Ätiologie und Pathogenese der meisten Formen des Hochdrucks scheinen noch weitgehend ungeklärt zu sein. Eine Ausnahme machen nur einige besondere Formen der Hypertonie, z. B. das Phäochromozytom, der einseitige sog. reno-vasculäre Hochdruck mit nachgewiesener vermehrter Reninproduktion und die seltene Form der hypokaliämischen Hypertonie.

Die Therapie des Hochdrucks kann daher vorerst nur symptomatisch sein. Daß aber die Drucksteigerung als solche, gleich welcher Genese, behandlungsbedürftig ist, steht außer Zweifel. Dies kann dadurch belegt werden, daß bei der unkomplizierten essentiellen Hypertonie nach einem mehr oder weniger langen Zeitraum der Manifestation sich die Folgen und Komplikationen des Hochdrucks am Herzen, den Nieren, den Augen und dem

Gehirn entwickeln. Damit ruft der Hochdruck irreversible, arteriosklerotisch bedingte anatomische Läsionen an diesen Organen hervor. Ein vielleicht noch besserer Beleg für die Notwendigkeit der Drucksenkung ergibt sich aus der langjährigen Beobachtung von Kranken mit der besonderen Form des malignen Hochdrucks. Diese, anatomisch durch Arteriolosklerose und Arteriolonekrose der Nieren und anderer Organe gekennzeichnete Hochdruckform entwickelt sich in etwa 90% der untersuchten Fälle als Folge einer längere oder kürzere Zeit bestehenden exzessiven Drucksteigerung. Ein dem menschlichen malignen Hochdruck sehr ähnliches Bild kann auch im Tierexperiment (Drosselungshochdruck) bei Kaninchen produziert werden, wie WILSON u. PICKERING bereits vor 30 Jahren zeigten. Daß die Druckerhöhung für diese Veränderungen entscheidend ist, geht aus einseitigen Drosselungsversuchen von WILSON u. BYROM (1939) hervor, bei denen ubiquitär Intima- und Medianekrosen erzeugt wurden, aber allein die gedrosselte Niere frei blieb. Mein Mitarbeiter SCHÄFER hat für die Entstehung der besonderen klinischen Form des malignen Hochdrucks einen Autoaggressionsmechanismus diskutiert, da er fluoreszenzfärbbare Immunniederschläge in der Arteriolenwand der Nieren solcher Kranken nachweisen konnte. Das Antigen entsteht dabei möglicherweise durch Intimaläsionen infolge des exzessiv erhöhten Blutdrucks. Allerdings vermag eine immunosuppressive Therapie den raschen Fortschritt dieser Hochdruckform, der üb-

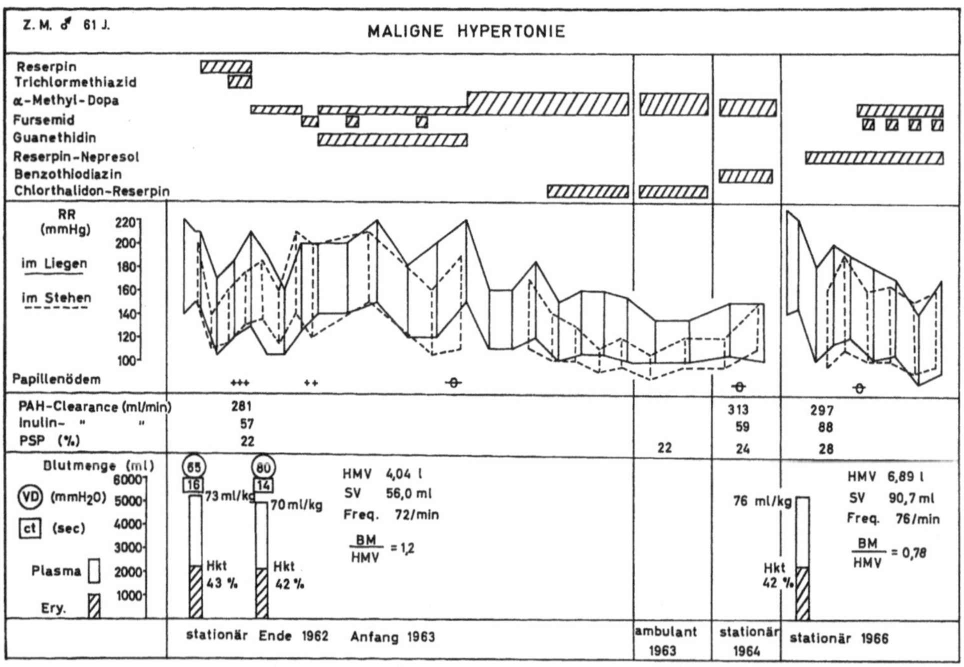

Abb. 1. Krankheitsverlauf bei einem 61jährigen Patienten mit maligner Hypertonie unter verschiedener hypotensiver Therapie. Beobachtungszeit über 4 Jahre. Verschwinden des Papillenödems unter langdauernder Drucksenkung, geringe Besserung der renalen Funktionsgrößen (aus: WOLLHEIM, E.: Proc. 9th Int. Congr. Life Ass. Med., Tel Aviv 1967, KARGER, Basel/New York 1968, 241).

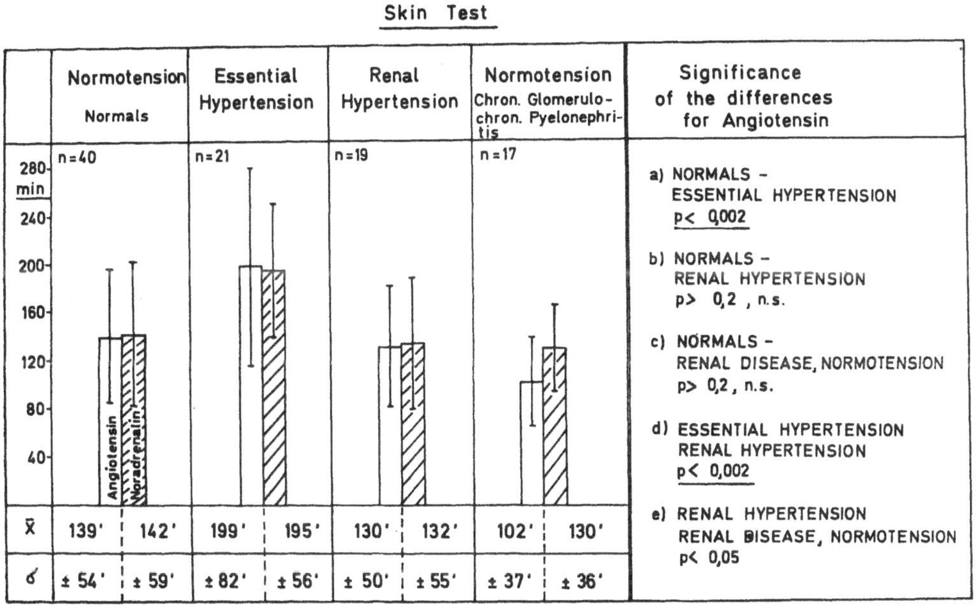

Abb. 2. Zeitdauer der Quaddelreaktion nach intrakutaner Gabe von 0,1 µg Angiotensin resp. 0,8 µg Noradrenalin bei normotonen, essentiellen und renalen Hypertonien (nach: PIPPIG, L. und M. IMHOFF: IV. Symp. Ges. Nephrol., Springer Berlin/Heidelberg/New York 1966, 7.27)

licherweise in wenigen Monaten zum Tode in Urämie und/oder Herzinsuffizienz führt, nicht aufzuhalten. Dagegen kann eine intensive blutdrucksenkende Behandlung, gleich welcher Art, zu einem eindeutigen Rückgang des charakteristischen Papillenödems, zu einer eindeutigen Verlängerung des Lebens und sogar unter Umständen zu einer leichten Besserung der Nierenfunktionswerte führen, wie ein Beispiel unserer eigenen Beobachtung zeigt. Es handelt sich um einen 61jährigen Patienten, der über 4 Jahre beobachtet werden konnte und während dieser Zeit mit den verschiedensten hypotensiven Pharmaka behandelt wurde (Abb. 1).

Aus diesem über Jahre erfolgreich behandelten Fall läßt sich auch ablesen, daß die drucksenkenden Effekte durch Pharmaka mit den verschiedensten Angriffspunkten auslösbar sind. Gleichartige Drucksenkungen lassen sich bei allen Hochdruckformen ebenso durch zentral angreifende Substanzen, z. B. die Rauwolfia-Alkaloide, durch peripher angreifende Ganglion- oder Sympathikusblocker oder durch Saluretica erzielen. Dies hat häufig dazu verführt, unberechtigte Schlüsse aus den therapeutischen Angriffspunkten auf die Pathogenese des Hochdrucks zu ziehen. Eine differenzierende funktionelle Diagnose sollte in allen Fällen vor der Therapie erfolgen.

Für die größte Gruppe der Hypertonien, den essentiellen Hochdruck, etwa 80–90% aller Hypertoniker, der zur Zeit die häufigste Erkrankung des Menschen ist, kann bezügl. der Pathogenese folgendes als gesichert gelten:

1. Die Krankheit ist genetisch bedingt (vergleiche WOLLHEIM u. MOELLER »Hypertonie« im Handbuch der Inneren Medizin 1960, Bd. IX/5 und mein Referat vor der Deutschen Gesellschaft für Kreislaufforschung, Bad Nauheim 1962). Die Vererbung

erfolgt nach unseren Feststellungen entsprechend den Mendel'schen Regeln. Ob ein oder mehrere genetische Faktoren eine Rolle spielen, ist noch unklar. Für die frühere oder spätere Manifestation der Erbanlage können Umwelteinflüsse entscheidend sein.

2. Bei der essentiellen Hypertonie lassen die peripheren Widerstandsgefäße, die Arteriolen, eine besondere Kontraktionsbereitschaft auf Reize der verschiedensten Art erkennen. Dies kann u. a. – allerdings mit großer individueller Streuung – durch einen einfachen intrakutanen Quaddeltest mit Angiotensin und Noradrenalin nachgewiesen werden (PIPPIG u. NOWICKI) (Abb. 2).

3. Hämodynamische Untersuchungen unserer Arbeitsgruppe (mit SCHNEIDER, HOCHREIN, PIPPIG u. a.) ergaben, wie inzwischen vielfach bestätigt, ein charakteristisches Verhalten des essentiellen Hochdrucks, im Gegensatz zu anderen untersuchten Hochdruckformen. Im Stadium kardiovasculärer und renaler Kompensation ist das aktive Blutvolumen, gemessen mit Evans-blue, Jod 131-Albumin oder Chrom 51, um 10–15% gegenüber der Norm verkleinert. Mehr als 90% aller untersuchten Hypertoniker zeigen normale oder etwas erniedrigte Herzminutenvolumina (Abb. 3). Mit zunehmendem Lebensalter tritt eine Verkleinerung des Herzschlag und -minutenvolumens ein. Eine Gruppe von 9% der Untersuchten, meist jugendliche Patienten, hatte über die Norm

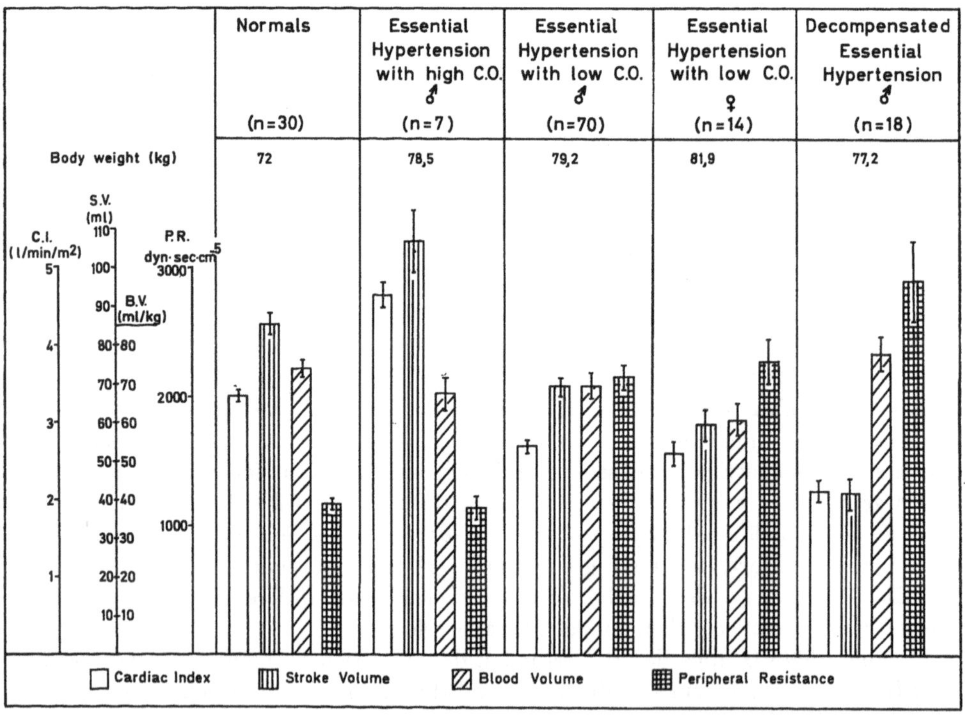

Abb. 3. Herzindex (HMV/Körperoberfläche), Herzschlagvolumen, aktives Blutvolumen und peripherer Widerstand bei 30 Normalen, 91 kompensierten essentiellen Hypertonikern und 18 dekompensierten essentiellen Hypertonikern. Bestimmung des HMV mittels Cardiogreen und Farbstoffverdünnungskurven, des aktiven Blutvolumens mit Jod 131-Albumin.

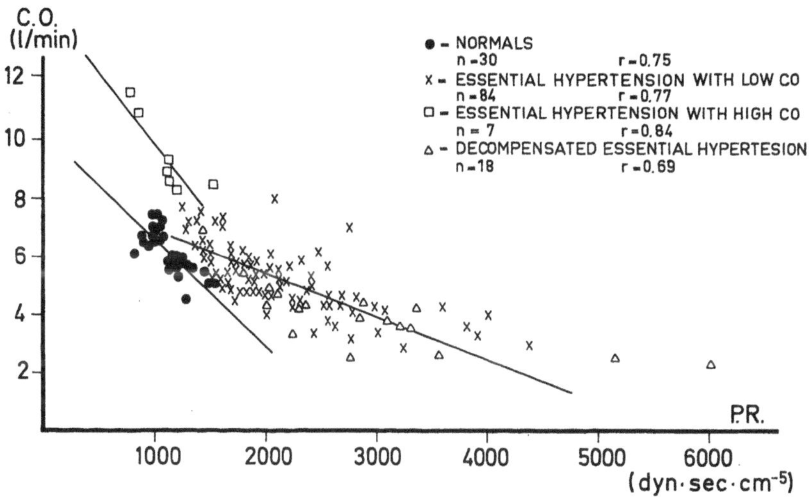

Abb. 4. Korrelation zwischen Herzminutenvolumen und peripherem Widerstand bei den in Abb. 3 wiedergegebenen Patientengruppen. Der periphere Widerstand ist in Relation zum Herzminutenvolumen für alle Gruppen der essentiellen Hypertonie mit Ausnahme der 2 Grenzfälle mit höchstem Herzminutenvolumen zu hoch.

erhöhte Herzschlag und -minutenvolumina. Es konnte aber ausgeschlossen werden, daß es sich hier etwa um Anfangsstadien des Hochdrucks handelt. Diese besondere Gruppe von Hochdruckkranken ist aber offenbar nicht identisch mit den 12% von Patienten, bei denen mein Mitarbeiter KUSCHKE, sowie STURM jun. u. a. eine erhöhte Ausscheidung von Katecholaminen oder deren Metaboliten fanden. In allen Altersgruppen, bei den 84 Patienten mit normalen oder niedrigen Herzminutenvolumina ebenso wie bei den 7 Patienten mit erhöhtem Herzminutenvolumen, war der periphere Gesamtwiderstand im Vergleich zu den Normalen erhöht. Mit dem Eintritt kardio-vasculärer Dekompensation nimmt das Blutvolumen zu, das Herzminutenvolumen ab und der periphere Gesamtwiderstand steigt weiterhin an. Aus diesen Untersuchungen ergab sich eindeutig für die essentielle Hypertonie das wesentliche Merkmal eines erhöhten peripheren Gesamtwiderstandes (Abb. 4).

4. Vielfach, insbesondere von LOSSE, wurde ein erhöhter Natriumgehalt der Gefäßwand als Kennzeichen des essentiellen Hochdrucks beschrieben. Es ist aber nicht zu bezweifeln, daß alle Hochdruckformen, auch solche experimenteller Art, bei vermehrter Natriumzufuhr eine Drucksteigerung erkennen lassen. Umgekehrt wirkt der Natriumentzug, sei es durch diätetische Maßnahmen, sei es durch Diuretica, drucksenkend. Es handelt sich also hier m. E. im Gegensatz zu den ersten 3 Punkten nur um ein sekundäres Merkmal des Hochdrucks.

Welcher genetische Faktor oder welche Faktoren letzten Endes die Ursache des essentiellen Hochdrucks sind, läßt sich noch nicht sicher sagen. Damit entfällt bisher die Möglichkeit einer wirklich kausalen Therapie. Wir sind allerdings damit beschäftigt, frühere Beobachtungen von mir, die beim essentiellen Hochdruck ein Defizit an einem beim Normalen reichlich im Harn ausgeschiedenen Polypeptid nachgewiesen haben,

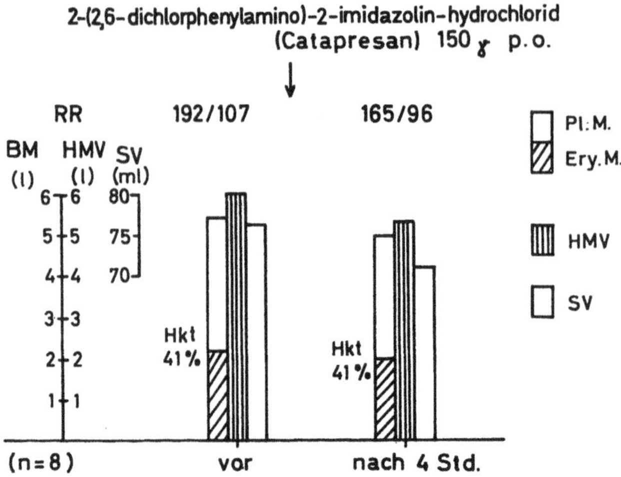

Abb. 5a. Wirkung von 150 gamma2-(2,6-dichlorphenylamino)-2-imidazolin-hydrochlorid = Catapresan® auf arteriellen Blutdruck, Blutvolumen, Herzminutenvolumen und Schlagvolumen (Mittelwert von 8 Untersuchungen) an essentiellen Hypertonikern.

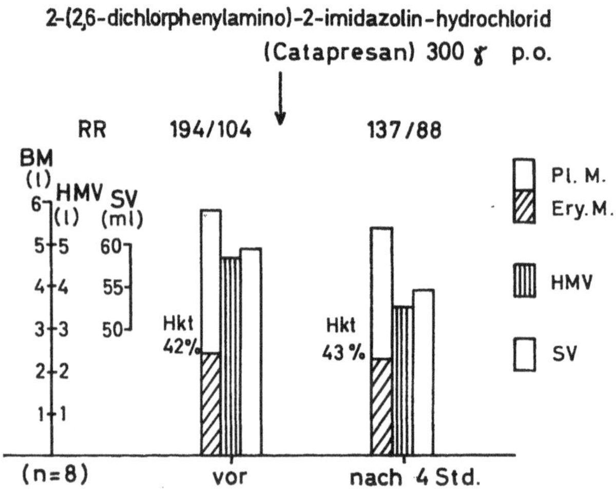

Abb. 5b. Wirkung von 300 gamma 2-(2,6-dichlorphenylamino)-2-imidazolin-hydrochlorid = Catapresan® auf arteriellen Blutdruck, Blutvolumen, Herzminutenvolumen und Schlagvolumen (Mittelwert von 8 Untersuchungen an essentiellen Hypertonikern). [Abb. 5a und b nach Befunden von SCHNEIDER, K. W. und W. GATTENLÖHNER; Dtsch. med. Wschr. 91 (1966), 35, 1533].

weiterzuführen. Es gelang uns, mit meinen Mitarbeitern Dr. NAST und Dr. ZIMMERMANN vom Physiologisch-Chemischen Institut der Universität Würzburg, mittels Reinigung durch Sephadex, Elektrophorese und Dünnschicht-Chromatographie aus Harn von Normalen 2 hochwirksame Faktoren zu isolieren. Die Konzentration dieser Stoffe im Harn von Kranken mit essentieller Hypertonie ist sehr niedrig. Dies vasodilatierende Polypeptid ist eindeutig unterschieden von der Kallikrein-Gruppe und den Kininen und hat selbstverständlich auch keinerlei Beziehungen zu dem neuerdings in Amerika gefundenen Nephromedullin, einem Lipoid.

Ebenso ungeklärt wie die Pathogenese des essentiellen Hochdrucks ist die Entstehung der Drucksteigerungen bei den meisten renalen Hochdruckformen, insbesondere bei der Pyelonephritis und chronischen Glomerulonephritis.

Für die bisher allein mögliche symptomatische Therapie der verschiedenen Hochdruckformen ist für alle zur Verfügung stehenden Substanzen der limitierende Faktor zunächst in den speziellen Nebenwirkungen dieser Stoffe zu sehen, z. B. bei den zentral angreifenden Rauwolfia-Alkaloiden in Depressionen bei hoher Dosierung und längerem Gebrauch, bei den Ganglienblockern und Sympathikusblockern durch starke orthostatische Nebenwirkungen und andere vegetative Störungen, bei Alpha-Methyl-Dopa durch Müdigkeit und Wasserretention, bei den Saluretica durch etwa durch sie provozierte Hypokaliämien und als deren Folge Herzrhythmusstörungen oder durch die Provokation eines latenten Diabetes.

Der zweite limitierende Faktor der drucksenkenden Therapie liegt im Grad der sekundären, oder bei den renalen Hochdruckformen, primären Einschränkung der Nierenfunktion. Schließlich kann die zentrale und kardiale Durchblutung bei allzu brüsker Drucksenkung gefährdet sein.

Es erschien uns daher sinnvoll, Substanzen aus den verschiedenen Wirkungsgruppen in ihren akuten und chronischen Effekten auf die Hämodynamik wie auf die Nierenfunktion näher zu untersuchen. Dabei ergaben sich eindeutige Unterschiede zwischen

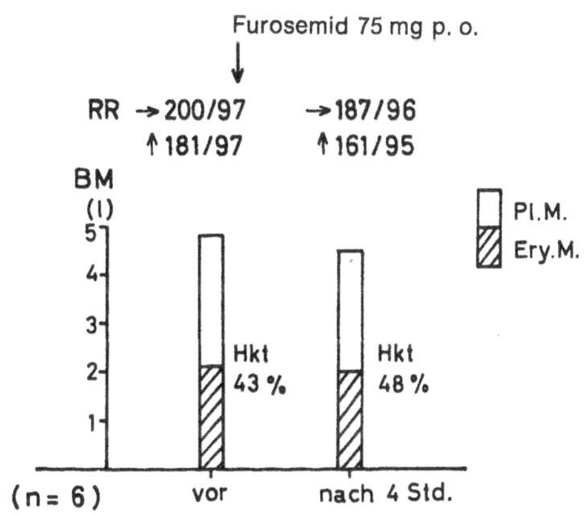

Abb. 6a. Wirkung von 75 mg Furosemid per os auf die Blutmenge, arteriellen Blutdruck und Blutvolumen bei Hypertonikern.

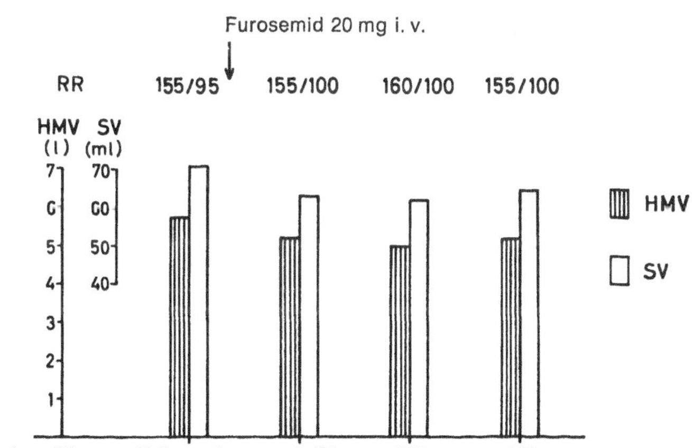

Abb. 6b. Wirkung von 20 mg Furosemid intravenös auf arteriellen Blutdruck, Herzminutenvolumen und Herzschlagvolumen (Mittelwert von 9 Untersuchungen). [Abb. 6a und b nach Befunden von Wölfer, Schneider, Gattenlöhner und Günther. Münch. med. Wschr. 106 (1964), 40, 1767].

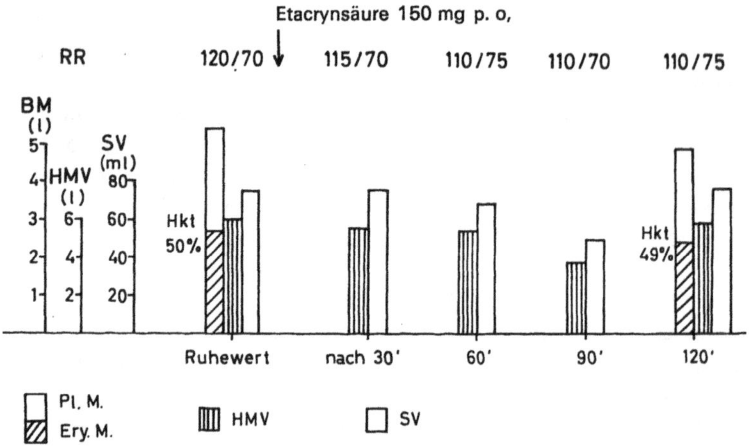

Abb. 7. Akute hämodynamische Wirkung von 150 mg Etacrynsäure p. o. auf arteriellen Blutdruck, Blutvolumen, Herzminutenvolumen und Schlagvolumen bei einem Normotoniker. (Nach K. W. SCHNEIDER, Münch. med. Wschr. 1966, 2571).

den akuten Wirkungen und den Effekten längerdauernder Behandlung. Die nun zu referierenden Beobachtungen entstammen Untersuchungen unserer nephrologischen Arbeitsgruppe mit den Herren HEIDLAND und KLÜTSCH und der kardiologischen Arbeitsgruppe mit den Herren SCHNEIDER, HOCHREIN, PIPPIG, GATTENLÖHNER u. a.

Als akute hämodynamische Wirkung ergibt sich bei intravenöser Applikation einer drucksenkenden Dosis bei den verschiedensten Substanzen als typisch eine Verkleinerung des aktiven Blutvolumens und eine entsprechende Verminderung des Herzschlag- und -minutenvolumens. Dies gilt für das Alpha-Methyl-Dopa ebenso wie für 2-(2,6-dichlorphenylamino)-2-imidazolin-hydrochlorid (Catapresan) (Abb. 5a und b), für die verschiedenen Thiazide ebenso wie für Furosemid (Abb. 6a und b) und für Etacrynsäure (Abb. 7). Unterschiedlich sind die Effekte auf das Blutvolumen nur darin, daß nach

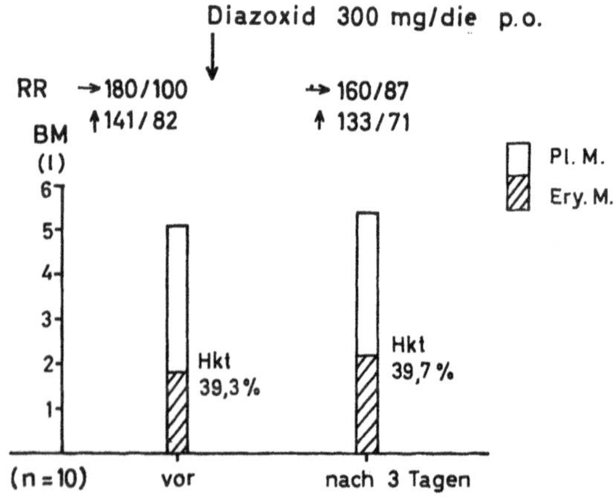

Abb. 8a. Wirkung von 300 mg Diazoxid p. o. auf arteriellen Blutdruck und Blutvolumen (Mittelwert von 10 Untersuchungen an essentiellen Hypertonien).

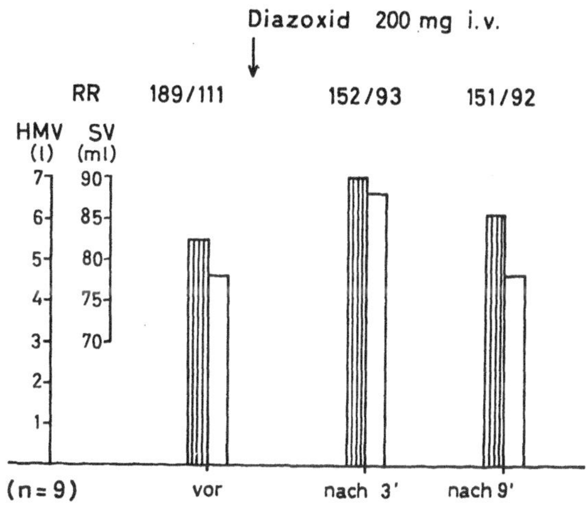

Abb. 8b. Akute Wirkung von 200 mg Diazoxid i. v. auf arteriellen Blutdruck, Herzminutenvolumen und Herzschlagvolumen (Mittelwert aus 9 Untersuchungen) (Abb. 8a und b nach Befunden von WÖLFER, SCHNEIDER und HOCHREIN, Arzneimittel-Forschg. 13 (1963), 748).

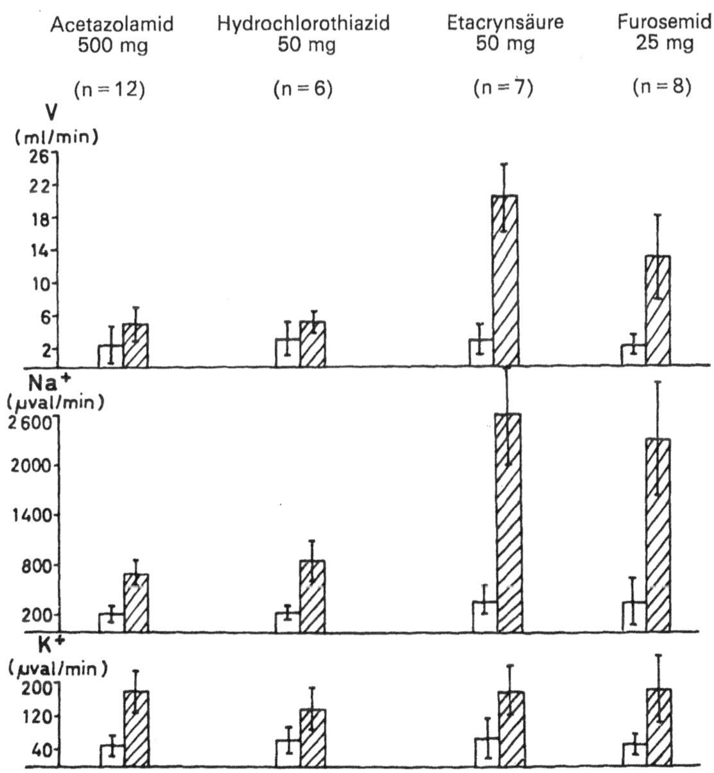

Abb. 9. Harnvolumen, Natrium- und Kaliumausscheidung nach Acetazolamid, Hydrochlorothiazid, Etacrynsäure und Furosemid (nach Untersuchungen von HEIDLAND).

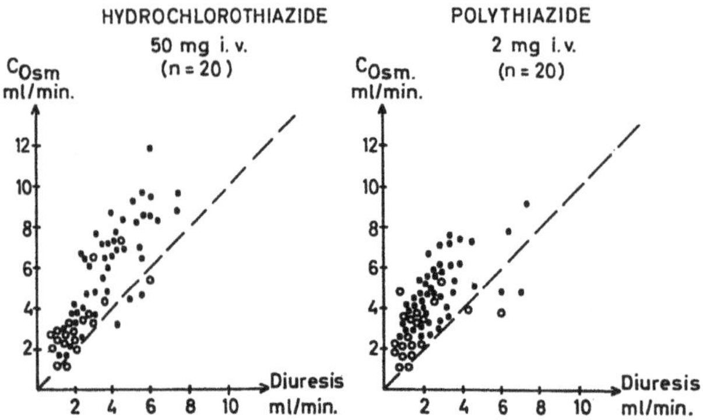

Abb. 10. Korrelation zwischen Diurese und osmolarer Clearance nach intravenöser Gabe von Hydrochlorothiazid, Polythiazid (offene Kreise: vor Verabreichung, Punkte: nach Verabreichung) [nach KLÜTSCH, HEIDLAND und SUZUKI. Atti della Arc. Med. Lombarda. 18 (1963) 1255].

Furosemid und Etacrynsäure allein das Plasmavolumen abnimmt, während unter 2-(2,6-dichlorphenylamino)-2-imidazolin-hydrochlorid (Catapresan) bei unverändertem Hämatokrit, Erythrozyten- und Plasmamenge gleichmäßig kleiner werden. Ein gegensätzliches Verhalten (Zunahme von Blutmenge und Herzminutenvolumen) zeigt nur das Diazoxid (Abb. 8a und b), das auch sonst, wie Herr ARNOLD in seinem Referat näher ausführen wird, in seinen Wirkungen von den anderen Thiaziden grundsätzlich abweicht.

Als akute renale Wirkungen ergaben sich für Azetazolamid ebenso wie für Hydrochlorothiazid eine Zunahme des Harnvolumens, der Natrium- und Kaliumexkretion. Etacrynsäure und Furosemid zeigen gleichartige Effekte in einem stärkeren Ausmaß (Abb. 9). Dabei ergab die Korrelation zwischen osmolarer Clearance und Diurese für zwei typische Thiazide (Hydrochlorothiazid und Polythiazide) eine quantitativ stärkere osmolare Clearance im Verhältnis zur Diurese (Abb. 10): Die offenen Zirkel sind die Werte vor Anwendung der Substanzen, die geschlossenen Punkte die Werte nach intravenöser Verabreichung der betreffenden Substanzen). Für verschiedene Dosen von Furosemid (Abb. 11) ergab sich dagegen ebenso wie für Etacrynsäure (Abb. 12) eine gleichmäßige Zunahme der osmolaren und Wasser-Clearance. Die Prüfung des Glomerulumfiltrats

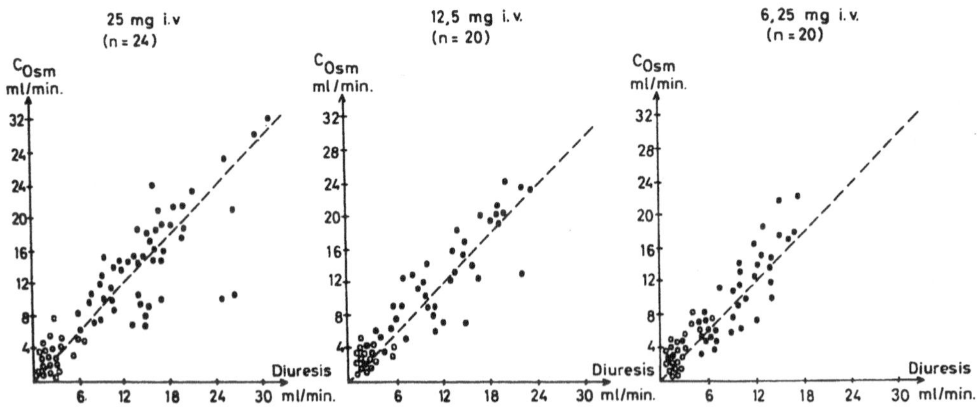

Abb. 11. Korrelation zwischen osmolarer Clearance und Diurese nach Verabreichung von Furosemid [nach HEIDLAND, KLÜTSCH und SUZUKI, Arzneimittel-Forschg. 14 (1964), 713].

(Inulin-Clearance) ergibt für Azetazolamid und Hydrochlorothiazid eine geringe Abnahme, für Furosemid und Etacrynsäure eine geringe Zunahme. Die effektive Nierendurchblutung (PAH-Clearance) nimmt unter Azetazolamid, Hydrochlorothiazid und Etacrynsäure unwesentlich ab, unter Furosemid ein wenig zu (Abb. 13).

Bei chronischer Verabreichung von Alpha-Methyl-Dopa, 2-(2,6-dichlorphenylamino)-2-imidazolin-hydrochlorid (Catapresan), der verschiedenen Thiazide, Furosemid und Etacrynsäure ergab sich aber bei fortdauender Drucksenkung ein Wiederanstieg von Blutvolumen, Herzschlag- und -minuten-Volumen auf die Ausgangswerte.

Als Beispiel der renalen Wirkung eines Thiazids bei 2 bis 3wöchiger Verabreichung sei die Wirkung von Cyclopenthiazid gezeigt (Untersuchungen von HEIDLAND). Bei statistisch signifikant drucksenkendem Effekt ist das Plasmavolumen bei kardiovasculär kompensierten Hypertonikern fast unverändert, die Inulin-Clearance nimmt signifikant

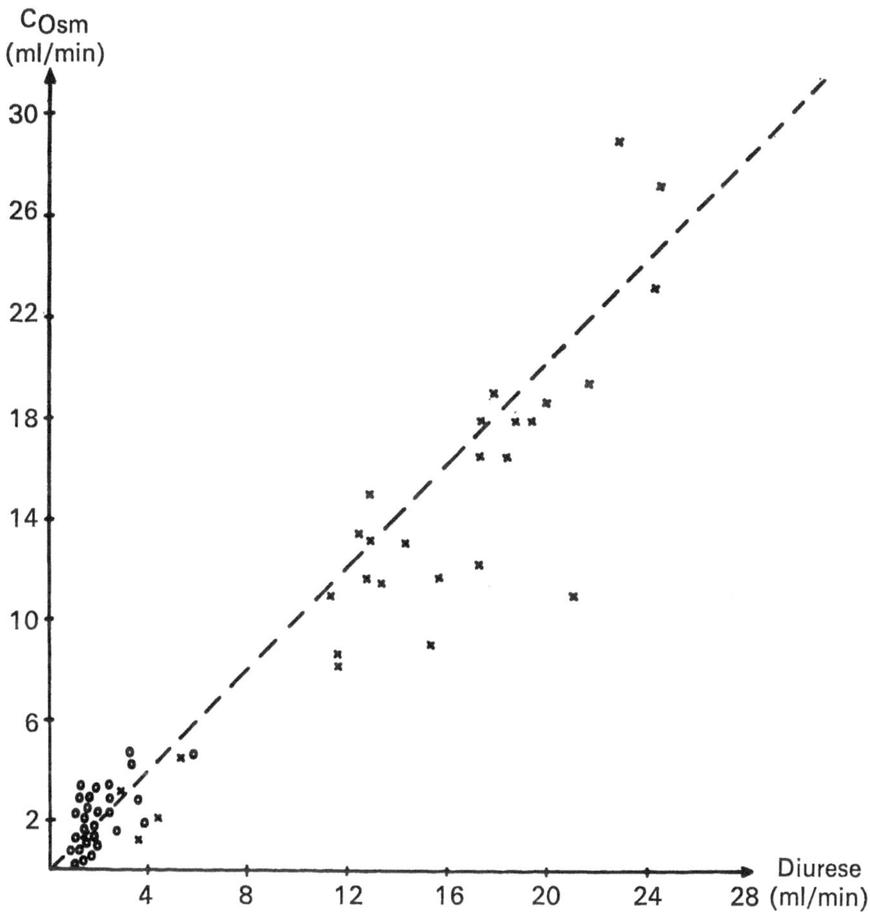

Abb. 12. Korrelation zwischen osmolarer Clearance und Diurese nach 50 mg Etacrynsäure (Kreise: vor Verabreichung, Kreuze: 45 min nach Gabe; n = 28) (LÖWENHEIM, URSULA, Inaug. Diss. Würzburg 1968).

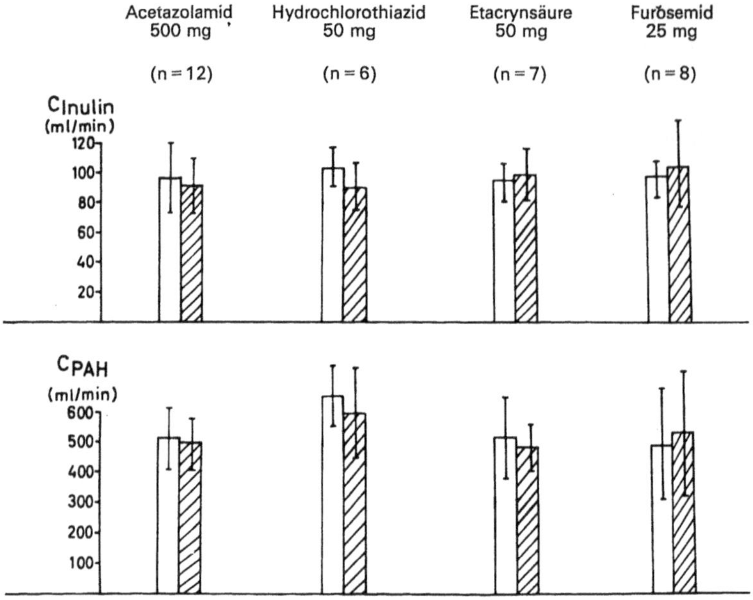

Abb. 13. Effektive Nierendurchblutung (PAH-Clearance) und Glomerulumfiltrat (Inulin-Clearance) vor und nach Acetazolamid, Hydrochlorothiazid, Etacrynsäure und Furosemid (nach HEIDLAND und Mitarb., unpubliziert).

ab, die PAH-Clearance nicht signifikant zu. Bei kardio-vasculär dekompensierten Hypertonien sind die renalen Effekte gleichartig, hier nimmt aber das vorher erhöhte Plasmavolumen – allerdings nicht signifikant – ab (Abb. 14). Für das Kombinationspräparat Adelphan-Esidrix, für Furosemid und Etacrynsäure verfügen wir nur über ein kleines Beobachtungsmaterial, danach sind aber die Veränderungen der Inulin- und PAH-Clearance mit denen der eben gezeigten nach Cyclopenthiazid gleichsinnig (Abb. 15).

Eine einheitliche Deutung der drucksenkenden Wirkung der verschiedenen Substanzen ist schwierig. Einerseits können eindeutige drucksenkende Effekte sowohl bei akuter wie chronischer Applikation ohne vermehrte Natriurese ausgelöst werden. Für Substanzen dieser Art (Alpha-Methyl-Dopa und Catapresan) muß eine Wirkung auf den peripheren Gesamtwiderstand mit unmittelbarem Angriff an der Gefäßperipherie als wahrscheinlich diskutiert werden. Daneben kommen auch zentralnervöse Wirkungen in Frage. Für alle Thiazide, Furosemid und Etacrynsäure wurde bei längerdauernder Behandlung der Hochdruckpatienten neben der Natriurese eine Abnahme des Glomerulumfiltrates bei Konstanz oder Erhöhung der Nierendurchblutung gefunden. Dies Phänomen läßt verschiedene Deutungsmöglichkeiten zu. Unwahrscheinlich ist, daß allein die Drucksenkung zu einer Herabsetzung des Filtrationsdruckes im Glomerulum bei konstanter Nierendurchblutungsgröße führt, zumal nach anders angreifenden drucksenkenden Pharmaka wie z. B. Alpha-Methyl-Dopa das Glomerulumfiltrat unverändert bleibt. Diskutabel sind einige andere Möglichkeiten:

1. Eine Widerstandsabnahme allein im vas efferens könnte zu einer Herabsetzung des Glomerulumfiltrates bei gleichbleibender oder steigender Nierendurchblutungsgröße

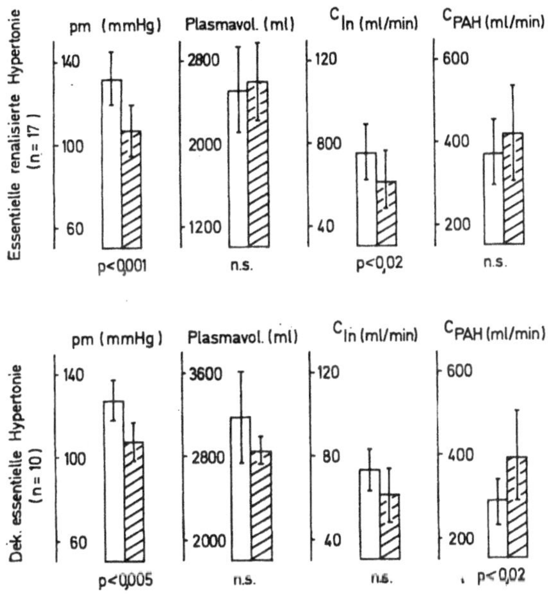

Abb. 14. Arterieller Blutdruck, Plasmavolumen, Inulin- und PAH-Clearance vor und nach 2–3wöchiger Verabreichung von Cyclopenthiazid (500 mg/die) bei 17 essentiellen renalisierten Hypertonien und 10 dekompensierten Hypertonien (nach HEIDLAND, KLÜTSCH, SCHNEIDER und SUZUKI. Klin. Wschr. 17 (1964), 831).

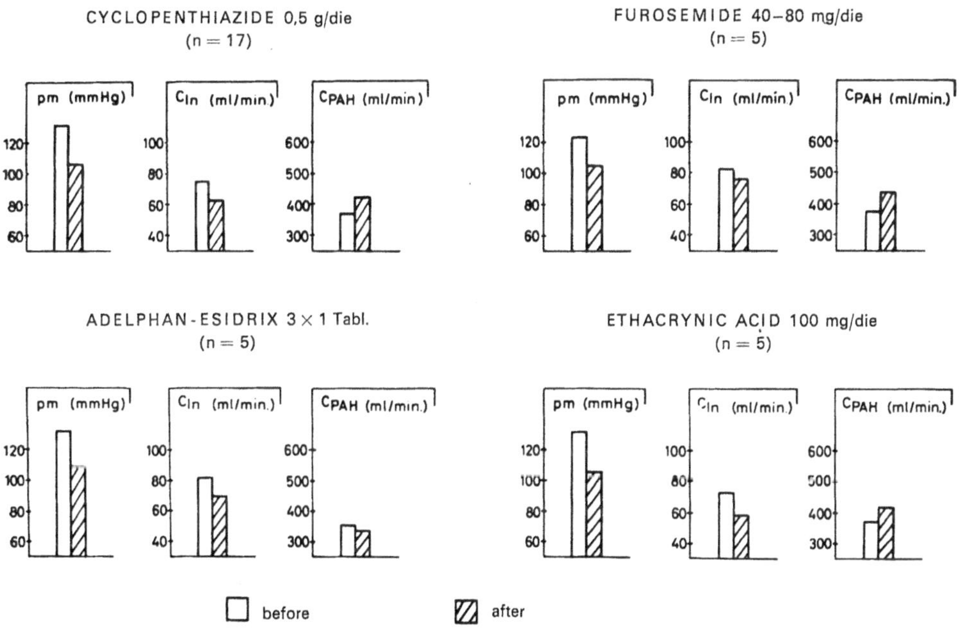

Abb. 15. Arterieller Blutdruck, Inulin- und PAH-Clearance nach Cyclopenthiazid, Furosemid, Adelphan-Esidrix und Etacrynsäure (nach E. WOLLHEIM; Proc. 9th Int. Congr. Life Ass. Med., Tel Aviv 1967, Karger, Basel/New York 1968, 241).

führen. Dies Phänomen läßt sich vielleicht aus Arbeitsergebnissen der Thurauschen Gruppe erklären, die eine höhere Reninkonzentration im vas afferens als im vas efferens gefunden hat, stimuliert durch den Natriumverlust.

2. Eine Abnahme des Glomerulumfiltrates bei konstanter oder leicht erhöhter Nierendurchblutungsgröße würde auch eintreten, wenn ein partieller intravasaler Shunt zwischen vas afferens und vas efferens eröffnet würde. GRANBERG, LAGERGREN u. LJUNGQVIST haben unter Kombination mikroangiographischer und histologischer Methoden in der normalen menschlichen Niere zwar nicht an den Glomerula der Rinde, aber im juxtamedullären Bereich Shunts zwischen vas afferens und vas efferens darstellen können. Auch aus der Klinik verfügen wir über Erfahrungen, die die Möglichkeit einer solchen Shunt-Bildung, zumindest unter pathologischen Bedingungen, nicht ausschließt.

Bei einer Patientin mit glomerulo-nephritischer Schrumpfniere, die in der Urämie verstorben ist, zeigte das histologische Präparat bei der Verödung praktisch aller Glomerula erstaunlich gut erhaltene Tubuli (Prof. ALTMANN, Pathol. Institut der Universität Würzburg). Dieser Befund konnte sich nur bei der Existenz eines unter den speziellen Umständen dieses Krankheitsfalles geöffneten intrarenalen Shunts erklären lassen. Bei der 7 Monate komplett anurischen Patientin war die Masse der Glomerula jedenfalls für Blut nicht mehr durchgängig.

Wie aber auch immer die Erklärung der Wirkung der verschiedenen blutdrucksenkenden Pharmaka sein mag, für ihre praktische Anwendung hat sich als weiterer wichtiger Gesichtspunkt ergeben, daß die Kombination von Substanzen mit verschiedenen Angriffspunkten zu einer eindeutigen Herabsetzung der für die Blutdrucksenkung notwendigen Einzeldosen führt. Damit werden die eingangs als erstes Limit jeder Therapie bezeichneten toxischen Nebenwirkungen der einzelnen Stoffe ebenfalls vermindert. Über die Vorteile dieser heute allgemein akzeptierten kombinierten Behandlung des Hochdruckes wird Herr ARNOLD ausführlicher sprechen.

Zusammenfassend ist festzustellen, daß bei den meisten Hochdruckformen eine kausale Therapie noch nicht möglich ist. Für die symptomatische Behandlung stehen Substanzen mit verschiedenen zentralen und peripheren Angriffspunkten zur Verfügung, unter ihnen nehmen die Thiazide, Furosemid, Mefrusid und Etacrynsäure als Natriuretica eine wichtige Stellung ein. Nur im akuten Effekt konnten hämodynamische Veränderungen nach diesen Substanzen nachgewiesen werden. Die gefundene Verkleinerung des aktiven Blutvolumens und entsprechende Abnahme des Herzminutenvolumens scheint mir aber nicht eine ausreichende Erklärung für die Drucksenkung zu ergeben. Dies um so weniger, als bei längerdauernder Behandlung die genannten hämodynamischen Faktoren auf die Ausgangswerte zurückkehren, während der blutdrucksenkende Effekt weiter manifest ist. Die Wirkung dieser Stoffe läßt sich also nur über ihre mit der Natriurese verbundene Herabsetzung des peripheren Gesamtwiderstandes erklären. Die bei der Untersuchung der Nierenfunktion erhobenen Befunde geben in dieser Hinsicht eindeutige Hinweise. Für die praktische Therapie hat sich zur Verminderung unerwünschter Nebenwirkungen die Kombinationsbehandlung mit Substanzen differenter Angriffspunkte bewährt.

Literatur / References

1. GRANBERG, P.-O., C. LAGERGREN and A. LJUNGQVIST: Micro-Angiographic Aspects of Some Renal Physiologic Problems; Proc. of the second Intern. Congr. of Nephrology, Prag, 26.–30. Aug. 1963, Excerpta Med. Foundation, Amsterdam/New York/London/Milan/Tokyo, S. 65.
2. HEIDLAND, A., K. KLÜTSCH und F. SUZUKI: Nierenhämodynamik, Wasser- und Elektrolytausscheidung nach 4-Chlor-N-(2-furylmethyl)-5-sulfamoyl-anthranilsäure; Arzneimittel-Forsch. 14, **6,** 713 (1964).
3. HEIDLAND, A., K. KLÜTSCH, K. W. SCHNEIDER und F. SUZUKI: Thiaziddiuretica und Nierenfunktion bei Hypertonie und kardialer Dekompensation; Klin.Wschr. **17,** 831 (1964).
4. HOCHREIN, H., K. W. SCHNEIDER und G. SCHULTE-TIGGES: Das Verhalten des Herzminuten- und Schlagvolumens sowie des peripheren Gesamtwiderstandes bei der essentiellen Hypertonie; Z. Kreislaufforsch. **52,** 779 (1963).
5. KLÜTSCH, K., A. HEIDLAND, F. SUZUKI: Cambiamenti comparativi nella clearance dell'acqua libera dopo somministrazione di idroclorotiazide, politiazide, e fursemid; Atti della Acc. Med. Lombarda **18,** 1255 (1963).
6. LÖWENHEIM, URSULA: Fraktionelle Flüssigkeitselimination nach Ethacrinsäure bei eingeschränkter Nierenfunktion; Inauguraldisseration, Würzburg **1968.**
7. PIPPIG, L. und L. NOWICKI: Untersuchungen zum »Angiotensin-Hauttest«; Z. Kreislaufforsch. **53,** 587 (1964).
8. PIPPIG, L. und M. IMHOFF: Aktuelle Probleme der Nephrologie, Renale Hypertonie und Angiotensin-Hauttest; IV. Symp. Ges. Nephrol., Springer Berlin/Heidelberg/New York 1966, 727.
9. SCHÄFER, E. und A. SCHÄFER: Aspekte zur Immunpathogenese der malignen Hypertonie, Med.Welt 1965, 1144.
10. SCHNEIDER, K.W.: Hämodynamische Wirkung von Diuretika; Münch. med.Wschr. **108,** 51, 2571 (1966).
11. SCHNEIDER, K. W. und W. GATTENLÖHNER: Hämodynamische Untersuchungen nach St 155 (2-(2,6-Dichlorphenylamino)-2-imidazolin-Hydrochlorid) beim Menschen; Dtsch. med.Wschr. **91,** 35, 1533 (1966).
12. WILSON, C. und G. W. BYROM: Renal changes in malignant hypertension, experimental evidence; Lancet **1,** 136 (1939).
13. WILSON, C. and G. W. PICKERING: Acute arterial lesions in rabbits with experimental renal hypertension; Clin. Sci. **3,** 343 (1938).
14. WÖLFER, H. J., K. W. SCHNEIDER und H. HOCHREIN: Klinische und hämodynamische Untersuchungen über eine neue antihypertensive Substanz aus der Thiazidreihe ohne diuretische Wirkung; Arzneimittel-Forsch. **13,** 748 (1963).
15. WÖLFER, H. J., K. W. SCHNEIDER, W. GATTENLÖHNER und J. GÜNTHER: Behandlung der arteriellen Hypertonie mit Fursemid; Münch. med.Wschr. **106,** 40, 1767 (1964).
16. WOLLHEIM, E. und J. MOELLER: Hypertonie – Hypotonie; in: Handbuch der Inneren Medizin, Bd. IX, Teil 5, Springer, Berlin/Göttingen/Heidelberg 1960.
17. WOLLHEIM, E.: Die essentielle Hypertonie als nosologische Einheit und ihre Differentialdiagnose; Verh. dtsch. Ges. Kreislaufforsch. 28, 59 (1963).
18. WOLLHEIM, E.: Hämodynamik und Organdurchblutung beim Hochdruck; in HEILMEYER und HOLTMEIER: Hochdruckforschung, Thieme, Stuttgart 1965, S. 136.
19. WOLLHEIM, E.: Saliurese – aktueller Weg zur Ödem- und Hypertoniebehandlung; Münch. med. Wschr. 108, 51, 2561 (1966).
20. WOLLHEIM, E.: Die essentielle Hypertonie und andere Hochdruckformen; 17th Gen. Ass. Japan Med. Congr. 1.–3.4.1967. Nagoya, Spec. Lect. **4,** 543 (1967).
21. WOLLHEIM, E.: Risiken der Behandlung mit antihypertensiven Pharmaka; Proc. 9th int. Congr. Life Ass. Med., Tel Aviv 1967, Karger. Basel/Mew York 1968: 241.

The Treatment of Hypertension with Diuretics

Zur Behandlung der Hypertonie mit Diuretica

O. H. ARNOLD

Summary: Depletion of body sodium pool as achieved by diet or pharmacological saluresis depresses high blood pressure
a) by a weak direct mechanism not well known yet,
b) by enhancing the effect of all known hypotensive compounds.

During the first and second week after onset of therapy, the effect of saluretics upon blood pressure is quantitatively paralleled by a negative sodium balance. The effect is reversed by administration of sodium chloride using a dose sufficient to level the deficit. After this initial phase, the hypotensive effect of the saluretic agent persists although exchangeable sodium, extracellular fluid and plasma volume remain normal. It is controversial whether intracellular sodium content or distribution is altered by long term administration of saluretics.

The enhancing effect of saluretics upon hypotension caused by other drugs is understood in two ways:
a) By increasing the sympathetic tone which is augmented to compensate for the decreased plasma volume (antihypertensive agents acting by interference with the adrenergic system are more effective if sympathetic tone is high).
b) By inhibiting increase of plasma volume consecutive to the augmented capacity of the vascular system resulting from the reduction of sympathetic nerve activity.

This effect, however, increases orthostatic fall in blood pressure which mostly occurs if combined therapy is used. Reduction of sympathetic activity is followed by a diminished ability to regulate variations in blood pressure which are caused by changes in blood volume.

The side effects of long term administration of saluretic agents are discussed. Finally, antihypertensive action of desamylbenzothiazide (diazoxide) is described. It is used to overcome hypertension refractory to conventional antihypertensive agents. This drug is considered to have a "direct" effect upon arteriolar tone which is independent from alterations in sodium metabolism, and a more hypothetical one upon sympathetic nervous system.

1956 wurde durch NOVELLO und SPRAGUE das erste oral stark wirksame Salureticum Chlorothiazid synthetisiert. Die Einführung dieser neuen Verbindungen in die Hochdrucktherapie durch HOLLANDER und WILKINS sowie FREIS und WILSON 1957 leitete eine neue Periode der Hochdrucktherapie ein. Ich möchte also das Aperçu von Herrn Dr. BEYER aufgreifen, der in der Einleitung zu seinem Referat sagte, man müsse in der medikamentösen Hochdrucktherapie eine Vor- und eine Nach-Chlorothiazid-Ära unterscheiden.

Schon seit 1850 wußte man, daß das Ödem durch kochsalzarme Kost zu beeinflussen war. ALLEN führte 1920 die kochsalzarme Kost in die Behandlung der Hypertonie ein. Durch die zuverlässigere und einfachere Methode der medikamentösen Salurese gelang es, die an sich gleichartigen Effekte des diätetischen Kochsalzentzuges so zu verstärken, daß damit die Therapie des Hochdrucks einfacher, wirksamer und für den Kranken weniger belastend wurde.

Der Kochsalzentzug wirkt

1. selbständig blutdrucksenkend, außerdem
2. verstärkt er die Wirkung besonders der Antihypertensiva, die über eine Hemmung des sympathischen Nervensystems wirksam werden;
3. dadurch können diese Medikamente niedriger dosiert und so deren Nebenwirkungen verringert werden.

Daß es möglich ist, mit strengem diätetischem Kochsalzentzug einen großen Teil der Hypertoniker, auch solche mit schwerem Hochdruck, sehr erfolgreich zu behandeln, zeigte u. a. KEMPNER 1948 bei seinen Versuchen mit der allein durch Natriumentzug wirkenden Reis-Frucht-Diät; er hatte damit eine Erfolgsquote von ca. 60%. FINNERTY und Mitarb. (1959) fanden nach Chlorothiazid allein – allerdings nur bei mittelschweren Hypertonien – eine deutliche Blutdrucksenkung in 50%; hierbei war die Wirkung gleichwertig einer Kombination von Hydralazine und Reserpin.

Ich verzichte darauf, hier ausführlich alle Beweise für die Wirksamkeit der medikamentösen Salurese auf die arterielle Hypertonie vorzulegen; sie sind allgemein bekannt und auch durch statistisch gut kontrollierte Studien erwiesen.

SMITH et al. (1964) (U. S. Public Health Studie) studierten im Doppeltblindversuch 381 Patienten, die den Blutdruck zu Hause über einen Monat mit Therapie, ohne Therapie und bei Placebomedikation maßen. Es zeigte sich, daß der Chlorothiazideffekt, in seinem Ausmaß abhängig von der Höhe des Ausgangsblutdrucks, statistisch signifikant war (Abb. 1).

In der bekannten Studie der Veterans Administration unter FREIS (1962), die mit einer etwas anderen Methodik erarbeitet wurde, wurden ähnliche Ergebnisse erzielt. Gegenüber der Placeboperiode bewirkten 2 × 500 mg Chlorothiazid tägl. eine Blutdrucksenkung von 7,9/3,8 mm Hg, in Kombination mit Reserpin von 14/11 mm Hg. Die Unterschiede gegenüber der Studie von SMITH (Public Health Service) entstanden durch die unter verschiedenen Umständen gewonnenen Kontrollwerte vor Beginn der beiden Untersuchungen: Bei der erstgenannten Studie waren es die Blutdruckwerte während stationärer Behandlung, während in der zweiten von SMITH die von den Patienten selbst zu Hause gemessenen Werte, die durchschnittlich 12/5 mm Hg höher liegen als die Werte in der Klinik, zugrunde gelegt wurden.

Eine weitere wichtige Bedeutung für die Hochdrucktherapie haben die Saluretica in der Prophylaxe der Schwangerschaftstoxikose (FINNERTY und BEBKO 1966).

Grundsätzlich wirken alle Saluretica blutdrucksenkend, gleichgültig welche chemische Konstitution sie haben, also die Sulfonamidderivate ebenso wie die Etacrynsäure, Triamteren wie Spironolacton. Die Unterschiede ergeben sich aus der Verschiedenheit der Wirkungsstärke pro Gewichtseinheit und besonders auch der Wirkungsdauer (Tab. 1). Wird auf diese Besonderheiten der einzelnen Präparate geachtet, ist die Wirkung auf den Blutdruck gleich, was z. B. DOLLERY et al. (1964) beim Vergleich der nur 6–8 Stunden wirkenden Etacrynsäure mit dem 10–12 Stunden wirkenden Hydrochlorothiazid nachgewiesen haben; sie fanden 50 mg Hydrochlorothiazid und 100 mg Etacrynsäure gleich stark wirksam auf den Blutdruck. Diese Erörterungen ändern nichts an der Tatsache, daß aus praktischen Gründen die lang wirkenden Saluretica, wie z. B. Chlorthalidon mit einer Wirkungsdauer von 60–72 Stunden, vorzuziehen sind. Hier genügt meist eine Dosis von 100 mg jeden 2. bis 3. Tag, während Hydrochlorothiazid streng genommen 2mal und Etacrynsäure oder Furosemid 3mal täglich gegeben werden müßten, wenn ein optimaler Effekt erwartet wird. Es hat sich jedoch aus der praktischen Erfahrung ergeben, daß auch eine diskontinuierliche Salurese bei vielen Hypertonikern ausreicht, um in Kombination mit anderen Antihypertonika eine kontinuierliche Senkung des Blutdruckniveaus zu gewährleisten.

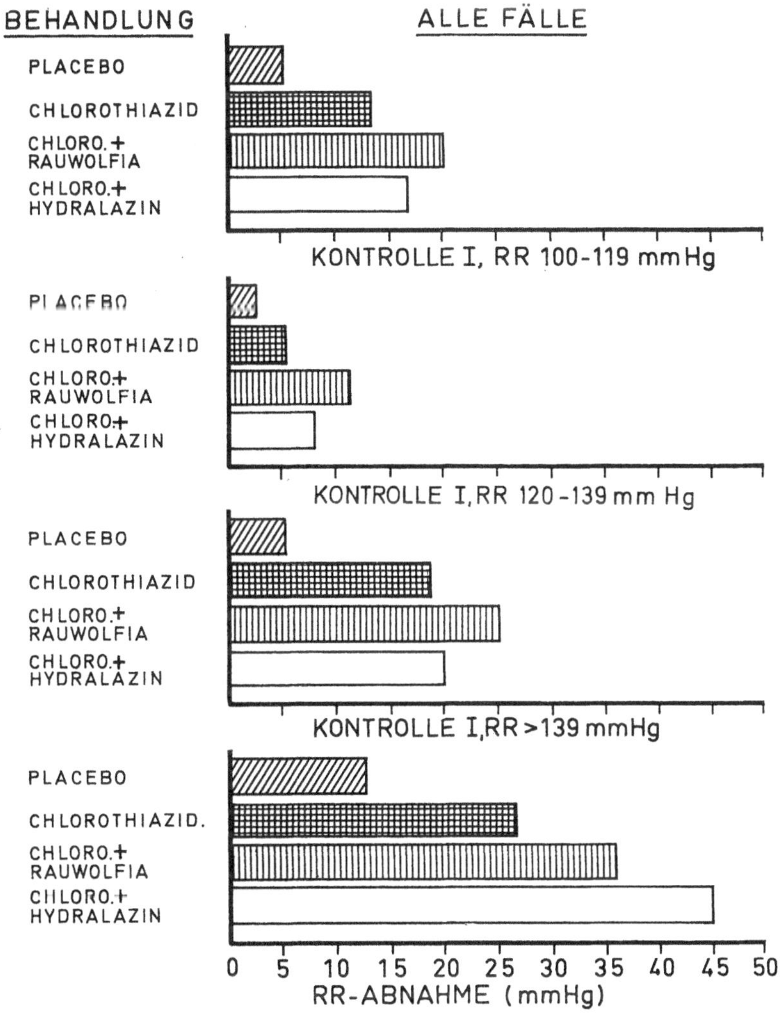

Abb. 1. Durchschnittliche Abnahme des mittleren arteriellen Druckes zwischen 1. Kontrolle und dem letzten Monat während ambulanter Druckmessung. Die Ergebnisse sind getrennt nach verschiedenen therapeutischen Maßnahmen aufgeführt. Es sind jeweils Gruppen entsprechend dem Blutdruck während Kontrolle I gebildet (nach SMITH, W. M. et al: Ann. intern. Med **61**, 829 (1964).

Tab. 1. Einzeldosis und Dosisbereich, Wirkungsmaximum, Wirkungsdauer einiger Saluretica. [Nach F. KRÜCK: Fortschr. Med. **8**, 354 (1968)].

	Einzeldosis (mg)	Dosisbereich (mg)	Max. Wirkung (Stunden)	Wirkungsdauer (Stunden)
Hydrochlorothiazid (Esidrix®)	25	25 – 100	4 – 6	10 – 12
Cyclopenthiazid (Navidrex®)	0,5	0,25 – 2	4 – 6	10 – 12
Chlorthalidon (Hygroton®)	100	50 – 200	2 – 20	60 – 72
Mefrusid (Baycaron®)	25	25 – 100	6 – 12	>12
Etacrynsäure (Hydromedin®)	50	50 – 200	½	6 – 8
Furosemid (Lasix®)	40	40 – 160	1	4 – 6

Die *klinisch-pharmakologische* Analyse der Wirkungsweise des medikamentösen Kochsalzentzuges auf den erhöhten Blutdruck hat bisher noch nicht zu eindeutigen Ergebnissen geführt. Der Kochsalzentzug durch Saluretica vom Typ des Chlorothiazids oder auch Saluretica anderer chemischer Konstitution wie übrigens auch durch Diät hat eine *zweiphasige Wirkung* auf den Blutdruck:

In der *ersten* Phase, ungefähr 1–3 Wochen nach Beginn der Therapie, ist die Blutdrucksenkung ursprünglich durch eine *Verminderung des Herzzeitvolumens infolge Abnahme des Plasmavolumens* erklärt worden, die parallel zu einer Abnahme des extrazellulären Flüssigkeitsvolumens und des austauschbaren Natriums verläuft (DUSTAN et al. 1959, FREIS 1960). FINNERTY et al. (1968) haben jedoch neuerdings gezeigt, daß die *Blutdrucksenkung der negativen Natriumbilanz parallel* geht, nicht der Verminderung des Plasmavolumens, dessen Abnahme im Einzelfall in keiner direkten Beziehung zum blutdrucksenkenden Effekt des Saluretieums stand; es wurden Furosemid und Hydrochlorothiazid zur Salurese verwendet. Die Blutdrucksenkung kann durch ausreichende Zulage von Kochsalz wieder rückgängig gemacht werden (s. a. JOHNSON et al. 1962). Plasmaexpander gleichen die Blutdrucksenkung nicht aus, wie früher schon HOLLANDER et al. (1960) gezeigt hatten. Sie erklären den Unterschied ihrer Ergebnisse gegenüber FREIS (1960) und DUSTAN et al. (1959) damit, daß die Patienten dieser Autoren während der Versuche unter Antihypertensiva standen, die die Reaktion auf Plasmaentzug bzw. -expansion ändern. Wegen des verminderten Plasmavolumens nach Saluretica wird der periphere Widerstand in dieser ersten Phase leicht erhöht (GIFFORD 1961, DUSTAN et al. 1959, VILLARREAL et al. 1962). Beim nierenlosen Hund bleibt Chlorothiazid im akuten Versuch ohne Wirkung auf Blutdruck, Wassergehalt des Gewebes oder die Gewebselektrolyte.

In der *zweiten* Phase wird bei Fortsetzung der Therapie mit Saluretica ein weiterer Verlust von Natrium durch die Nieren verhindert; *die Werte für das Plasmavolumen, den interstitiellen Flüssigkeitsraum und das Schlag- bzw. Herzzeitvolumen gehen wieder in den Normbereich zurück.* Trotzdem bleibt die Blutdrucksenkung bestehen. Der *periphere*

Widerstand ist in dieser Phase deutlich vermindert (DUSTAN et al. 1959, WILSON und FREIS 1959, FROHLICH et al. 1960, VILLARREAL et al. 1962). Eine Erhöhung des Blutvolumens durch Zufuhr von Plasma beeinflußt den gesenkten Blutdruck nicht (CONWAY und LAUWERS 1960, VARNAUSKAS et al. 1961). CONWAY und PALMERO (1963) fanden eine Abnahme des Gefäßwiderstandes am Unterarm um 18%.

Der Kochsalzentzug führt auch zu einer Änderung der renalen Hämodynamik. Gleichgültig, ob durch diätetischen Entzug oder durch Saluretica hervorgerufen, führt er zu einer Abnahme des renalen Plasmastroms und der glomerulären Filtration, die im Verhältnis zur Durchblutung stärker reduziert ist. Damit kann ein Anstieg des Harnstoffs verbunden sein.

Es ist versucht worden, die Wirkung der Saluretica beim Hypertonus darauf zurückzuführen, daß eine für diese Krankheit spezifische abnorme Vermehrung von Natrium im ganzen oder in bestimmten Substraten des Organismus, z. B. der Gefäßwände, ausgeschwemmt werden; dadurch könnte der Arteriolentonus vermindert oder auch ein Intimaödem beseitigt werden (WELLER und HOOBLER 1959).

Für das *extrazelluläre Natrium* ist dies unwahrscheinlich; es ist nachgewiesen, daß beim Hypertoniker das gesamte Körperwasser, der Extrazellularraum, das Plasmavolumen, das austauschbare Natrium und die Halbwertszeit von ^{22}Na normal sind (WINER 1959, HOLLANDER et al. 1961, DAHL et al. 1966). Die Blutdrucksenkung in der ersten Phase ist demnach wahrscheinlich ein für den Hypertoniker unspezifischer Effekt der Kochsalzausschwemmung.

Von einer Reihe von Autoren wurde jedoch nachgewiesen, daß bei der primären Hypertonie der *intrazelluläre Gehalt* an Natrium, z. B. der Erythrozyten (LOSSE et al. 1962), erhöht ist. Für die Gefäßwände konnte dies von mehreren Autoren bei Hypertonie verschiedener Art gezeigt werden (TOBIAN und BINION 1952, 1954, ROSS 1956, TOBIAN et al. 1961, VILLAMIL et al. 1963, DOUGLAS et al. 1967). Bei chronischer Anwendung bleibt der Kochsalzbestand des Körpers normal, wie GIFFORD (1961) bei Isotopenstudien zeigen konnte. Die Meinungen hierzu sind allerdings nicht einhellig; LAUWERS und CONWAY (1960) und FRIEDMANN et al. (1960) sowie auch spätere Autoren fanden nach Chlorothiazid eine Abnahme des Wasser- und Natriumgehaltes der Zellen. Diese Elektrolytverschiebungen zwischen extra- und intrazellulärem Raum können jedoch auch, wie dies für das abnorme Verhalten der Niere des Hypertonikers bei i. v. Kochsalzbelastungen erwiesen ist (COTTIER 1960), Folge der Hypertonie sein (HOLLANDER et al. 1966).

Bei der Widersprüchlichkeit der Befunde und Ansichten hat man nach anderen Möglichkeiten gesucht, die Wirkung der Saluretica auf den peripheren arteriellen Widerstand zu erklären. SELLER et al. (1965) sahen eine direkte Beziehung zwischen der Blutdrucksenkung durch Chlorothiazid und dem Verhältnis zwischen intrazellulärem Kalium und Magnesium in den Erythrozyten.

Die Thiazide schwächen den pressorischen Effekt der Katecholamine z. B. beim Phäochromozytom ab (HUVOS und HOLLANDER 1966). Dies entspricht auch den Ergebnissen tierexperimenteller Studien (PREZIOSI et al. 1959, BOCK und GROSS 1960). Dieser Effekt hängt nach der Ansicht von FINNERTY et al. (1968) ebenso wie die Blutdrucksenkung nicht von einer Verminderung des Plasmavolumens, sondern von der Negativität der Natriumbilanz ab. Die Autoren konnten zeigen, daß die volle Reaktivität des Gefäßsystems auf Noradrenalin nicht durch Plasmaexpansion mit Dextran, sondern nur durch

5% NaCl-Lösung wiederhergestellt werden kann. Am Aortenstreifenpräparat fand Rubin (1963) eine Unterdrückung des Effektes von Noradrenalin, Angiotensin, Serotonin und Azetylcholin durch Thiazide, Acetazolamid, Aminoisotetradine und auch Quecksilberdiuretica. Am isolierten Muskel wirkt Chlorothiazid durch Änderung der transmembranen Ionengradienten. Es fördert die Natriumaufnahme, ohne einen gleichzeitigen Kaliumverlust zu erzeugen.

Die zur Zeit mit der experimentellen Evidenz am besten zu vereinbarende Deutung der Wirkung der Saluretica auf den peripheren arteriellen Widerstand ist, daß intrazelluläre Änderungen des Ionenbestandes der Gefäßmuskulatur erzeugt werden, die von der renalen Elimination von Natrium und somit von der Bruttobilanz des gesamten Organismus abhängig sein können. Diese Ionenverschiebungen wirken entweder direkt oder durch Abschwächung des Noradrenalineffektes auf die Zelle tonusvermindernd. Ein spezifischer, von Wirkungen auf den Ionenstoffwechsel unabhängiger vaskulotroper Effekt der Saluretica durch direkte Interaktion des Moleküls mit der glatten Muskulatur ist unwahrscheinlich, weil Saluretica verschiedenster chemischer Konstitution dieselbe Wirkung ausüben können.

In diesem Zusammenhang ist auch zu diskutieren, ob die zweiphasige Wirkung der Saluretica nicht Ausdruck einer Adaptation der Regelung des Kreislaufs an eine Änderung des Natriumgehaltes des Organismus bzw. des interstitiellen Flüssigkeitsraumes und des Blutvolumens ist: Nicht nur der Kochsalzentzug führt zu einer zweiphasigen Änderung der Kreislaufregulation; auch die Kochsalzretention bewirkt eine Umstellung der Hämodynamik, die das Spiegelbild dessen ist, was wir bei der Salurese sehen. Borst und Borst de Geus (1963) fanden nach Natriumbelastung, z. B. mit Succus liquiritiae, folgenden Ablauf: Hochdruck durch Herzzeitvolumenvermehrung bei hohem Plasmavolumen, der nach einiger Zeit von einem Hochdruck durch Erhöhung des peripheren Widerstandes abgelöst wurde. Man kann also annehmen, daß plötzliche Änderungen des Verhältnisses von Plasmavolumen zur Gefäßkapazität durch eine Änderung des Herzzeitvolumens ausgeglichen werden, langfristige durch Änderung des arteriolären Widerstandes.

Man könnte vermuten, daß dieser hämodynamischen Umschaltung ein typisches Verhalten der arteriellen Peripherie zugrunde liegt, die den Sinn hat, die Durchströmung der Organe trotz Änderung des Perfusionsdrucks konstant zu erhalten.

Aus den bis heute bekannt gewordenen Befunden ergibt sich, daß die blutdrucksenkende Wirkung besteht:

1. In einem selbständigen Effekt, der den peripheren arteriellen Widerstand herabsetzt. Diese Wirkung der Saluretica auf den Blutdruck wird nur bei chronischer Verabreichung wirksam, sie ist schwach.
2. In einem zweifach unterstützenden Effekt, der die Wirkung der auf den Sympathikus hemmend wirkenden Antihypertonica verstärkt:

a) Die Saluretica steigern indirekt den Sympathikustonus, da dieser reflektorisch erhöht wird, wenn das Blutvolumen abnimmt. Die Antihypertonica wirken bei erhöhtem Sympathikustonus jedoch stärker als bei niedrigem.

b) Der verstärkende Effekt auf die sympathikuswirksamen Antihypertonica ist an die Salurese und die Verminderung des Plasmavolumens oder besser die Verhinderung seines Anstieges gebunden, die kompensatorisch eintritt, wenn die blutdrucksenkenden

Medikamente die Gefäßkapazität erhöhen und damit den venösen Rückfluß und das Herzzeitvolumen vermindern. Er wird durch Zufuhr großer Kochsalzmengen aufgehoben oder wenn ein kochsalzretinierendes Medikament gegeben wird.

Der Synergismus mit den über den Sympathikus wirkenden Hypotensiva ist für die Therapie des Hochdrucks die wichtigere von den beiden Wirkungskomponenten der Saluretica.

Wie einleitend schon vorweggenommen, erleichtert die Kombination mit Saluretica die Einstellung des Blutdrucks ganz wesentlich. Die notwendigen Dosen der Hypotensiva sind kleiner, Nebenwirkungen treten dadurch zurück. Da diese unterstützende Wirkung jedoch, wie eben dargelegt, über die Beeinflussung des Blutvolumens und des extrazellulären Flüssigkeitsraums erfolgt, wird dieser Vorteil mit einer Verstärkung der orthostatischen Blutdrucksenkung bezahlt. Unter dem Einfluß der sympathikuswirksamen Antihypertensiva werden die Hypertoniker bekanntlich gegen absolute und auch relative Änderungen des Blutvolumens sehr anfällig (Tab. 2). Die Gruppe von Freis und

Tab. 2. Faktoren, die den blutdrucksenkenden Effekt sympathikuswirksamer Medikamente verstärken.

I. Erweiterung der arteriellen Peripherie	*II.* Verminderung des Blutvolumens
Körperliche Ruhe – Schlaf	Kochsalzverarmung (z. B. durch Saluretica oder strenge Diät)
Stehende Position	Flüssigkeitsverluste
Körperliche Tätigkeit	Blutungen
Nahrungsaufnahme	Anämie
Alkohol und andere Vasodilatantien	
Hitze, Fieber	
Sedativa, Narkose	

Mitarb. hat 1951 zuerst darauf hingewiesen, daß nach vorausgehender Sympathikusblockade schon durch Aderlässe von 250–500 ml hochgradige Blutdrucksenkungen erzielt werden können. Auch diejenigen Antihypertonica wie Reserpin oder Dichlorphenylaminoimidazolin (DCAI Chlonidinhydrochlorid), die, allein gegeben, nur eine geringe orthostatische Blutdrucksenkung verursachen, bewirken, zusammen mit Saluretica gegeben, oft eine deutliche orthostatische Hypotension. Noch stärker wirkt sich dies selbstverständlich bei der Kombination mit den adrenergischen Neuronenblockern aus, wie z. B. Guanethidin, deren initiale blutdrucksenkende Wirkung in kleinen und mittleren therapeutischen Dosen fast ausschließlich über eine Herzzeitvolumenverminderung infolge einer Verminderung des venösen Rückstroms bewirkt wird.

Die *Nebenwirkungen* der Therapie des Hochdrucks mit Saluretica sollen hier nur insoweit besprochen werden, als sie bei der jahre- und jahrzehntelangen Anwendung in der Hochdrucktherapie bedeutungsvoll werden können.

Ich möchte die Diskussion über die Frage der *Verminderung des gesamten austauschbaren Kaliums* unter chronischer Behandlung mit Thiaziden nicht wieder neu aufgreifen; es wurde in dem Referat von Dr. Wilkinson ausführlich darüber berichtet und anschließend auch darüber diskutiert. Praktisch gesehen spielt diese Frage in der Hochdrucktherapie nach unserer Erfahrung keine große Rolle. Vorausgesetzt, daß keine schwere

Nierengefäßerkrankung bei maligner Hypertonie vorliegt, die zu einem sekundären Hyperaldosteronismus führt, oder daß nicht zusätzlich Kalium durch enterale Verluste, Ausschwemmung von größeren Ödemmengen, Inanition, Fieber oder Steroidtherapie verlorengeht, ist eine Substitution von Kalium oder die Zulage von antikaliuretischen Präparaten nicht nötig, wenn man, wie wir es tun, mit möglichst geringen Mengen von Saluretica, wie z. B. 0,5 mg Cyclopenthiazid täglich oder 100 mg Chlorthalidon jeden 2. Tag, auszukommen sucht. Ich meine, man sollte den Hypertonikern, die ja für sehr lange Fristen auf eine möglichst konstante Arzneikombination eingestellt werden müssen, jedes nicht unbedingt notwendige Medikament ersparen. Eine Ausnahme machen digitalisierte Kranke, bei denen selbstverständlich eine sehr sorgfältige Überwachung nötig ist. Hier genügt schon eine stärkere Verschiebung des extra-intrazellulären Ionengradienten ohne absolute Kaliumverarmung des gesamten Organismus, um Rhythmusstörungen auszulösen.

Über die Wirkung der Saluretica auf den Kohlehydrathaushalt nur einige kurze Bemerkungen. Bei genügender Sorgfalt in der Überwachung entstehen keine Gefahren für den Kranken, die ursprünglich deshalb überbewertet wurden, weil übersehen worden war, daß die primäre Hypertonie sehr häufig mit einem Altersdiabetes zusammen auftritt. FREIS (1964) fand in einer Langzeitstudie bei einem gleichartigen Krankengut von Hypertonikern, bei dem alle manifesten und subklinischen Diabetiker ausgeschlossen waren, nach drei Jahren bei 4,8% der Placebogruppe und 3,1% der mit Saluretica behandelten Gruppe einen Diabetes mellitus. HEIMSOTH und HARTMANN (1965) haben eine Gruppe von 113 Patienten systematisch untersucht und 14mal Störungen des Kohlehydrathaushaltes, die auf das Saluretícum bezogen werden konnten, gefunden (s. Tab. 3).

Tab. 3. Zahl der aufgetretenen Kohlenhydrat-Toleranzstörungen bei Hypertonikern, die bis zu vier Jahren mit 25–125 mg Hydrochlorothiazid behandelt wurden. [Nach HEIMSOTH und HARTMANN (1965).]

Zahl der Fälle			Zahl der Störungen
1. Stoffwechselgesunde	73	79	3
2. Potentieller Diabetes	6		1
3. Latenter Diabetes		12	3
4. Manifester Diabetes		22	7
Summe:		113	14

Wenn auch, wie WOLFF und LINDEMAN (1966) einwandfrei erwiesen haben, bei Hypertonikern unter Saluretica sowohl der Nüchternblutzucker als auch die Kohlehydrattoleranz sich verschlechtern und in einzelnen Fällen der Seruminsulinspiegel nach Glukosebelastung nur noch geringfügig ansteigt (BRECKENRIDGE 1967), braucht bei sorgfältiger Überwachung in der Hochdrucktherapie auf die Saluretica nicht verzichtet zu werden. Ohne sie wäre bei dem heutigen Stand der Dinge eine befriedigende Therapie des Hochdrucks in der überwiegenden Zahl der Fälle unmöglich.

Die vermehrte tubuläre Harnsäureretention unter Saluretica bringt in der Langzeitbehandlung keine Schwierigkeiten. Gicht tritt wahrscheinlich nur beim dazu Disponierten auf. Im Verlauf der Langzeittherapie nimmt die durch Saluretica hervorgerufene Hyperurikämie oft ab. HEIMSOTH und HARTMANN (1965) fanden, daß die Hyperurikämie zunehmend seltener wird; nach sechs Monaten hatten 48%, nach zwölf Monaten 17% und nach längerer Behandlung nur noch 9% eine Hyperurikämie. Die höchsten Gipfel, 8–9 mg% bei 11 Patienten, lagen um den dritten Monat und sanken dann ab, wobei allerdings der Ausgangswert nicht erreicht wurde. Die Harnsäuresteigerung ist nicht dosisabhängig.

Eine Gicht tritt in einem Prozentsatz von 5–10 auf (HOLLANDER und WILKINS 1966). Bei der Hälfte der betroffenen Patienten dieser Autoren war der Harnsäurespiegel schon vor der Thiazidtherapie hoch, ¾ hatten eine Koronarerkrankung und einen hohen Cholesterolspiegel über 250 mg%. Auf die große Häufigkeit der Hyperurikämie bei Hypertonikern überhaupt hat auch BRECKENRIDGE (1966) hingewiesen. Er fand ohne Behandlung bei 27% erhöhte Harnsäurewerte. Auch er sah bei diesen Kranken eine Häufung von atherosklerotischen Komplikationen und auch eine Hypercholesterolämie. Bei der Gicht nach Saluretica sind Frauen viel häufiger betroffen als bei der spontanen Form.

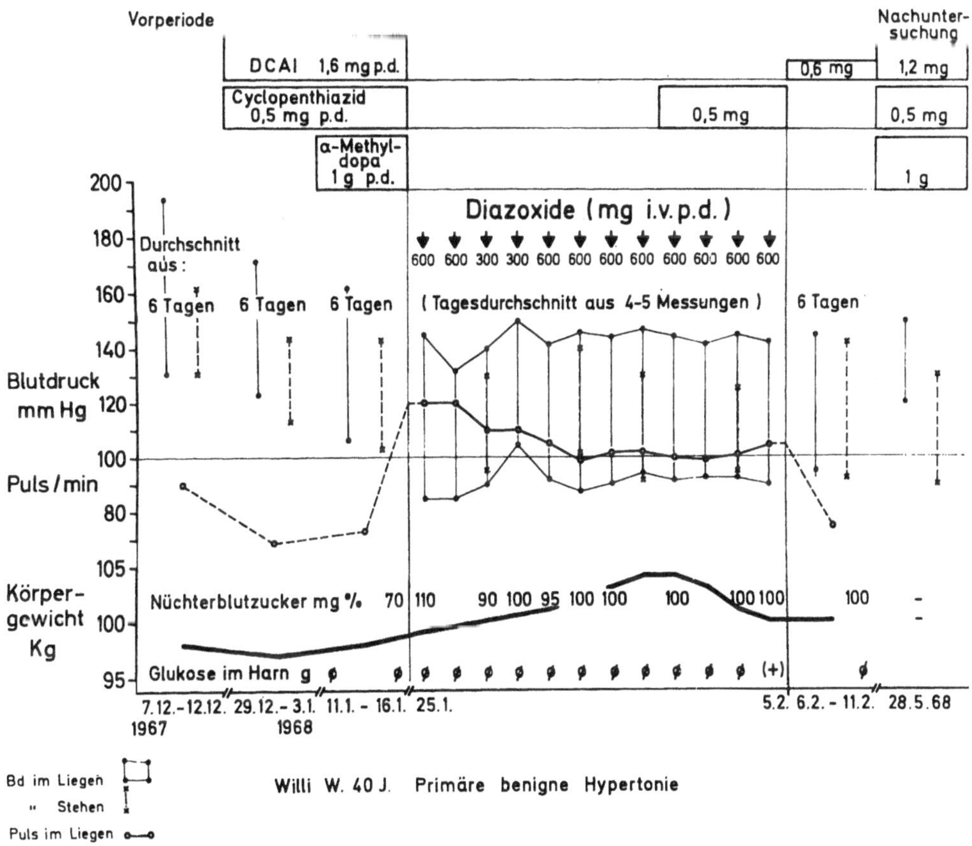

Abb. 2.

Zum Schluß sei noch auf eine interessante Verbindung eingegangen, die – streng genommen – mit meinem Thema nichts mehr zu tun hat, wohl aber mit dem dieses Symposions. *Desamylbenzothiazin (Diazoxid)*, also das Molekül des Chlorothiazids ohne Sulfonamidgruppe, ist ein stark wirkendes Antihypertonikum, ohne saluretisch zu wirken, im Gegenteil, die Substanz ist ein an den Tubuli der Nieren angreifendes Antinatriureticum (TAYLOR 1963).

Die Blutdrucksenkung wird, wie aus Abb. 2 hervorgeht, durch die starke antidiuretische Wirkung, die sich an der erheblichen Gewichtszunahme erkennen läßt, nicht aufgehoben und auch nicht wesentlich verstärkt, wenn durch Saluretica das retinierte Wasser wieder ausgeschieden wird. Die Wirkung auf den Blutdruck ist offensichtlich von einer Veränderung der Plasmamenge und des extrazellulären Flüssigkeitsraumes unabhängig. Diese interessante Tatsache weist auf eine direkte, vom Sympathikus unabhängige, isolierte Wirkung des Diazoxids auf den Arteriolentonus hin. Im klinischen Versuch wird diese Vermutung bestätigt:

a) durch die Beobachtung, daß Diazoxid keine orthostatische Blutdrucksenkung verursacht und

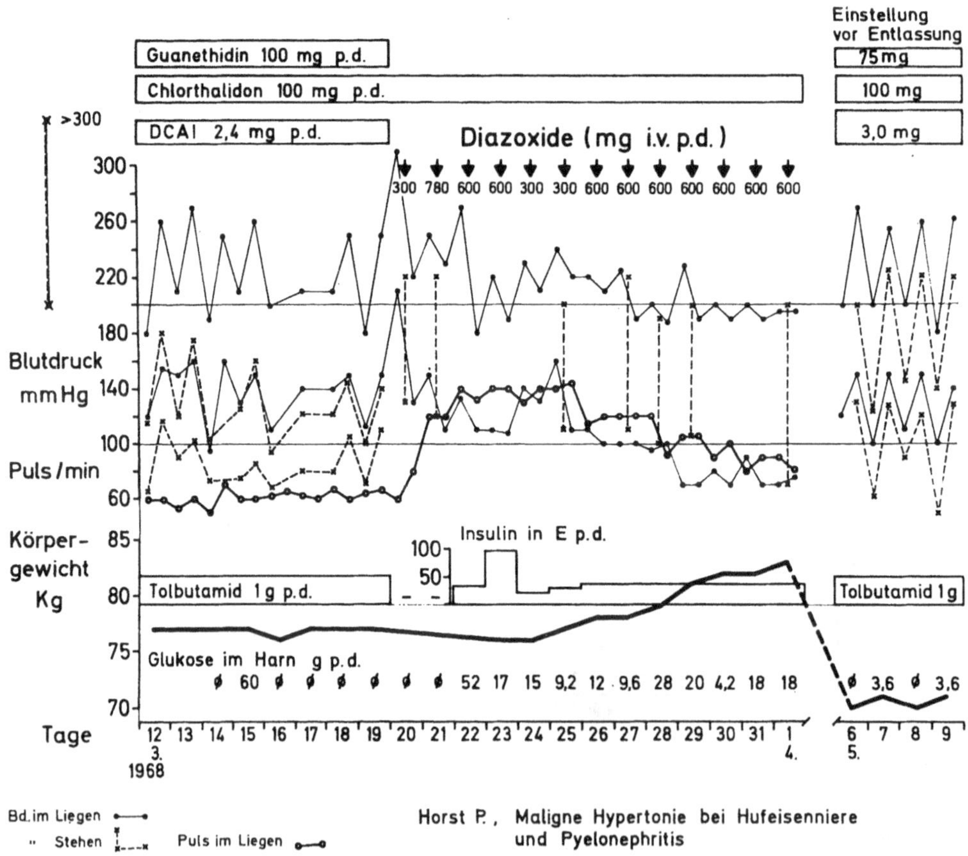

Abb. 3.

b) daß die Blutdrucksenkung mit einer starken, im Verlauf der Therapie langsam abklingenden Tachykardie verläuft; das Herzzeitvolumen nimmt auch durch Vermehrung des Schlagvolumens zu (RUBIN et al. 1963, HAMBY et al. 1968).

Diazoxid wird zur Zeit in Dosen von 300–600 mg schnell in 15–30 Sekunden intravenös bei Hochdruckkrisen injiziert und dazu verwendet, um die Resistenz schwerer Hypertoniker gegen die medikamentöse Therapie mit sympathikuswirksamen Antihypertonica zu durchbrechen (Abb. 3). Da regelmäßig eine Hyperglykämie und später oft auch eine manifeste diabetische Stoffwechselstörung auftritt, verbietet sich die langfristige Anwendung von Diazoxid. Bei einer Anwendung über maximal 20 Tage haben FINNERTY und Mitarb. (1967) und HAMBY und Mitarb. (1968) keine nachteiligen Folgen für die Kranken beobachtet; der arterielle Mitteldruck wurde im Kollektiv von HAMBY und Mitarbeitern um 26% gesenkt. Die zur Einstellung des Blutdrucks notwendigen Dosen waren nach der Senkung des Blutdrucks durch Diazoxid erheblich kleiner. Wir selbst haben bei unserer allerdings noch zu kleinen Zahl von Patienten diesen günstigen langfristigen Effekt der intensiven Blutdrucksenkung mit intravenösen Dosen von Diazoxid noch nicht erreicht. Die Blutdruckwerte stiegen nach eindrucksvoller Senkung unter der intravenösen Therapie langsam wieder auf die ursprünglichen Werte an bzw. es wurden später wieder die gleichen Mengen von Antihypertonica gebraucht wie vor der Diazoxidanwendung.

Ich habe in diesem Vortrag versucht, Ihnen darzulegen, daß die direkte Wirkung der Saluretica verschiedener Konstitution auf den Arteriolentonus wahrscheinlich mit Ionenverschiebungen zwischen Zelle und Interstitium zusammenhängt und daß wegen der Verschiedenartigkeit der chemischen Konstitution der hochdruckwirksamen Saluretica eine direkte vaskulotrope Wirkung nicht wahrscheinlich ist. Nach der bis jetzt verfügbaren Evidenz scheint Diazoxid grundsätzlich anders als die Saluretica auf den »myogenen« Anteil des Arteriolentonus zu wirken. Diese Verbindung ist deshalb theoretisch so interessant, weil mit ihr ein stark wirkendes Hypotensivum gefunden wurde, wie wir es für die Hochdrucktherapie theoretisch postulieren: Ein Präparat, das nicht über eine Hemmung der sympathischen Innervation, sondern durch eine direkte Beeinflussung der Arteriolenkontraktur wirkt, die das Wesen der chronischen Hypertonie auszumachen scheint.

Literatur / References

ALLEN, F. M.: Arterial hypertension. J. Amer. med. Ass. **71,** 652 (1920).

ALLEN, F. M. and J. W. SHERRILL: The treatment of arterial hypertension. J. metab. Res. **2,** 429 (1922).

BOCK, K. D. und F. GROSS: Abschwächung pressorischer Wirkungen durch Sali-Diuretica. Naunyn-Schmiedeberg's Arch. exp. Path. Pharmak. **238,** 339 (1960).

BORST, J. G. G. and A. BORST DE GEUS: Hypertension explained by Starling's theory of circulatory homoeostasis. Lancet **1963 I,** 677.

BRECKENRIDGE, A.: Hypertension and hyperuricaemia. Lancet **1966 I,** 15.

BRECKENRIDGE, A., T. A. WELBORN, C. T. DOLLERY and R. FRASER: Glucose tolerance in hypertensive patients on long-term diuretic therapy. Lancet **1967 I,** 61.

CONWAY, J. and P. LAUWERS: Hemodynamic and hypotensive effects of long-term therapy with chlorothiazide. Circulation **21,** 21 (1920).

CONWAY, J. and H. PALMERO: The vascular effect of the thiazide diuretics. Arch. intern. Med. **111,** 203 (1963).

COTTIER, P.: Renale Hämodynamik, Wasser- und Elektrolytausscheidung bei Hypertonie. Helv. med. acta **27**, Suppl. 39 (1960).

DAHL, L. K., L. C. LAX, C. R. YOUNG, E. SCHACKOW and K. D. KNUDSEN: Failure to confirm a prolongation of the biological half-life of ^{22}Na in hypertensive patients. Circulat. Res. **19**, 750 (1966).

DOLLERY, C. T., E. H. O. PARRY and D. S. YOUNG: Diuretic and hypotensive properties of ethacrynic acid: A comparison with hydrochlorothiazide. Lancet **1964 I**, 947.

DOUGLAS, B. H., O. CARRIER and L. GARRET: Electrolyte changes in aortas of hypertensive pregnant and nonpregnant animals. Amer. J. Obstet. Gynec. **97**, 1092 (1967).

DUSTAN, H. P., G. R. CUMMINGS, A. C. CORCORAN and I. H. PAGE: A mechanism of chlorothiazide anhancing effectiveness of hypertensive ganglionoplegic drugs. Circulation **19**, 360 (1959).

FINNERTY, F. A. jr., J. H. BUCHHOLZ, J. TUCKMAN, G. T. HAJJAR and G. DE CARLO MASSARO: Evaluation of chlorothiazide alone in the treatment of moderately severe and severe hypertension. Circulation **20**, 1037 (1959).

FINNERTY, F. A. and F. J. BEBKO jr.: Lowering the perinatal mortality and the prematurity rate; the value of prophylactic thiazides in juveniles. J. Amer. med. Ass. **195**, 429 (1966).

FINNERTY, F. A. jr., M. DAVIDOV and N. KAKAVIATOS: The long-term effect of rapid repeated reductions of arterial blood pressure with diazoxide. Amer. J. Cardiol. **19**, 377 (1967).

FINNERTY, F. A. jr., M. DAVIDOV and N. KAKAVIATOS: Relation of sodium balance to arterial pressure during drug induced saluresis. Circulation **37**, 175 (1968).

FREIS, E. D., J. R. STANTON, F. A. FINNERTY jr., H. W. SCHNAPER, R. L. JOHNSON, C. E. RATH and R. W. WILKINS: The collapse produced by venous congestion of the extremities or by venesection following certain hypotensive agents. J. clin. Invest. **30**, 435 (1951).

FREIS, E. D. and J. M. WILSON: Potentiating effect of chlorothiazide (Diuril) in combination with antihypertensive agents: Preliminary report. Med. Ann. D. C. **26**, 468, 516 (1957).

FREIS, E. D.: Mechanism of antihypertensive effects of diuretics; possible role of salt in hypertension. Clin. Pharmacol. Ther. **1**, 337 (1960).

FREIS, E. D.: Double-blind control of antihypertensive agents. II.: Further report on the comparative effectiveness of reserpine, reserpine and hydralazine, and three ganglion blocking agents, chlorisondamine, mecamylamine, and pentolinium tartrate. Arch. intern. Med. **110**, 222 (1962).

FREIS, E. D.: Benzothiadiazines and diabetes mellitus. J. Amer. med. Ass. **187**, 462 (1964).

FRIEDMAN, S. M., N. NAKASHIMA and C. L. FRIEDMAN: Relation of saluretic and hypotensive effects of hydrochlorothiazide in the rat. Amer. J. Physiol. **198**, 148 (1960).

FROHLICH, E. D., H. W. SCHNAPER, J. M. WILSON and E. D. FREIS: Hemodynamic alterations in hypertensive patients due to chlorothiazide. New Engl. J. Med. **262**, 1261 (1960).

GIFFORD, R. W.: Use of diuretics in hypertension. J. Amer. med. Ass. **177**, 70 (1961).

HAMBY, W. M., G. J. JANKOWSKI, J. M. POUGET, G. DUNEA and C. L. GANTT: Intravenous use of diazoxide in the treatment of severe hypertension. Circulation **37**, 169 (1968).

HEIMSOTH, V. und F. HARTMANN: Klinische Bewertung der Kohlenhydratstoffwechselstörungen durch Saluretica. Dtsch. med. Wschr. **90**, 1467 (1965).

HEIMSOTH, V. und F. HARTMANN: Untersuchungen zur Störung des Harnsäurestoffwechsels nach Saluretica-Verabreichung. Dtsch. med. Wschr. **90**, 1905 (1965).

HOLLANDER, W. and R. W. WILKINS: A new type of drug for treatment of arterial hypertension. Boston med. Quart. **8**, 69 (1957).

HOLLANDER, W., A. V. CHOBANIAN and R. W. WILKINS: Role of diuretics in the management of hypertension. Ann. N. Y. Acad. Sci. **88**, 975 (1960).

HOLLANDER, W., A. V. CHOBANIAN and B. A. BURROWS: Body fluid and electrolyte composition in arterial hypertension. I.: Studies in essentiel, renal and malignant hypertension. J. clin. Invest. **40**, 408 (1961).

HOLLANDER, W., D. M. KRAMSCH, S. YAGI and I. M. MADOFF: Metabolic and hemodynamic factors in the increased aslt and water content of hypertensive arteries. In: L'hypertension artérielle. Première réunion du club international sur l'hypertension artérielle. Paris: L'expansion scientific française 1966, p. 305.

HOLLANDER, W. and R. W. WILKINS: The pharmacology and clinical use of rauwolfia, hydralazine, thiazides and aldosterone antagonists in arterial hypertension. Progr. cardiovasc. Dis. **8**, 291 (1966).
HUVOS, A. and W. HOLLANDER: The effects of thiazide diuretics and the levels of blood glucose on arterial pressure in pheochromocytoma. Clin. Res. **14**, 379 (1966).
JOHNSON, O. D., H. RUCHELMAN and R. V. FORD: Diuretics and hypertension: Effect of sodium balance. New Engl. J. Med. **267**, 336 (1962).
KEMPNER, W.: Treatment of hypertensive vascular disease with rice diet. Amer. J. Med. **4**, 545 (1948).
LAUWERS, P. and J. CONWAY: Effect of long-term treatment with chlorothiazide on body fluids, serum electrolytes and exchangeable sodium in hypertensive patients. J. Lab. clin. Med. **56**, 401 (1960).
LOSSE, H., H. ZUMKLEY und H. WEHMEYER: Untersuchungen über den Elektrolyt- und Wassergehalt von Erythrozyten bei arterieller Hypertonie. Z. Kreislaufforsch. **51**, 43 (1962).
NOVELLO, F. C. and J. M. SPRAGUE: Benzothiadiazine dioxides as novel diuretics. J. Amer. chem. Soc. **79**, 2028 (1957).
PREZIOSI, P., A. BIANCHI, B. LOSCALZO and A. F. DE SCHAEPDRYVER: On the pharmacology of chlorothiazide, with special regard to its diuretic and antihypertensive effects. Arch. in Pharmacodyn. **118**, 467 (1959).
ROSS, E. J.: Total exchangeable sodium in hypertensive patients. Clin. Sci. **15**, 81 (1956).
RUBIN, A. A.: Hemodynamic aspects of certain antihypertensive agents. Angiology **14**, 74 (1963).
SELLER, R. H., O. RAMIREZ-MUXO, A. N. BREST and J. H. MOYER: Magnesium metabolism in hypertension. J. Amer. med. Ass. **191**, 654 (1965).
SMITH, W. M., A. N. DAMATO, N. J. GALLUZZI, C. F. GARFIELD, O. G. HANOWELL, W. H. STIMSON, R. H. THURM, J. J. WALSH and L. BROMER: The evaluation of antihypertensive therapy. Cooperative clinical trial method. I.: Double-blind control comparison of chlorothiazide, rauwolfia serpentina and hydralazine. Ann. intern. Med. **61**, 829 (1964).
TAYLOR, R. M.: Renal aspects of certain antihypertensive agents. Angiology **14**, 79 (1963).
TOBIAN, L. jr. and J. T. BINION: Tissue cations and water in arterial hypertension. Circulation **5**, 754 (1952).
TOBIAN, L. jr. and J. T. BINION: Artery wall electrolytes in renal and DCA hypertension. J. clin. Invest. **33**, 1407 (1954).
TOBIAN, L., J. JANECEK, A. TOMBOULIAN and D. FERREIRA: Sodium and potassium in the walls of arterioles in experimental renal hypertension. J. clin. Invest. **40**, 1922 (1961).
VARNAUSKAS, E., G. CRAMER, R. MALMCRONA and L. WERKÖ: Effect of chlorothiazide on blood pressure and blood flow at rest and on exercise in patients with arterial hypertension. Clin. Sci. **20**, 407 (1961).
VILLAMIL, M. F., N. YEYATI, M. A. ENERO, C. RUBIANES and A. C. TAQUINI: Effect of long-term treatment with hydrochlorothiazide on water and electrolytes of muscle in hypertensive subjects. Amer. Heart J. **65**, 294 (1963).
VILLARREAL, H., J. E. EXAIRE, A. REVOLLO and J. SONI: Effects of chlorothiazide on systemic hemodynamics in essential hypertension. Circulation **26**, 405 (1962).
VILLARREAL, H., A. REVOLLO, J. E. EXAIRE and F. LARRONDO: Effects of chlorothiazide on renal hemodynamics: Comparative study of acute administration in normotensive and hypertensive subjects. Circulation **26**, 409 (1962).
WELLER, J. M. and S. W. HOOBLER: Salt metabolism in hypertension. Ann. intern. Med. **50**, 106 (1959).
WILSON, J. M. and E. D. FREIS: Relationship between plasma and extracellular fluid volume and antihypertensive effect of chlorothiazide. Circulation **20**, 1028 (1959).
WINER, B. M.: Studies of the content and distribution of sodium, potassium and water in hypertension. In: Hypertension. Ed.: J. H. MOYER. Philadelphia: W. B. Saunders 1959, p. 268.
WOLFF, F. W. and R. D. LINDEMAN: Effects of treatment in hypertension. J. chron. Dis. **19**, 227 (1966).

Krecke: Bei der Frage nach dem Verhalten der renalen Hämodynamik unter Etacrynsäure hatten Sie festgestellt, daß sich nach einmaliger intravenöser Injektion von 50 mg weder die glomeruläre Filtrationsrate noch der effektive Plasmastrom im Mittel ändern. Wir selber haben kürzlich, gemeinsam mit Krück, Uhse und Klein, über ähnliche Experimente an insgesamt 20 normo- und hypertensiven Patienten berichtet (Verh. Dtsch. Ges. inn. Med. **74**, 588 1968), die unter Clearance-Bedingungen im akuten Versuch initial 50 mg Etacrynsäure i. v. und unmittelbar danach eine Dauerinfusion von 50 mg/Std. erhielten. Zur Kontrolle dienten vor der Etacrynsäure-Applikation 3 Clearance-Perioden, denen sich 6 eigentliche Versuchsperioden von jeweils etwa 15 Minuten Dauer anschlossen. Unter diesen Voraussetzungen zeigten 8 Probanden (= Gruppe A) einen erheblichen kontinuierlichen Abfall und 7 (= Gruppe B) einen, allerdings nur auf die ersten 30–45 Minuten beschränkten, wesentlichen Anstieg der glomerulären Filtrationsrate. Der effektive Plasmastrom verhielt sich im großen ganzen gleichsinnig. Bei näherer Analyse ergibt sich zunächst, daß die Ausgangs-GFR beider Gruppen im Mittel nicht sicher voneinander abweicht. Statistisch signifikante Differenzen bestehen jedoch beim arteriellen Mitteldruck und bei der damit wahrscheinlich eng gekoppelten Natriumausscheidung im Urin, da die Gruppe A ausschließlich Hochdruckkranke betrifft, die zu Beginn nahezu immer eine absolute Natriumausscheidung von weit über 300 µÄq/min hatten, während Gruppe B fast ausschließlich Normotensive sind, deren basale Natriumexkretion nur wenig um einen Mittelwert von 270 µÄq/min streut. Von besonderem Interesse ist ferner, daß die fraktionale Natriumelimination $\left(\frac{C_{Na}}{C_{In}}\right)$ und das Harnzeitvolumen *während* des Versuchs, d. h. *unter* Etacrynsäure, in Gruppe A eindeutig höher liegen als in Gruppe B. Aus diesen Befunden glauben wir schließen zu dürfen, daß das Absinken der GFR bei den Probanden der Gruppe A in erster Linie auf einer *stärker* negativen Natrium- und Wasserbilanz mit konsekutiver Hypovolämie beruht, die am peripheren Blutdruck (unblutig nach Riva-Rocci) allerdings nicht objektiviert werden konnte. Die *kumulativ* negative Flüssigkeitsbilanz kam am *Ende* des Experiments anscheinend auch in Gruppe B zum Tragen, da sich hier etwa von der 45. Minute an eine deutliche Tendenz zum Wiederabsinken der GFR bemerkbar machte. Warum es in diesen Fällen von weniger akzentuierten renalen Natriumverlusten (Gruppe B), die, wie gesagt, vor allem Patienten mit normalem bzw. fast normalem Blutdruck betreffen, nach intravenöser Gabe von Etacrynsäure *zu Beginn* zu einem eindeutigen Anstieg der GFR kommen kann, muß jedoch nach wie vor offen bleiben.

Herms: Soll man auch bei Patienten mit maligner Hypertonie und hochgradig eingeschränkter Nierenfunktion mit einem Glomerulumfiltrat um oder unter 20 ml/min intensiv antihypertonisch behandeln ?

Wollheim: Wir senken den Blutdruck gerade auch bei der malignen Hypertonie und auch in Fällen mit Niereninsuffizienz. Nur hat die Drucksenkung hier sehr viel vorsichtiger zu erfolgen. Wir würden uns bei eingeschränkter Nierenfunktion mit Blutdruckwerten von 160/95 glücklich fühlen, während wir beim Nierengesunden tiefer gehen. Die Gefahren einer exzessiven Drucksteigerung sind sicherlich größer als die der Niereninsuffizienz.

Schwiegk: Die Selbstmessung des Blutdrucks durch den Patienten stößt immer wieder auf den Widerstand der Ärzte die befürchten, daß damit Blutdruck-Hypochonder erzeugt werden. Ich glaube aber, daß man eine rationale Hochdrucktherapie ohne Selbstmessung nicht durchführen kann, da der Blutdruck zu verschiedenen Tageszeiten und unter verschiedenen Belastungen geprüft werden muß. Weiterhin stellt sich die Frage, ob nun alle Hypertoniker auch mit Diuretica behandelt werden sollen. Herr Arnold hat sich dafür eingesetzt. Vielleicht liegen weitere Erfahrungen dazu vor ? Auf jeden Fall möchte ich die Notwendigkeit einer Frühbehandlung des Hypertonus betonen.

Reubi: Ich möchte ein Wort zur Blutdruckmessung zuhause sagen. Ich bin ganz Ihrer Ansicht. Wir haben die Selbstmessung schon vor vielen Jahren in Bern eingeführt, und die Erfolge sind sehr gut. Der Patient wird nicht zum Hypochonder, sondern er hat selbst den

Eindruck, daß er die Krankheit beherrscht, indem er die Therapie nach entsprechenden Vorschriften anpassen kann. Er braucht dazu nicht einmal sehr intelligent zu sein, wenn er nur gewissenhaft ist. Wir verfügen heute über so wirksame Medikamente, daß ohne häufige Blutdruckmessung eine Hochdrucktherapie aber völlig illusorisch ist. Die einzige Möglichkeit ist, daß der Patient soweit gebracht wird, daß er seinen Blutdruck selbst mißt. – Zur Frage der Behandlung der malignen Hypertonie mit Niereninsuffizienz: Wir wissen, daß solche Patienten in kurzer Zeit zugrundegehen, wenn man sie nicht behandelt. Die Niereninsuffizienz verschlechtert sich rasch, oder die Patienten gehen an cerebralen oder Herzkomplikationen zugrunde. Wenn man bei solchen Patienten den Blutdruck senkt, läßt sich ein Anstieg des Bluthamstoffes nicht vermeiden. Das kann soweit gehen, daß der Patient anurisch wird. Wir befinden uns dann in der Situation der präterminalen Niereninsuffizienz, es muß also entweder chronisch dialysiert oder transplantiert werden. Wenn man Glück hat, kann man die kritische Phase mit einzelnen Peritonealdialysen überbrücken. Die akute Wirkung der blutdrucksenkenden Therapie geht zwar mit einer Verminderung des Herzminutenvolumens und auch der Nierendurchblutung einher. Später zeigt sich jedoch wieder eine gewisse Tendenz zur Vasodilatation, sodaß der Bluthamstoff nach einem initialen Anstieg trotz gleichbleibenden Blutdrucks wieder absinkt und vielleicht die Diurese wieder in Gang kommt. Das Verhalten ist aber von Fall zu Fall verschieden.

BAETHMANN: Ist eine anti-hypertonische Wirkung der Diuretica auch bei nephrektomierten Tieren oder Patienten nachweisbar?

ARNOLD: Nein. Es handelt sich allerdings um akute Versuche, in denen man nur die erste Phase der Diureticawirkung prüfen kann.

KLEINFELDER: Im Referat von Herrn ARNOLD wurde mitgeteilt, daß eine Hyperurikämie bei diuretischer Therapie im Laufe einer längeren Behandlung wieder zurückgeht. Wir haben bei einer großen Zahl von Hypertonikern, die mit Diuretica behandelt wurden, den Harnsäurespiegel bestimmt und – ähnlich wie bei BRECKENRIDGE – ihn in über 50% der Fälle erhöht gefunden. Es gibt nun autoptische Befunde von GONICK und Mitarb., nach denen es bei chronischer Hyperurikämie zu Nierengefäßveränderungen kommt. Ich möchte daher zur Diskussion stellen, ob die chronische Harnsäureerhöhung beim Hypertoniker, der mit Salidiuretica behandelt wird, nicht doch einen nachteiligen Einfluß auf die Nierengefäße hat.

ARNOLD: Das ist sicherlich nicht ganz auszuschließen, und man wird bei exzessiven Hyperurikämien mit Allopurinol behandeln. Der Harnsäurespiegel ist aber bei Hypertonikern auch ohne Behandlung häufig erhöht, so daß man einen solchen Befund nicht nur auf die Diuretica-Therapie zurückführen soll.

HOLZGREVE: Sie haben gezeigt, daß Diazoxid die Glukose-Konzentration im Blut erhöht und antinatriuretisch wirkt. Wie verhält sich die Kaliumausscheidung nach Diazoxid? Da die nach Verabreichung von Diuretica auftretenden Störungen des Kohlehydratstoffwechsels auf den Kaliummangel zurückgeführt worden sind, wäre es interessant zu wissen, ob das chemisch mit den Thiaziden verwandte Diazoxid auch ohne Kaliumverluste Störungen im Kohlehydrathaushalt verursachen kann.

ARNOLD: Diazoxid wirkt leicht kaliuretisch.

KRAMER: Wir haben beobachtet, daß bei natriumarm ernährten Hunden das Hydrochlorothiazid höchstens einen Tag lang natriuretisch wirkt. Wie lange hält die Wirkung beim Menschen an, und könnte man nicht bei natriumfreier Diät auf diese Mittel verzichten?

WOLLHEIM: Eine natriumfreie Ernährung ist beim Menschen nicht durchführbar. Selbst die Kempner'sche Reisdiät enthält noch eine gewisse Menge Kochsalz.

Arnold: Das zweite wesentliche Argument für die Anwendung der Diuretica beim Hypertonus besteht darin, daß wir die Wirkung der anderen Antihypertonika verstärken. Das ist überhaupt die entscheidende Indikation.

Baer: In animal experiments you get an excretion of salt which is followed by retention. The balance over 24 hours or longer looks as if nothing is happening.

Krück: Wenn Diuretica in Kombination mit streng kochsalzfreier Kost gegeben werden, ist die Gefahr eines iatrogenen sekundären Aldosteronismus besonders groß. Von einem bestimmten Zeitpunkt an wirken die Diuretica dann nicht mehr natriuretisch; es kommt vielmehr zu Kaliumverlusten.

The Importance of Diuretics for the Treatment of Hypertension

Bedeutung der Diuretica für die Hypertoniebehandlung

H. KAMPFFMEYER, J. CONWAY

In der Universität von Michigan hat die Abteilung für Hypertonie im Department of Internal Medicine humanpharmakologische Untersuchungen über die antihypertensive Wirkung von Diuretica durchgeführt. Einige Ergebnisse sind auf der Tabelle wiedergegeben. Die Versuchsplanung und die damit gewonnenen Ergebnisse dürften von Interesse sein.

Zwölf ambulante Hypertoniker, mit Hydrochlorothiazid vorbehandelt, erhielten 3 Wochen lang Placebo, danach bekam jeder Patient für 3 Wochen Hydrochlorothiazid oder Amilorid oder eine Kombination beider Diuretica. Die zeitliche Reihenfolge der Medikation wurde nach Zufall in lateinischen Quadraten verteilt und war doppelt blind. Aufgrund dieser Versuchsplanung konnten wir durch Varianzanalyse und orthogonalen Kontrast für viele gemessene Parameter die Null-Hypothese ablehnen, was bei Verwendung von T-Testen nur mit 2–3 mal so viel Patienten möglich gewesen wäre (Tab. 1).

Was die Blutdruckmessungen betrifft, hing der Erfolg des Versuches von der Zuverlässigkeit der Patienten ab. Die Patienten bestimmten ihren morgendlichen Blutdruck zu Hause selbst. Wir setzten dann die Mittelwerte der letzten 5 Behandlungstage jeder Periode in die Analyse ein.

Die Mittel des morgendlichen diastolischen Blutdrucks am Ende beider Behandlungsperioden mit Hydrochlorothiazid allein waren gleich groß. Amilorid allein beeinflußte den systolischen und diastolischen Blutdruck nur wenig; mit Hydrochlorothiazid zusammen war die zusätzliche Erniedrigung des diastolischen Druckes durch Amilorid innerhalb der Fehlerbreite der statistischen Methode.

Die von der Schwester gemessenen Blutdrucke waren etwas höher. Diese Daten hatten eine größere Streuung weshalb es nicht möglich war, Unterschiede zwischen den Behandlungen zu zeigen.

Am Ende jeder Behandlungsperiode entnahmen wir Blut, zentrifugierten sofort und sandten das Serum zu einem Laboratorium, dessen Analysenwerte eine kleine Streuung haben.

Nach dreiwöchiger Behandlung mit 10 mg Amilorid 2mal täglich war die Kaliumkonzentration im Serum erhöht. Die Kombination von Amilorid mit konventioneller Dosierung von Hydrochlorothiazid verhinderte die bei Anwendung von Hydrochlorothiazid allein beobachtete Hypokaliämie. Amilorid bewirkt in dieser Dosierung nicht seine größtmögliche Natriurese, wie wir in anderen Versuchen feststellten.

Tab. 1. Patienten mit mäßiger essentieller Hypertonie wurden für 3 Wochen mit Hydrochlorothiazid [HC] (100 mg/Tag) und Amilorid [AM] (20 mg/Tag) und beiden Pharmaka zusammen (Cb) behandelt. Die zeitliche Reihenfolge der Behandlungsperioden wurde für die Individuen in lateinischen Quadraten nach Zufall bestimmt.

	Vor-behand-lung	Placebo	Behandlung in den lateinischen Quadraten			F-Werte der Varianz-Analyse					
			AM	HC	Cb	Behand-lungs-Perioden F (2,14)	AM gegen HC+Cb F (1,14)	HC gegen Cb F (1,14)	Gruppen F (3,14)	Patien-ten F (8,14)	Zeit-perioden F (8,14)
Blutdruck syst.	147	162	156	149	143	27[3])	43[3])	13[2])	20[3])	71[3])	3,3[1])
zu Hause diast.	93	99	98	93	91	12[3])	22[3])	3.2	40[3])	27[3])	1,8
(mm Hg)											
Blutdruck in syst.	161	174	159	157	157	0,2	0,4	<0,1	3	8,3[3])	1,7
der Klinik diast.	102	106	100	96	97	0,9	1,8	<0,1	6,3[1])	6,7[2])	1,2
Körpergewicht	78	79	78	78	76	4,5[1])	4,5	4,5	335[3])	102[3])	0,9
Serum											
Kalium [mEq]	3,6	4,3	4,7	3,5	4,2	28[3])	39[3])	16[2])	0,5	2,0	0,7
Natrium	149	148	145	147	143	9,2[2])	<0,1	18[3])	0,5	2,4	1,2
Chlorid	103	107	108	101	101	56[3])	113[3])	0,5	4,1[1])	3,1[1])	1,3
Kreatinin	1,3	1,1	1,3	1,2	1,4	4,2[1])	0,5	7,9[1])	19,6[2])	2,3	2,6
Rest-N [mg%]	22,4	16,6	18,8	19,5	23,1	5,8[1])	4,6[1])	6,9[1])	7,5[2])	3,5[1])	2,3
Glucose	106	93	95	108	107	2,9	5,7[1])	<0,1	0,9	0,5	1,2
Harnsäure	7,1	6,2	6,7	7,4	7,5	3,2	6,5[1])	<0,1	8,7[2])	5,7[2])	0,8

1 = P < 0,05 2 = P < 0,01 3 = P < 0,001

Mittelwerte und F-Werte der Varianz-Analyse von zwölf ambulanten Hypertonikern.

Amilorid beeinflußte weder die Chlorionenkonzentration noch die Blutzucker- und Harnsäurekonzentration. Die Wirkung von Hydrochlorothiazid auf diese Parameter wurde von Amilorid in Kombination mit Hydrochlorothiazid nicht beeinflußt.

In den letzten 3 Säulen der Tab. 1 sind F-Werte aufgeführt, welche bei der Varianzanalyse für die 4 Gruppen von Patienten, für die Patienten untereinander, und für die 3 Zeitperioden errechnet wurden. Die Ermittlung der Daten für diese F-Werte erleichtert einen statistischen Vergleich zwischen den Behandlungsperioden.

Ich habe versucht, die Vorteile einer Versuchsplanung nach statistischen Gesichtspunkten an diesem Beispiel hervorzuheben. Solche Vorteile sollten in den ersten beiden Stadien humanpharmakologischer Untersuchungen voll genutzt werden, um bei den Prüfungen auf Toxizität und Wirksamkeit von Verbindungen unbekannter Wirkung am Menschen an einer kleinen Zahl von Personen zu einem Urteil zu gelangen.

The Importance of Diuretics for the Treatment of Hypertension

In my brief presentation, I would like to demonstrate some data in this table of our experiments in the Hypertension Unit of the University Hospital, Ann Arbor, Michigan about antihypertensive effects of diuretic agents. The design of the experiment and the results obtained may be of some interest.

Twelve patients already under treatment with hydrochlorothiazide (HC) for moderate established essential hypertension were placed on placebo for three weeks, semiblindly. Thereafter, the patients received amiloride (AM) (20 mg per day) alone, HC (100 mg per day) alone, or a combination of both for a period of three weeks. The treatment periods were randomized in double blind fashion, 3 patients per group in four Latin squares. The patients took one capsule and one tablet twice daily throughout the whole trial; the formulation of the placebo appeared identical (Table 1).

The data for the whole treatment period over 9 weeks have been analyzed by the analysis of variance for a group of Latin squares. The two degrees of freedom for the three single treatment periods were broken down for orthogonal comparison. By this statistical method rejection of the null-hypothesis for many parameters was possible. As many as three times the number of patients used would have been required.

In respect to measurements of the blood pressure the outcome of the experiment was dependent on the reliability of the patients. The patients had been trained by the clinic nurse to take their own blood pressure in recumbent position at home and to list the data. For analysis the mean values of the blood pressure in the morning over the last 5 days of each period were entered into each box of the analysis.

The means of the diastolic blood pressures at the end of the pre-treatment period with HC and the treatment period with HC alone were the same. AM alone had only little effect on the systolic blood pressure and when coadministered with HC the additional fall of the diastolic pressure was within the error of the statistical method.

The blood pressure taken by the nurse was slightly higher than the pressure recorded at home. The nurse's data were more variable and hence it was not possible to detect differences among treatment periods from her data.

Table 1. Mean Values and F-Values of Analysis of Variance on Twelve Hypertensive Outpatients Treated Randomly for Three Week Periods with Hydrochlorothiazide [HC] (100 mg/d), or Amiloride [AM] (20 mg/d) or Both Drugs (Cb) Coadministered.

		Pretreatment HC	Placebo	Treatments in Latin Sq.			F-Values of Analysis of Variance					
				AM	HC	Cb	Among Treatments F (2,14)	AM vs HC+Cb F (1,14)	HC vs Cb F (1,14)	Sq F (3,14)	Pt F (8,14)	Time Periods F (8,14)
Home blood pressure (mm Hg)	syst.	147	162	156	149	143	27[3]	43[3]	13[2]	20[3]	71[3]	3.3[1]
	diast.	93	99	98	93	91	12[3]	22[3]	3.2	40[3]	27[3]	1.8
Clinic blood pressure	syst.	161	174	159	157	157	0.2	0.4	<0.1	3	8.3[3]	1.7
	diast.	102	106	100	96	97	0.9	1.8	<0.1	6.3[1]	6.7[2]	1.2
Body weight (Kg)		78	79	78	78	76	4.5[1]	4.5	4.5	335[3]	102[3]	0.9
Serum												
Potassium [mEq]		3.6	4.3	4.7	3.5	4.2	28[3]	39[3]	16[2]	0.5	2.0	0.7
Sodium		149	148	145	147	143	9.2[2]	<0.1	18[3]	0.5	2.4	1.2
Chloride		103	107	108	101	101	56[3]	113[3]	0.5	4.1[1]	3.1[1]	1.3
Creatinine		1.3	1.1	1.3	1.2	1.4	4.2[1]	0.5	7.9[1]	19.6[2]	2.3	2.6
BUN [mg%]		22.4	16.6	18.8	19.5	23.1	5.8[1]	4.6[1]	6.9[1]	7.5[2]	3.5[1]	2.3
Glucose		106	93	95	108	107	2.9	5.7[1]	<0.1	0.9	0.5	1.2
Uric acid		7.1	6.2	6.7	7.4	7.5	3.2	6.5[1]	<0.1	8.7[2]	5.7[2]	0.8

1 = $P < 0.05$ 2 = $P < 0.01$ 3 = $P < 0.001$

On the day of each visit in the outpatient department, at the end of each treatment period, a blood sample was drawn and centrifuged immediately. The serum was sent to a laboratory producing data with a small standard deviation.

After three weeks of treatment with 10 mg of AM twice daily the serum potassium concentration was elevated. The combination of AM together with a conventional dose of HC prevented the potassium lowering effect of HC when given alone. At this dose AM does not produce its greatest natriuretic effect as indicated by other experiments. AM did not alter the chloride nor the glucose and uric acid concentrations. The effects of HC on these parameters were not influenced by AM when both drugs were administered together.

In the last three columns of Table 1 F-values are listed which have been calculated for the 4 groups of patients, among all patients and between the three time periods, respectively. The calculations for these F-values facilitate a comparison among groups of treatment whereas in t-tests these variances are included in the total variance of an inhomogeneous sample.

By this presentation I have attempted to emphasize the benefits of a useful experimental design which can be carried out with cooperation of the patients.

The advantages are obvious, especially in designing drug trials during phase one and phase two studies in man planned for evaluation of toxicity and effectiveness, respectively.

Literatur / References

KAMPFFMEYER, H. and J. CONWAY: Clin. Pharmacol. and Therap. **9**, 350–354 (1968).

Natriuresis in Arterial Hypertension During Treatment with Saluretics

Natriurese bei arterieller Hypertonie unter der Wirkung von Saluretica

D. P. MERTZ, P. SCHWOERER

Beim Hypertoniker findet sich eine funktionelle Störung der Fähigkeit der Niere, Natrium während osmotischer Diurese oder während Wasserdiurese adäquat zu konservieren (siehe bei MERTZ 1966 a, b; MERTZ und SCHINDERA 1967). Bei Diskussion des Problems, wie die Natriumbilanz bei Patienten mit arterieller Hypertension reguliert wird (MERTZ 1967), blieb die von physiologischer Seite gestellte Frage (FLECKENSTEIN, pers. Mitteilung) nach dem Verhalten der Natriumausscheidung solcher Kranker unter der Wirkung von Saluretica unbeantwortet. Auch fanden wir in der Literatur keine beweiskräftigen Unterlagen darüber, ob Saluretica bei Patienten mit arterieller Hypertension im Vergleich zu Gesunden eine beschleunigte und verstärkte Natriumausscheidung bewirken. Die Klärung dieser Frage schien uns sowohl von praktisch-klinischem Interesse als auch von prinzipiell theoretischer Bedeutung zu sein. Wir untersuchten daher den zeitlichen Ablauf der Wirkung einer intravenösen Injektion von 20 mg Furosemid auf die renale Eliminierung von Natrium und Wasser bei einem Kollektiv von Hypertonikern, deren Nierenfunktion nicht oder in nicht nennenswertem Umfang eingeschränkt war. Die Befunde wurden denjenigen, die unter vergleichbaren Bedingungen bei einer normotensiven nierengesunden Vergleichgruppe erhoben worden waren, gegenüber gestellt.

In die Untersuchungen waren 5 normotensive Männer und 3 normotensive Frauen im Alter zwischen 17 und 47 Jahren sowie 4 hypertensive Männer und 3 hypertensive Frauen im Alter zwischen 35 und 71 Jahren einbezogen. Bei 4 dieser Kranken lag eine essentielle Hypertension, bei den restlichen 3 eine Hypertension bei chronisch-rezidivierender Pyelonephritis vor.

Alle Versuche fanden morgens am liegenden, über 12 Stunden gefasteten Patienten statt. Eine Stunde nach Trinken von 15–20 ml Flüssigkeit/kg Körpergewicht innerhalb von 30 Minuten folgten vier 20 min dauernde Versuchsperioden, in denen mittels Blasenkatheterung kontinuierlich Harn und am Ende jeder Periode Blut gewonnen wurden. Am Ende der ersten Versuchsperiode, die als Kontrollperiode diente, injizierten wir jeder Versuchsperson 20 mg Furosemid intravenös. In allen Blut- und Urinproben wurden die Konzentrationen von Inulin (nach ROE et al. 1949) und Natrium (flammenphotometrisch) bestimmt. Die intravenöse Dauerinfusion von Inulin erfolgte mit 1 ml/min einer physiologischen Kochsalzlösung. Alle für Harnzeitvolumen (V), Clearance von Inulin (C_{In}) bzw. von Natrium (C_{Na}) und Natriumausscheidung (A_{Na}) ermittelten Werte wurden auf 1,73 m^2 Körperoberfläche bezogen. Weiterhin bestimmten wir das Konzentrationsverhältnis von Natrium zwischen Urin und Plasma (U/P_{Na}) sowie die tubuläre Rejek-

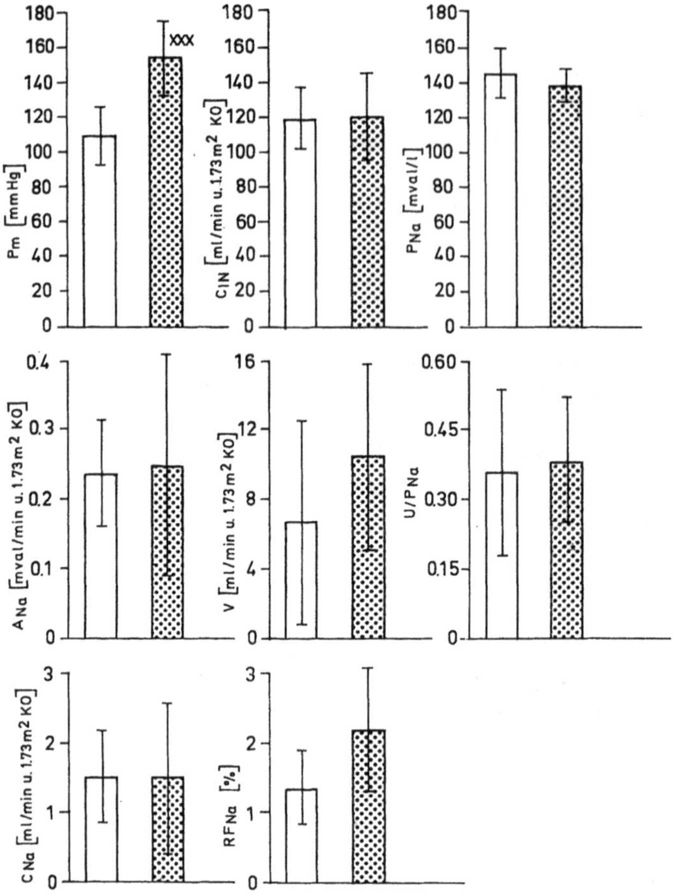

Abb. 1. Basalwerte der renalen Behandlung von Natrium und Wasser bei Normotonikern (n = 8) und Hypertonikern (n = 7).

Fig. 1. Basal values of renal function dealing with sodium and water in normotensives (n = 8) and hypertensives (n = 7).

× × × $P < 0{,}001$	× × × $P < 0.001$
□ Normotones Vergleichskollektiv	Normotensive control group
░ Hypertoniker	Hypertensive
P_m Mitt. art. Blutdruck.	Mean arterial pressure
$C_{In,\,Na}$ Clearance von Inulin, Natrium	Clearance of Inulin, sodium
P_{Na} Plasmanatrium Konzentration	Plasma sodium concentration
A_{Na} Natriumausscheidung	Sodium excretion
V Harnzeitvolumen	Urine volume during a given time
RF_{Na} Tubuläre Rejektionsfraktion von Natrium	Tubular rejection fraction of sodium
U/P_{Na} Natrium Konz. verh. zwischen Urin und Plasma	Sodium concentration relation between urine and plasma

tionsfraktion von Natrium (RF_{Na}) als prozentuale Ausscheidung der glomerulär filtrierten Menge. Die Differenzen der Mittelwerte jeder Meßgröße wurden nach der t-Verteilung (Student) statistisch bearbeitet.

Nach Abb. 1 unterscheidet sich die normotensive von der hypertensiven Gruppe hier nur im Hinblick auf das Niveau des mittleren arteriellen Blutdruckes (Pm). Die Basalwerte der renalen Behandlung von Natrium und Wasser sind bei beiden Versuchsgruppen in vergleichbarer Größenordnung und statistisch nicht unterschiedlich. In bei-

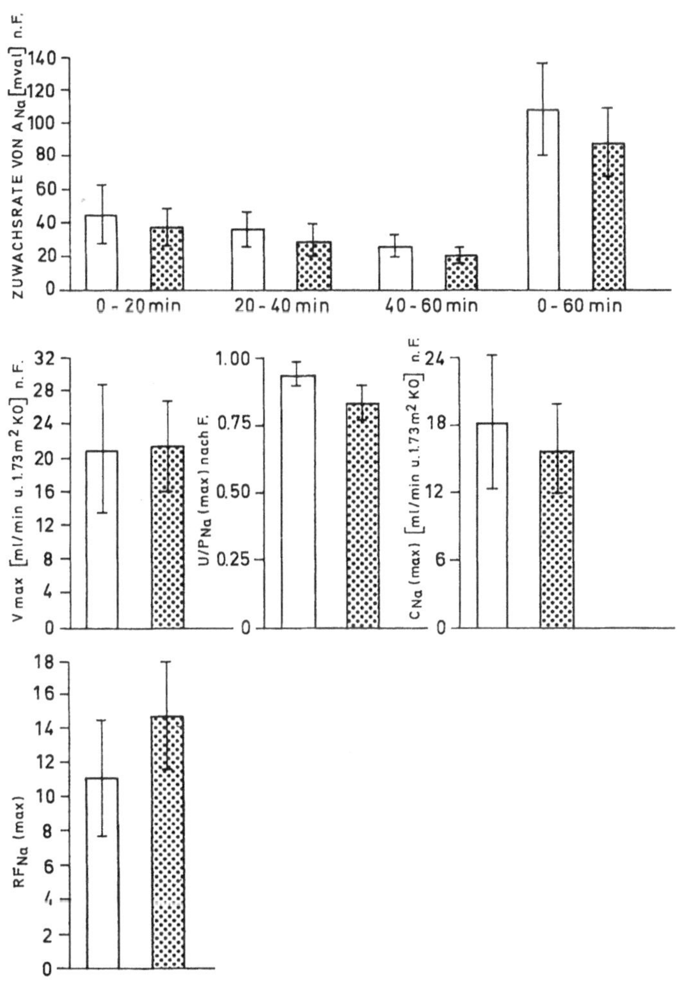

Abb. 2. Zuwachsraten bzw. Maximalwerte der renalen Ausscheidung von Natrium und Wasser nach intravenöser Injektion von 20 mg Furosemid (F) bei Normotonikern □ und Hypertonikern ░. Zuwachsrate von A_{Na} (mval) nach Furosemid.

Fig. 2. Rates of increase and maximal values of renal excretion of sodium and water after intravenous injection of 20 mg furosemid (F) in normotensives □ and hypertensives ░. Rate of increase of A_{Na} (mval) after furosemide.

den Kollektiven nehmen alle gemessenen oder errechneten Werte für die Ausscheidung von Natrium und Wasser unter der Wirkung von Furosemid hochsignifikant zu. Abb. 2 zeigt, daß sich für die Differenzen der unter dem Einfluß von Furosemid erzielten Mittelwerte aller renalen Parameter zwischen der normotensiven Gruppe und den Hochdruckkranken keine statistische Sicherung erbringen läßt. Hypertoniker reagieren also im Hinblick auf eine durch Saluretica induzierte osmotische Diurese qualitativ und quantitativ wie Normotoniker, zumindest solange ihre Nierenfunktion nicht nennenswert eingeschränkt ist.

Bis jetzt ist nicht bekannt, ob die vorgegebene reabsorptive Kapazität des Tubulusepithels bei Hypertonikern durch einen hypothetischen humoralen natriuretischen Faktor (Johnston et al. 1967; Krück 1967) oder durch eine erhöhte intrazelluläre Natriumkonzentration (Kramer 1965; Reinhardt und Behrenbeck 1967; Behrenbeck und Reinhardt 1967) im Vergleich zu Normotonikern vermindert ist. Unabhängig von seiner Natur wird der sonst zur Hypernatriurese führende Mechanismus bei Hochdruckkranken durch die abundante saluretische Wirkung von Furosemid entweder überspielt oder kommt überhaupt nicht zur Wirkung. Für die Praxis ist dieses Resultat insofern von Bedeutung, als Saluretica beim Hypertoniker keine überschießende oder beschleunigte Natriumausscheidung im Vergleich zu Normotonikern bewirken können.

Natriuresis in Arterial Hypertension During Treatment with Saluretics

In hypertension there is a functional disturbance of the capacity of the kidneys to adequately preserve sodium during osmotic diuresis or during water diuresis (Mertz, 1966 a, b; Mertz and Schindera, 1967). In the discussion of the problem of how the sodium balance is regulated in patients with arterial hypertension (Mertz, 1967) there was no reply to the question raised by a physiologist (Fleckenstein, personal communication) as to the behaviour of sodium excretion under treatment with saluretics. Nor did we find any conclusive evidence in the literature on whether saluretics cause an acceierated and increased sodium excretion in patients with arterial hypertension as compared with healthy persons. The clarification of this question seemed to us of practical clinical interest as well as of fundamental theoretical importance. We therefore examined the course of action of an intravenous injection of 20 mg furosemide on the renal elmination of sodium and water in a sample of hypertensive patients whose renal function was not, or not significantly, impaired. The results were compared with those found under comparable conditions in a control group of people with normal blood pressure and healthy kidneys.

Included in the investigation were 5 men and 3 women with normal tension, aged 17 to 47, and 4 men and 3 women with hypertension, aged 35 to 71. Four of these patients had essential hypertension, the remaining three hypertension with chronic recurrent pyelonephritis.

All tests were carried out in the morning, the patient lying down and having had no food for 12 hours. One hour after drinking 15–20 ml fluid per kg body weight within 30 minutes, four test periods followed of 20 min duration each, during which urine was taken continuously by bladder catheterization, and blood at the end of each period. At the end of the first test period, which served as control, each test subject was injected with 20 mg furosemide intravenously. In all blood and urine samples the concentration of Inulin (acc. to ROE et al., 1949) and of sodium (flame-photometrically) was determined. Intravenous drip infusion of Inulin was done with 1 ml normal saline per min. All values of urine time volume (V), clearance of Inulin (C_{In}), sodium (C_{Na}) and of sodium excretion (A_{Na}) were related to 1.73 m^2 body surface. We also determined the difference in sodium concentration between urine and plasma (U/P_{Na}) and the tubular rejection fraction of sodium (RF_{Na}) as percentual excretion of the amount filtered by the glomeruli. The differences of the mean values of each parameter were statistically evaluated according to t-distribution (Student).

As seen in Fig. 1, the normotensive group differs from the hypertensive only with regard to the level of mean arterial pressure (Pm). The basic values of the renal function in dealing with sodium and water are of a comparable order and statistically indistinguishable. In both groups all measured or calculated values of sodium and water excretion increased highly significantly under the effect of furosemide. Fig. 2 shows that there is no statistical support for the differences of the mean values of all renal parameters resulting from the effect of furosemide between the normotensive group and the hypertensive. Hypertensive patients thus react qualitatively and quantitatively like normotensives as regards osmotic diuresis induced by saluretics, at least as long as their renal function is not significantly impaired.

It is not yet known whether the alleged re-absorptive capacity of the tubular epithelium in hypertensives is reduced in comparison with normotensives by a hypothetical humoral natriuretic factor (JOHNSTON et al., 1967; KRÜCK, 1967) or by increased intracellular sodium concentration (KRAMER, 1967; REINHARDT, and BEHRENBECK, 1967; BEHRENBECK and REINHARDT, 1967). Independently of its nature, the mechanism in other cases leading to hypernatriuresis is in hypertensive patients either overcome by the abundant saluretic effect of furosemide or does not come into play at all. In practice, this result is important insofar as saluretics can produce no excessive or accelerated sodium excretion in hypertensives in contrast to normotensives.

Literatur / References

BEHRENBECK, D. W. und H. W. REINHARDT: Untersuchungen an wachen Hunden über die Einstellung der Natriumbilanz. II. Postprandiale Elektrolyt- und Wasserbilanz bei unterschiedlicher Kochsalzzufuhr. Pflügers Arch. ges. Physiol. **295**, 280 (1967).

FLECKENSTEIN, A.: pers. Mitteilung.

JOHNSTON, C. I., J. O. DAVIS, S. S. HOWARDS and F. S. WRIGHT: Cross-circulation experiments on the mechanism of the natriuresis during saline loading in the dog. Circul. Res. **20**, 1 (1967).

KRAMER, K.: Diskussionsbemerkung. In: »Aktuelle Probleme der Nephrologie«. IV. Symposion der Gesellschaft für Nephrologie 1965 (herausgegeben von F. KRÜCK). S. 421. Springer, Berlin/Heidelberg/New York 1966.

KRÜCK, F.: Biologischer Nachweis eines humoralen natriuretischen Prinzips im Urin gesunder Menschen. Klin. Wschr. **45**, 30 (1967).

MERTZ, D. P.: Über den Mechanismus einer beschleunigten Natriumausscheidung während intravenöser Zufuhr stark hypertonischer Kochsalzlösungen bei Patienten mit essentieller Hypertonie. I. Glomeruläre Faktoren. Klin. Wschr. **44**, 233 (1966a).

MERTZ, D. P.: Über den Mechanismus einer beschleunigten Natriumausscheidung während intravenöser Zufuhr stark hypertonischer Kochsalzlösungen bei Patienten mit essentieller

Hypertonie. II. Tubuläre Faktoren. Vermutliche funktionelle Zusammenhänge. Klin. Wschr. **44,** 244 (1966b).

Mertz, D. P. und F. Schindera: Beschleunigte Natriurese bei arterieller Hypertonie während akuter Änderungen im Säure-Basen-Haushalt. Klin. Wschr. **45,** 1024 (1967).

Mertz, D. P.: Zur Regulierung der Natriumbilanz bei arterieller Hypertonie. Vortrag. Freiburger Medizinische Gesellschaft. 21.11.1967.

Reinhardt, H. W. und D. W. Behrenbeck: Untersuchungen an wachen Hunden über die Einstellung der Natriumbilanz. I. Die Bedeutung des Extracellulärraumes für die Einstellung der Natrium-Tagesbilanz. Pflügers Arch. ges. Physiol. **295,** 266 (1967).

Roe, J. H., J. H. Epstein and N. P. Goldstein: A photometric method for the determination of inulin in plasma and urine. J. biol. Chem. **178,** 839 (1949).

Diuretic Therapy in Patients with Cirrhosis

SHEILA SHERLOCK

Summary: The mechanism of ascites formation in patients with cirrhosis is outlined. Control requires rigid dietary sodium chloride restriction, limitation of fluid intake and diuretics in various doses and combinations.

One hundred and thirty seven patients with cirrhosis and ascites were treated with dietary sodium restriction and various diuretics alone and in combination. Ascites could be controlled in 130 patients. Failures were in those with particularly severe hepato-cellular failure. In mild cases frusemide alone was adequate. In more severe cases of fluid retention the combination of frusemide with amiloride proved satisfactory. Potassium chloride supplements were given as required. Complications of diuretic therapy included hypokalaemia, hyponatraemia, hypochloraemic alkalosis and azotaemia. The incidence of hypochloraemic alkalosis and of precoma was low when amiloride was used with frusemide.

The importance of adjusting the dose and frequency of diuretic administration is stressed. If large doses of potent diuretics are given to patients with cirrhosis renal failure may be precipitated.

The problems of diuretic therapy in patients with cirrhosis and ascites are much greater than in any other form of fluid retention. Sodium is excreted in the urine with much more difficulty, larger doses of the diuretic and stricter control of dietary salt intake are necessary. Complications are consequently more frequent.

The mechanism of ascites of liver disease is complex, (Fig. 1) (SHERLOCK, 1968). The two most important factors are failure of the liver to synthesise albumin, and hence a lowered plasma osmotic pressure and portal venous hypertension. More fluid enters the peritoneal cavity than leaves it and ascites develops. This results in depletion of the effective body fluids, which causes the renal tubules to retain sodium and water. The mechanism of the action on the proximal tubules is uncertain although "third factor" must be considered. The distal tubular effect is presumably through aldosterone. In some instances renal blood flow and glomerular filtration rate may be reduced, adding to the sodium retention. By these various methods sodium and water are retained, body fluids are again replete, more ascites is formed and the whole cycle starts again. An active role of the peritoneal capillary membrane in controlling the passage of fluid is possible. The hepatic venous outflow block, due to nodule formation in cirrhosis, may stimulate the formation of hepatic lymph and add to the ascites.

Treatment can be directed to the primary event. The serum albumin level can be raised by infusions of salt-poor human albumin. The colloid osmotic pressure is maintained at normal levels by weekly injections of approximately 25–100 grams. Patients certainly feel better for a few days after the infusions. When compared to a control group, however, there is no difference in diuretic needs, life expectancy, working ability or capacity to manufacture albumin when the infusions are stopped (WILKINSON and

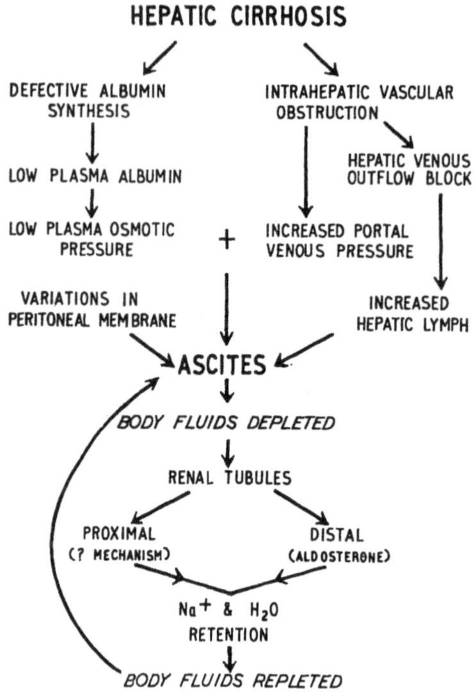

Fig. 1. The possible mechanisms of ascites in portal cirrhosis (SHERLOCK and SHALDON, 1963).

SHERLOCK, 1962). The portal pressure may be reduced by end-to-side or preferably side-to-side portacaval shunt. Ascites however always implies defective hepato cellular function and the mortality of porta caval anastomosis in cirrhotics with ascites is very high, 35.2 per cent in one series (WELCH et al. 1964). Post-operatively, neuropsychiatric complications of varying degree are extremly frequent in these patients. Treatment is therefore directed to the secondary events of sodium and water retention. This paper is based on the results of therapy, using dietary and diuretic means, of 137 patients with cirrhosis and ascites. A salt restricted diet to less than 22 mEq and preferably less than 10 mEq sodium daily is essential. Fluid intake is restricted to one litre. Although in other forms of fluid retention the newer, more potent diuretics may compensate for extra dietary salt this is not so in cirrhosis. Sodium retention is too avid. The usual patient excretes less than 5 mEq sodium daily in the urine. In some patients bed rest and sodium and fluid restriction will be sufficient to initiate a diuresis. This may occur in the alcoholic cirrhotic who is deprived of alcohol and put to bed on this regime (Fig. 2). It is also so in the patient with cirrhosis and a large portal-systemic circulation who has developed a huge natural portal-systemic shunt and lence a normal portal pressure. Fuid retention develops in the legs and on bed rest and dietary sodium restriction the oedema disappears rapidly. If such patients had been given diuretics the fluid loss might have been so enormous that electrolyte imbalance, even renal failure and hepatic precoma, might have been precipitated. No patient with cirrhosis and ascites should be given diuretics until they have had at least four days bed rest while receiving a sodium and fluid restricted intake. During this period the urine output and body weight are recorded daily.

If at the end of four days the weight loss has not been at least one kilogram diuretics should be added. The most satisfactory is probably frusemide 80 mg on waking in the morning and before food is taken. This is a rapidly acting diuretic which causes loss of both sodium and potassium at a proximal tubular level. Ethacrynic acid is an alternative to frusemide. It should be given in a dose of 25 mg daily. It is probably the most potent diuretic now available but has certain disadvantages in patients with cirrhosis. Complications are more frequent (Table 1). The continuation of action, even for 48 hours after one dose, may be disastrous in a patient with cirrhosis who is passing into pre-coma following a large diuresis. It should therefore always be given intermittently. One of the thiazides, such as bendrofluothiazide or chlorothiazide would be alternative if a less expensive diuretic is required.

In all instances potassum supplements must be given, as the chloride (KASSIRER et al., 1965). Potassium will not be retained unless chloride is adequate and a non-chloride supplement will not correct the alkalosis that often accompanies hypokaläemia. Unfortunately, most chloride preparations are unpalatable. The effervescent potassium tablet (potassium bicarbonate and potassium acid tartrate) is of no value as it does not contain chloride. The potassium chloride may be given as an enteric coated tablet (6.5 mEq K per

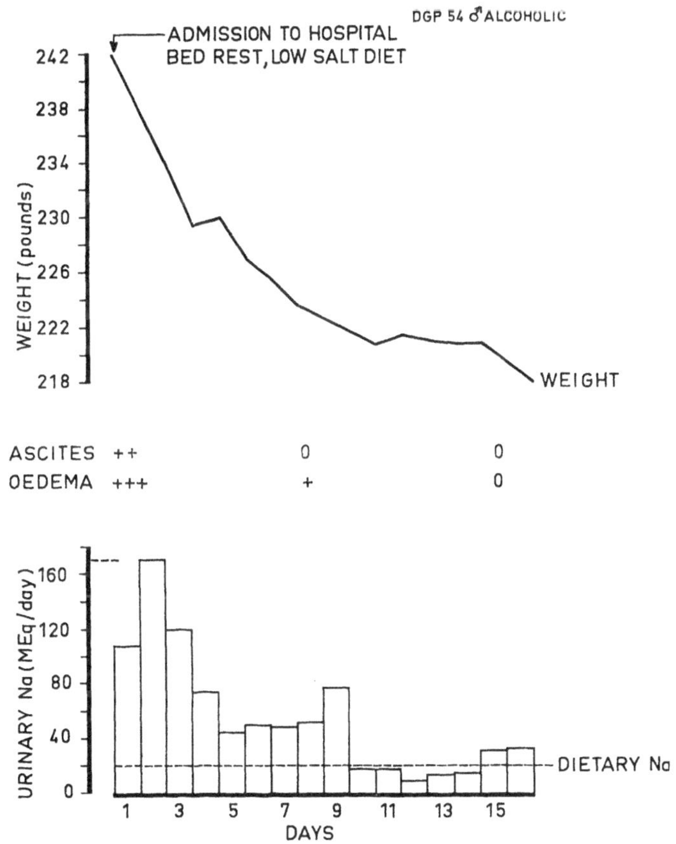

Fig. 2. Cirrhosis of the alcoholic. A diuresis follows simple dietary sodium restriction, bed rest and alcohol abstention.

tablet). This does however carry a small risk of intestinal ulceration and stenosis. Alternatively, slow release potassium chloride may be given (8 mEq K per tablet). The potassium is in a wax matrix which releases potassium slowly. The best one however may be an effervescent potassium chloride tablet (KLOREF) containing trimethylglycine hydrochloride and potassium bicarbonate (6.5 mEq per tablet) (Cox Continental Ltd.). The preparation is quite palatable. The dose of all these tablets must be tailored to the patients needs, but about 8–32 tablets a day are usually required.

If after four days on this regime a diuresis does not ensue then a further diuretic should be added. This should be one that acts not only on the proximal-tubular natriuresis but also distally, conserving potassium. Three diuretics fall into this category, spironolactone, triamterene and amiloride. Spironolactone (100 mg daily) may be added to the frusemide (Fig. 3). This is an efficient, non-toxic aldosterone antagonist. In a patient with cirrhosis and ascites it rarely produces a diuresis when given alone but does so in combination with other diuretics. The combination results in a synergistic action with significant sodium loss and less potassium diuresis. Supplements of potassium chloride 100–150 mEq daily are required. There is a 24–48 hour delay before spironolactone acts so that the frusemide is omitted on the first day of therapy to avoid increasing potassium loss. Spironolactone has the disadvantage of causing gynaecomastia in some patients with cirrhosis. The successful use of frusemide and spironolactone is shown in Fig. 3. Triamterene may be used as an alternative to spironolactone. It is not a true aldosterone

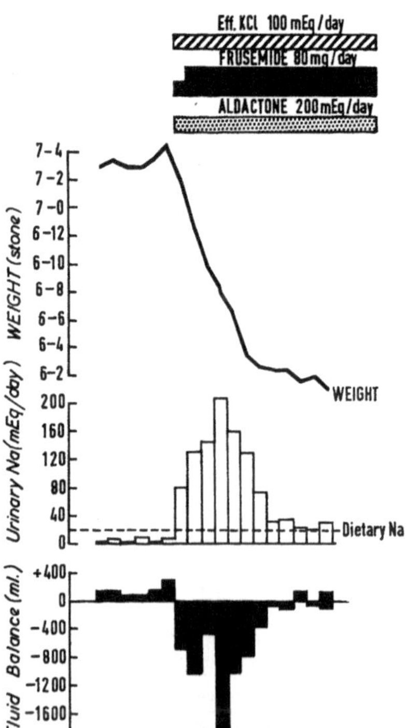

Fig. 3. Before treatment this patient with hepatic cirrhosis and ascites excreted less than 10 mEq sodium daily in the urine and was in positive fluid balance. He was treated with frusemide 80 mg and aldactone 200 mg a day with extra potassium chloride 100 mEq a day. A marked natriuresis ensued. Fluid balance became negative and body weight dropped 15 lbs. in 2 weeks.

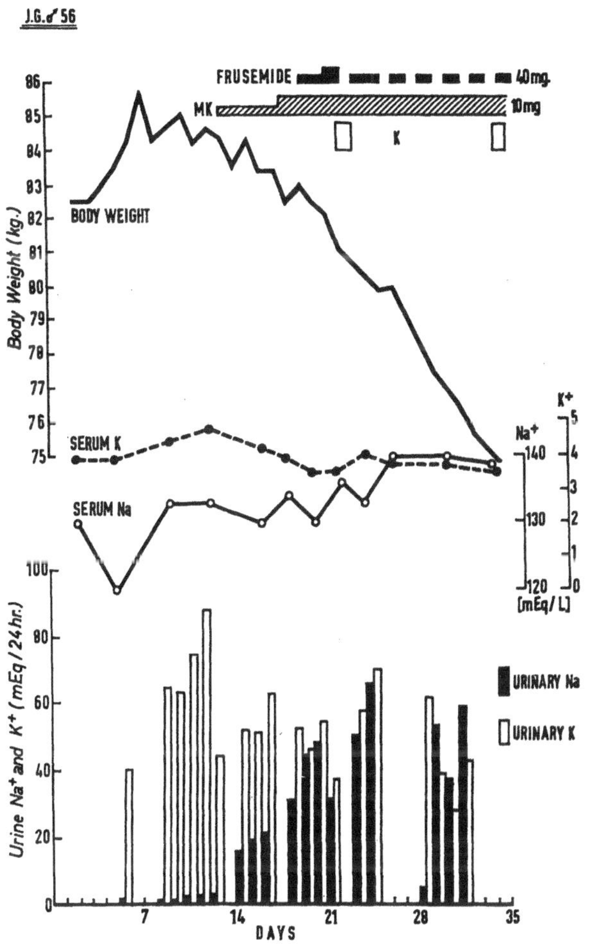

Fig. 4. Hepatic cirrhosis with ascites. Before treatment the urinary sodium was less than 5 mEq and potassium greater than 60 mEq per 24 hours, reflecting marked secondary hyperaldosteronism. The patient was first treated with amiloride 5–10 mg a day. When this was combined with frusemide 40–80 mg every other day a profound natriuresis ensued but urinary potassium did not increase. Body weight fell 9 kg in 3 weeks. Potassium supplements (K) were given on only two occasions. The serum potassium level did not fall below 3.5 mEq/litre.

antagonist. Occasionally azotaemia, due to a fall in glomerular filtration rate, complicates therapy. This is completely reversible if the triamterene is given intermittently. Amiloride (MK 870) is the most efficient potassium sparer of the group and in most instances potassium supplements are not needed when it is combined with frusemide (Fig. 4). Using this combination, in one series 20 of 24 patients with cirrhosis had a successful diuresis (Senewiratne and Sherlock, 1968). The diuresis was unpredictable, sometimes moderate and sometimes massive, one patient losing 238 mEq sodium in a urine volume of 4 litres.

If this combination fails then the dose of frusemide may be increased to 160 to 200 mg daily. Alternatively two distal tubular potassium sparers may be added to the frusemide. For instance, if frusemide and spironolactone are being combined then amiloride may be given in addition (Figs. 5 and 6). The amiloride and the spironolactone have different mechanisms of action on the distal tubule and seem to potentiate one another.

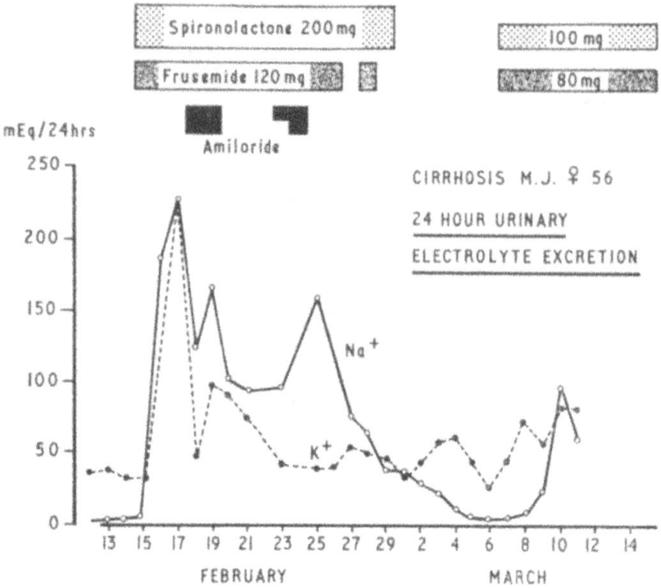

Fig. 5. Cirrhosis with ascites: The diuresis was induced by frusemide and spironolactone. The addition of amiloride, on two occasions, caused a marked fall in urinary potassium excretion. The natriuresis persisted.

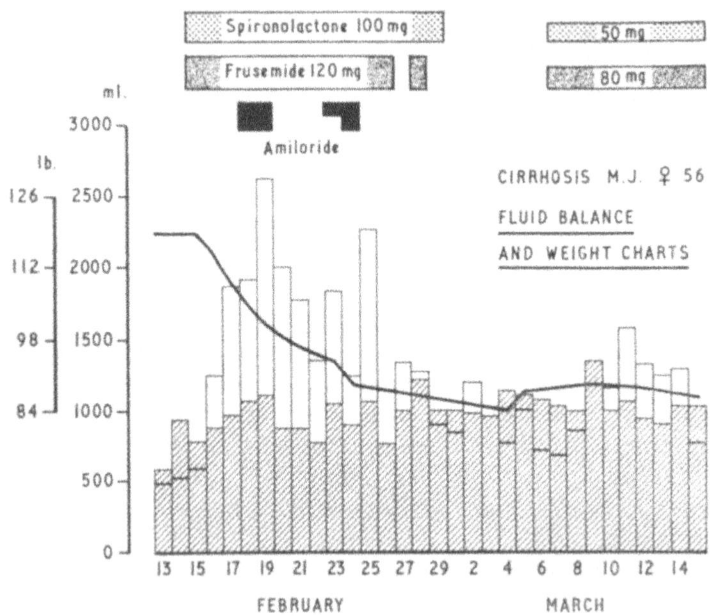

Fig. 6. Cirrhosis with ascites (same patient as in Fig. 5). The diuresis was augmented by the addition of amiloride to the combination of frusemide and spironolactone. The body weight falls progressively as the diuresis continues.

General Results

Using the regime outlined above, a diuresis with ultimate control of ascites was achieved in 130 of 137 patients with cirrhosis (SHERLOCK et al., 1966; SENEWIRATNE and SHERLOCK, 1968). These results include successful treatment of 24 of 25 patients using frusemide and amiloride. It must be emphasised that these results were only achieved when patients were hospitalised for at least three weeks. Also that the combination and dose of diuretics were varied according to the patient's response. From time to time the diuretics need to be stopped for a few days. In a few patients, on discharge from hospital, diuretics were no longer required. In the majority, however, the dietetic and diuretic regime had to be continued as an outpatient, the diuretics being given in varying doses and at different intervals according to the individual needs of the patient.

The failures were usually in those with very poor underlying hepatocellular function. All 7 died within 6 months of starting therapy. In the majority, varying combinations of diuretics were given but all had to be withdrawn because of intractable uraemia, hypotension or hepatic coma.

Table 1. Proportion (%) of patients developing serum-electrolyte changes or encephalopathy after diuretic therapy (Data, with additions, taken from SHERLOCK et al. 1966 and SENEWIRATNE and SHERLOCK 1968).

Diuretic	No. treated	Encephalopathy	Hypokalaemia*	Hyponatraemia**	Azotaemia***	Hypochloraemic**** Alkalosis
Chlorothiazide	31	22	55	40	22	6
Chlorothiazide + Spironolactone	39	28	16	49	31	0
Frusemide	17	26	64	43	43	9
Frusemide + Amiloride	25	4	16	40	40	5
Ethacrynic acid	16	53	50	56	56	59

* Serum potassium less than 3.1 mEq per litre.
** Serum sodium less than 130 Eq per litre.
*** Blood urea greater than 40 mg per 100 ml.
**** Serum chloride less than 90 mEq per litre. Serum-bicarbonate greater than 35 mEq/l.

Potassium Changes

Hypokalaemia is most frequent when chlorothiazide, frusemide or ethacrynic acid are given alone. The combination with either spironolactone or amiloride remarkably lowers the incidence of hypokalaemia. This emphasises the value of adding a potassium-sparing drug when potassium conservation is required. Patients with cirrhosis and ascites have low body potassium stores (CASEY et al., 1965). There is much to be said for giving supplements of potassium chloride (100 mEq daily) for the four control days before any diuretic is started. Care must be taken however that the blood urea level is normal. If potassium deficiency follows amiloride or frusemide it may be due to enhancement of the secondary hyperaldosteronism found in cirrhosis and ascites. In two patients given amiloride and frusemide a negative potassium balance developed which was corrected by spironolactone (SENEWIRATNE and SHERLOCK, 1968).

Hyponatraemia

Hyponatraemia reflects urinary excretion of sodium in excess of water in patients on a greatly restricted sodium intake. In the particularly ill terminal case it may also indicate the passage of sodium into the cells. It more usually reflects the potency of the newer diuretics. It is therefore more frequent the more effective the diuretic combination. As an isolated event it is not serious and may correct itself. If treatment is necessary then the diuretic is stopped and fluid intake further restricted to 500 ml daily. If necessary prednisolone (30 mg daily for about 7 days) may be used as a water diuretic. Terminal hyponatraemia with hypotension is untreatable (HECKER and SHERLOCK, 1956).

Azotaemia

This is most frequent the more potent the diuretic. It results in poor renal plasma flow rather than any lesion of the parenchyma (LANCESTREMERE et al., 1962). Renal cortical vasoconstriction is combined with increased medullary blood flow (SCHROEDER et al., 1967). A brisk diuresis results in contraction of the extracellular fluid volume and accentuates the tendency towards azotaemia in the cirrhotic patient. The effectiveness of the main diuretic decreases as the glomerular filtration rate falls. Blood urea should be estimated frequently while the patient is in hospital and at least every 4–5 weeks as an outpatient. It is also advisable to ask the patient to return if there is no diuresis after taking the drug or if body weight increases. The rise in blood urea and serum creatinine values is a serious disadvantage of all potent diuretics including the combination of amiloride with frusdemie. However increases are usually corrected by stopping diuretics and progression to the terminal stage of "renal failure" in cirrhotic patients is unusual. However a low incidence of serious renal complications can only be hoped for if the diuretics are given cautiously and withdrawn rapidly if azotaemia develops (SENEWIRATNE and SHERLOCK, 1968).

Hypochloraemic Alkalosis

This is surprisingly rare. Ethacrynic acid, given alone, was associated with the highest incidence of alkalosis. This is due to urinary sodium chloride loss with normal tubular reabsorption of bicarbonate which leads to contraction of the sodium chloride but not the bicarbonate extra cellular space (LIEBERMAN and REYNOLDS, 1965). It is corrected by giving chloride supplements but not by potassium alone. Amiloride given with frusemide was shown to have a particularly low association with hypochloraemic alkalosis but in the study reported chloride supplements had been given (SENEWIRATNE and SHERLOCK, 1968).

Precoma and Coma

Neuropsychiatric changes following the use of thiazide diuretics have been associated with hypokalaemia (READ et al., 1959). In the present series hypokalaemia was not closely associated with hepatic precoma. This may not be as important a precipitant of hepatic coma as was originally thought. The incidence of hepatic encephalopathy was only 4 per cent in the group treated with frusemide and amiloride compared with 30 per cent in a similar group of patients treated with potent diuretics but excluding amiloride.

These improved results might be related to a reduced incidence of alkalosis. Alkalosis is known to precipitate hepatic coma and ammonia ionises more and passes the blood brain barrier better in the presence of an alkalosis (WARREN et al., 1960). It is interesting that the administration of ethacrynic acid alone was associated with the highest incidence of precoma and also of hypochloraemic alkalosis. The lowered incidence of hepatic coma in cirrhotic patients receiving amiloride is an important therapeutic advance. Hepatic precoma may be prevented by increasing diuretic dosage gradually and if necessary giving the drugs intermittently. A massive uncontrolled diuresis should not be allowed to develop. Patients on diuretics should be examined repeatedly for sings of hepatic encephalopathy, particularly a flapping tremor, confusion and stupor. If these are detected the diuretic must be stopped immediately. Potassium chloride supplements may be needed.

References

CASEY, T. H., W. H. J. SUMMERSKILL and A. L. ORVIS: Gastroenterology **48**, 198 (1965).

HECKER, R. and S. SHERLOCK: Lancet **11**, 1121 (1956).

KASSIRER, J. P., P. M. BERKMAN, D. R. LAWRENZ and W. B. SCHWARTZ: Amer. J. Med. **38**, 172 (1965).

LANCESTREMERE, R. G., P. L. DAVIDSON, L. E. EARLY, J. J. O'BRIEN and S. PAPPER: J. clin. Invest. **41**, 1922 (1962).

LIEBERMAN, F. L. and T. B. REYNOLDS: Gastroenterology, **49**, 531 (1965).

READ, A. E., R. M. HASLAM, J. LAIDLAW and S. SHERLOCK: Clin. Sci. **18**, 409 (1959).

SCHROEDER, E. T., L. SHEAR, S. M. SANCETTA and G. J. GABUZDA: Amer. J. Med., **43**, 887 (1967).

SENEWIRATNE, B. and S. SHERLOCK: Lancet **I**, 120 (1968).

SHEAR, L., P. W. HALL III and G. J. GABUZDA: Amer. J. Med., **39**, 199 (1965).

SHERLOCK, S.: Diseases of the liver and biliary system. 4th edition. Blackwell, Oxford, p. 138 (1968).

SHERLOCK, S. and S. SHALDON: Gut, **4**, 95 (1963).

SHERLOCK, S., B. SENEWIRATNE, A. SCOTT and J. G. WALKER: Lancet **I**, 1049 (1966).

WARREN, K. S., F. L. IBER, W. DÖLLE and S. SHERLOCK: J. Lab. clin. Med., **56**, 678 (1960).

WELCH, H. F., C. S. WELCH and J. H. CARTER: Surgery **56**, 75 (1964).

WILKINSON, P. and S. SHERLOCK: Lancet **II**, 1125 (1962).

DÖLLE: Prof. SHERLOCK, I would like to comment on the complications of diuretic treatment in patients with cirrhosis, especially on hyponatremia. There are two situations in which we observe hyponatremia. The first situation occurs if we treat the patient too long. This situation can be handled very easily: you stop the treatment. The second situation occurs in patients who do not respond to the diuretic treatment or who develop hyponatremia during the treatment even if they lose weight. Usually, we see this hyponatremia associated with hyperkalemia and azotemia. You comment in your paper on the frequency of complications in relation to the different drugs. In think one should look into this problem in terms of the severity of the disease. You said that the frequency of azotemia reflects the potency of the drugs, especially of ethacrynic acid, and I think this means that it reflects also the severity of the disease because we have to use the most potent drugs in the most severe cases. One could make the statement that we really do not need more potent drugs for the therapy of ascites in cirrhosis. – My second comment deals with albumin infusions. You said albumin infusions are not recommendable in patients with ascites. I think this is true, but after ascites and edema have been removed, what we call the 2nd phase of treatment begins. We try to build up the patient's protein stores and to elevate his serum-albumin concentration, and in this phase albumin infusions have their place.

SCHWIEGK: Wenn man bei schweren Fällen besonders stark wirksame Mittel anwendet, so ist das eigentlich nicht das richtige Prinzip. Die schweren Fälle bedürfen meiner Meinung nach immer einer besonders schonenden Behandlung.

JAHRMÄRKER: Zum Natriumspiegel möchte ich sagen, daß wir im Gegensatz zu früher eine leichte Hyponatriämie von 130–120 mval/l nicht mehr so schwer bewerten, und daß bei schweren Fällen mit kombinierter diuretischer Therapie und Cortison-Substitution manchmal ein solcher Bereich durchschritten wird und sich dann von selbst wieder bessert. Kritisch wird die Situation bei tieferen Werten und terminalen Zuständen.

GESSLER: Machen Sie auch dann keine Albumininfusionen, wenn die Gesamteiweiß- und Albumin-Werte im Serum sehr stark abgesunken sind? Wir haben beobachtet, daß Patienten erst nach einer solchen Infusionsbehandlung wieder auf Diuretica ansprachen.

REUBI: I would like to ask you, Mrs. SHERLOCK, whether you do not see an indication for the use of salt-poor albumin in those cases in which high doses of diuretics have produced a reduction of the plasma volume. Of course, in the nephrotic syndrome we never use salt-poor albumin, because it is excreted almost immediately and there is only a transient effect on the urine output. But I always thought that liver cirrhosis might be an indication for this medicament. I can believe that there is no longlasting effect. But if you give salt-poor albumin in order to prevent diminution in the plasma-volume or to restore it to normal values, I wonder whether you might diminish the incidence of azotemia observed in your cases. It is well-known that the renal plasma-flow strongly depends on the plasma volume and also the electrolyte composition of the body. In ascites we meet rather special conditions because the ascitic fluid represents a more or less separate compartment. If we give diuretics, we promote excretion of salt and water from the whole body, but presumably not in the first place from the ascitic compartment.

SHERLOCK: We did a controlled trial of intravenous albumin infusions in which we kept up the patient's serum albumin level artificially by giving 800–1000 g over a period of 10 days and then maintained it by infusions once a week. There was absolutely no difference between the treated and control groups (WILKINSON, P. and S. SHERLOCK 1962, Lancet **II**, 1125). What is important for the patient is his own albumin synthesis.

Now, Dr. REUBI is on an entirely different line. He is saying, if the azotemia is due to decreased renal-plasma-flow, why do we not increase the plasma volume? Well, you could, you might use albumin, you might use dextran or mannitol. These are unspecific methods of increasing plasma volume. I do not think this therapy is necessary because the azotemia goes once the diuretic is stopped, but there would be a theoretical reason for giving albumin under those circumstances.

I quite agree about serum sodium concentration. Hyponatremia in cirrhosis has a lot of different significances. About 13 years ago HECKER and I (HECKER, R. and S. SHERLOCK: Lancet **II**, 1121 [1956]), described the terminal state in liver disease in which hyponatremia is very profound and in which these dilutional effects cannot be corrected. Clearly, this is an entirely different hyponatremia from the one Dr. JAHRMÄRKER is mentioning where it has followed the diuretic and is usually of very little significance. The serum sodium returns to normal even sometimes without stopping the diuretic.

MULLER: I would like to ask two questions. Do you have evidence that when you treat your patients suffering from cirrhosis and ascites with diuretics that they live longer than when you leave the ascites as it is, except in the very rare cases where the ascites is so extensive that the patient cannot move anymore? Secondly: How do you explain that amiloride combined with a diuretic prevents complications more readily than, let's say, chlorothiazide with spironolactone? Theoretically, there shouldn't be a difference between the two substances or do you think that spironolactone as a substance is more toxic than amiloride.

SHERLOCK: I don't think we have clear evidence that the patients do live longer when ascites is controlled. In fact, when we analyzed our complications and results, we wondered whether it wouldn't be justifiable to run a controlled trial, one group having diuretics and the other not. I don't think we have any clear proof that the patients live longer, but I think they are kept more comfortable.

As regards the lower incidence of encephalopathy when amiloride is added to furosemide. This may be related to the reduced urinary loss of chloride as well as less potassium, compared to the use of spironolactone.

MULLER: We made a retrospective study on 180 patients with cirrhosis who all came to autopsy, part of them were treated with diuretics, part of them were treated without diuretics. After 24 months we found about the same number of survivors out of these 180 patients. When we looked on the complications with and without diuretic therapy, diuretics were used intermittently, again there was not much difference between the two groups.

LEPPLA: Prof. SHERLOCK, in your paper you stressed the hazards of metabolic alkalosis in cirrhotic patients. Could you comment also on respiratory alkalosis in cirrhosis patients and on possible combinations between metabolic and respiratory alkalosis with regard to increased ammonium toxicity?

SHERLOCK: There is no doubt that patients with cirrhosis do have a respiratory alkalosis which is particularly marked in the terminal stages. Alkalosis increases the permeability of the blood-brain barrier to the ammonia ion. Once we measured the arterial pH in the cirrhotics in coma and we found that it tended toward the alkaline side. We gave them infusions of hydrochloride acid and brought the pH back to normal. This certainly reduced the ammonia level both in the arterial blood and in the cerebrospinal fluid but it didn't influence very much their coma (WARREN, K. S., F. L. IBER, W. DOLLE and S. SHERLOCK [1960], J. lab. clin. Med. **56,** 687).

KRÜCK: You mentioned the gynaecomastia as a side effect of spironolactone. How can you make sure that this effect is really caused by the drug alone and not by the original liver disease?

SHERLOCK: Patients with cirrhosis have a tendency towards gynaecomastia anyway, although it is not very common. There is little doubt, however, that patients with cirrhosis who have no gynaecomastia before they start spironolactone will develop it on the drug. This is a painful and embarrassing complication. I suppose this is due to the fact that the liver is not very good in handling spironolactone which is a steroid. The nephrotic patient will manage perfectly well on spironolactone but the cirrhotic will not.

JAHRMÄRKER: Für das Problem einer medikamentenbedingten Gynäkomastie ist vielleicht von Interesse, daß auch unter Herzglykosiden, die ja auch Steroide sind, gelegentlich eine Gynäkomastie auftritt.

SCHWIEGK: Aus meiner eigenen Erfahrung möchte ich sagen, daß seit Verwendung von Spirolactonen ein grundsätzlicher Wandel eingetreten ist, während uns früher die Ascitesfälle große Schwierigkeiten bereitet haben. Das Schwinden des Ascites unter Aldosteron-Antagonisten bei der Leberzirrhose war mir immer sehr eindrucksvoll. – Darf ich dann noch eine Frage stellen. Wir glaubten früher, daß die deletäre Folge einer diuretischen Therapie mit Ausgang ins Koma auf die Hypokaliämie zurückzuführen sei. Verstehe ich Sie richtig, daß es weniger die Hypokaliämie als die Alkalose ist, die ja so gut wie immer mit der Hypokaliämie verbunden ist?

KOCZOREK: Eigentlich überrascht es mich selbst immer wieder, wenn wir bei unseren Diskussionen um das Für und Wider der kombinierten diuretischen Therapie vergessen zu haben scheinen, wie außerordentlich gut gerade die dekompensierten Leberzirrhosen oft auch auf die alleinige Anwendung von Spirolactonen ansprechen können. In diesem Zusammenhang möchten wir kurz die Beobachtung eines extrarenalen Effektes von Aldadiene-Kalium, einem intravenös wirksamen Spirolacton-Derivat, mitteilen. Wir sahen nämlich unter der Injektion dieser Substanz bei Patienten mit dekompensierter Leberzirrhose im hepatischen Koma mehrfach eine deutlich reproduzierbare, passagere Aufhellung ihres Bewußtseins (KOCZOREK und EISENBURG; bisher unveröffentlichte Beobachtungen 1967 und 1968). Dieser Effekt von Aldadiene-Kalium verdient sicherlich auch weiterhin Beachtung. – Zur Frage der verlängerten Überlebenszeit von Leberzirrhotikern nach diuretischer Therapie möchte ich einen Patienten mit einer bioptisch gesicherten dekompensierten Leberzirrhose erwähnen, bei dem wir etwa 1 ½ Jahre größte Schwierigkeiten hatten, seinen extremen Aszites zu kontrollieren. Nachdem es uns jedoch durch multipel und wechselnd kombinierte Maßnahmen dennoch gelungen war, diesen Aszites zu beseitigen, lebt dieser Patient jetzt schon 5 Jahre lang überraschend beschwerdearm und ohne je wieder einen stärkeren Aszites zu entwickeln.

SHERLOCK: I think we have all seen patients like that. We wish there were more of them. Had the patient's serum albumin level risen? Had the portal venous pressure fallen?

KOCZOREK: Der Serum-Albumin-Spiegel des Patienten ist in der Zwischenzeit tatsächlich wieder angestiegen, wenn auch nicht in den Bereich der Norm. Messungen des Pfortaderdrucks wurden bei dem Patienten nicht vorgenommen.

SCHWIEGK: Mein Mitarbeiter EISENBURG hat die frühere und jetzige Lebenserwartung bei Zirrhose verglichen. Danach scheint eine gezielte Therapie doch zu einer Lebensverlängerung zu führen. Vor allem geht es den Patienten unter dieser Therapie wesentlich besser.

LEPPLA: I would like to come back to alkalosis again: Would you think it is possible that, besides an increase in ammonia, cerebral hypoxia induced by alkalosis could contribute to the encephalopathy in cirrhotic patients?

SHERLOCK: Yes, I am sure that is possible. I would not like you to believe that the coma following diuretics is just due to alkalosis. I think it is much more complex. It's not just simply explained by hypokalemia or hypochloremic alkalosis, or what have you. In many instances there is no change in arterial ammonia. The induction of coma must be related to the state of the brain in the cirrhotic patient which is not normal. We know that cirrhotic patients will show EEG changes following drugs such as morphine that would have absolutely no effect on a normal person (LAIDLAW, J., A. E. READ and S. SHERLOCK [1961] Gastroenterology, **40,** 389). If alkalosis produces mild cerebral hypoxia, that will also send him into coma. There are countless ways in which the patient with liver disease reaches the end-picture of coma. As regards diuretics, it is very difficult to place quite such emphasis on potassium as I did 10 years ago (READ, A. E., J. LAIDLAW, R. M. HASLAM and S. SHERLOCK [1959] Clin. Sci. **18,** 409). It now seems that alkalosis may be more important, but it could equally well be one of a multitude of different factors.

The Administration of Diuretics and the Metabolism of Aldosterone in Liver Disease

Zur Diuretica-Anwendung und zum Aldosteron-Stoffwechsel bei Erkrankungen der Leber

F. DÜRR, W. KAUFMANN, B. STEINER

Bei 14 Kranken mit Leberzirrhose wurde der Aldosteronstoffwechsel untersucht. Die Aldosteronanalysen erfolgten nach der Doppelisotopenmethode von KLIMAN und PETERSON.

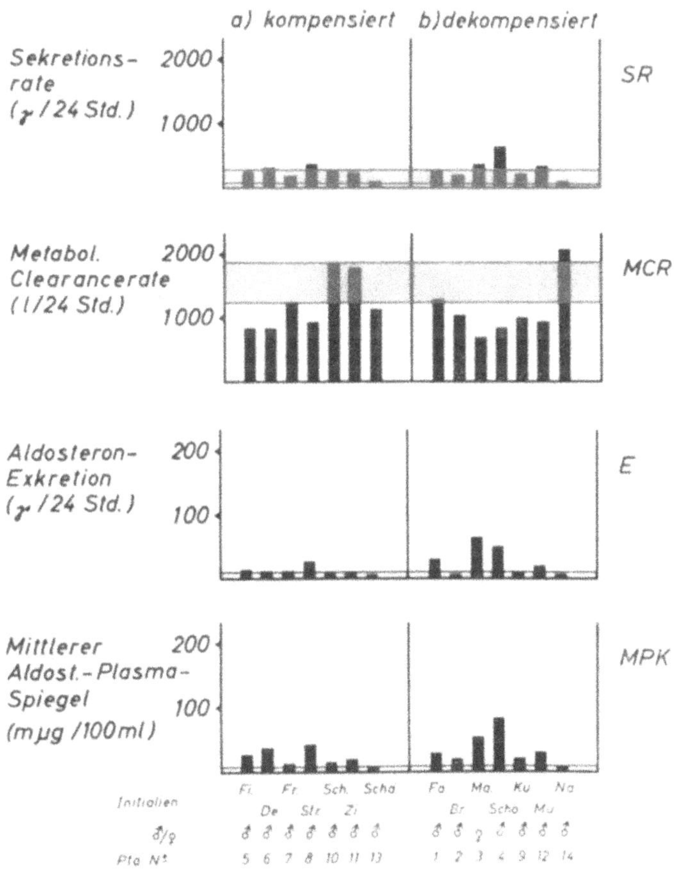

Abb. 1. Verhalten der einzelnen Parameter des Aldosteronstoffwechsels bei 7 Kranken mit kompensierter Leberzirrhose und bei 7 Fällen mit dekompensierter Leberzirrhose (Ascites!) in der behandlungsfreien Vorperiode.

Fig. 1. The behaviour of various parameters of the aldosterone-metabolism in 7 patients with compensated cirrhosis of the liver and in 7 patients with decompensated cirrhosis of the liver (ascites!) in the medication-free pretreatment period.

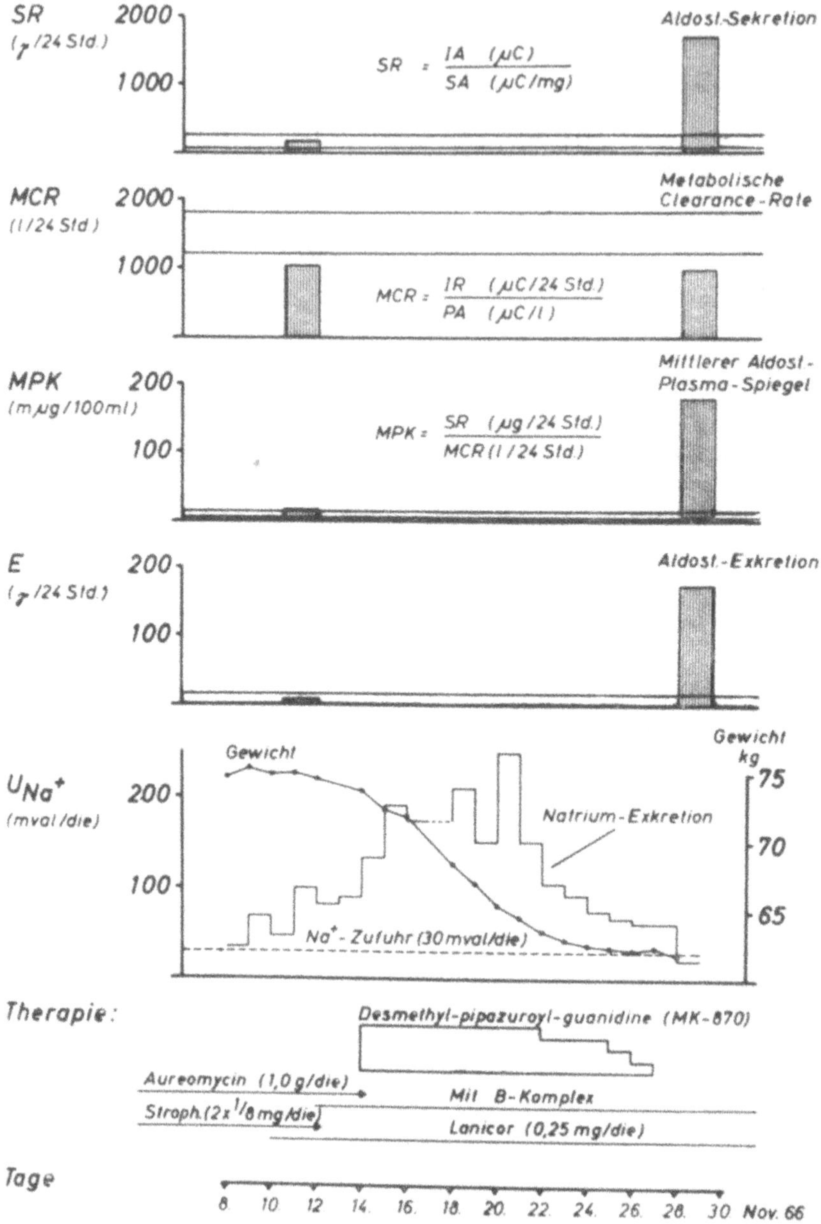

Abb. 2. Br. H., 73 J., dekompensierte Leberzirrhose mit Ascites. Ansteigen der Aldosteronsekretion – und -exkretion, sowie der mittleren Plasmakonzentration des Aldosterons unter einer durch Amilorid (MK 870) induzierten negativen Natriumbilanz.

Fig. 2. Br. H., 73 year-old-patient with decompensated cirrhosis of the liver with ascites. Increase of aldosterone-secretion and -excretion; rise of mean plasma concentration of aldosterone during a negative sodium balance induced by amiloride (MK 870).

Im einzelnen wurden bestimmt:

renale Exkretion (E γ/24 Std.),
Sekretionsrate (SR γ/24 Std.),
Metabolische Clearance-Rate (MCR in l/24 Std.),
Mittlere Aldosteron-Plasmakonzentration (MPK in mμg/100 ml).

Die Ergebnisse dieser Untersuchungen bei 7 Kranken mit kompensierter Leberzirrhose und bei 7 Kranken mit dekompensierter Leberzirrhose mit Ascites sind in Abb.1 dargestellt. Bei den 7 Kranken mit kompensierter Leberzirrhose war die Sekretionsrate und die Aldosteronexkretion nur bei einem Fall leicht erhöht. 6 Kranke hatten normale Werte. Durch Erniedrigung der metabolischen Clearance-Rate war bei allen Fällen die mittlere Aldosteronplasmakonzentration leicht erhöht. Auch bei den Fällen mit dekompensierter Leberzirrhose war eine Steigerung der Aldosteronsekretion in der Vorperiode d. h. bei positiver Natriumbilanz – nur in 3 Fällen nachweisbar mit einem Maximum von 650 γ/24 Std. Die Aldosteronexkretion lag gegenüber der Vergleichsgruppe jedoch höher, auch die mittlere Plasmakonzentration, die bei 6 von 7 Fällen erhöht war.

Die Kranken mit dekompensierter Leberzirrhose wurden in der Folge unter standardisierten Bilanzbedingungen mit Salidiuretica behandelt, wobei insbesondere Amilorid und Etacrynsäure verwendet wurden.

Abb.2 zeigt den Effekt von Amilorid-HCl auf Natriumexkretion, Körpergewicht und Aldosteronstoffwechsel. Die durch die Amilorid-Medikation induzierte negative Natriumbilanz führte zu einer erheblichen Steigerung der Aldosteronsekretion von 180 γ/24 Std. der Vorperiode auf 1700 γ/24 Std. und zu einer Erhöhung der Aldosteronexkretion von 6 γ/24 Std. der Vorperiode auf 210 γ/ 24 Std. Die mittlere Plasmakonzentration des Aldosteron steigt bei gleichbleibender metabolischer Clearance-Rate von 17 mμg/100 ml auf 180 mμg/100 ml an. Ähnliche Beobachtungen wurden bei den übrigen Kranken unter dem Einfluß von Etacrynsäure, z. T. in Kombination mit Amilorid gemacht.

Die Untersuchungen zeigen, daß selbst bei der dekompensierten Leberzirrhose meist erst unter den Bedingungen der medikamentös bedingten negativen Natriumbilanz eine Steigerung der Aldosteronsekretion hervortritt, während die in der Vorperiode als Zeichen des Hyperaldosteronismus nachweisbare leichte Erhöhung der mittleren Aldosteronplasmakonzentration nicht so sehr auf eine erhöhte Sekretionsrate, sondern vielmehr auf die verzögerte Aldosteroninaktivierung – erniedrigte metabolische Clearance-Rate! – zurückzuführen ist.

Das gezeigte Beispiel läßt darüber hinaus erkennen, daß die Wirkung von Amilorid nicht an das Vorliegen eines sekundären Hyperaldosteronismus gebunden ist, wie dies auch aus tierexperimentellen Untersuchungen bekannt ist. Es muß allerdings betont werden, daß ein so ausgeprägter natriumeliminierender Effekt – wie der in Abb.2 gezeigte – durch Amilorid nur sehr selten erzielt wurde.

The Administration of Diuretics and the Metabolism of Aldosterone in Liver Disease

Aldosterone metabolism was investigated in 14 patients suffering from cirrhosis of the liver. The analysis of aldosterone was carried out according to the isotope method of Kliman and Peterson. The following parameters in particular were determined:

Renal excretion (E γ/24 hrs),
Secretion rate (SR γ/24 hrs),
Metabolic clearance rate (MCR in l/24 hrs),
Mean aldosterone plasma concentration (MPC in mμg/100 ml).

The results of these investigations of 7 patients suffering from compensated cirrhosis of the liver and of 7 patients suffering from decompensated cirrhosis with ascites are shown in Fig. 1. Secretion rate and aldosterone excretion in the 7 patients suffering from compensated cirrhosis of the liver were slightly increased in one case only. 6 patients had normal values. Due to lowering of the metabolic clearance rate mean aldosterone plasma concentration was slightly raised in all cases.

In decompensated cirrhosis of the liver an increase of aldosterone secretion was demonstrable initially, i. e. at positive sodium balance, in 3 cases only with a maximum of 650 γ/24 hrs. Compared with the control group aldosterone excretion was higher, as was the mean plasma concentration, which was increased in 6 out of 7 patients.

The patients with decompensated cirrhosis of the liver were treated subsequently under standardized balance conditions with saluretics, particularly with amiloride and ethycrynic acid.

Fig. 2 shows the effect of amiloride on sodium excretion, body weight and aldosterone metabolism. The negative sodium balance, induced by administration of amiloride, caused a great increase of aldosterone secretion from 180 γ/24 hrs initially to 1700 γ/24 hrs and of aldosterone excretion from 6 γ/24 hrs initially to 210 γ/24 hrs. The mean plasma concentration of aldosterone increased at a constant metabolic clearance rate from 17 mμg/100 ml to 180 mμg/100 ml. Similar observations were made in the other patients who were under the influence of ethacrynic acid or of a combination of ethacrynic acid and amiloride.

The investigations showed that an increase of aldosterone secretion occurred even in decompensated cirrhosis of the liver usually only under conditions of a negative sodium balance due to medication, while the minor initial rise of mean aldosterone plasma concentration, indicating hyperaldosteronism, was due not so much to an increase in secretion rate but to delayed inactivation of aldosterone (reduced metabolic clearance rate).

This example moreover demonstrates that the action of amiloride-HCl is not tied to the presence of secondary hyperaldosteronism, as is well known from animal experiments. It must be pointed out, however, that such a pronounced effect on sodium elimination by amiloride as shown in Fig. 2 was seen only very rarely.

Clinical Application of Diuretics in Renal Disease

Klinische Anwendung der Diuretica bei Erkrankungen der Niere

F. REUBI

Summary: 1. The main factors influencing the effectiveness of diuretics in patients with renal diseases are the basal sodium reabsorption and the glomerular filtration. The influence of the glomerular filtration is of a complex nature as shown by studies performed with merallurid, chlorothiazide, furosemide and ethacrynic acid. We should like to assume that in cases of chronic renal insufficiency, decrease in the number of functioning nephrons causes a reduction of the proximal water and sodium reabsorption in the unaffected tubules. In distal sections, a larger fraction of the tubule-urine is reabsorbed corresponding to the increased load. Presumably, diuretics block a fixed fraction of this reabsorption.

2. In acute experiments, furosemide and ethacrynic acid increase the renal blood flow and sometimes even the glomerular filtration rate.

3. The main indication for diuretics in renal disease is the nephrotic syndrome. Even in azotemia, ethacrynic acid and furosemide are effective diuretic agents; whereby, however, the increased diuresis does not cause a lowering of the elevated blood urea values.

Die Bedeutung der Nierenfunktion für die diuretische Therapie ergibt sich aus zwei Tatsachen:

1. Viele Nierenkrankheiten führen zu Wasser- und Salzretention und/oder zur Hypertonie, was den Einsatz von Diuretica nahelegt.
2. Diuretica besitzen in erster Linie einen renalen Angriffspunkt, indem sie die tubuläre Natrium- und Wasserrückresorption hemmen. Da der diuretische Effekt sowohl von der glomerulären Filtration als auch von der basalen tubulären Rückresorption abhängig ist, ist bei primären Nephropathien und bei sekundären Nierenstörungen ein verändertes Ansprechen auf Diuretica zu erwarten.

Im folgenden werden wir uns auf drei Aspekte der diuretischen Therapie bei Nierenkrankheiten beschränken:

I. Faktoren, welche die Wirksamkeit der Diuretica beeinflussen.
II. Sonderstellung des Furosemid und der Etacrynsäure.
III. Klassische und umstrittene Indikationen.

I. Faktoren, welche die Wirksamkeit der Diuretica beeinflussen

Es ist jedem Kliniker bekannt, daß viele nephrotische Patienten, auch solche mit normaler glomerulärer Filtration, auf Diuretica sehr schlecht reagieren (15, 16). Bei diesen Kranken ist die basale Natriumausscheidung äußerst gering; mit anderen Worten, die tubuläre Natriumrückresorption ist sehr stark erhöht. Dies stellt den ersten limitierenden Faktor für den diuretischen Effekt dar. Da die Natriumrückresorption vorwiegend extrarenal gesteuert wird, wird übrigens eine ähnliche Situation auch bei Krankheiten mit hartnäckigen Ödemen angetroffen, die primär mit der Niere nichts zu tun haben: Herzinsuffizienz, Leberzirrhose mit Ascites. Die geringe Wirkung der Diuretica erklärt sich dadurch, daß diese Mittel in der Regel die basale Ausscheidung um einen bestimmten Koeffizienten erhöhen: ist diese stark erniedrigt, bleibt sie auch nach Medikamentverabreichung trotz relativer Zunahme doch absolut unbedeutend, so daß es zu keiner Diurese kommt (15).

Ebensogut bekannt ist die Tatsache, daß ödematöse Patienten mit Azotämie sich schlecht entwässern lassen. Dies läßt eine Beziehung der diuretischen Wirkung zum Glomerulumfiltrat vermuten. Beim Tier führt die akute Drosselung des Nierenblutstromes zu einer parallelen Abnahme des Filtrates und des diuretischen Effektes (5, 13). Beim Menschen mit permanenter Einschränkung der glomerulären Filtration sind die Verhältnisse komplexer. Wir möchten auf diesen Punkt kurz eingehen.

Unsere ersten Untersuchungen wurden vor einigen Jahren mit *Chlorothiazid*, 500 mg i. v., und *Merallurid*, 176 mg i. v., bei ödemfreien Nierenpatienten durchgeführt (15, 18). Dabei kann ein merkwürdiges Verhalten des diuretischen und natriuretischen Effektes bei den verschiedenen Filtrationsgrößen zum Vorschein. Solange die Inulinclearance mehr als 30% der Norm betrug, blieb – trotz Reduktion des Filtrates – die Wirkung des Diureticums auf Wasser-, Natrium- und Chlorausscheidung fast unverändert (Abb. 1). Erst in einem sehr niedrigen Filtrationsbereich (< 25 ml/min) wurde die Abhängigkeit des diuretischen Effektes von der Filtrationsgröße eindeutig. Hingegen schien die kaliuretische Wirkung im ganzen Filtrationsbereich eine lineare Funktion der Inulinclearance darzustellen.

Die relative Unabhängigkeit der diuretischen und natriuretischen Wirkung von der glomerulären Filtration in einem weiten Bereich ist auf den ersten Blick überraschend.

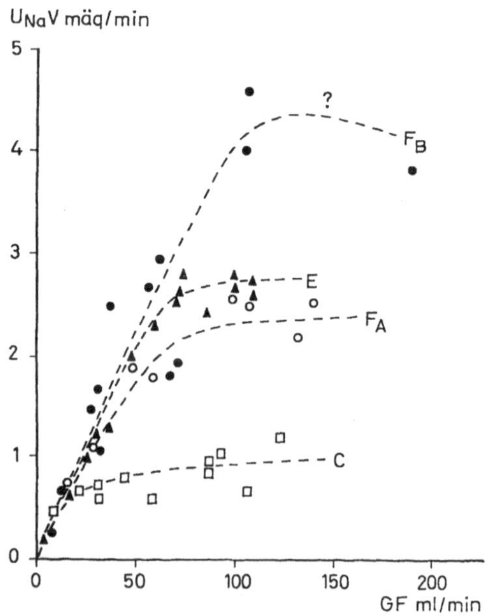

Abb. 1. Maximale Natriurese als Funktion der glomerulären Filtration nach i. v. Verabreichung von Chlorothiazid (C, □), Etacrynsäure (E, ▲) und Furosemid (F) in zwei verschiedenen Dosierungen (A, ○ und B, ●).

Man muß annehmen, daß bei permanenter Einschränkung der Filtration eine tubuläre Anpassung dazu führt, daß innerhalb bestimmter Grenzen sowohl die basale Kochsalz- und Wasserausscheidung als auch das Ansprechen auf Diuretica normal bleiben (18). Das Phänomen ließ sich sowohl mit Quecksilber-Diuretica als auch mit Chlorothiazid nachweisen, obschon diese Substanzen einen verschiedenen Angriffspunkt besitzen. Es war deshalb von Interesse, zu prüfen, wie sich Furosemid und Etacrynsäure diesbezüglich verhalten. Entsprechende Untersuchungen wurden von meinem Mitarbeiter VORBURGER durchgeführt (17, 19, 24).

Mit Furosemid wurden zwei verschiedene Dosierungen angewandt (Abb. 1). Mit Dosierung A (40 mg i.v.) wurde im Filtrationsbereich 70–150 ml/min ein beinahe konstanter saluretischer Effekt erzeugt, der etwa 2–3mal stärker war als mit Chlorothiazid. Unterhalb 70 ml/min wurde eine der Filtrationsgröße ungefähr proportionale Abnahme des saluretischen Effektes beobachtet. Mit Dosierung B (12,5 mg i.v., dann konstante intravenöse Infusion von 1 mg/min) ließ sich die Proportionalität zwischen Salurese und Glomerulumfiltrat zwischen 5 und 109 ml/min Inulinclearance verfolgen. Für höhere Filtratwerte schien keine weitere Zunahme des saluretischen Effektes einzutreten; allerdings war die Zahl der entsprechenden Beobachtungen klein. Die maximale Wirkung war etwa 5mal stärker als mit Chlorothiazid.

Mit Etacrynsäure ließ sich nach einer einmaligen intravenösen Injektion von 50 mg ein ähnliches Verhalten beobachten wie mit 40 mg Furosemid (Abb. 1). Von 70 ml/min Inulinclearance aufwärts blieb der saluretische Effekt beinahe konstant. Unterhalb dieses Grenzwertes nahm er ungefähr proportional zu der Filtration ab.

Obschon man den Eindruck hat, daß Furosemid in der Dosierung B sich prinzipiell anders verhält als Chlorothiazid und Merallurid, braucht es nicht unbedingt der Fall zu sein, wie aus dem Verlauf der Kurven Furosemid A und Etacrynsäure hervorgeht. Der scheinbare Unterschied könnte lediglich auf der stärkeren Wirkung des Mittels beruhen. Wie dem auch sei, müssen wir annehmen, daß bei chronisch eingeschränkter Filtration die meisten Diuretica eine größere Fraktion der tubulären Rückresorption blockieren (17, 19). Diese Fraktion ist jedoch quantitativ limitiert. Für Natrium beträgt sie mit Chlorothiazid etwa 30% der filtrierten Menge, mit Furosemid mehr als 45%. Um diese Eigenart der diuretischen Wirkung bei Nierenkranken zu verstehen, müssen wir zunächst die Verhältnisse unter basalen Bedingungen näher betrachten.

Der ödemfreie Nierenkranke scheidet unter basalen Bedingungen trotz Einschränkung der glomerulären Filtration meistens die gleiche Menge Wasser, Natrium und Chlor wie das normale Individuum aus. Die funktionelle Adaptation der kranken Niere besteht in einer Verminderung der tubulären Rückresorption, d. h. in einer Vermehrung des nichtresorbierten Anteils der filtrierten Menge (sog. »tubular rejection«). Beträgt die glomeruläre Filtration 100 ml/min und der nicht-resorbierte Anteil 3%, wird der Patient 3 ml/min Harn ausscheiden. Bei einer glomerulären Filtration von 10 ml/min ist eine Diurese von 3 ml/min nur möglich, wenn der nicht resorbierte Anteil auf 30% ansteigt. Eine ähnliche Überlegung gilt für das Natrium und das Chlor.

Die Wirkung der Diuretica wird weitgehend durch die Ausgangslage bestimmt. Die Diuretica scheinen nicht in erster Linie einen fixen Anteil der tubulären Rückresorption, der z. B. nur von der Dosis abhängig wäre, zu hemmen. In erster Annäherung möchten wir postulieren, daß sie den basalen nicht-resorbierten Anteil um einen bestimmten

Koeffizienten oder Multiplikationsfaktor verändern. Diese vereinfachte Formulierung ist nicht ganz zutreffend; immerhin wird die Demonstration klarer, wenn wir von vereinfachten zahlenmäßigen Beispielen ausgehen.

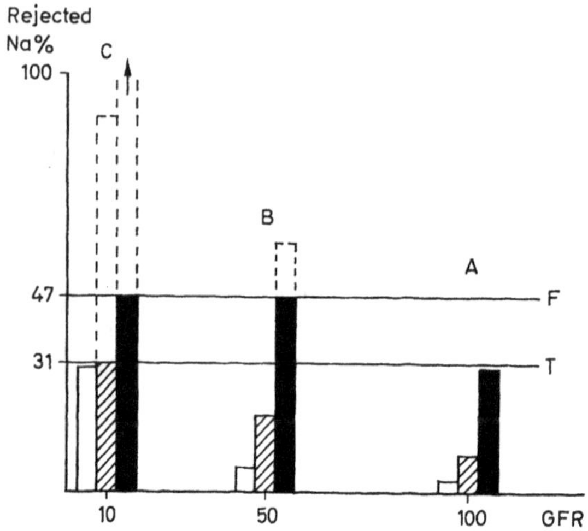

Abb. 2. Schematische Darstellung der Wirksamkeit von Thiazid-Diuretica (T) und Furosemid (F) bei eingeschränkter glomerulärer Filtration. K = Kontrollwerte = leere Säulen T = schattierte Säulen F = schwarze Säulen

Vergleichen wir zunächst die Wirkung von Chlorothiazid und Furosemid bei *ödemfreien* Patienten, welche alle die gleiche normale Natriumausscheidung aufweisen (Abb. 2). Für Chlorothiazid wird der Multiplikationsfaktor mit 3 willkürlich angesetzt, für Furosemid mit 10. Das Maximum des nicht resorbierten Anteils liegt für Chlorothiazid um 31%, für Furosemid um 47% (experimentelle Daten). Beim Patienten A mit der glomerulären Filtration von 100 ml/min bewirkt Chlorothiazid eine Erhöhung des nicht resorbierten Natriumanteils von 3% auf 9%, Furosemid auf 30%. Furosemid ist somit ca. 3,3mal wirksamer als Chlorothiazid. Beim Patienten B mit einer glomerulären Filtration von 50 ml/min erhöht Chlorothiazid den nicht resorbierten Anteil von 6% auf 18%. Die natriuretische Wirkung ist somit die gleiche wie beim Patienten A. Theoretisch sollte Furosemid den nicht resorbierten Anteil von 6% auf 60% erhöhen. Dies ist aber nicht möglich, da das Maximum der hemmbaren Rückresorption bei 47% liegt und nicht überschritten wird. Furosemid ist somit weniger wirksam als bei Patient A, und nur ca. 2,5mal wirksamer als Chlorothiazid.

Beim Patienten C mit der glomerulären Filtration von 10 ml/min beträgt der basale nicht-resorbierte Anteil bereits 30%. Da das Maximum der Chlorothiazid-Wirkung bei 31% liegt, bleibt in diesem Fall die natriuretische Wirkung aus. Dagegen wird Furosemid den nicht-resorbierten Anteil doch noch auf 47% erhöhen können (19, 24).

Bei Patienten *mit Ödemen* sind die Verhältnisse weniger übersichtlich. Es scheint jedoch festzustehen, daß die natriuretische Wirkung in grobem Verhältnis zur eingeschränkten basalen Natriumausscheidung steht, und daß sie deshalb wesentlich schwächer bleibt als bei ödemfreien Patienten. Wie sich das Maximum der hemmbaren Rückresorption verhält, ist zur zeit nicht bekannt.

Für den Physiologen ist es allerdings schwer zu verstehen, wie ein Diureticum, das einen Teil der Rückresorption hemmt, seine Wirkung in direktem Verhältnis zum nichtrückresorbierten Anteil entfalten kann. Wir möchten deshalb versuchen, den postulierten Vorgang in einer mehr physiologischen Denkweise auszudrücken.

Der Mechanismus der verminderten Wasser- und Salzrückresorption bei Patienten mit reduzierter Filtration ist nicht bekannt. Bei den meisten chronischen Nephropathien geht die Abnahme der glomerulären Filtration mit einer entsprechenden Reduktion der Zahl der funktionierenden Nephren einher. Die nicht zerstörten Nephren sollen nach der meistverbreiteten Ansicht eine beinahe normale Leistungskapazität behalten (3, 14). Als Folge der eingetretenen Anpassung an den Verlust anderer Einheiten werden sie aber die eigene Wasser- und Salzrückresorption vermindern müssen. Ob der Adaptationsvorgang renal oder extrarenal gesteuert wird, entzieht sich unseren Kenntnissen.

Immerhin spricht Einiges dafür, daß vorwiegend die *proximale* Rückresorption vermindert wird. Tierexperimentell ist bekannt, daß osmotische Diurese, Salzdiurese und Wasserdiurese die proximale Rückresorption vermindern (8). Bei nierenkranken Menschen dürfte bei unveränderter Tätigkeit der Einzelnephren und unveränderter Wasser- und Natriumzufuhr eine Verkleinerung der Gesamtpopulation aktiver Einheiten einer Salzwasserbelastung gleichkommen. Um Retention zu vermeiden, wird – wie im Tierexperiment – die proximale Rückresorption vermindert, jedoch vermutlich nicht unter einer bestimmten Grenze.

Nach der heutigen Auffassung gibt es aber in der Niere einen weiteren Kompensationsmechanismus, wonach bei verminderter proximaler Rückresorption die Rückresorption in der Henle'schen Schleife zunimmt (8). Mit anderen Worten, was der proximale Tubulus durchläßt, wird bis zu einem gewissen Teil weiter distal kompensatorisch aufgenommen. *An einer gegebenen Stelle der tubulären Passage ist somit der rückresorbierte Anteil vom perfundierenden Angebot abhängig.* Diese Stelle ist nicht unbedingt mit der Henle'schen Schleife identisch. Möglicherweise nehmen das distale Segment des proximalen Tubulus, sowie das proximale Segment des distalen Tubulus am Kompensationsmechanismus auch teil. Versuchen wir die eigenartige Wirkungsweise der Diuretica bei Nierenkranken auf diese basalen Vorgänge zu beziehen, besteht offenbar nur eine Möglichkeit: Die Diuretica müssen ausschließlich oder teilweise auf den zweiten Rückresorptionsvorgang einwirken. Sie blockieren einen fixen Anteil dieser distalen Rückresorption, welche vom perfundierenden Angebot abhängig ist. Nur so kann die diuretische Wirkung in einem bestimmten Bereich vom Filtrat unabhängig bleiben. Im tieferen Filtratbereich ergibt sich die Abhängigkeit zwischen Filtrat und Diurese daraus, daß die proximale Rückresorption nicht unter einem Minimum gehemmt werden und das Angebot pro Nephron nicht mehr zunehmen kann.

Diese Annahme scheint besonders für das Chlorothiazid und für die Quecksilberdiuretica zuzutreffen. Auf Abb. 1 ist nämlich das obere Kurvensegment für beide Substanzen beinahe horizontal. Für die Etacrynsäure und das Furosemid läßt sich nicht mit Sicherheit entscheiden, ob das obere Kurvensegment waagrecht oder schräg verläuft. Ein schräger Verlauf würde sich theoretisch aus der Kombination zweier Mechanismen ergeben: der bereits besprochene und die zusätzliche Hemmung eines fixen Anteils der proximalen Rückresorption.

II. Sonderstellung der Etacrynsäure und des Furosemid

Den Kliniker interessiert vor allem die starke Wirksamkeit dieser Medikamente, welche besonders bei hoher Dosierung zur Geltung kommt und auf einer Hemmung der Natriumrückresorption in der Henle'schen Schleife beruht (4, 6, 7, 22). Für den Nephrologen ist ein besonderer Punkt ebenfalls von Bedeutung: Im Gegensatz zu den Thiaziddiuretica führen im akuten Experiment Furosemid und Etacrynsäure zu einer Zunahme der Nierendurchblutung und manchmal zu einer Zunahme der glomerulären Filtration (9, 20, 24). Besonders bei eingeschränkter Filtration läßt sich beim Menschen eine Vermehrung der Inulin- und PAH-Clearances beobachten [(17), Abb. 3]. Verschiedene Autoren haben von einem einfachen »washout«-Effekt gesprochen (22). Dies trifft sicher nicht zu, da bei einer so erheblichen Diurese der Nieren-Nierenbecken-Harnleiter-Totraum nach wenigen Minuten bereits ausgespült ist. Die Filtrationszunahme kann aber 1–2 Stunden anhalten. Übrigens konnte mein Mitarbeiter VORBURGER beim narkotisierten Hund mit Hilfe eines auf die A. renalis aufgesetzten elektromagnetischen Durchflußmessers nach intravenöser Injektion von 0,4–0,6 mg/kg Furosemid eine Hyperämie der Niere beobachten (25). Unmittelbar nach der Injektion trat eine passagäre, ca. 5–10 sec dauernde, leichte Abnahme der Durchblutung auf, die von einer regelmäßigen Zunahme gefolgt war. Das Maximum der Durchblutungssteigerung trat 8–12 Minuten nach der Injektion auf. In den ersten 10 Minuten nach Furosemid lag die Durchblutung im Mittel um 29,7%, in den folgenden 10 Minuten um 21,6% und in der dritten 10-Minuten-Periode um 9,1% über dem Ausgangswert (Abb. 4). Diese im Akutversuch beobachteten Veränderungen traten regelmäßig auch im chronischen Experiment an nicht narkotisierten Hunden auf.

Auch mit *Etacrynsäure* konnten neuerdings BIRTCH und Mitarb. (2) eine transitorische Vermehrung der Gesamtdurchblutung beobachten. Möglicherweise kommt es außerdem innerhalb der Niere zu einer Änderung der Blutverteilung, welche nach diesen Autoren mit dem diuretischen Effekt in Zusammenhang stehen dürfte.

Es scheint somit erwiesen, daß Etacrynsäure und Furosemid eine direkte Wirkung auf die Nierengefäße ausüben. Das Verhalten der glomerulären Filtration nach Verabreichung eines potenten Diureticums ist jedoch von einem weiteren Faktor abhängig: die

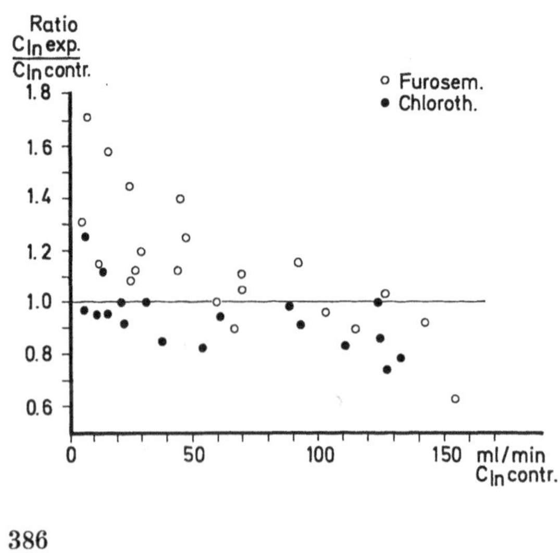

Abb. 3. Verhältnis zwischen C_{In} exp. (Inulinclearance nach Diureticum) und C_{In} kontr. (basale Inulinclearance) als Funktion der basalen Inulinclearance. Nach Furosemid nimmt besonders im niedrigen Filtratbereich die Inulinclearance zu.

starke Salurese kann zu einer Kontraktion des extrazellulären Raumes führen, und diese Veränderungen gehen in der Regel mit einer Verminderung der Nierendurchblutung und der glomerulären Filtration einher. Bei ödemfreien Patienten mit normaler Filtration kann infolge der hier besonders starken Diurese die medikamentös bedingte Nierenhyperämie ausbleiben und das Filtrat progressiv abnehmen. Bei primär eingeschränkter Filtration ist der Wasser- und Salzverlust weniger groß, so daß die spezifische gefäßerweiternde Wirkung des Diureticums deutlicher zum Vorschein kommt (17).

Aus diesen Beobachtungen läßt sich unschwer ableiten, daß die Azotämie an sich keine Kontraindikation für die Anwendung von Furosemid oder Etacrynsäure darstellt, wenn allzu große Volumenverschiebungen und Elektrolytstörungen vermieden werden können. Diese Mittel sind deswegen bei schlechter Nierenfunktion anderen Diuretica vorzuziehen.

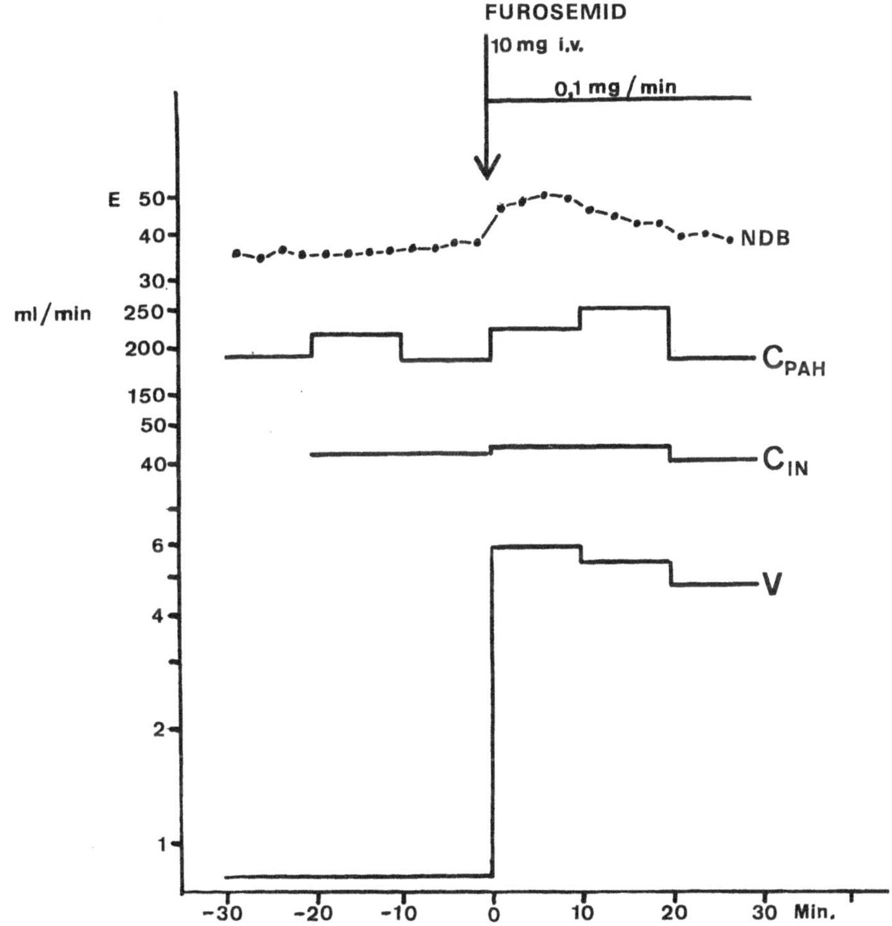

Abb. 4. Akute Wirkung von Furosemid auf die direkt gemessene Nierendurchblutung (elektromagnetischer Flow-meter), sowie auf die Inulin- und die PAH-Clearance und die Diurese beim Hund (nach VORBURGER, unveröffentlichte Daten).

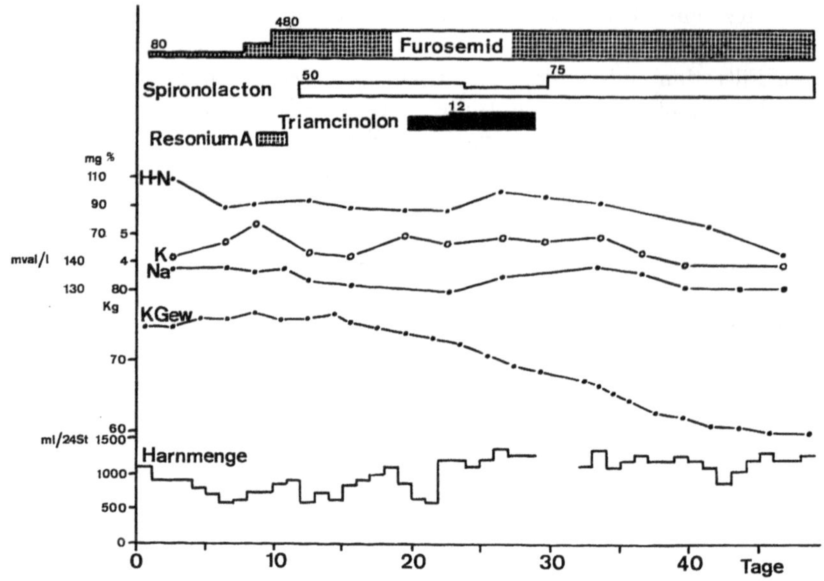

Abb. 5. Erfolgreiche Entwässerung eines azotämischen Patienten mit ausgedehnten nephrotischen Ödemen durch die kombinierte Anwendung von Furosemid, Spironolacton und Triamcinolon.

III. Klassische und umstrittene Indikationen

Die heute gebräuchlichsten Diuretica, welche in der Nephrologie zur Anwendung kommen, sind:

1. Die Thiaziddiuretica und das Chlorthalidon.
2. Die stark wirksamen Furosemid und Etacrynsäure.
3. Die kaliumsparenden Spirolactone, Triamteren und Amilorid.
4. Die Glucocorticoide.
5. Das osmotische Diureticum Mannit.

Die klassischen Indikationen der diuretischen Therapie bei Nierenkrankheiten umfassen das nephrotische Syndrom jeder Genese, die cardio-renalen Ödeme der chronischen Nephritis und den nephrogenen Diabetes insipidus (letztere Indikation wird im Referat von BUCHBORN noch ausführlich besprochen). Auch bei der akuten Glomerulonephritis können Diuretica die Ödemausschwemmung beschleunigen. Beim akuten Nierenversagen ist in den ersten 24 Stunden nach Anuriebeginn ein Versuch mit Mannit gerechtfertigt.

Bei Fällen von nephrotischem Syndrom, welche auf Corticosteroide ansprechen (z. B. die klassische Lipoidnephrose), kann mit Prednison oder Triamcinolon allein eine vollständige Ödemausschwemmung erreicht werden, wobei gleichzeitig die Proteinurie meistens abnimmt oder sogar verschwindet (16). Der Wirkungsmechanismus der Glucocorticoide ist bis heute ungeklärt. Zu Beginn müssen sie hoch dosiert werden (60–100 mg Prednison, bzw. 40–60 mg Triamcinolon). Die Diurese setzt meistens zwischen dem 10. und dem 20. Behandlungstag ein. Die Therapie wird dann mit kleineren Dosen über

Wochen oder Monate fortgesetzt, wobei eine totale Remission des nephrotischen Syndroms angestrebt wird.

Bei steroidrefraktären Fällen von nephrotischem Syndrom sind Diuretica im engeren Sinn indiziert. Auch bei Fällen von Lipoidnephrose mit schweren Ödemen ist neben der Steroidtherapie die palliative Anwendung von Diuretica empfehlenswert. Diese Zustände verlangen meistens hohe Dosen. In der Regel kombinieren wir Furosemid oder Etacrynsäure mit einem Aldosteronantagonisten, z. B. 200–300 mg Furosemid und 150 mg Aldactone-A, unter Umständen noch größere Mengen. Mit dieser Kombination ist keine Hypokaliämie zu befürchten. Wenn jedoch die Mittel in hohen Dosen und über längere Zeit ohne gleichzeitige Steroidbehandlung verabreicht werden, kann sich eine Hyponatriämie entwickeln. In solchen Fällen empfehlen wir – auch bei steroidrefraktären Fällen – die zusätzliche Gabe von Triamcinolon in kleineren Dosen (12–20 mg). Es hat sich nämlich gezeigt, daß damit die Hyponatriämie behoben und die Wirkung der übrigen Diuretica potenziert werden kann (10, 11). Abb. 5 belegt den günstigen Effekt einer solchen Kombination bei einem azotämischen Patienten mit einem nephrotischen Syndrom.

Bei Nierenkranken mit leichter Tendenz zu Wasser- und Salzretention genügen meistens die üblichen Thiaziddiuretica.

Bei Patienten mit akuter Anurie werden intravenöse 25%ige Mannit-Infusionen empfohlen (1). Mannit soll die Diurese wieder in Gang bringen, wobei der Wirkungsmechanismus nicht bekannt ist. Es könnte sich sowohl um eine Besserung der Nierendurchblutung als auch um eine Hemmung der pathologisch erhöhten Rückresorption handeln. Tierexperimentell läßt sich eine günstige Wirkung belegen (12, 23). Beim Menschen ist es äußerst schwierig, den Effekt zu objektivieren.

Die Tatsache, daß sogar bei Patienten mit Harnstoff-N-Werten über 100 mg% Etacrynsäure und Furosemid einen gewissen – wenn auch bescheidenen – diuretischen Effekt entfalten, und daß im allgemeinen die Harnstoffclearance mit der Diurese etwas zunimmt, ließ den Gedanken aufkommen, daß sich diese Diuretica für die palliative Behandlung der chronischen Niereninsuffizienz eignen könnten (21). Es wurden dabei Furosemid-Dosen bis 2 g täglich empfohlen (26). Unsere eigenen Untersuchungen ergaben jedoch keine positiven Resultate. 7 Patienten mit chronischer Niereninsuffizienz und Serum-Harnstoff-N-Werten von 103–166 mg% erhielten während 2–10 Tagen täglich intravenöse Furosemid-Dosen von 480–2000 mg (Tab. 1). Die Diurese nahm bei 6 Patienten zu. Bei 2 Patienten blieb der Serum-Harnstoff unverändert, bei den übrigen stieg er an, ebenso das Serum-Kreatinin. Das Serum-Natrium nahm meistens etwas ab, einmal sehr deutlich. Bei 6 Patienten mußte nach dem erfolglosen Furosemid-Versuch eine Peritonealdialyse vorgenommen werden. Im Fall M. H., welcher den tiefsten Ausgangswert für Harnstoff-N aufwies (103 mg%), wurden die Ödeme während der Furosemid-Behandlung zwar ausgeschwemmt (Abb. 6), gleichzeitig nahm jedoch der Serum-Harnstoff bis zu 160 mg% zu, vielleicht z. T. als Folge der Blutdrucksenkung (von 205/110 auf 175/95). Die Blutdrucksenkung selbst war vorwiegend auf das Salureticum zurückzuführen, da nach Absetzen des Furosemid der Blutdruck trotz Erhöhung der Catapresan-Dosis auf 200/105 wieder anstieg.

Es ist nicht zu bezweifeln, daß Etacrynsäure und Furosemid bei Patienten mit mäßiger Azotämie die Harnausscheidung fördern, während andere Mittel sich als unwirksam erweisen. In einer eigenen Serie von Nierenkranken mit Filtrationswerten

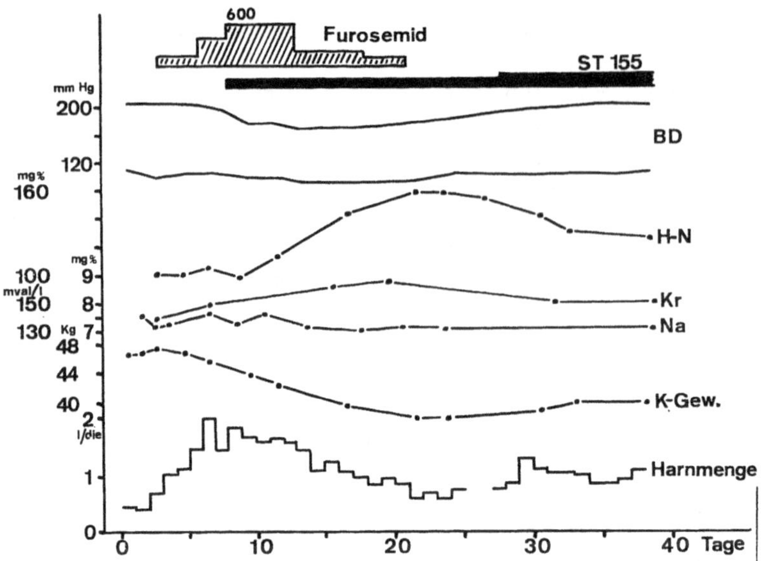

Abb. 6. Effekt hoher Furosemid-Dosen bei einer azotämischen Patientin: Zunahme der Diurese, jedoch Anstieg des Bluthamstoffs.

zwischen 5,1 und 16,7 ml/min bewirkte *Chlorothiazid* im Durchschnitt eine 64%ige Zunahme der Natriurese. Unter gleichen Bedingungen betrug nach *Furosemid* die Zunahme der Natriurese 260% (17, 24). Es wäre jedoch verfehlt, die Zunahme der Diurese mit der Besserung der Nierenfunktion zu verwechseln. Unseres Erachtens haben auch die stärksten Diuretica keinen Platz in der Behandlung der Azotämie.

Tab. 1. Diurese und Blutchemismus unter hochdosierter Furosemid-Behandlung bei 7 Fällen von chronischer Niereninsuffizienz.

Patient	Werte *vor* Therapie				Werte *während* Furosemid Therapie			Werte *nach* Therapie		
	Urin	Serum			Dosis	Dauer	Urin	Serum		
	Menge/ 24h*) ml	H-N mg%	Kreatinin mg%	Natrium mval/l	mg/ Tag	Tage	Menge/ 24h**) ml	H-N mg%	Kreatinin mg%	Natrium mval/l
1. E.J.	500	166	22,5	134	2 000	4	700	200	23,5	129
E.J.	300	120	20,0	135	1 600	2	425	146	23,0	130
2. M.H.	550	103	7,5	143	550	7	1 650	143	8,6	135
3. M.R.	750	134	—	—	1 000	4	850	140	—	—
4. R.W.	1 300	122	—	139	1 000	6	2 100	122	—	115
5. R.F.	500	130	18,5	135	1 200	10	1 400	162	19,6	139
6. P.L.	500	150	14,7	—	480	8	750	150	—	—
7. W.R.	300	146	—	132	600	2	250	156	—	138

*) Durchschnitt von 3 Tagen
**) Durchschnitt während Behandlung

Literatur / References

1. BARRY, K. G. and J. P. MALLOY: Oliguric renal failure. Evaluation and therapy by the intravenous infusion of mannitol. – J. Amer. med. Ass. **179,** 510 (1962).
2. BIRTCH, A. G., R. M. ZAKHEIM, L. G. JONES and A. C. BARGER: Redistribution of renal blood flow produced by Furosemide and ethacrynic acid. – Circul. Res. **21,** 869 (1967).
3. BRICKER, N. S., P. A. F. MOVRIN and S. W. KIME: The pathologic physiology of chronic Bright's disease. – Amer. J. Med. **28,** 77 (1960).
4. BUCHBORN, E. und S. ANASTASAKIS: Angriffspunkt und Wirkungsmechanismus von Furosemid am distalen Nephron des Menschen. – Klin. Wschr. **42,** 1127 (1964).
5. DAVIDSON, D. G., N. G. LEVINSKY and R.W. BERLINER: Maintenance of potassium excretion despite reduction of glomerular filtration during sodium diuresis. – J. clin. Invest. **37,** 548 (1958).
6. DEETJEN, P.: Mikropunktionsuntersuchungen zur Wirkung von Furosemid. – Pflüger's Archiv **284,** 184 (1965).
7. EARLEY, L. E. and R. M. FRIEDLER: Renal tubular effects of ethacrynic acid. – J. clin. Invest. **43,** 1495 (1964).
8. GIEBISCH, G. and E. E. WINDHAGER: Renal tubular transfer of sodium chloride and potassium. – Amer. J. Med. **36,** 643 (1964).
9. HEIDLAND, A., K. KLÜTSCH und F. SUZUKI: Nierenhämodynamik, Wasser- und Elektrolytausscheidung nach Furosemid. – Arzneimittelforschg. **14,** 713 (1964).
10. HEIDORN, G. H. and P. R. SCHEMM: The clinical use of corticotropin and adrenal corticosteroids in the therapy of intractable edema. – Amer. J. Med. Sci. **229,** 611 (1955).
11. JICK, H.: The use of glucocorticoids for diuresis in patients with fluid retention not resulting from renal disease. – Ann. New York Acad. Sci. **139,** 512 (1966).
12. PARRY, W. L., J. A. SCHAEFER and C. B. MULLER: Experimental studies of acute renal failure. – J. Urol. **89,** 1 (1963).
13. PITTS, R. F. and J. J. DUGGAN: The relationship between glomerular filtration rate, proximal tubular reabsorption of sodium and efficacy of mercurials. – J. clin. Invest. **29,** 365 (1950).
14. PLATT, R.: Structural and functional adaptation in renal failure. – Brit. med. J. 1952, **I,** 1313 und 1372.
15. REUBI, F.: Die Anwendung von Diuretica bei Nierenkranken. In: SCHWIEGK, H., E. BUCHBORN und K. D. BOCK: Diurese und Diuretica. Springer, Berlin (1959).
16. REUBI, F.: Nierenkrankheiten. Huber, Bern und Stuttgart (1960).
17. REUBI, F.: Clinical use of Furosemide. – Bull. New York Acad. Sci. **139,** 433 (1966).
18. REUBI, F. and P. COTTIER: Effects of reduced glomerular filtration rate on responsiveness to Chlorothiazide and mercurial diuretics. – Circulation **23,** 200 (1961).
19. REUBI, F. und C. VORBURGER: Wirkung der Diuretica bei eingeschränkter Nierenfunktion. – In: HEILMEYER, L.: Diureseforschung. Thieme, Stuttgart (1967).
20. SCHIRMEISTER, J. und H. WILLMANN: Über die Harnsäure- und andere Clearances nach Gabe von Furosemid beim Menschen. – Klin. Wschr. **42,** 623 (1964).
21. SCHREINER, G. E.: Chlorothiazide in renal disease. – Ann. New York Acad. Sci. **71,** 420 (1958).
22. SUKI, W., F. C. RECTOR and D.W. SELDIN: The site of action of Furosemide and other sulfonamide diuretics in the dog. – J. clin. Invest. **44,** 1458 (1965).
23. TESCHAN, P. E. and N. L. LAWSON: Studies in acute renal failure. Prevention by osmotic diuresis. – Nephron **3,** 1 (1966).
24. VORBURGER, C.: Die akute Wirkung des Diureticums Furosemid auf das Glomerulumfiltrat, die renale Hämodynamik, die Wasser-, Natrium-, Chlorid- und Kaliumausscheidung und auf den Sauerstoffverbrauch der Nieren. – Klin. Wschr. **42,** 833 (1964).
25. VORBURGER, C.: Unveröffentlichte Daten.
26. Persönliche Mitteilung der Farbwerke Hoechst.

HOLZGREVE: Ich glaube, daß man auf Grund von Mikropunktionsuntersuchungen folgende allgemeine Feststellungen über den Einfluß von Diuretica auf die glomeruläre Filtrationsrate machen kann:

1. Im akuten Versuch bei normalem Hydratationszustand sehen wir nach Gabe von Diuretica immer eine Tubulusdilatation, die auf einem Anstieg des intratubulären Druckes beruht. Dieser Druckanstieg verringert den effektiven Filtrationsdruck (eff. Filtrationsdruck = glom. Kapillardruck – intratubulärer Druck – koll. osm. Druck). Man muß daher erwarten, daß jedes Diureticum mit ausschließlich tubulärer Wirkung die glomeruläre Filtrationsrate vermindert. Das ist in der Tat bei den meisten Diuretica der Fall.

Für Furosemid trifft das aber nicht zu. Obwohl der intratubuläre Druck ansteigt, bleibt die glomeruläre Filtrationsrate gleich oder nimmt sogar zu. OCHWADT und Mitarb. (Pflügers Arch. ges. Physiol., **295**, 80, 1967) haben gefunden, daß der glomeruläre Kapillardruck nach Gabe von Furosemid ansteigt. Gleichzeitiger, entsprechender Anstieg des glomerulären Filtrationsdruckes und des intratubulären Druckes lassen den effektiven Filtrationsdruck, und damit auch das Glomerulumfiltrat, unverändert. Furosemid scheint demnach außer einem tubulären Effekt auch noch einen Einfluß auf die renale Hämodynamik zu haben und bildet unter den Diuretica hinsichtlich des Einflusses auf das Glomerulumfiltrat eine Ausnahme.

2. Bei chronischer Diureticagabe oder bei vermindertem Hydratationszustand trifft alles das zu, was Sie über die hämodynamischen Veränderungen und ihren Einfluß auf die glomeruläre Filtrationsrate gesagt haben. Eine gewisse Rolle könnte auch noch die Zunahme des kolloidosmotischen Druckes bei Dehydratation spielen.

GESSLER: Geben Sie auch beim akuten Nierenversagen Diuretica? Wir machen es grundsätzlich so, daß wir bei jedem akuten Nierenversagen, bei dem noch eine Restdiurese von 100–200 ccm besteht, zuerst mit Mannitol und dann mit Furosemid behandeln. Man hat den Eindruck, daß bei einigen Patienten die Diurese daraufhin sofort in Gang kommt. Haben Sie auch solche Beobachtungen?

OELERT: Die Verbesserung einer herabgesetzten Filtrationsrate durch die modernen Diuretica läßt sich auch nach operativen Eingriffen am Menschen beobachten. Wenn bei oder nach einer Operation der Harnfluß absinkt und als Ursache dafür eine Verminderung der GFR gemessen wird, ist nach Gabe von Furosemid oder Etacrynsäure wieder ein Anstieg von Harnfluß und GFR zu beobachten. Bisher hatte man dies damit zu erklären versucht, daß Eiweiß- oder Hämoglobinzylinder aus den Nierenkanälchen ausgewaschen werden. Ich glaube aber, daß diese Vorstellung nicht länger zutreffend ist, wenn man Ihre Untersuchungen betrachtet.

KRECKE: Aus Ihrem Referat geht hervor, daß Sie die von anderer Seite beschriebene günstige Wirkung von Furosemid bei Azotämien an Ihren eigenen Patienten nicht bestätigen konnten. Soweit ich Ihren Abbildungen entnahm, kam es aber in einigen dieser Fälle zu einer Zunahme der *Absolut*ausscheidung von Harnstoff im Urin. Wenn Sie dennoch kein Absinken des Serum-Harnstoffspiegels feststellten, so läßt sich das meines Erachtens nur durch eine Abnahme des extrazellulären Flüssigkeitsvolumens oder einen erhöhten Eiweißumsatz erklären. Oder haben Sie dafür eine andere Interpretation?

REUBI: Bei der akuten Niereninsuffizienz verabreichen wir routinemäßig eine Mannitolinfusion, aber nur, wenn wir sicher sind, daß die Anurie nicht länger als 24 Stunden besteht. Nach unserer Erfahrung sind alle Versuche zu einem späteren Zeitpunkt wirkungslos. Leider kommen die Patienten meistens später. Sie wissen genauso wie ich, wie schwierig es ist zu beurteilen, ob die Diurese wieder spontan in Gang kommt, oder ob das auf einen diuretischen Effekt zurückzuführen ist. – Die Überlegungen bezüglich der Harnstoffkonzentration sind richtig. Nur haben wir nicht gefunden, daß die Harnstoffausscheidung signifikant zunimmt. Es handelte sich nur um einen sehr bescheidenen diuretischen Effekt. Dementsprechend änderte sich auch der Harnstoffspiegel nicht.

SCHELER: Es ist bekannt, daß mit zunehmender Verminderung des GFR die Wirkung der Diuretica abnimmt. Vor allem Furosemid und Etacrynsäure (ES) sind in der Lage, bis zu einem GFR um 10 ml/min eine deutliche Wirkung zu entfalten.

Im akuten Versuch haben wir bei 19 Patienten mit Serum-Kreatinin-Werten von 2 bis 10 mg% festgestellt, daß mit 100 mg ES i. v. die Na-Ausscheidung auf 50 bis 200 μval/min gesteigert werden kann, gleichzeitig kommt es zu einer Mehrausscheidung von K in der Größenordnung von 15 bis 80 μval/min. Während die natriuretische Wirkung durch MK 870 nicht signifikant verstärkt werden kann, läßt sich der K-Verlust praktisch aufheben. Im Extremfall kann durch 100 mg ES i. v. der prozentuale Anteil des Urinvolumens vom GFR von 25% auf 55% erhöht werden. Eine signifikante Veränderung der Harnstoff- oder Kreatininausscheidung ließ sich nicht feststellen; die Kreatininausscheidung nahm eher zu.

Bei 7 Patienten mit Serum-Kreatinin-Werten zwischen 5 bis 20 mg% wurden über 5 Tage täglich 100 μval $NaHCO_3$ und 100 mg ES i.v. verabreicht. Im Vergleich zu 5 Pat. mit Serum-Kreatinin-Werten zwischen 3–11 mg%, die nur $NaHCO_3$ erhielten, ließen sich keine signifikanten Änderungen auf pH Standardbicarbonat und pCO_2 nachweisen. Es konnte lediglich die Na-Retention verringert werden, ohne daß es zu K-Verlusten kam.

Bei 20 Patienten mit Serum-Kreatinin-Werten zwischen 2–10 mg% konnte die durch 100 mg ES oral erreichte Steigerung der Urin- und Na-Ausscheidung durch 10 mg MK 870 oder durch 300 mg Aldadiene K i. v. geringfügig gesteigert werden. Sowohl die zusätzliche natriuretische Wirkung als auch die antikaliurische Wirkung war unter MK 870 am deutlichsten.

The Influence of Diuretics on the Fractional Fluid and Electrolyte-Excretion in Renal Insufficiency

Der Einfluß von Diuretica auf die fraktionelle Flüssigkeits- und Elektrolytexcretion bei eingeschränkter Nierenfunktion

A. HEIDLAND, K. KLÜTSCH, H. HENNEMANN, U. LÖWENSTEIN, H. J. KUSCHKE

Summary: In patients with renal insufficiency, ethacrynic acid and furosemide effect a more potent filtrate-dependent diuresis than in healthy renal subjects. This effect is demonstrable up to a reduction of filtrate to 10 ml/min. Under azetolamide, only in cases of moderate limitation of renal function (GFR 80–40 ml/min), a relative increase of effect could be shown.

Hydrochlorothiazide does not cause a definite change of effect in the individual filtrate-sectors.

Humoral factors, among others, might be discussed as the origin of the varying filtrate-dependent excretion. To explicate the foregoing: Increases by the 1.3 to 10.0 fold of the control value were seen in determinations of the pyrocatechin amines in the urine after application of 20 mg furosemide, whereby the rise was registered as directly proportional to the glomerulum filtration and to the absolute fluid excretion.

In addition, furosemide and ethacrynic acid caused direct activation of the renin/angiotensin-system which is at its maximum at the peak of diuresis.

It is assumed that the antidiuretic and sodium-retaining properties of pyrocatechin amines and angiotensin diminish the effect of the diuretic on the nephron. This effect ought to present itself more extensively in healthy renal subjects due to a higher total fluid excretion and stronger activation of humoral factors than in patients with renal insufficiency, who, in addition are "protected" by an osmotic diuresis.

Bei chronischer Niereninsuffizienz nehmen fraktionelle Flüssigkeits- und Elektrolytausscheidungen progressiv zu, wodurch auch bei extremer Filtratreduktion noch eine Konstanz des extrazellulären Flüssigkeitsvolumens möglich ist. Als Ursache des gesteigerten tubulären Perfusionsvolumens werden folgende Faktoren diskutiert:

1. glomeruläre Hyperfiltration und Azotämie (BRICKER u. Mitarb., 1964),
2. gesteigerte Aktivität des hypothetischen natriuretischen Hormons (DE WARDENER u. Mitarb., 1961, DIRKS u. Mitarb., 1965, JOHNSTON und DAVIS, 1966),
3. veränderte Geometrie des proximalen Tubulus (BRUNNER u. Mitarb., 1966, RECTOR u. Mitarb., 1966) sowie
4. tubuläre Defekte (BIBER u. Mitarb., 1968).

Alle Diuretica werden mit fortschreitender Filtratabnahme weniger effektiv. Ihr Wirkungsverlust beruht vorwiegend auf dem Ausfall von Nephronen. Weiterhin kommen ungenügender transtubulärer Diureticatransport sowie Defekte natriumresorbierender

Tab. 1

	GFR	Pat. (n)	C_{In} v	ml/min n	$V/C_{In} \times 100$ v	n	$C_{Na}/C_{In} \times 100$ v	n	$C_K/C_{In} \times 100$ v	n
Acetazol-	> 80	12	102,0 ± 18,3	91,9 ± 11,1	2,3 ± 1,7	5,3 ± 2,1	1,6 ± 0,9	5,5 ± 1,2	13,3 ± 4,2	56,4 ± 20,3
amid	80–40	12	59,8 ± 11,3	51,6 ± 14,0	4,7 ± 2,5	10,0 ± 3,3	3,7 ± 1,9	9,5 ± 3,5	21,1 ± 12,0	61,8 ± 18,9
500 mg	< 40	5	27,6 ± 10,6	26,6 ± 11,3	12,2 ± 11,9	15,0 ± 10,5	5,5 ± 2,5	10,1 ± 4,5	42,1 ± 20,6	78,7 ± 15,6
Hydrochlo-	> 80	6	102,0 ± 13,6	89,3 ± 15,4	3,3 ± 1,8	6,2 ± 1,5	2,1 ± 0,6	7,3 ± 1,9	16,5 ± 8,8	40,1 ± 15,5
rothiazid	80–40	8	64,6 ± 11,2	60,7 ± 12,8	2,9 ± 1,3	6,4 ± 2,6	1,9 ± 0,6	6,9 ± 4,0	20,4 ± 11,8	46,4 ± 15,3
50 mg	< 40	5	22,2 ± 6,2	19,8 ± 5,8	9,4 ± 2,7	12,3 ± 3,0	8,3 ± 3,1	12,7 ± 4,3	45,3 ± 13,9	58,6 ± 9,1
Etacryn-	> 80	7	94,3 ± 12,6	98,0 ± 16,9	3,2 ± 1,7	20,8 ± 3,2	2,9 ± 1,5	19,2 ± 4,8	17,6 ± 6,7	45,1 ± 14,9
Säure	80–40	12	63,1 ± 7,4	75,8 ± 9,8	3,7 ± 2,0	23,3 ± 6,4	3,0 ± 1,2	21,7 ± 8,1	19,6 ± 10,6	52,1 ± 26,2
50 mg	< 40	13	25,1 ± 9,9	26,3 ± 11,7	8,4 ± 3,9	37,4 ± 11,4	6,1 ± 2,5	29,1 ± 11,3	53,5 ± 22,0	114,7 ± 50,7
Furosemid	> 80	8	94,3 ± 11,4	103,0 ± 3,2	2,3 ± 0,9	14,8 ± 3,3	2,4 ± 1,1	16,3 ± 4,8	12,6 ± 6,0	43,1 ± 19,2
25 mg	80–40	15	64,1 ± 12,4	73,6 ± 18,3	4,2 ± 2,3	21,5 ± 8,0	3,1 ± 1,7	19,4 ± 7,9	21,2 ± 9,5	62,3 ± 17,7
	< 40	5	19,6 ± 8,9	25,6 ± 14,3	7,9 ± 2,6	29,2 ± 8,7	6,5 ± 3,3	24,2 ± 8,4	43,9 ± 10,5	86,8 ± 19,8

Mechanismen am Angriffspunkt des Diureticums in Betracht. Osmotische Faktoren können eine Furosemid- und Etacrynsäure-Diurese steigern, wie Untersuchungen in Mannitoldiurese gezeigt haben (BUCHBORN u. ANSTASAKES 1964, EDEL u. Mitarb., 1965). Quecksilberdiuretica sollen dagegen eine Mannitoldiurese abschwächen (PORUSH u. ABRAMSON, 1965).

Zur Prüfung der Frage, ob die Wirkungscharakteristik eines Diureticums durch die genannten osmotischen, regulativen und tubulären Faktoren quantitativ oder qualitativ verändert wird, haben wir Acetazolamid, Hydrochlorothiazid, Etacrynsäure und Furose-

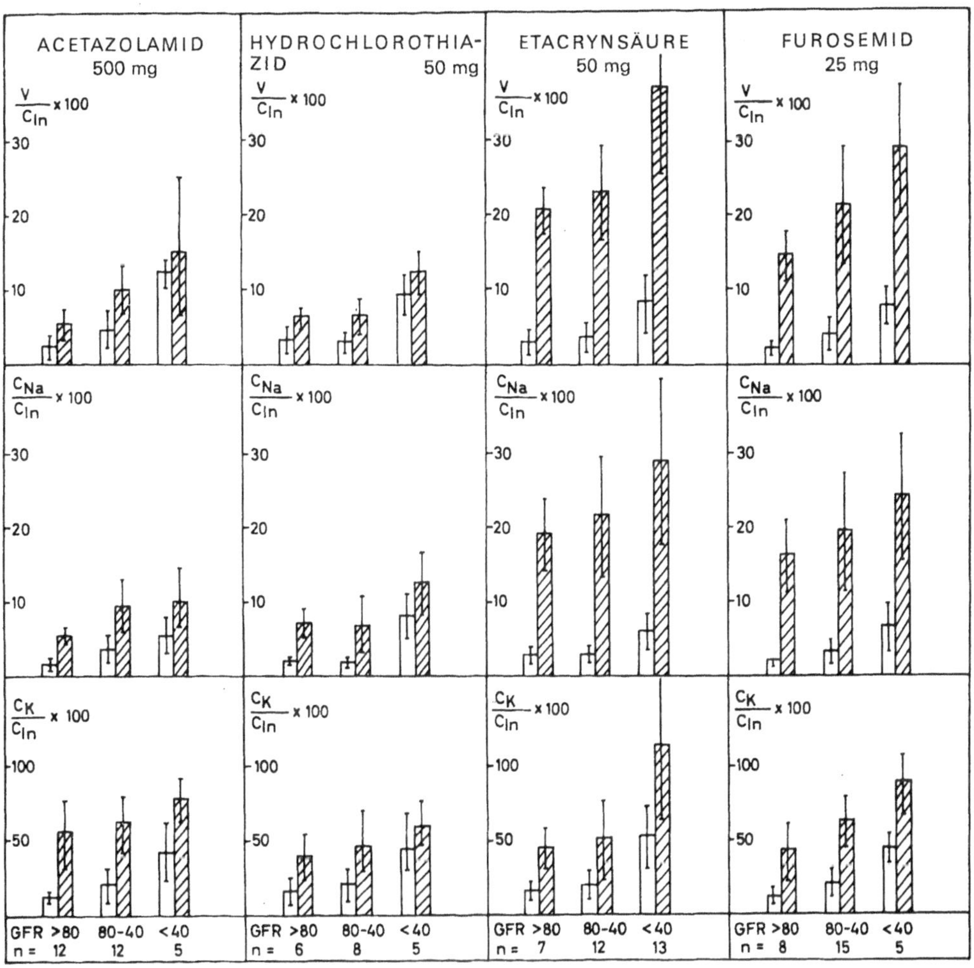

Abb. 1. Fraktionelle Flüssigkeitsausscheidung ($V/C_{In} \times 100$), Natrium- und Kalium-Rejektion ($C_{Na}/C_{In} \times 100$, $C_K/C_{In} \times 100$) vor (weiße Säulen) und nach (gestrichelte Säulen) Acetazolamid, Hydrochlorothiazid, Etacrynsäure und Furosemid. Das 1. Säulenpaar entspricht Patienten mit einem Glomerulumfiltrat (GFR) über 80 ml/min, das 2. Filtratwerten zwischen 80–40 ml/min und das 3. Filtratwerten unter 40 ml/min.

mid in therapeutischer Dosierung an chronisch niereninsuffizienten Patienten geprüft und mit Normalpersonen verglichen. Die Untersuchungen erfolgten unter Clearancebedingungen mittels Dauerinfusionsmethode. Als Bezugsgröße des effektiv wirksamen Nierenparenchyms diente das mittels Inulin bestimmte Glomerulumfiltrat (GFR), (chemische Analysen nach ROE u. Mitarb., 1949).

Die Wirkungsstärke wurde als fraktionelle Flüssigkeits-, Natrium- und Kaliumelimination definiert ($V/C_{In} \times 100$, $C_{Na}/C_{In} \times 100$, $C_K/C_{In} \times 100$). Die Patienten gliederten sich in 3 Untersuchungsgruppen auf:

Gruppe I diente mit einer GFR über 80 ml/min als Kontrollgruppe, Gruppe II wies eine Einschränkung der Filtration auf Werte zwischen 80–40 ml/min und Gruppe III auf Werte zwischen 40 und 10 ml/min auf.

Ergebnisse:

500 mg Acetazolamid bewirkten eine Zunahme der fraktionellen Flüssigkeitsausscheidung um 2,9% in Gruppe I, um 5,3% in Gruppe II und um 2,7% in Gruppe III (vgl. Tab. 1, Abb. 1). Gleichzeitig stieg die Natriumrejektion um 3,7, 5,3 bzw. 4,7% an, während die Kaliumrejektion um 43,1, 40,6 bzw. 36,6% zunahm.

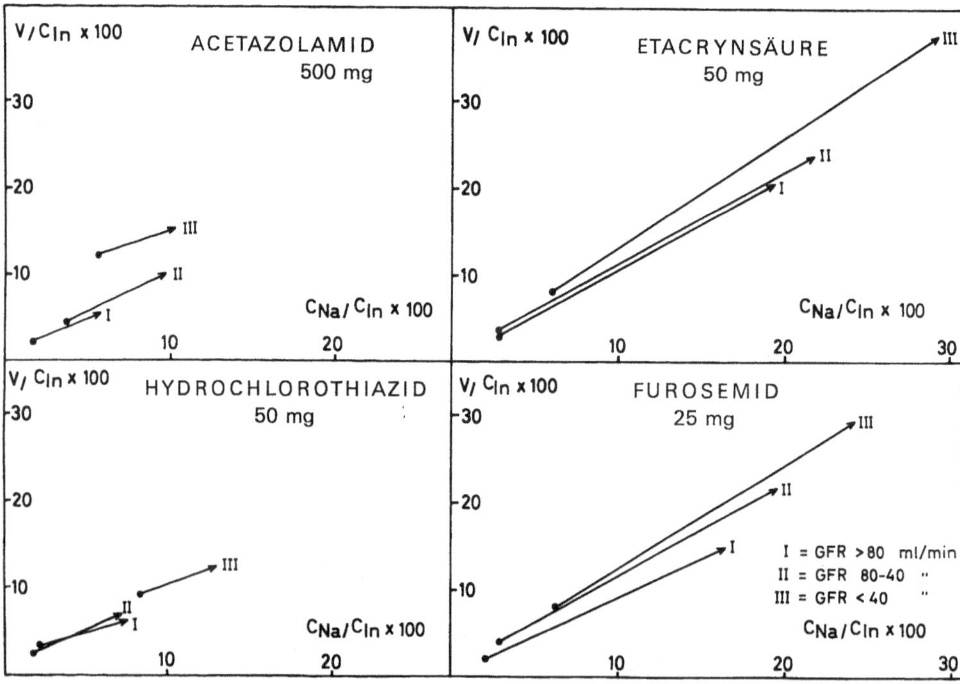

Abb. 2. Korrelation von fraktioneller Flüssigkeitsausscheidung ($V/C_{In} \times 100$) und Natriumrejektion ($C_{Na}/C_{In} \times 100$) nach Acetazolamid, Hydrochlorothiazid, Etacrynsäure und Furosemid. Die Symbole I, II und III repräsentieren die einzelnen Untersuchungsgruppen mit einem Filtrat über 80 ml/min, 80–40 ml/min und unter 40 ml/min. Wie ersichtlich, führen Etacrynsäure und Furosemid in Gruppe III zu stärkerer fraktioneller Flüssigkeitselimination.

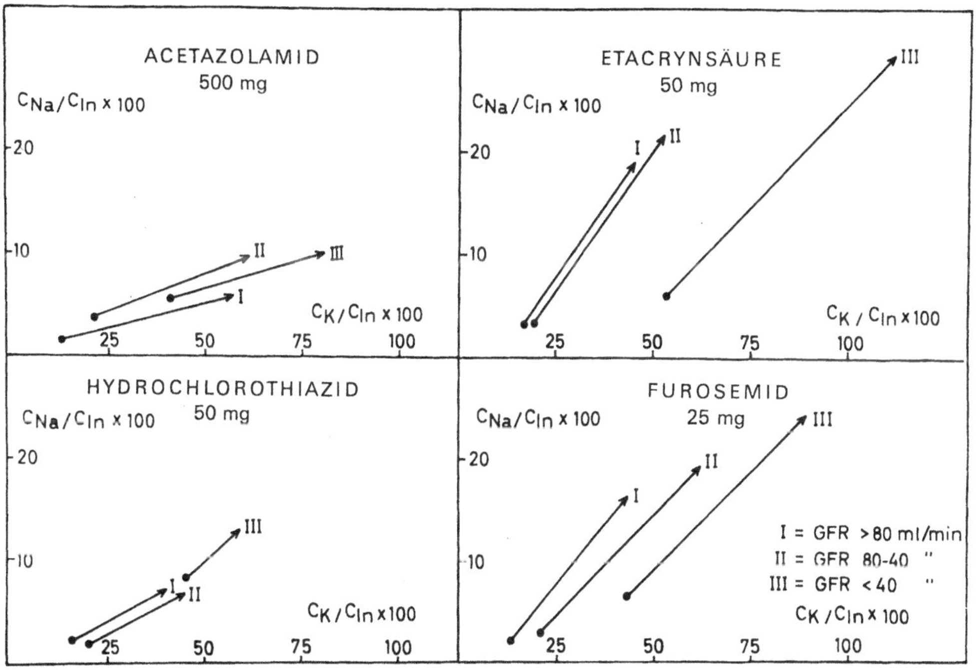

Abb. 3. Korrelation von Natrium- und Kalium-Rejektion ($C_{Na}/C_{In} \times 100$, $C_K/C_{In} \times 100$) nach Diuretica bei Patienten mit unterschiedlichem Glomerulumfiltrat. Nach Etacrynsäure besteht in Gruppe III eine vergleichsweise stärkere Zunahme der Kaliumrejektion.

50 mg Hydrochlorothiazid führten zu einer Steigerung von $V/C_{In} \times 100$ um 2,8% in Gruppe I, 3,5% in Gruppe II und 2,9% in Gruppe III. Die Natriumrejektion zeigte dabei eine Zunahme um 5,2, 4,9 bzw. 4,4%, die von Kalium um 22,6, 25,9 bzw. 13,4%.

Nach 50 mg Etacrynsäure nahm die fraktionelle Flüssigkeitsausscheidung um 17,6 in Gruppe I, 19,6% in Gruppe II und 29% in Gruppe III zu. Die entsprechenden Zunahmen der Natriumrejektion betrugen 16,3, 18,7 und 23,0%. Die Kaliumrejektion zeigte einen Anstieg um 22,2, 32,5 und 41,2%.

Nach 25 mg Furosemid stieg der Anteil der Diurese am Filtratvolumen um 12,5% in Gruppe I, 17,2% in Gruppe II und 21,4% in Gruppe III an. Die fraktionelle Natriumausscheidung wies eine Steigerung um 13,6, 16,3 bzw. 17,6% auf, während die Kaliumrejektion um 34,6, 44,1 bzw. 43,2% zunahm.

Die Korrelation von fraktioneller Flüssigkeitsausscheidung mit der Natriumrejektion (Abb.2) ergab nach Acetazolamid und Hydrochlorothiazid in allen Filtratbereichen ein paralleles Verhalten, das heißt, es bestand eine unveränderte Wirkungscharakteristik bei den niereninsuffizienten Patienten. Demgegenüber führten Etacrynsäure und Furosemid in Gruppe III zu einer vergleichsweise stärkeren fraktionellen Flüssigkeitselimination.

Die Korrelation von Natrium- und Kaliumrejektion (Abb.3) ergab nach Acetazolamid und Hydrochlorothiazid in allen Gruppen ebenfalls parallele Kurvenverläufe. Nach Etacrynsäure bestand dagegen in Gruppe III eine vergleichsweise stärkere Zunahme der Kaliumrejektion.

Diskussion

Die nach Furosemid und Etacrynsäure beobachtete umgekehrte Proportion zwischen Glomerulumfiltrat und fraktioneller Flüssigkeits- und Natriumausscheidung entspricht Befunden von REUBI und VORBURGER (1966), die bei reduziertem Filtrat ebenfalls eine stärkere Hemmung der tubulären Reabsorption feststellten. Auch DEETJEN und Mitarb. (1965, 1967) fanden bei der Ratte im extrem eingeschränkten Filtratbereich eine relative Wirkungszunahme von Furosemid und Etacrynsäure. Sie konnten daneben unter diesen Bedingungen mittels Mikropunktionstechnik einen proximal tubulären Angriffspunkt dieser Substanzen sichern.

Beim Menschen nimmt jedoch in einem Filtratbereich unter 10 ml/min die tubuläre Flüssigkeitsrejektion wieder ab – offenbar infolge ungenügender Diureticasekretion in das Tubuluslumen, die nach DEETJEN (1966) eine Voraussetzung ihrer Wirkung ist. In diesen Fällen kann durch eine pharmakologische Maximaldosis und damit erhöhter Diuretica »filtered load« noch ein Anstieg von V/GFR erzielt werden. So fanden wir bei 10 chronisch urämischen Patienten mit einem Filtrat um 3 ml/min nach Infusion von 1000 mg Furosemid eine statistisch signifikante Zunahme der filtratbezogenen Diurese von 43 auf 68% und der Natriumrejektion von 26 auf 61% (HEIDLAND und Mitarb. 1967).

Als Ursache der differenten relativen Wirkungsstärke in den einzelnen Filtratbereichen können u. E. humorale Faktoren diskutiert werden. FRASER und Mitarb. (1965), MEYER und Mitarb. (1966) u. a. haben nach Furosemid bzw. Etacrynsäure im akuten Versuch innerhalb weniger Minuten eine gesteigerte Reninfreisetzung festgestellt, die nach ROSENTHAL und Mitarb. (1967) auf dem Höhepunkt der Diurese am stärksten ist. Der Reninanstieg wird offen-

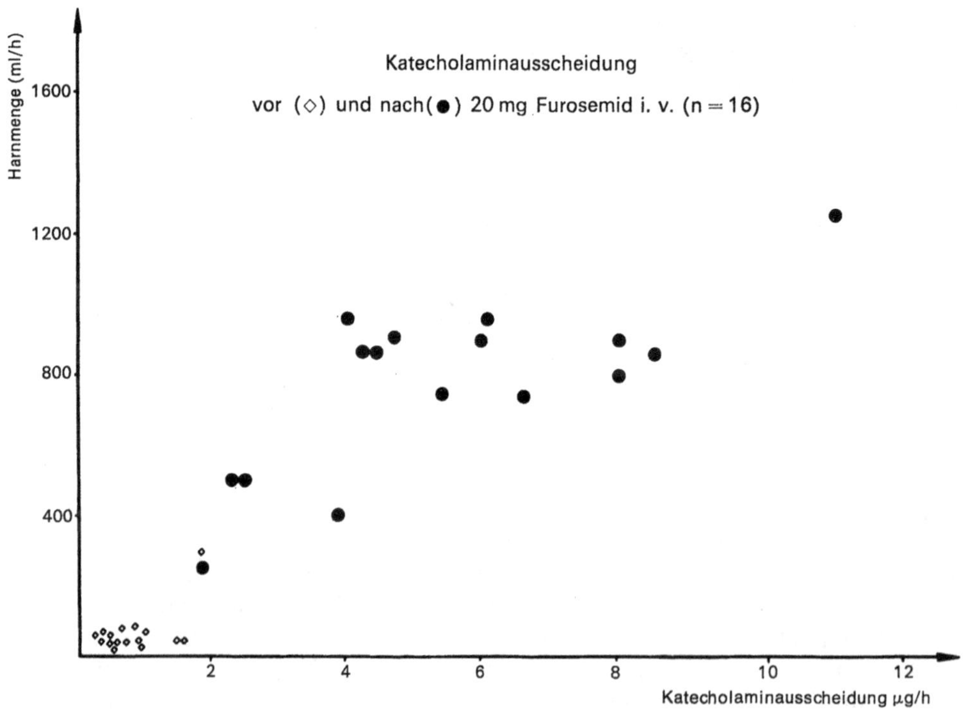

Abb. 4. Beziehungen zwischen Diurese/Stunde und Katecholaminausscheidung/Stunde bei 16 Pat. mit normaler und eingeschränkter Nierenfunktion.

bar vornehmlich durch eine negative Natriumbilanz induziert, da eine gleichzeitige NaCl-Substitution den diureticabedingten Reninanstieg verhindert (KLAUS und BOCSKOR 1968).

Unterstellt man, daß Nierengesunde infolge stärkerer absoluter Flüssigkeits- und Natriumausscheidung auch eine stärkere Reninfreisetzung aufweisen, so könnte das hierdurch entstehende Angiotensin über einen direkten tubulären Effekt und/oder verminderte Natrium filtered load (THURAU 1968) zu einer Interferenz mit der natriuretischen Wirkung des Diureticums führen. Bei niereninsuffizienten Patienten wäre demgegenüber eine geringere Reninfreisetzung und damit geringere Angiotensinwirkung zu erwarten. Allerdings kann der dosisabhängige antidiuretische und antinatriuretische Effekt von Angiotensin II (BOCK und Mitarb. 1958) bei Hypertonikern eine Wirkungsumkehr erfahren (BROWN und PEART 1962).

Akute Hypovolämien führen zu einem Anstieg der Brenzkatechinaminausscheidung (KUSCHKE und HERZER 1963, GORDON und Mitarb. 1967). Eine ähnliche Aktivierung des sympatico-adrenalen Symstems kann auch nach Diuretica auftreten, wie NICOLOSI und SANTORO (1964) nach Thiaziden erstmals feststellten. Eigene Bestimmungen der Brenzkatechinamine im Harn (Methode von EULER und FLODING 1955) ergaben nach Furosemid (20 mg i. v.) an 16 untersuchten Personen innerhalb von 60 Minuten eine Zunahme um das 1,3–10fache des Kontrollwertes. Der Anstieg stand in direkter linearer Korrelation zu Glomerulumfiltrat und Harnausscheidung (Abb. 4). Unter der Voraussetzung, daß Katechinaminbestimmungen im Harn unter den gewählten Bedingungen repräsentativ für ihre Plasmakonzentration sind, würden die antidiuretischen und natriumretinierenden Eigenschaften von Adrenalin und Noradrenalin (NICKEL und Mitarb. 1954, LARAGH 1962) wiederum bei Normalpersonen stärker sein als bei niereninsuffizienten Patienten. Nach VANDER (1965) sowie WATHEM und Mitarb. (1965) sollen Brenzkatechinamine zudem eine gesteigerte Reninfreisetzung bewirken.

Literatur / References

BIBER, Th., M. MYLLE, A. P. BAINES, C. W. GOTTSCHALK, J. OLIVER and McDOWELL: Study by micropuncture and microdissection of acute renal damage in rats. Am. J. Med. **44**, 664 (1968).

BOCK, K. D., H. DENGLER, H. J. KRECKE und G. REICHEL: Untersuchungen über die Wirkung von synthetischem Hypertensin II auf Elektrolythaushalt, Nierenfunktion und Kreislauf beim Menschen. Klin. Wschr. **36**, 808 (1958).

BRICKER, N. S., S. KLAHR and R. E. RIESELBACH: The functional adaptation of the diseased kidney. J. Clin. Invest. **43**, 1915 (1964).

BROWN, J. J. and W. S. PEART: The effect of angiotensin on urine flow and electrolyte excretion in hypertensive patients. Clin. Sci. **22**, 1 (1962).

BRUNNER, F. P., F. C. RECTOR and D. W. SELDIN: Mechanism of glomerular-tubular balance. J. Clin. Invest. **45**, 590 (1966).

BUCHBORN, E. und S. ANASTASAKIS: Angriffspunkt und Wirkungsmechanismus von Furosemid am distalen Nephron des Menschen. Klin. Wschr. **42**, 22, 1127 (1964).

DEETJEN, P.: Mikropunktionsuntersuchungen zur Wirkung von Furosemid. Pflügers Arch. ges. Physiologie **284**, 184 (1965).

DEETJEN, P.: Micropuncture studies on site and mode of diuretic action of furosemide. Ann. New York Acad. Sci. **139**, 408 (1966).

DEETJEN, P., W. E. BÜNTIG, K. HARDT and R. RHODE: Diuretic effect of ethacrynic acid in the rat: A micropuncture study of the relationship of site and mode of action. 5. Symp. f. Nephrologie, Lausanne 1967.

DIRKS, J. H., W. J. CIRKSENA and R. W. BERLINER: The effect of saline infusion on sodium reabsorption by the proximal tubule of the dog. J. Clin. Invest. **44**, 1160 (1965).

EDEL, H. H., J. EIGLER und E. RENNER: Zum Wirkungsmechanismus der Etacrynsäure. Klin. Wschr. **44**, 8, 421 (1966).

FRASER, R., V. H. T. JAMES, J. J. BROWN, P. ISAAC and A. F. LEVER: Effect of angiotensin and of frusemide on plasma aldosterone, corticosterone, cortisol, and renin in man. Lancet **II**, 989 (1965).

GORDON, R. D., O. KÜCHEL, G. W. LIDDLE and P. ISLAND: Role of the sympathetic nervous system in regulating renin and aldosterone production in man. J. Clin. Invest. **46** 4 (1967).

HEIDLAND, A., K. KLÜTSCH, T. TAKUMA und E. SCHEITZA: Funktionelle Aspekte der chronischen Niereninsuffizienz mit Urämie. 5. Symp. Ges. f. Nephrologie, Lausanne 1967.

JOHNSTON, C. L. and J. O. DAVIS: Evidence from cross circulation studies for a humoral mechanism in the natriuresis of saline loading. Proc. Soc. exp. Biol. (N. Y.) **121,** 1058 (1966).

KLAUS, D. und D. BOCSKOR: Zur Regulation der Reninsekretion beim Menschen. Verhandl. dtsch. Ges. inn. Med. 1968 im Druck.

KUSCHKE, H. J. und R. HERZER: Die Brenzkatechinaminausscheidung bei essentieller Hypertonie unter orthostatischer Belastung. Verh. Dtsch. Ges. Kreislauff. **28,** 232 (1963).

LARAGH, J. H.: Interrelationship between angiotensin, norepinephrine, epinephrine, aldosterone secretion and electrolyte metabolism in man. Circulation **25,** 203 (1962).

MEYER, PH., J. MENARD, J. M. ALEXANDRE and P. MILLIEZ: Variations de l'activité rénine plasmatique après injection d'acide éthacrynique. J. Urol. Néphrol. **72,** 619 (1966).

NICOLOSI, G. and R. SANTORO: La eliminazione urinaria de catecholamine réel corso di deplezione idrosalina. Prog. med. (Napoli) **20,** 289 (1964).

NICKEL, J. F., P. B. LOWRANCE, E. LEIFER and S. E. BRADLEY: Renal function, electrolyte excretion and body fluids in patients with chronic renal insufficiency before and after sodium deprivation. J. Clin. Invest. **32,** 68 (1953).

PORUSH, J. G. and R. G. ABRAMSON: The effects of hypertonic mannitol on renal sodium excretion in hydropenic man. Clin. Sci. **29,** 475 (1965).

RECTOR, C. F., J. C. SELLMAN, M. MARTINEZ-MALDONADO and D. W. SELDIN: The mechanism of suppression of proximal tubular reabsorption by saline infusions. J. Clin. Invest. **46,** 1 (1967).

REUBI, F. C.: Clinical use of furosemide. Ann. New York Acad. Sci. **139,** 433 (1966).

REUBI, F. und C. VORBURGER: Wirkung der Diuretica bei eingeschränkter Nierenfunktion. In: Diureseforschung IV. Symp. Freiburg 1966, Georg Thieme Verlag Stuttgart.

ROSENTHAL, J., R. BOUCHER, W. NOWACYNSKI and J. GENEST: Acute changes in plasma volume, renin activity and free aldosterone levels in healthy subjects following furosemide administration. Can. J. Physiol. Pharmacol. **46,** 85 (1966).

THURAU, K.: Intrarenale Wirkung des Angiotensins. In: Renaler Transport und Diuretica. Springer, Berlin, Heidelberg, New York 1969.

VANDER, A. J.: Effect of catecholamines and the renal nerves on renin secretion in unanesthetized dogs. Am. J. Physiol. **209,** 659 (1965).

WATHEM, R. L., W. S. KINGSBURY, D. A. STOUDER, E. G. SCHNEIDER and H. H. ROSTORFER: Effects of infusion of catecholamines and angiotensin II on renin release in unanesthetized dogs. Amer. J. Physiol. **209,** 1012 (1965).

Symptomatic Diuretic Therapy of the Nephrotic Edema with the Fixed Combination Ethacrynic Acid/Amiloride

Symptomatische diuretische Behandlung des nephrotischen Ödems mit dem Kombinationspräparat Etacrynsäure/Amilorid

W. HOLLER

Summary: The combination of the diuretics ethacrynic acid and amiloride have proven very effective in our studies involving patients with nephrotic syndrome. Even after longterm administration and in patients with extensive diuresis, we did not observe a single case of hypokalemia. In two cases with renal insufficiency, a hyperkalemia developed demanding a lower amiloride-concentration of the combination. In the presence of a severely reduced plasma albumin-level, a complete diuretic effect could only be obtained by correction of the hypovolemia and the oncotic pressure with plasma- or hyperoncotic dextran infusion.

With the exception of the mentioned case of hyperkalemia and temporary muscle cramps in another patient with a massive diuresis (4 liters per day), no other side effects were observed.

Die Notwendigkeit einer symptomatischen diuretischen Behandlung des nephrotischen Syndroms ergibt sich immer wieder, wenn im Vordergrund des klinischen Bildes ausgeprägte Ödeme bestehen und der Erfolg einer speziellen Therapie mit Corticosteroiden oder Cytostatica nicht abgewartet werden kann (3, 7). Die hierbei üblicherweise verwandten Saluretica (Thiazide, Furosemid, Etacrynsäure) bewirken eine gesteigerte Kaliurese. Diese Kaliumverluste müssen zur Vermeidung einer Hypokaliämie durch orale Kaliumsubstitution oder gleichzeitige Gabe von Spironolacton ausgeglichen oder vermieden werden. Beide Methoden haben ihre Gefahren und Nebenwirkungen (2, 4, 10), auf die hier nicht näher eingegangen werden kann.

In der Kombination eines Salureticums (Etacrynsäure) mit einer kaliumretinierenden Substanz [Amilorid (1, 5, 6, 9)] im Verhältnis 5:1 oder 10:1 stand uns ein Diureticum zur Verfügung, dessen Wirksamkeit unter anderen auch an 8 Patienten mit nephrotischem Syndrom erprobt wurde.

Methode: Bei 7 der 8 Patienten, über deren diuretische Behandlung mit dem neuen Kombinationspräparat hier berichtet werden soll, lag dem nephrotischen Syndrom eine chronische membranöse bzw. perimembranöse Glomerulonephritis zu Grunde.

Die histologischen Diagnosen verdanken wir Herrn Prof. Dr. BOHLE, Patholog. Institut der Universität Tübingen. Ein Patient war ein halbes Jahr vor der hiesigen stationären Aufnahme linksseitig wegen funktionsloser Nieren nephrektomiert worden. Die histologische Untersuchung hatte damals eine Nierenvenenthrombose ergeben. Bei der Aufnahme bei uns bestand ein ausgeprägtes nephrotisches Syndrom mit schweren Ödemen.

Tab. 1.

Patient	Diagnose	Ödeme	Kreatinin i. Serum	Therapie	Diuretische Therapie	Behandlungs-dauer	Gewichts-abnahme	Diuretische Wirkung	Neben-wirkungen
D. A. 38 J. ♂ Kb. Nr. 415	Nephrot. Syndrom bei chron. membranöser (perimembranöser) Glomerulonephritis	++	0,8 mg%	ACTH Prednisolon Imurel	täglich 50 mg Etacrynsäure 10 mg Amilorid	4 Monate	5,5 kg	sehr gut	keine
S. E. 46 J. ♂ KB. Nr. 1149	Nephrot. Syndrom bei Exacerbation einer chron. membranösen Glomerulonephritis	+++	0,9 mg%	Prednisolon	jeden 2. Tag 100 mg Etacrynsäure 20 mg Amilorid	4 Wochen	9 kg	sehr gut	keine
K. M. 19 J. ♂ Kb. Nr. 385	Nephrot. Syndrom bei chron. membranöser Glomerulonephritis	+++	0,7 mg%	ACTH Prednisolon	jeden 2. Tag 100 mg Etacrynsäure 20 mg Amilorid	17 Tage	15 kg	sehr gut	Muskelkrämpfe
J. K. 63 J. ♂ Kb. Nr. 1375	Nephrot. Syndrom bei chron. membranöser (perimembranöser) Glomerulonephritis	+++	1,8 mg%	Prednisolon	jeden 2. Tag 100 mg Etacrynsäure 20 (10) mg Amilorid	6 Wochen	9,6 kg	sehr gut	Hyperkaliämie
N. K. 67 J. ♂ Kb. Nr. 1096	Nephrot. Syndrom bei Verd. Nierenvenen-thrombose re. Restniere	+++	4,1 mg%	Antikoagulant. Imurel	jeden 2. Tag 100 mg Etacrynsäure 20 (10) mg Amilorid	2 Monate	16,5 kg	sehr gut	Hyperkaliämie
U. R. 53 J. ♀ Kb. Nr. 819	Nephrot. Syndrom bei chron. membranöser Glomerulonephritis	+	0,6 mg%	Indcmethacin Prednisolon Imurel	jeden 2. Tag 50 mg Etacrynsäure 10 mg Amilorid	4 Monate	2 kg	gering	keine
S. E. 56 J. ♀ Kb. Nr. 205	Nephrot. Syndrom bei chron. perimembranöser Glomerulonephritis	+	0,8 mg%	ACTH Prednisolon Imurel	jeden 2. Tag 100 mg Etacrynsäure 10 mg Amilorid	4 Wochen	3,5 kg	gut	keine
N. R. 53 J. ♀ Kb. Nr. 444	Nephrot. Syndrom bei chron. membranöser Glomerulonephritis	+	0,9 mg%	ACTH Prednisolon	täglich 50 mg Etacrynsäure 10 mg Amilorid	7 Tage	3,4 kg	gut	keine

Unsere Verdachtsdiagnose »nephrotisches Syndrom bei Verdacht auf Nierenvenenthrombose der rechten Restniere« ließ sich aber bis jetzt nicht sicher bestätigen. Röntgenologisch hatte sich die untere Hohlvene glattwandig dargestellt.

Alle Patienten hatten Ödeme verschiedenen Schweregrades. Bei 2 Patienten lag eine Retention harnpflichtiger Substanzen mit Serumkreatininwerten von 1,8 mg% und 4,1 mg% (Tab. 1) vor. Es wurde eine kochsalzarme, ca. 50 mval Natrium/die enthaltende Diät gegeben.

Folgende Serumwerte wurden in regelmäßigem Abstand überprüft: Harnstoff, Harnsäure, Kreatinin, Natrium, Kalium und Chlorid. Die K^+-Bestimmung im Serum erfolgte jeden 3. Tag. Vor, während und nach der diuretischen Behandlung wurden die Leberwerte: Bilirubin im Serum, Transaminasen, alkalische Phosphatase und BSP-Retention bestimmt; ebenso Nüchternblutzucker, Thrombozytenzahl, rotes und weißes Blutbild und Hämatokrit. Die Patienten wurden täglich gewogen. Vom täglichen 24-Stunden-

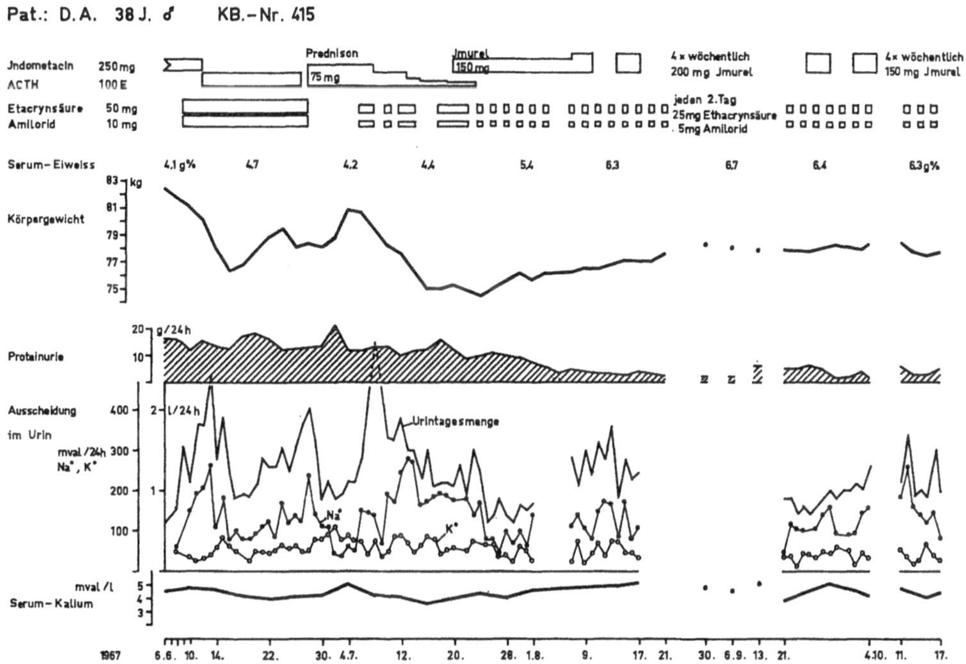

Abb. 1. Patient D. A., 38 Jahre. Diagnose: Nephrotisches Syndrom bei chronisch membranöser (perimembranöser) Glomerulonephritis. Die Behandlung des nephrotischen Syndroms war bei diesem Patienten zunächst mit Indometacin über 4 Wochen erfolglos durchgeführt worden, ebenso erbrachte die ACTH- und anschließende Prednisolonbehandlung keinen Rückgang der Proteinurie. Erst nach Cytostatica kam es zum Rückgang der Proteinurie und zum Anstieg des Gesamteiweißes im Serum. Nach Verordnung von täglich 50 mg Etacrynsäure und 10 mg Amilorid wurden die Ödeme, die vor allem im Bereich des Halses als beengend empfunden wurden, ausgeschwemmt. Die Steigerung der Urintagesmenge und der Natriurese bei gleichbleibender Kaliurese ist aus der Abbildung zu ersehen. Trotz Verabreichung des Diureticums über 4 Monate blieb der Serumkaliumwert im Normbereich.

Urin wurde Gesamtvolumen, Eiweiß-, Kalium- und Natrium-Ausscheidung gemessen. Über die Dosierung des Diureticums sowie die gleichzeitige spezielle Therapie des nephrotischen Syndroms unterrichtet die Tabelle 1.

Ergebnisse:

1. Bei allen Patienten konnten die Ödeme zum Verschwinden gebracht werden. Als zuverlässigster Maßstab wurde die Abnahme des Körpergewichtes in der Tab. 1 angegeben. Es ist erwähnenswert, daß der Patient J. H. 63 Jahre, KB.-Nr. 1375 zuvor 12 Tage lang täglich mit 6 Dragées Aldactone-A und 100 mg Chlorthalidon ohne Erfolg behandelt worden war. Nach Gabe des Kombinationspräparates Etacrynsäure + Amilorid stieg

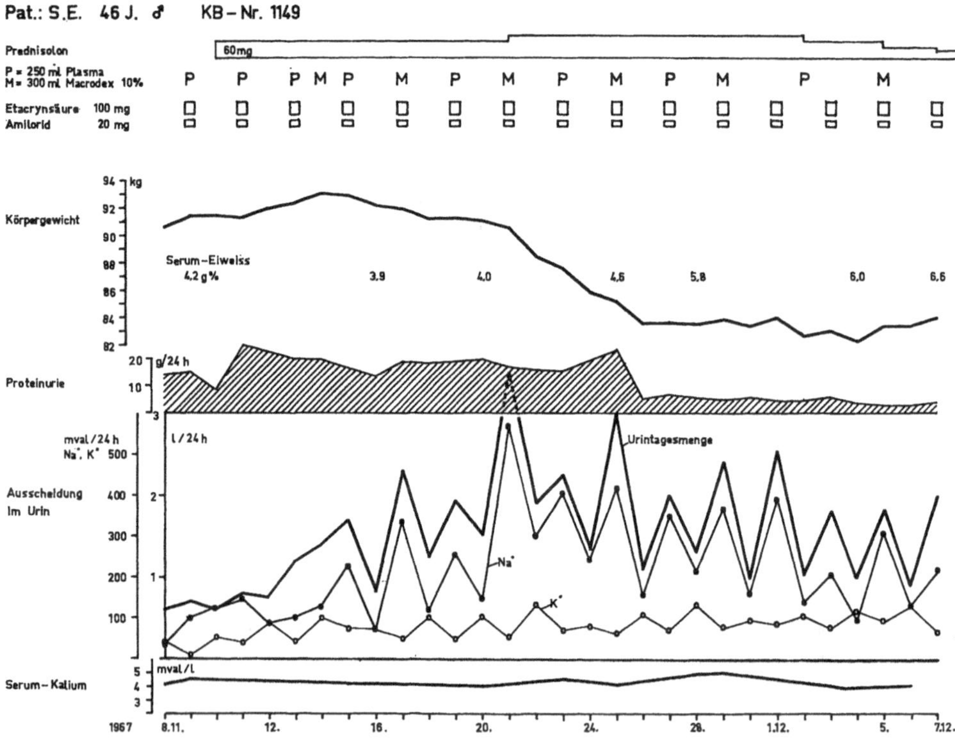

Abb. 2. Patient S. E., 46 Jahre. Diagnose: Nephrotisches Syndrom bei Exacerbation einer chronischen membranösen Glomerulonephritis. Bei einem Serum-Gesamteiweiß von 4,2 g% und einer Hypoalbuminämie von 1,4 g% kam es trotz Gabe von 100 mg Etacrynsäure und 20 mg Amilorid an jedem 2. Tag erst nach einer »onkotischen« Therapie mit Plasma und hyperonkotischer Dextranlösung (Macrodex 10%) zu einer wirksamen Diurese mit Rückgang des Körpergewichtes um 9 kg und zum Verschwinden der Ödeme. Bei der intermittierenden Verabreichung des Diureticums an jedem 2. Tag läßt sich in der Abbildung 2 die Zunahme der Diurese und Natriurese bei leichtem Rückgang der Kaliumausscheidung an den Tagen der Diureticumverabreichung erkennen. Auch hier blieb das Serumkalium im Normbereich.

die Diurese an und das bei ihm bestehende extreme, über kindskopfgroße Scrotalödem bildete sich vollständig zurück.

2. Bei gleichbleibender Kaliurese steigerte sich die Natriumausscheidung bis maximal auf das 7- bis 8fache des Ausgangswertes.
3. Bei allen Patienten mit uneingeschränkter oder nur geringfügig eingeschränkter Nierenfunktion blieb der Serumkaliumwert bei einer Kombination von Etacrynsäure + Amilorid im Verhältnis 5:1 im Normbereich. Bei 2 Patienten (Patient J. K. und Patient N. K.) mit einer kompensierten Retention kam es zu einer Hyperkaliämie von 6,8 mval/l und 5,9 mval/l. Nach einer mehrtägigen Pause erfolgte Weiterbehandlung mit 100 mg Etacrynsäure und 10 mg Amilorid jeden 2. Tag ohne weitere Komplikationen.
4. Ein Einfluß der diuretischen Therapie auf das Kreatinin, den Harnstoff und die Harnsäure im Serum wurde nicht festgestellt.

Zusammenfassend läßt sich in der hier gebotenen Kürze sagen, daß sich die Anwendung des Kombinationspräparates Etacrynsäure + Amilorid bei der symptomatischen Behandlung des nephrotischen Ödems sehr gut bewährt hat. Es kam trotz massiver Ödemausschwemmungen nie zu Hypokaliämien. Bei stärker eingeschränkter Nierenfunktion mit beginnender Retention harnpflichtiger Substanzen ist allerdings eine Reduktion des Amiloridanteils in dem Kombinationspräparat wegen der Gefahr der Hyperkaliämie angezeigt (1, 5). Eine regelmäßige Kontrolle des Serumkaliums ist in diesen Fällen unerläßlich. Bei stark herabgesetztem Serumalbumin wird eine volle diuretische Wirkung erst nach Korrektur der Hypovolämie und des onkotischen Drukkes durch Plasma- oder hyperonkotischen Plasmaersatz-Infusionen erreicht (8). Besonders bewährte sich eine gleichzeitige Verabreichung von Plasma bzw. Macrodex 10% und 100 mg Etacrynsäure + 20 mg Amilorid an jedem 2. Tag.

Außer der erwähnten Hyperkaliämie bei eingeschränkter Nierenfunktion und vorübergehenden Muskelkrämpfen, die in einem Fall wohl infolge der Elektrolytverschiebungen bei einer Tagesdiurese von über 4 Litern auftraten, wurden von uns keine Nebenwirkungen beobachtet.

Literatur / References

1. Brunner, F. B.: Klinische Erfahrungen mit dem neuen kaliumsparenden Diureticum Amilorid (Moduretic, Colectril, MK-870). Schw. med. Wschr. **97**, 1542 (1967).
2. Clark, E. J.: Amer. Med. Ass. **193**, 163 (1965).
3. Cottier, P. and C. Vorburger: Die diuretische Behandlung des nephrotischen Syndroms. In: Das nephrotische Syndrom. Hrsg. Reubi, F. und H. Pauli. Thieme Stuttgart 1963.
4. Gantt, C. L. and R. E. Ecklund: Amer. J. Med. **33**, 490 (1962).
5. Heidland, A., K. Klütsch und A. Moormann: Zur renalen Kaliumretention nach Verabreichung von Amilorid-HCl. Arzneim.-Forsch. (Drug Res.) **17**, 1314–1318 (1967).
6. Hitzenberger, G., H. Kampffmeyer and J. Conway: The diuretic effect of desmethylpipazuroyl-guanidine (MK-870) in man. Clin. Pharm. a. Ther. (1968) Vol. **9**, No. 1, 71–79.
7. Sarre, H.: Nierenkrankheiten. Thieme Stuttgart, 3. Aufl. 1967.
8. Schreiner, G. E.: The nephrotic syndrome. In: Diseases of the kidney. Little, Brown and Company, Boston 1963.
9. Senewiratne, B. and Sheila Sherlock: Amiloride (MK-870) in patients with ascites due to cirrhosis of liver. Lancet 120 (1968).
10. Wagner, A.: Kaliuminduzierte Dünndarmulcera. Med. Klin. **63**, Nr. 24, 941 (1968).

The Application of Diuretics in Diabetes Insipidus

Die Anwendung von Diuretica bei Diabetes Insipidus

E. BUCHBORN

Summary: In cases of neurohypophyseal and nephrogenic diabetes insipidus the longterm therapy with diuretics leads independent from ADH to continuous increase of osmolality and sodium-concentration in the urine as a consequence of a partial inhibition of the sodium transport in the distal nephron. Therefore, the ingested solutes, especially NaCl can be excreted in a relatively smaller fluid volume than with maximal dilution of urine. Due to the fact that diabetes insipidus is an isolated imbalance of the urine-concentration mechanism but with normal osmoregulation, a perfect fluid balance and an increased fluid turnover is a prerequisite. By application of diuretics, it is possible to maintain the isotonicity of body fluids in spite of lacking ADH-effect by means of a reduced fluid turnover; i. e.: polydipsia and polyuria are decreasing. This primarily renal effect may secondarily, on an extra-renal basis be favourably influenced by an initial increase of natriuresis in connection with a reduction of the extracellular space and, thus, be maintained by a dietetic sodium restriction; conversely, it can be revoked by increased sodium intake.

Ein »paradoxer«, nämlich ein antidiuretischer Effekt von Diuretica bei Patienten mit Diabetes insipidus wurde erstmals bereits 1905 nach Theophyllin-Injektionen (7) und dann ein Jahr nach Einführung des ersten intravenös applizierbaren Quecksilber-Diureticums 1924 beschrieben (1). Praktische Bedeutung erlangte diese diuresehemmende Behandlung zunächst jedoch nicht, weil sie ständige Injektionen erforderte und toxische Hg-Nebenwirkungen befürchten ließ.

Nach Entwicklung der oral wirksamen Thiazide wurde diese antidiuretische Diureticawirkung 1959 von Reerink und Mitarb. (2) bei hereditärem, nephrogenem Diabetes insipidus und wenig später von Crawford und Kennedy (3) auch für den neurohypophysären Diabetes insipidus wiederentdeckt.

Seither ist diese Beobachtung durch umfangreiche klinische Kasuistik bestätigt. Dabei findet sich regelmäßig schon am ersten Tag der Behandlung mit therapeutischen Saluretica-Dosen, z. B. 2×25 mg Hydrochlorothiazid als primär renale Wirkung eine prompte Steigerung der Natriurese und damit auch der osmolalen Clearance. Innerhalb der nächsten 2–4 Tage nimmt die Natriurese langsam wieder ab und unterschreitet schließlich nicht selten die Ausgangswerte der Vorperiode. Gleichzeitig wird der antidiuretische Effekt immer deutlicher, bis die Diurese bei Fortsetzung der saluretischen Therapie auf $^1/_2$ bis $^2/_3$ der initialen Polyurie reduziert bleibt (Abb. 1).

Die Harnosmolalität nimmt dabei gegenüber der Vorperiode von etwa 100 mosm/kg auf mehr als das Doppelte zu – ebenso die Natriumkonzentration im Harn (z. B. von 17–40 auf 30–90 mval/l) – ohne daß jedoch die Plasmaisotonie in der Regel überschritten wird. Eine echte Antidiurese mit Bildung eines hypertonen Harns liegt somit, auch nach hohen Diureticadosen, nicht vor.

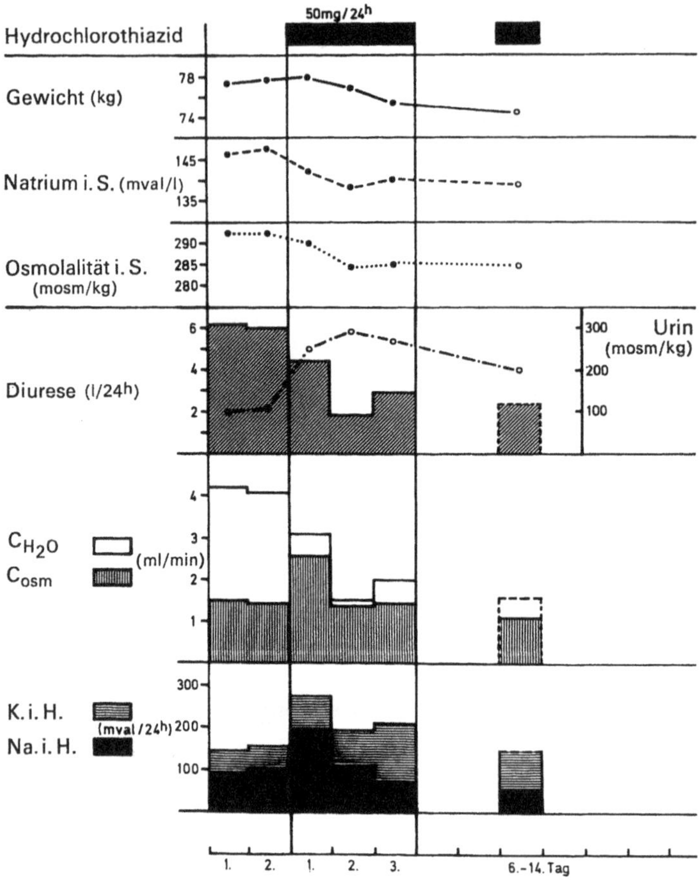

Abb. 1. Saluretica-Therapie bei Diabetes insipidus.

Sekundär zu dieser primär renalen Diureticawirkung kommt es regelmäßig zur Abnahme von Natriumspiegel und Serumosmolalität um 3–10 mosm/kg und damit zur Verminderung von Durstgefühl und Trinkmenge. Die gleichzeitige Herabsetzung des Körpergewichts um 2–4 kg bzw. des extrazellulären Raums weisen überdies auf eine negative Natriumbilanz mit Verminderung des Gesamtnatriumbestandes hin. Oft nimmt während dieser Phase die Kaliumausscheidung stärker zu, und der Na/K-Quotient im Harn kann als Ausdruck eines sekundären Aldosteronismus bis unter 1,0 absinken. Dementsprechend führen jetzt zusätzlich zum Saluretieum verabfolgte Aldosteronantagonisten zu erneuter Natriurese mit Wiederanstieg des Na/K-Quotienten (4).

Wesentlich für den Dauereffekt der Behandlung ist zunächst die anhaltende Erhöhung der Osmolalität bzw. der Natriumkonzentration im Endharn auf ca. das Doppelte, die vom antidiuretischen Hormon unabhängig ist. Hierdurch können die nutritiv zugeführten, osmotisch wirksamen Mineralien, vor allem NaCl in einem relativ kleineren Wasservolumen ausgeschieden werden als bei maximaler Harnverdünnung (5). Die Homoiostase der Isotonie im Körpermilieu kann damit, trotz Fehlen von ADH durch einen geringeren Wasserumsatz gewährleistet werden als bei unbehandeltem Diabetes insipidus. Damit könnte die zunächst paradox erscheinende Gleichzeitigkeit von Saluresa und Antidiurese durch den renalen Effekt der Diuretica erklärt werden. Die einzelnen Saluretica eignen sich hierfür je nach Wirkungsstärke und -dauer unterschiedlich.

Weiterhin mitentscheidend für eine erfolgreiche Dauerbehandlung ist es, die initiale Verminderung des Gesamtnatriumbestandes durch eine mäßige Natriumrestriktion aufrechtzuerhalten. Steigert man die tägliche Natriumzufuhr mit der Nahrung auf mehr als 4 g NaCl, dann läßt nach den Befunden von CUTLER u. Mitarb. (6) der diuresehemmende Diuretica-Effekt unter erneutem Anstieg des Körpergewichts sowie der Osmolalität und des Natriumspiegels im Serum bald wieder nach; ebenso wenn man andere osmotisch wirksame Mineralien anstelle von NaCl vermehrt zuführt.

Dagegen vermindert die Kombination von mittleren Dosen möglichst lang wirkender Saluretica und einer mäßigen Natriumrestriktion die Harn- und Trinkmenge um maximal 50%. Das bedeutet für die Patienten erhebliche Erleichterung, z. B. im Berufsleben, bei sonstigen sozialen Kontakten und meist auch in Form einer ungestörten Nachtruhe. Dies gilt besonders für den nephrogenen Diabetes insipidus, der – anders als die neurohypophysäre Form – einer hormonalen Substitutionsbehandlung wegen seiner distaltubulären ADH-Refraktärität nicht zugänglich ist.

Der *Wirkungsmechanismus* dieser diuresehemmenden Therapie bei Diabetes insipidus läßt sich am ehesten vom primär renalen Effekt her verstehen: Klinische Beobachtungen und tierexperimentelle Mikropunktionsbefunde stimmen darin überein, daß Saluretica bei Diabetes insipidus die Natriumkonzentration sowohl im Endharn wie auch am Ende der Henle'schen Schleife, vermutlich also entlang des ganzen distalen Nephron gegenüber unbehandelten Kontrollen oder forcierter Wasserdiurese erhöhen. Ob dieser Anstieg der frühdistalen Natriumkonzentration Folge eines erhöhten Einstroms aus dem proximalen Konvolut oder nur Folge einer partiellen Hemmung des Natriumtransportes im aufsteigenden Schleifenschenkel ist, bleibt vorerst offen.

Daneben können aber Ausmaß und Dauer des Therapieeffektes durch sekundäre extrarenale Wirkungen auf den Natriumhaushalt, z. B. durch diätetische Natriumrestriktion modifiziert werden. So begünstigt die initial negative Natriumbilanz mit Verminderung von Osmolalität, Natriumkonzentration und Menge der extrazellulären Flüssigkeit, evtl. auch mit geringer Herabsetzung des Glomerulumfiltrates die Persistenz des primär renalen Effektes, wie dieser umgekehrt durch vermehrte nutritive Natriumzufuhr wieder abgeschwächt oder aufgehoben werden kann.

Literatur / References

1. BAUER, J. and B. ACHNER: Die therapeutische Wirkung des Novasurols bei Diabetes insipidus. – Zbl. inn. Med. **1924**, 682.
2. REERINK, H., E. E. BRONGERS and H. SCHOUTEN: Use of chlorothiazide in treatment of three cases of nephrogenic diabetes insipidus. – Ned. T. Geneesk. **103**, 2347 (1959).
3. CRAWFORD, J. D. and G. C. KENNEDY: Chlorothiazide in Diabetes insipidus. – Nature (Lond.) **183**, 891 (1959).
4. EARLEY, L. E. and J. ORLOFF: The mechanism of antidiuresis associated with the administration of hydrochlorothiazide to patients with vasopressin-resistant diabetes insipidus. – J. clin. Invest. **41**, 1, 988 (1962).
5. BUCHBORN, E.: Klinik der Harnkonzentrierung und -verdünnung. – In: Diurese und Diuretica, S. 39ff. Berlin/Göttingen/Heidelberg, Springer 1959.

6. CUTLER, R. E., C. R. KLEEMAN, M. H. MAXWELL and T. DOWLING: Physiologic studies in nephrogenic diabetes insipidus. – J. clin. Endocr. **22**, 827 (1962).
7. MEYER, E.: Über Diabetes insipidus und andere Polyurien. Dtsch. Arch. klin. Med. **83**, 1 (1905).

HERMS: Zur Erklärung eines möglichen Wirkungsmechanismus der Diuretica möchte ich auf Befunde von SENFT u. Mitarb. (Naunyn-Schmiedebergs Arch. Pharmak. exp. Path. **255** (1966), 369 hinweisen, die nach Gabe von Chlorothiazid und auch Furosemid eine signifikante Abnahme der Aktivität der Phosphodiesterase im Gewebe feststellen konnten. Es ist natürlich verlockend, den möglichen antidiuretischen Effekt als Folge einer erhöhten Konzentration des 3,5-AMP in der Niere mit konsekutiv erhöhter Wasserpermeabilität der Sammelrohrepithelien in der Niere zu erklären. Das würde allerdings nur für den zentralen Diabetes insipidus gelten.

ULLRICH: Wir haben vor einiger Zeit die Wasserpermeabilität des distalen Konvolutes von Diabetes insipidus-Ratten unter Furosemid gemessen. (Annals of the New York Acad. Science **139**, 416 [1966].) Ein eindeutiger Effekt von Furosemid auf die Wasserpermeabilität wurde nicht beobachtet. Es wäre nach dem, was Herr BUCHBORN ausgeführt hat auch schwer zu verstehen, da man den Effekt der saluretischen Sulfonamide auf die Wasserausscheidung bei Diabetes insipidus durch Zulage von extra NaCl zur Diät rückgängig machen kann.

KLAUS: Stehen Ihre Untersuchungen in Übereinstimmung mit den Befunden von HELLER, nach denen der osmotische Gradient im Nierenmark unter Hydrochlorothiazid bestehen bleibt, unter Furosemid aber aufgehoben wird? Sind mit Hydrochlorothiazid bessere Erfolge zu erzielen als mit Furosemid?

BUCHBORN: Nach SENFT ist die Wirkung der Diuretica dem Adiuretin-Effekt insofern ähnlich, als die Bildung von 3',5'-AMP in ähnlicher Weise beeinflußt, nämlich gesteigert wird. Es erscheint aber fraglich, ob man das zur Erklärung heranziehen kann. Dies wäre eigentlich nur dann überzeugend, wenn wirklich ein hypertoner Urin, also ein ADH-ähnlicher Effekt durch die Diuretica erzielt wird, da ja 3',5'-AMP für die Steigerung der Wasserpermeabilität in den Sammelrohren verantwortlich sein soll. Ich versuchte aber gerade zu zeigen, daß dies nicht der Fall ist. Wir beobachten niemals einen hypertonen Urin, d. h. eine echte Harnkonzentrierung. – Was Herr ULLRICH sagte, bestätigt meine Auffassung, daß die distale Wasserpermeabilität bei Diabetes insipidus durch Diuretica nicht beeinflußt wird. Dagegen glaube ich nicht, daß die Wirkungsweise der Diuretica bei Diabetes insipidus ungeklärt ist! Wie ich zeigte, handelt es sich primär um eine partielle Hemmung des Na-Transportes im distalen Nephron, die zur Erhöhung der Na-Konzentration im Endharn führt. Hierdurch kann das nutritiv zugeführte NaCl in einem kleineren Wasservolumen ausgeschieden werden als ohne Behandlung. Damit kann die Isotonie des Körpermilieus durch einen kleineren Wasserumsatz, d. h. durch eine kleinere Trinkmenge aufrechterhalten werden als ohne Diuretica. Das ist auch der Grund, warum Änderungen der Na-Zufuhr den Saluretica-Effekt modifizieren können. – Die Kombination von ADH und Diuretica habe ich selbst nicht versucht. Ein additiver Effekt ist aber zu erwarten und in der Literatur mehrfach belegt. Praktisch versucht man allerdings gerade die Unbequemlichkeit der Substitutionsbehandlung mit ADH mittels der Diuretica zu umgehen, von der Wirkungslosigkeit der ADH-Substitution bei der nephrogenen Form abgesehen. – Die Beeinflussung des osmotischen Gradienten im Nierenmark scheint unabhängig davon zu sein, wie die Diuretica bei Diabetes insipidus wirken, nachdem wir von Herrn ULLRICH hörten, daß ein Einfluß auf die Wasserpermeabilität im distalen Nephron nicht nachweisbar und daher eine Beeinflussung der passiven Wasserrückdiffusion in das hypertone Nierenmark von Saluretica nicht zu erwarten ist. Bei der Auswahl des Mittels wird man diejenigen bevorzugen, die eine möglichst lange Wirkungsdauer haben. Hier ist das Chlorthalidon nach übereinstimmender Ansicht am zweckmäßigsten, da mit 100–150 mg, einmal am Tage gegeben, eine gleichmäßige Wirkung erzielt wird, während z. B. von Etacrynsäure 4×50 mg oder von Furosemid $4–5 \times 40$ mg hierzu erforderlich sind.

The Effect of Diuretics on the Extracorporeal Transplanted Kidney

Diureticawirkung an der extrakorporal transplantierten Niere

H. DOBBELSTEIN, H. H. EDEL

Summary: Action of diuretics on the extracorporeal transplanted kidney. During preservation of a cadaver kidney in a perfusion chamber designed by R. LAVENDER, functional data were collected over a 14^h period.

In addition, the influence of furosemide on the functional data was measured. After 14^h perfusion, the kidney was transplanted to the patient, who had the chamber mounted to his forearm. The next day GFR and RBF were again determined. The contralateral cadaver kidney of the same donor was immediately transplanted to another patient. Kidney function of the perfused kidney was compared with that of the immediately transplanted organ.

The kidney during extracorporeal perfusion showed a normal GFR, normal RBF and a normal response to furosemide. After transplantation it showed also normal function.

The perfusion chamber seems to be a good way to preserve cadaver kidneys until function and histocompatibility are tested. Moreover, if offers possibilities to solve pharmacological and physiopathologic problems.

Die von LAVENDER (1967) beschriebene Methode der extrakorporalen Nierentransplantation ermöglicht erstmals eine längere körperwarme Konservierung menschlicher Nieren in voll funktionstüchtigem Zustand. Für die Transplantation von Leichenorganen bedeutet diese Möglichkeit einen erheblichen Vorteil: sie stellt genügend Zeit zur Verfügung, um Histokompatibilitätstests durchzuführen und danach den geeignetsten Empfänger für ein verfügbares Transplantat auszuwählen. Auf diese Weise lassen sich die bisher der Leichennierentransplantation anhaftenden Nachteile vermeiden. Weiterhin kann die funktionelle Eignung des vorgesehenen Transplantats zuverlässig geprüft und gegebenenfalls durch bioptisch-histologische Untersuchungen ergänzt werden. Erfüllt das Transplantat die gestellten Bedingungen nicht, so kann es ohne Nachteile für den Patienten wieder aus dem Kreislauf ausgeschaltet werden. Andernfalls kann die endgültige Verpflanzung in Ruhe vorbereitet und unter optimalen chirurgischen Voraussetzungen vorgenommen werden.

Im Rahmen des Transplantationsprogramms der Münchner Kliniken wurde in enger Zusammenarbeit mit R. LAVENDER (Chicago) diese extrakorporale Perfusionstechnik wiederholt am Menschen angewandt. Dabei ergab sich u. a. die Gelegenheit, die Wirkung von Diuretica auf das extrakorporal transplantierte Organ zu untersuchen.

Methodik: Die Perfusion der unmittelbar nach dem Tod entnommenen menschlichen Niere erfolgt über einen besonders weitlumigen arteriovenösen Shunt, der wie der Scribner-Shunt zur Hämodialyse am Unterarm angelegt wird. Vor dem Einbringen in die

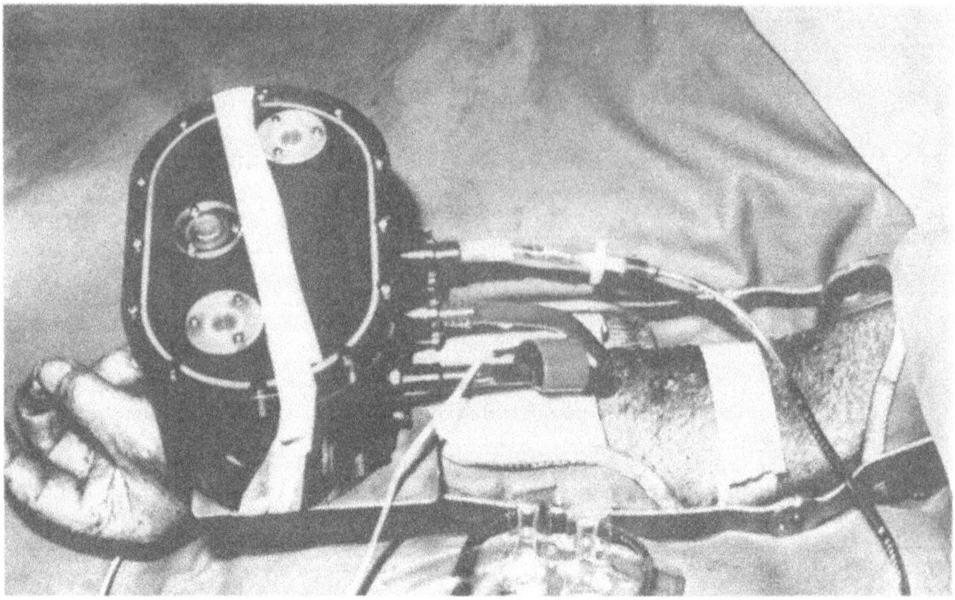

Abb. 1. Perfusionskammer in situ.

Kammer wird die Nierenarterie kanüliert und dann über eine Öffnung in der Kammer direkt an den arteriellen Schenkel des Shunts angeschlossen (Abb. 1). Das venöse Blut fließt dagegen frei in die Kammer, umspült die Niere und wird durch eine zweite Öffnung wieder in den venösen Schenkel des Scribner-Shunts zurückgeleitet. In der Kammer ist bei pulsatorischer Durchströmung eine schonende körperwarme Konservierung ohne Kompression des Organs und ein freier Abfluß von venösem Blut und Lymphe gewährleistet. Das Durchflußvolumen beträgt zwischen 400 und 800 ml/min. Der Ureter wird ebenfalls kanüliert und der Urin über eine dritte Öffnung in der Kammer in einen Plastikbeutel abgeleitet. Die Gerinnung des Blutes in der Plexiglaskammer wird durch Benzalkonium-Graphitbeschichtung der Innenwände und Heparinisierung des Blutes (in vergleichbarer Dosierung wie zur extrakorporalen Hämodialyse) verhindert. Bis zur Beendigung der Kompatibilitätstests und der Funktionsprüfungen ist an der perfundierten Niere die Möglichkeit zu experimentellen Untersuchungen gegeben. Dabei unterscheidet sich die extrakorporal transplantierte Niere aus folgenden Gründen vorteilhaft von der bereits implantierten:

1. Es können zuverlässige Clearance-Untersuchungen und Extraktionsbestimmungen vorgenommen und durch direkte Messung der Nierendurchblutung kontrolliert werden.
2. Perfusionsvolumen und der Perfusionsdruck lassen sich in gewissen Grenzen variieren und fortlaufend registrieren.
3. Die perfundierte Niere ist mit Gewißheit denerviert. Wegen der raschen Regeneration vegetativer Nerven erscheint es möglich, daß schon wenige Wochen nach der Transplantation eine teilweise Reinnervation erfolgt, so daß nervale Einflüsse auf transplantierte Nieren nicht sicher auszuschließen sind.

4. Auch wiederholte bioptische Untersuchungen können ohne Risiko für den Empfänger vorgenommen werden.

Ergebnisse:

Die Wirkung einer intraarteriellen Injektion von 0,6 mg Furosemid pro Minute nach 12stündiger Perfusion der Niere in der Kammer ist in Abb. 2 graphisch dargestellt: neben einer deutlichen Zunahme des Harnzeitvolumens von 5 auf 12 ml/min erkennt man einen Anstieg der osmolalen Clearance und eine erhebliche Zunahme der Natriurese. Den Befund im ersten Diagramm, die Abnahme der Inulin-Clearance unter Furosemid, darf als

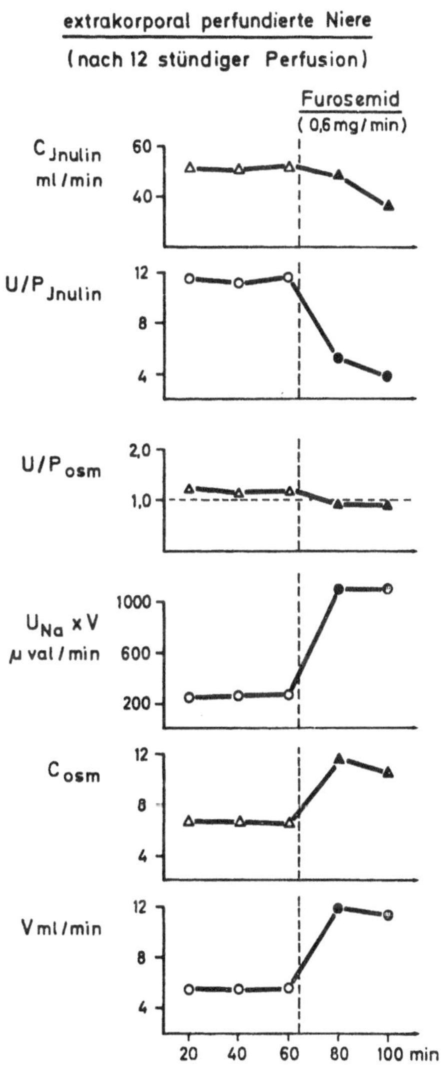

Abb. 2. Beeinflussung einzelner renaler Funktionsgrößen durch Furosemid (intraarterielle Injektion).

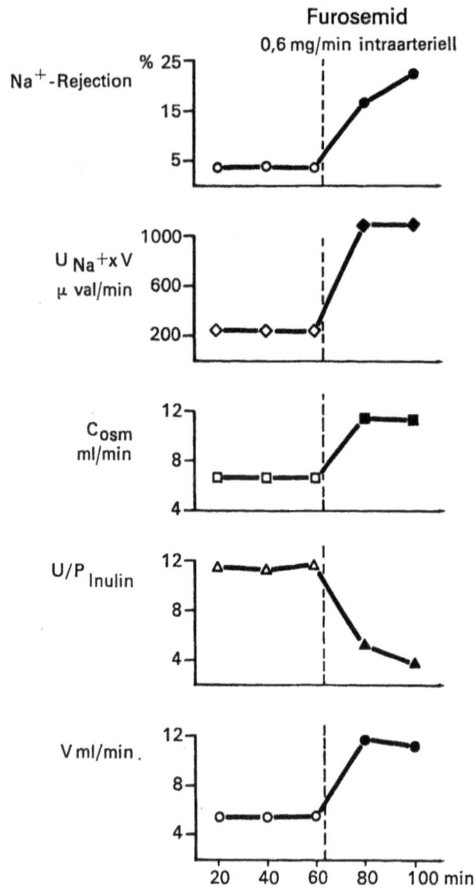

Abb. 3. Beeinflussung einzelner renaler Funktionsgrößen durch Furosemid (intraarterielle Injektion).

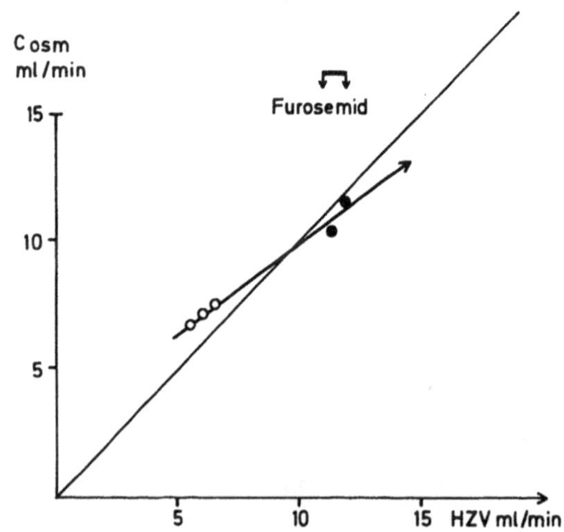

Abb. 4. Beziehung zwischen osmolarer Clearance (C_{osm}) und Harnzeitvolumen (HZV) vor und nach Furosemidgabe.

Einzelbefund nur mit Zurückhaltung betrachtet werden. Der Versuch mußte nach insgesamt 14stündiger Perfusionsdauer wegen des festgesetzten Transplantationstermins abgebrochen werden.

Neben den bereits genannten Daten zeigt Abb. 3, daß die Natrium-Rejection unter Furosemid von 3,8% auf 23% ansteigt. Korreliert man das Harnzeitvolumen, das sehr stark zunimmt, mit der osmolalen Clearance, die vergleichsweise weniger ansteigt, dann ergibt sich das Diagramm in Abb. 4: Auch an der extrakorporal perfundierten Niere verursacht Furosemid also einen hypotonen Diuresezuwachs. Es ist der gleiche Befund, den BUCHBORN u. Mitarb. (1964), EDEL u. Mitarb. (1966) auf Grund ihrer Untersuchungen mit Furosemid und Etacrynsäure an der gesunden Niere in situ erhoben. Der hypotone Diurese-Zuwachs bedeutet, daß nicht nur die Natriumrückresorption gehemmt wird, sondern auch die Wasserpermeabilität im distalen Tubulus beeinflußt werden muß.

Die übrigen Funktionsgrößen der perfundierten Niere vor der Gabe von Furosemid, gemessen am Ende einer 12stündigen Perfusionszeit sind in der Tabelle dargestellt:

Tab. 1. Funktionswerte während extrakorporaler Perfusion und nach Transplantation dieser Niere, im Vergleich dazu die entsprechenden Daten der kontralateralen Niere des gleichen Spenders, die unmittelbar einem zweiten Patienten transplantiert worden war.

	Niere extrakorporal	Niere *) transplantiert	kontralaterale Niere nach Transplantation
C_{Inulin} ml/min	51	33	35
$C_{Kreatinin}$ ml/min	53,6	26,3	51
$C_{Harnstoff}$ ml/min	31,2	18,9	30,4
RBF $\frac{C_{PAH}}{E_{PAH}}$	418	248	445
U/P_{Inulin}	11,4	22,8	13,4
U/P_{Osmol}	1,2	1,6	1,3
TC_{H_2O} ml/min	+1,09	+1,06	+1,12

* Mittelwerte aus 4 Einzelbestimmungen.

Die Durchblutung betrug etwa 400 ml/min, die Inulin-Clearance 51 ml/min, die Kreatinin-Clearance 53 ml/min, die Harnstoff-Clearance etwa 60% der Kreatinin-Clearance. Der U/P_{Inulin}- und der U/P_{Osm} unter einer endogenen osmotischen Diurese (infolge Azotämie und Natriurese) zeigt, daß die Niere eine gewisse Konzentrierungsfähigkeit hat. Dabei ist zu berücksichtigen, daß absichtlich eine Polyurie durch quantitativen Ersatz der ausgeschiedenen Flüssigkeits- und Elektrolytmengen aufrecht erhalten wurde. In der dritten Spalte sind zum Vergleich die Funktionswerte der kontralateralen Niere des gleichen Spenders aufgeführt, die einem anderen Patienten sofort transplantiert wurde. Sie zeigen, daß die funktionelle Leistung der perfundierten Niere z. T. diejenige der transplantierten Niere übertrifft. In der zweiten Spalte sind die Parameter der Nierenfunktion einen Tag nach der Transplantation der vorher in der Kammer perfundierten Niere aufgetragen. Die Abnahme der Durchblutung ist vermutlich vorgetäuscht, da nach der Transplantation die PAH-Extraktion nicht bestimmt werden konnte und die somit (unkorrigierte) C_{PAH} kein zuverlässiges Maß für die Durchblutung darstellt.

Die geschilderten Ergebnisse zeigen, daß die extrakorporale Perfusion einer menschlichen Niere mit Hilfe der geschilderten Methode eine normale Durchblutung, ein normales Glomerulumfiltrat und ein normales Ansprechen auf die Gabe von Furosemid ergeben kann.

Zum ersten Mal ist so eine Organkonservierung über viele Stunden und mit weitgehend normaler Funktion möglich geworden. Auch bioptisch-histologisch war nach 14stündiger Perfusion im gezeigten Fall kein pathologischer Befund festzustellen. Neben der Bedeutung für die klinische Nierentransplantation bietet sich mit der von LAVENDER angegebenen Perfusionstechnik ein geeignetes Modell für pathophysiologische Fragestellungen an.

Literatur / References

BUCHBORN, E. und S. ANASTASAKIS: Angriffspunkt und Wirkungsmechanismus von Furosemid am distalen Nephron des Menschen. Klin. Wschr. **42,** 1127 (1964).

EDEL, H., J. EIGLER und E. RENNER: Zum Wirkungsmechanismus der Etacrynsäure. II. Der Einfluß der Etacrynsäure auf das distale Nephron des Menschen. Klin. Wschr. **44,** 421 (1966).

LAVENDER, A. R.: Laboratory and Clinical Studies in Treatment of Chronic Renal Disease. Münchner Dialyse-Ärzte-Treffen, Band 4, S. 5 (1967).

REINHARDT: Sie haben die verhältnismäßig hohen Ausgangswerte von Harnvolumen und Natriumrejektion auf eine durch die Azotämie induzierte osmotische Diurese bezogen. Wäre es denkbar, daß diese Niere eine herabgesetzte Empfindlichkeit gegenüber ADH hat (etwa durch Verlust an 3,5-AMP), und daß zusätzlich eine Störung der Natriumrückgewinnung aufgrund der Ischämie-Zeit vorliegt ? Diese Frage scheint mir berechtigt zu sein, da bei unter ähnlichen Verhältnissen transplantierten Hundenieren (Ischämiezeit 3–5 Min.) das Harnzeitvolumen gegenüber der Kontrolle bei nicht erhöhter Natriurese trotz viel höherer Harnstoff-Plasma-Werte nur kurzfristig anstieg.

DOBBELSTEIN: Dazu ist zu sagen, daß man beim Hund durch Harnstoffinfusionen keine vergleichbare osmotische Diurese wie beim Menschen bekommt, und daß zweitens unser Patient eine subakute Glomerulonephritis mit Ödemen und wahrscheinlich auch einem Natriumüberschuß hatte, so daß dadurch und durch die hohen Harnstoffwerte die großen Ausgangswerte der Diurese zu erklären sind. Zweifellos kann eine Hemmung der proximaltubulären Natriumrückgewinnung zusätzlich bedingt sein durch die Ischämiezeit; sie betrug von der Herausnahme des Organs bis zur Durchströmung in der Kammer 11 min.

REUBI: Sie benötigen sehr dicke Kanülen und Schläuche. Wenn die Niere anschließend nicht transplantiert wird, bedeutet das einen ständigen Shunt von etwa 1 l/min.

DOBBELSTEIN: Das U-Rohr, mit dem der Shunt zwischenzeitlich kurzgeschlossen wird, ist konisch eingeengt, so daß das Durchflußvolumen nicht wesentlich über dem eines konventionellen Scribner-Shunt's liegt.

KRAMER: Wie bringen Sie aber die dicken Kanülen in die Gefäße?

DOBBELSTEIN: Man nimmt nicht die Arteria radialis, distal wie bei einem Scribner-Shunt, sondern kanüliert die Arteria ulnaris oder radialis weiter oben. Außerdem gibt es spezielle Dilatatoren, mit denen die Gefäße auf die erforderliche Weite aufgedehnt werden.

KRAMER: Ist es richtig, daß die Durchblutung der Niere nach der anschließenden Transplantation nur etwa halb so groß war wie vorher?

DOBBELSTEIN: Nach der Transplantation ist keine genaue Messung der Durchblutung möglich. Die rechnerische Verminderung der Durchblutung ist sicher z. T. vorgetäuscht, weil die Extraktion von PAH nur 0,6 betrug. Wenn man die gleiche Größe bei der transplantierten Niere einsetzt, würde sich wieder die ursprüngliche Durchblutung von 400 ml/min ergeben.

KRAMER: In Lüttich, bei Prof. NIZET, haben wir beobachtet, daß Nieren, die eine zeitlang am Hals angeschlossen waren, nach Re-Implantation eine Verschlechterung der Leistung zeigten.

DOBBELSTEIN: Ich darf dazu sagen, daß die Kreatinin-Clearance einen Tag später wieder auf 70–80 ml/min angestiegen ist und der Patient normale Harnstoffwerte hatte. Es handelte sich also um kein endgültiges Absinken der Leistung.

SCHWIEGK: Es ist hoffentlich klar geworden, daß dies keine nierenphysiologischen Experimente sind, sondern daß der Sinn des Verfahrens darin besteht, Zeit zu gewinnen, bis die Kompatibilitätsprüfungen durchgeführt sind und man entscheiden kann, ob diese Niere für den Patienten optimal verträglich ist. Außerdem ist es in der Chirurgie schwierig, zwei Transplantationen gleichzeitig durchzuführen, wenn bei einem Verstorbenen zwei Nieren entfernt werden. Es würde sehr viel einfacher sein, eine oder auch beide Nieren zunächst in eine solche Kammer zu bringen.

Diuretics in Cardiac Diseases

Diuretica bei Herzkrankheiten

A. F. MULLER, A. GRANDCHAMP, R. VEYRAT

Summary: Intermittent diuretic therapy is preferable; secondary hyperaldosteronism is less pronounced. Salt restriction is still the most important prophylactic and therapeutic tool. Interprotation of urinary aldosterone in cardiac patients must be done with circumspection. It does not always reflect the really decisive parameter, which is the biologically active blood level of aldosterone. Renal function, hepatic blood flow and conjugation are important contributing mechanisms. If the blood level cannot be measured directly, it can be calculated by determining the metabolic clearance rate and secretion rate.

The existence of a mineralocorticoid excess can be suspected either on the basis of a low Na/K ratio in the urine or the sweat, the latter is particularly useful in hypertensive patients without edema.

Nicht ohne Bedenken habe ich mich überzeugen lassen, über Diuretica-Therapie bei Herzpatienten zu sprechen. Diese Bedenken beruhen darauf, daß ich keine prinzipiell neuen Befunde vorlegen kann, und mit dem Einverständnis des Herrn Vorsitzenden werde ich mir daher erlauben, nur einige allgemein gültige Ausführungen zu machen.

Die erste Frage betrifft das Problem: Dauertherapie oder intermittierende Therapie? Ich muß gestehen, daß ich bis jetzt noch nie gezwungen war, bei einem Patienten eine Dauertherapie zu verschreiben, denn wir sind eigentlich immer mit einer intermittierenden Therapie ausgekommen. Natürlich unter der Voraussetzung, daß der Patient salzarm ernährt wird, bei salzarm meine ich wirklich salzarm, das heißt, wie heute morgen Frau SHERLOCK sagte, etwa 20 mval Natrium pro Tag. Unter diesen Bedingungen ist es möglich, wenn der Patient einmal seine Ödeme ausgeschwemmt hat, nur einen ganz schwachen Gewichtsanstieg zu verzeichnen, d. h. eine positive Natriumbilanz von etwa 10–15 mval pro Tag, was dann ja mehr als eine Woche verstreichen läßt bevor der Patient ein Kilo zugenommen hat!

Ein anderer Grund, warum wir so stark auf die salzarme Diät setzen, ist der, daß wir glauben, daß durch eine salzarme Diät *allein* der schwächste sekundäre Hyperaldosteronismus entsteht. Es ist bekannt, daß, wenn ein Patient seine Ödeme ausgeschwemmt hat, die Aldosteronproduktion öfters ansteigt, d. h. die Aldosteronexkretion liegt nachher höher als vorher. Dieser sekundäre Anstieg des Aldosterons, beruht sicher zum Teil auf dem Renin-Angiotensin-System. Dieser Anstieg ist um so stärker, je schneller, das heißt je plötzlicher oder je schroffer der Salzverlust eintritt. Nach unseren Erfahrungen ist es daher äußerst ratsam, außer in einer Notfallsituation, nie durch eine hochdosierte Diuretica-Therapie einen schnellen Ödemschwund herbeizuführen, gerade um diesen sekundären Hyperaldosteronismus, wenn möglich, abzuschwächen. Denn es ist klar, daß dieser sekundäre Hyperaldosteronismus in der Rekonvaleszenz-Phase den Patienten gerade dazu prädisponiert, seine Ödeme wieder zu bilden. Wenn Herzpatienten über Monate oder über Jahre verfolgt werden, so wird mit der Zeit der Hyperaldosteronismus immer stärker, und gleichzeitig nimmt die Natriumexkretion im Urin ab. Man kann sich daher fragen, ob es in den fortgeschrittenen, schweren Fällen, wo ein Hyperaldosteronismus sicher besteht, ratsam ist, die Patienten bis zur »Trockenheit«, wenn ich so sagen darf, zu behandeln, oder ob es nicht besser wäre, ein kleines Ödem beizulassen um damit den sekundären Hyperaldosteronismus abzuschwächen. Wenn wir uns auch vollkommen klar sind, daß das Aldosteron nicht der einzige Faktor ist, der zu den Ödemen beiträgt und noch andere Momente in Frage kommen, so scheint es uns dennoch wichtig, daß die Aldosteronproduktion so tief wie möglich gehalten wird.

Wenn zu einer Diuretica-Therapie geschritten werden muß, dann ist es sicher von Wichtigkeit und von Nutzen den Hyperaldosteronismus irgendwie erfassen zu können. Meistens kann man nicht warten, bis im Labor der Aldosteronwert bestimmt wird. Aus diesem Grunde müssen wir über eine Methode verfügen die es uns erlaubt, einen eventuellen Hyperaldosteronismus zu erkennen.

Bevor wir aber auf dieses Problem eingehen, noch einige Worte zur Interpretation des Aldosterons bei Herzpatienten.

Die Bestimmung des Aldosterons im Urin oder die Sekretionsrate sind die zwei Parameter, die bis heute hauptsächlich verfolgt wurden; sind beide erhöht, darf mit Sicherheit auf einen sekundären Hyperaldosteronismus geschlossen werden. Andererseits kennen wir Fälle wo die Urinausscheidung normal und nur die Sekretion erhöht ist. Mit anderen Worten: es gelingt nicht, durch die Urinbestimmung den Hyperaldosteronismus zu erfassen. Das ist einer der Gründe, warum wir uns anfänglich bei den überraschend

Tab. 1. Sekretionsrate, 24 Stunden-Aldosteronausscheidung und Urinnatrium bei 7 Herzpatienten mit generalisierten Ödemen.

			Sekretion µg/24 h	Ausscheidung µg/24 h	Natrium im Urin mÄq/24 h
1	♂	65 Jahre Arteriosklerose	259	8	7
2	♂	75 Jahre Arteriosklerose	170 458 476	4 11 13	45 2 2
3	♂	53 Jahre Koronardurchblutungsstörung	189 214	— —	— —
4	♂	65 Jahre Koronardurchblutungsstörung	134	13	74
5	♂	75 Jahre Syphilitisches Herzleiden	145	7	10
6	♀	52 Jahre Rheumatisches Herzleiden	360	18	<1
7	♀	55 Jahre Rheumatisches Herzleiden (Aszites)	660	27	2

Tab. 2. Herzinsuffizienzen (Nach LUETSCHER und Mitarbeiter – J. clin. Invest. **44**, 356 [1965]).

	Sekretionsrate µg/24 Std.	Metabolic Clearance Rate Liter	Mittlerer Plasma-Aldosteronwert mµg/100 ml
Leichte Fälle	50	1350	4
	103	1470	7
	130	1270	10
Mittelschwere Fälle	160	1610	10
	91	850	11
	288	1270	23
Schwere Fälle	50	630	8
	110	910	12
	110	600	18
	190	775	24
	270	630	43
	400	765	52

tiefen Aldosteronwerten im Urin über die Wichtigkeit des Aldosterons bei Herzpatienten täuschten. Der Grund liegt in einer Veränderung der Beziehung die normalerweise zwischen Exkretion und Sekretion besteht. Diese Situation liegt vor bei Patienten mit Niereninsuffizienz (1). Normalerweise finden wir zwischen 5 und 8% der Gesamtsekretion als 3-Oxoaldosteron im Urin. Bei Herzpatienten liegt dieser Prozentsatz tiefer. Tab. 1 zeigt sieben Herzpatienten mit Ödemen. Vergleicht man nun die Sekretion mit der Exkretion und dem Urinnatrium, so besteht eigentlich keine Korrelation; mit anderen Worten: bei 2 Patienten mit 13 γ Aldosteron im Urin kann sowohl eine Sekretionsrate von 134 als auch von 476 γ für 24 Stunden vorliegen. Auch die Korrelation mit dem Urinnatrium ist nicht durchwegs erhalten, dennoch darf man im allgemeinen bei einem tiefen Wert auf einen Hyperaldosteronismus schließen. Die Resultate in Tab. 1 zeigen jedoch eindeutig die Verschiebung zwischen Sekretion, Exkretion und Urinnatrium. Eine gewisse Niereninsuffizienz, wie sie bei Herzpatienten in Folge der Stauung und/oder der erniedrigten Nierendurchblutung vorliegt, kann dafür sicher teilweise verantwortlich gemacht werden.

Ein zweites Moment, das auch berücksichtigt werden muß, ist die sogenannte »metabolic clearance-rate«, d. h. die Menge Blut in der das durch den Gesamtorganismus pro 24 Stunden metabolisierte Aldosteron enthalten ist (2). Wie bei jeder Clearance-Berechnung wird die 24 Stunden-Menge einer Substanz durch ihren Blutspiegel dividiert, in unserem Falle wird die Aldosteron Sekretionsrate pro 24 Stunden durch den mittleren Plasma-Wert des Aldosterons dividiert. Das daraus resultierende Volumen entspricht der Leberdurchblutung pro 24 Stunden, mit anderen Worten der Blutspiegel des Aldosterons wird nicht nur durch die Sekretionsrate bestimmt, sondern hängt zugleich von der Leberdurchblutung ab. Da letztere bekanntlich bei Herzpatienten stark absinken kann, wird es leicht verständlich, daß bei Herzkranken eine verminderte Sekretionsrate und folglich auch eine erniedrigte Urinausscheidung mit einem erhöhten Aldosteronwert im Blut einhergehen können.

LUETSCHER (3) hat solche Fälle untersucht. Tab. 2 enthält einige Beispiele aus seiner Statistik. Bei schweren Herzinsuffizienzen sind die Sekretionsraten öfters vergleichbar mit den Werten die LUETSCHER bei relativ leichten Fällen gefunden hat; der Aldosteronblutspiegel liegt aber bedeutend höher. Der Grund liegt in der stark erniedrigten Leberdurchblutung. Diese Befunde zeigen eindeutig, welche Bedeutung der Leberdurchblutung bei Herzpatienten zugesprochen werden muß. Die früher bei Herzkranken als »normal« bezeichneten Aldosteron Sekretionsraten und Aldosteron Urinausscheidungen dürfen in dieser neuen Optik nicht mehr als ausschlaggebend bezeichnet werden.

Die dritte Möglichkeit, ebenfalls durch die Leber bedingt, die zu einer Diskrepanz der verschiedenen Aldosteronwerte führt, besteht in einer Verzögerung der Konjugationsprozesse. Damit kommt es zu einer Verlängerung der Halbwertszeit des biologisch aktiven Aldosterons, was zur Folge hat, daß trotz einer an sich normalen Urinausscheidung und Sekretionsrate der Blutspiegel erhöht sein kann. Es ist durchaus möglich, daß Herzpatienten sowohl eine verminderte »metabolic clearance-rate« als auch eine Verzögerung der Konjugation des Aldosterons in der Leber aufweisen. Diese Bemerkungen zeigen einmal mehr, wie notwendig es ist, den Hyperaldosteronismus direkt zu erfassen. Die Ideallösung wäre die mehrmalige Bestimmung des Aldosterons im Blut, was heute auf breiter Basis noch nicht realisierbar ist. Wir müssen uns somit mit indirekten Methoden begnügen:

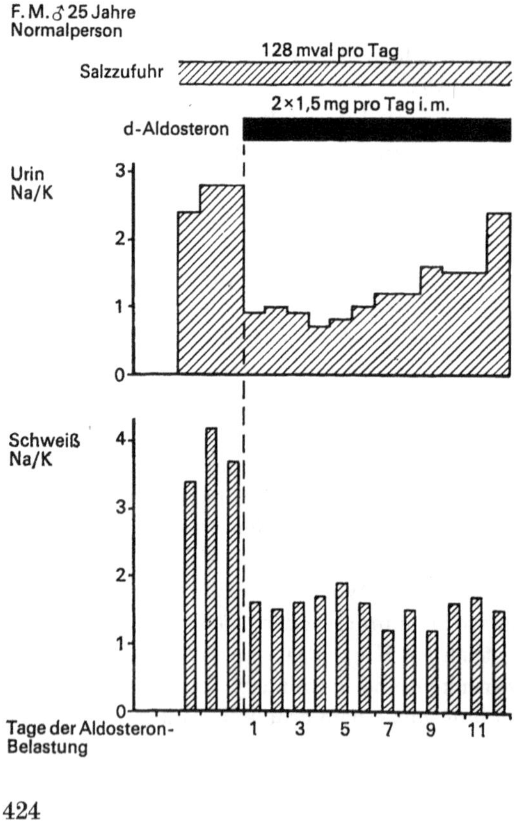

Abb. 1. Schweiß und Urin Na/K Quotient bei einer Normalperson unter Aldosteronbelastung.

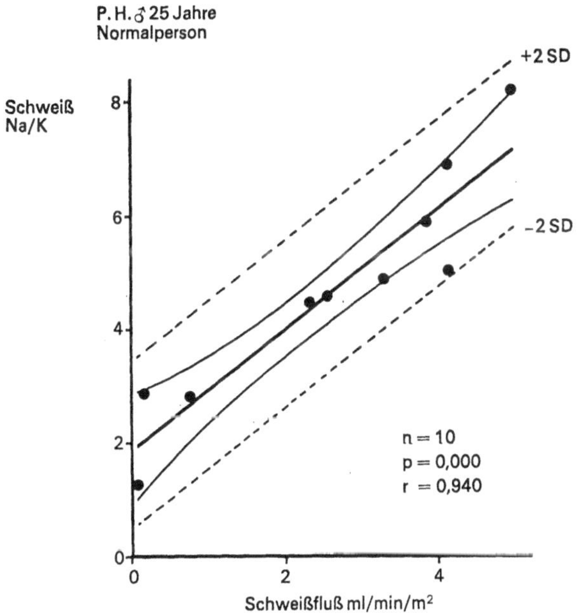

Abb. 2. Abhängigkeit des Na/K Quotienten vom Schweißfluß bei einer Normalperson. Der Schweißfluß wurde künstlich (Pilocarpin Ionophorese) variiert.

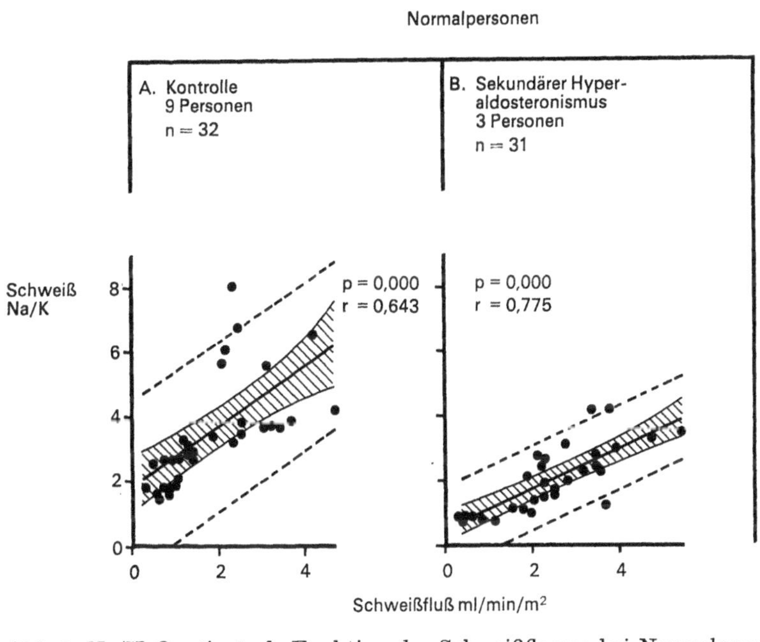

Abb. 3. Na/K Quotient als Funktion des Schweißflusses bei Normalpersonen, salzreich und salzarm (sekundärer Hyperaldosteronismus) ernährt.

Zwei Wege sind gangbar:
1. Die Bestimmung im Urin des Natriums und/oder des Na/K Quotienten.
2. Die Bestimmung im Schweiß des Na/K Quotienten als Funktion des Schweißflusses.

Beim normalen Individuum, wegen des sogenannten »escape phenomenon« (4), kann die Urinnatrium-Ausscheidung trotz vermehrter Aldosteronproduktion erhöht sein. Beim Ödempatienten hingegen besteht eine gewisse Korrelation zwischen dem Aldosteron und dem Urinnatrium, d. h. eine erhöhte Aldosteronproduktion geht mit einer erniedrigten Urinnatriumausscheidung einher. Andererseits ist aber nicht jede tiefe Natriumausscheidung unbedingt ein Beweis eines Hyperaldosteronismus. Wir haben schon vor Jahren darauf hingewiesen, daß die Urinnatrium-Konzentration zu einem gewissen Maße als prognostisches Zeichen der Ansprechbarkeit der Diuretica verwendet werden kann (5). Bei ein und demselben Patienten sinkt über die Jahre die Urinnatriumkonzentration um so tiefer, als sich die Tendenz zur Ödembildung verstärkt. Wenn am Anfang ein Herzpatient auf Salzentzug und Salidiuretica anspricht, so sind im späteren Verlauf Furosemid oder Etacrynsäure notwendig. Manchmal mußte sogar zur Kombinationstherapie mit Aldactone geschritten werden. Eines steht sicher fest: je höher die Urinnatriumausscheidung am Anfang, um so leichter und erfolgreicher wird jegliche Diuretica-Therapie sein. Von der Sicht des kritischen klinischen Pharmakologen dürften bei der Beurteilung der Wirksamkeit eines Diureticums, eigentlich nur diejenigen Resultate verglichen werden, die bei Patienten mit relativ tiefer Natriumausscheidung gewonnen wurden.

Als zweite Möglichkeit einen Aldosteronismus zu erfassen, dient die Elektrolytbestimmung im Schweiß (6). Diese Methode ist bedeutend zuverlässiger als die Natriumkonzen-

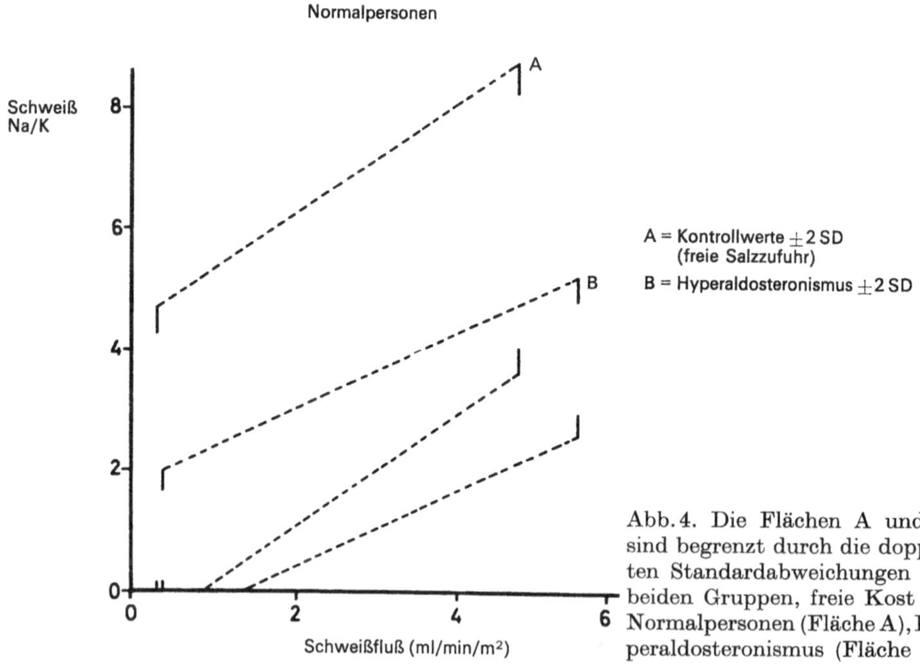

Abb. 4. Die Flächen A und B sind begrenzt durch die doppelten Standardabweichungen der beiden Gruppen, freie Kost bei Normalpersonen (Fläche A), Hyperaldosteronismus (Fläche B).

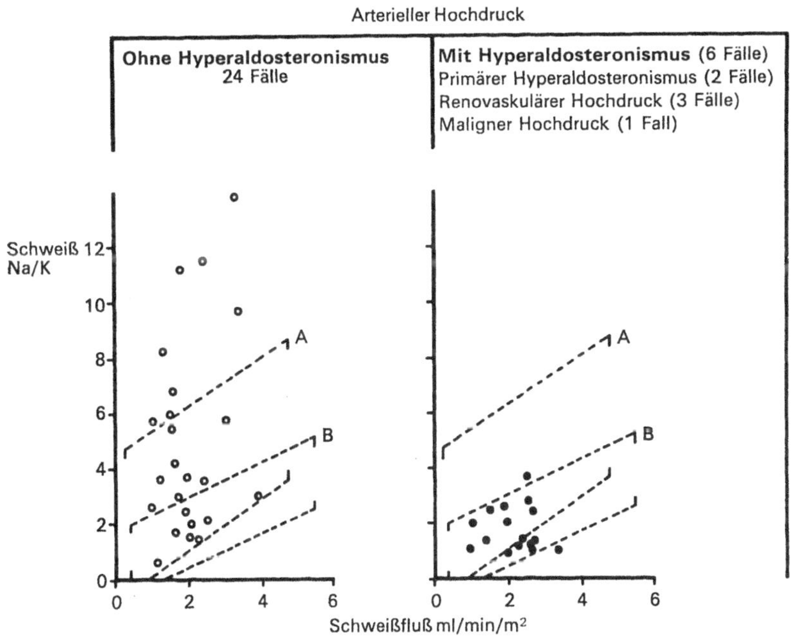

Abb. 5. Schweiß Na/K Quotienten bei Hochdruckkranken ohne Aldosteronismus (Aldosteronexkretion unter 14 µg/24 Std.) und 6 Fällen von sicherem Hyperaldosteronismus.

tration im Urin die von mehreren Faktoren abhängt. Besonders wertvoll sind die Schweißbestimmungen bei Patienten ohne Ödeme, die ja bekanntlich unter einer Mineralocorticoidbelastung im Urin das sogenannte »escape«-Phänomen aufweisen. Abb. 1 zeigt den Verlauf der Na/K Quotienten in Schweiß und Urin unter exogener Aldosteron-Zufuhr bei einer Normalperson. Anfänglich kommt es zu einem Abfall beider Quotienten; nach einigen Tagen nimmt die Urinnatriumausscheidung trotz der Aldosteron-Verabreichung wieder zu, was gleichzeitig zu einem Anstieg des Na/K Quotienten führt. Dank eines Kompensationsmechanismus entziehen sich die Nieren (escape) der Aldosteronwirkung, nicht aber die Schweißdrüsen (7). Es ist aber äußerst wichtig, nicht nur den Na/K Quotienten allein zu berücksichtigen, sondern als Funktion des Schweißflusses, wie Abb. 2 deutlich zeigt. Wenn bei der selben Person der Schweißfluß variiert, so wechselt auch der Na/K Quotient in gleichem Maße, was die direkte Abhängigkeit der beiden Werte beweist.

Abb. 3 zeigt die Resultate bei Normalpersonen mit und ohne Hyperaldosteronismus, d. h. bei salzarmer und normaler Kost. Die Regressionslinien mit ihren Hüllen (schraffierte Flächen) sind statistisch signifikant verschieden, hingegen die Flächen A und B die den beiden Doppelstandardabweichungen entsprechen, überschneiden sich teilweise (Abb. 4). Es ist somit mit dem Schweißtest nicht möglich, mit Sicherheit einen Hyperaldosteronismus zu diagnostizieren oder vorsichtiger ausgedrückt, einen Hypermineralocortizismus; denn andere Steroide wie z. B. Corticosteron haben neben ihrer Glucocorticoid-Wirkung auch einen mineralocorticoiden Effekt (8).

Es ist zu sagen, daß dieser Schweißtest vor allem im Hinblick auf Hochdruckkranke entwickelt wurde, wo man sich nicht auf das Urinnatrium verlassen kann (Abb. 5). Er ist aber ebenso zuverlässig bei Ödempatienten zusammen mit dem Urinnatrium Kalium Quotienten. Der Schweißtest ist aber bei jenen Ödempatienten ausschließlich verwendbar, die Diuretica bekommen haben. Damit kann ein unter Diuretica-Therapie verstärkter Hyperaldosteronismus jederzeit leicht erfaßt werden: Eine Erkenntnis die sowohl therapeutisch als auch prognostisch von Wichtigkeit sein kann.

Inwieweit Renin- oder sogar Angiotensinbestimmungen bei Herzpatienten Aufschluß geben können, muß noch abgewartet werden. In aller Wahrscheinlichkeit werden sie kaum den Aldosteronbestimmungen überlegen sein.

Zum Schluß darf sicher noch erwähnt werden, daß trotz Diuretica Digitalis verabreicht werden muß; besonders bei Rhythmusstörungen können sehr schöne Erfolge eintreten, ohne daß die salzarme Kost durch Diuretica verstärkt werden muß.

Eine andere Situation, wo Diuretica allein nicht zum Erfolg führen können, sind Patienten mit Cor pulmonale und starkem Sauerstoffmangel. Erst die künstliche Beatmung mit Korrektion des Sauerstoffdefizits verleiht den Diuretica wieder ihre Ansprechbarkeit. Manchmal sind sie sogar nicht mehr nötig (Abb. 6 und 7). (9).

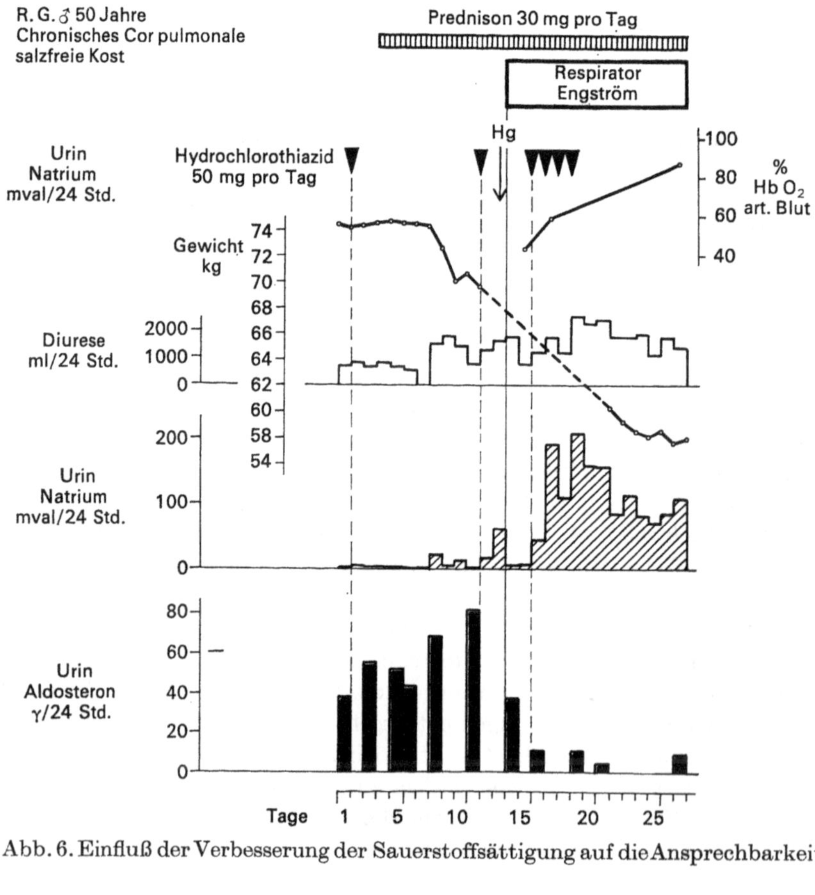

Abb. 6. Einfluß der Verbesserung der Sauerstoffsättigung auf die Ansprechbarkeit der Diuretica.

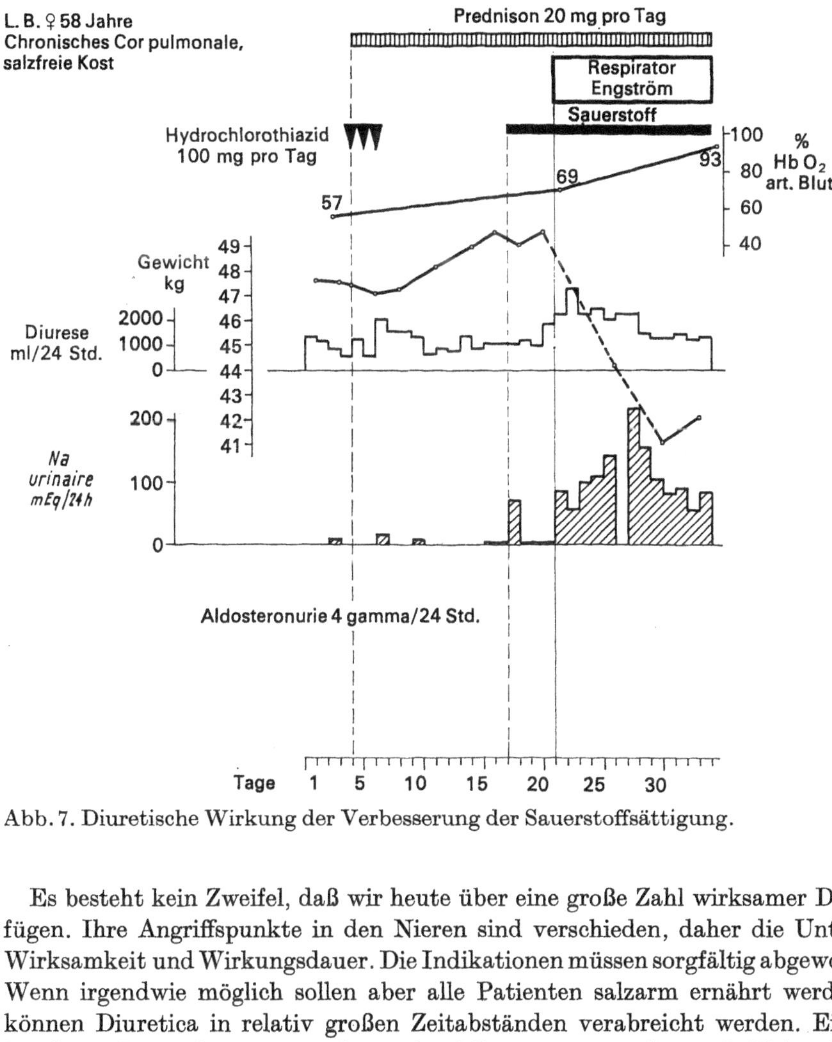

Abb. 7. Diuretische Wirkung der Verbesserung der Sauerstoffsättigung.

Es besteht kein Zweifel, daß wir heute über eine große Zahl wirksamer Diuretica verfügen. Ihre Angriffspunkte in den Nieren sind verschieden, daher die Unterschiede in Wirksamkeit und Wirkungsdauer. Die Indikationen müssen sorgfältig abgewogen werden. Wenn irgendwie möglich sollen aber alle Patienten salzarm ernährt werden, dadurch können Diuretica in relativ großen Zeitabständen verabreicht werden. Eine ununterbrochene Dauertherapie ist dann ebenfalls nie notwendig und Elektrolytstörungen können vermieden werden. Digitalis und, wenn nötig, Sauerstoff bleiben neben salzarmer Ernährung und Ruhe die Grundpfeiler jeder Therapie bei Herzpatienten.

Literatur / References

1. A. F. Muller and E. L. Manning: Structure and metabolism of corticoids. Academic Press, p. 147, 1964. Ed. J. R. Pasqualini and M. F. Jayle.
2. J. F. Tait, B. Little, S. A. S. Tait and C. Flood: J. clin. Invest. **41,** 2093 (1962).
3. C. A. Camargo, A. J. Dowdy, E. W. Hancock and J. A. Luetscher: J. clin. Invest. **44,** 356 (1965).
4. A. S. Relman and W. B. Schwartz: Yale J. biol. Med. **24,** 540 (1952).
5. R. Veyrat: Helv. med. Acta **29,** 311 (1962).

6. W. C. CAGE and R. L. DOBSON: J. clin. Invest. **44**, 1270 (1965).
7. F. MANTERO, A. QUOIDBACH, R. VEYRAT and R. S. MACH: Schweiz. med. Wschr. **97**, 1271 (1967).
8. A. GRANDCHAMP, J. R. SCHERRER, R. VEYRAT and A. F. MULLER: Helv. med. Acta, 1968 (im Druck).
9. A. CRUCHAUD, O. KORALNIK, A. F. MULLER et R. VEYRAT: Rev. méd. Suisse rom. **80**, 411 (1960).

KRÜCK: Ich möchte doch ein Wort zur Ehrenrettung des Natrium-Kalium-Quotienten bei der Diagnostik eines mit Flüssigkeitsretention einhergehenden sekundären Aldosteronismus sagen. Bei Ödemzuständen finden wir immer eine strenge umgekehrte Korrelation zwischen Aldosteron-Sekretionsrate bzw. Plasma-Aldosteron-Konzentration und Natrium-Kalium-Quotienten im Urin. Dies gilt nicht mehr, wenn ein »escape«-Phänomen eintritt, wie beim sekundären Aldosteronismus, bei Nierenarterienstenose und beim Conn-Syndrom. Dann liegt aber auch kein Ödem vor.

MULLER: Ich bin ganz einverstanden. Wir haben den ganzen Versuch im Hinblick auf das »escape«-Phänomen geplant, und ich habe mir erlaubt, diese Resultate hier »einzuschleichen«.

WESSELS: Wie wird die Schweißgewinnung durchgeführt ? Und dann vielleicht eine Ergänzung: Wir haben uns mit dem Kationenflux an Erythrozyten beschäftigt und unter anderem nach Behandlung mit Aldosteron eine deutliche Beschleunigung des Natriumein- und -ausstroms der Erythrozyten gefunden. Ein Hyperaldosteronismus könnte demnach evtl. auch durch die Analyse des Natriumtransportes der Erythrozyten diagnostiziert werden.

MULLER: Der Schweiß wird unter Standardbedingungen mittels Pilokarpin-Iontophorese gewonnen; die Reproduzierbarkeit der Methode ist sehr gut. Es ist allerdings erforderlich, den Schweißfluß mit in Betracht zu ziehen.

KRAMER: An den Speicheldrüsen hat man doch einen ähnlichen Indikator ? Dort ist die Flux-Abhängigkeit der Kationenkonzentrationen gut bekannt. Ändert sich eigentlich der Quotient, weil mehr Natrium zurückgehalten wird, oder weil mehr Kalium abgegeben wird ? Wie sind die Konzentrationen ?

MULLER: Maßgeblich für den Quotienten ist vor allem das Verhalten des Natriumgehaltes. Die Natriumkonzentration im Schweiß liegt bei den meisten Patienten zwischen 10 und 60 mval/l, gelegentlich bei Gesunden aber vor allem bei Mukoviszidose-Patienten auch höher.

BAETHMANN: Sie haben das »escape«-Phänomen bei Patienten nach 6–8 Tagen beobachtet. Wir haben an Ratten mit 6–7mal höheren Aldosteron-Dosen bereits nach 6 Std. ein »escape«-Phänomen gefunden. Beruht dies auf einer unterschiedlichen Ansprechbarkeit der Ratte gegenüber dem Aldosteron, im Vergleich zum Menschen ?

MULLER: Die Ratte kenne ich nur aus einer gewissen »Distanz«. Beim Menschen kann man das »escape«-Phänomen verstärken durch Pitressin, wie RELMAN zeigte, oder auch durch eine sehr hohe Natriumzufuhr.

KRAMER: Herr ELLINGHAUS hat in unserem Institut entsprechende Untersuchungen am Hund durchgeführt. Bei niedriger Natriumzufuhr tritt das »escape«-Phänomen etwa nach 4 Tagen, bei hoher Natriumzufuhr (15 mval/kg/Tg) bereits nach 1 oder 2 Tagen ein.

HUSMANN: Die Diskrepanz zwischen den Sekretionsraten und den Ausscheidungswerten von Aldosteron kann teilweise auch damit zusammenhängen, daß der Abbau des Aldosterons geändert sein könnte in Richtung Tetrahydro-Aldosteron. Haben Sie Untersuchungen angestellt, in denen auch Tetrahydro-Aldosteron mit erfaßt wurde?

MULLER: Wir haben nicht sehr viele Beobachtungen. Vielleicht kann Herr KOCZOREK etwas dazu sagen.

KOCZOREK: Wir haben bei unseren früheren Untersuchungen über den Einfluß von Störungen der Leberfunktionen auf das Ausscheidungsmuster der verschiedenen Aldosteronfraktionen im Urin das in der Leber durch enzymatische Hydrierung gebildete Tetrahydro-Aldosteron nicht mit erfaßt. Wir konnten aber durch differenzierte Bestimmungen des freien Aldosterons und des sog. Δ^4-3-Oxo-Konjugates bei Leberkranken im Vergleich zu gesunden Probanden und durch die Bestimmung des Ausscheidungsverhältnisses dieser beiden nicht metabolisierten Aldosteronfraktionen vor und nach exogen zugeführtem, synthetischen Aldosteron es wahrscheinlich machen, daß bei einer Beeinträchtigung des hepatischen Aldosteronmetabolismus mehr freies Aldosteron plus Δ^4-3-Oxo-Konjugat auf Kosten der Fraktion des Tetrahydroaldosterons (und vermutlich auch anderer Metaboliten) ausgeschieden wird. Metabolisch bedingte Veränderungen der einzelnen im Urin erfaßbaren Aldosteronfraktionen sind also durchaus möglich.

MULLER: Bei der Leberinsuffizienz kann es zu einem relativ starken Anstieg des 3-oxo-Konjugates auf Kosten des Tetrahydro-Aldosterons kommen. Bei den Fällen mit eingeschränkter Nierenfunktion fanden wir, daß die Parallelität im Verhalten des 3-oxo-Konjugates und des Tetrahydro-Aldosterons gewahrt war, d. h. wir hatten eine Ausscheidung im Urin von etwa 4–5mal mehr Tetrahydro-Aldosteron. Wir nehmen daher an, daß bei der Niereninsuffizienz beide Fraktionen im Verhältnis zur Sekretion vermindert ausgeschieden werden.

KOCZOREK: Bei den eben erwähnten Untersuchungen haben wir außerdem Befunde erarbeitet, die die Ausführungen von Herrn MULLER über die im Verhältnis zur Sekretion verminderte Elimination des Tetrahydro-Aldosterons und des Δ_4-3-Oxo-Konjugates bei Niereninsuffizienz durchaus ergänzen. Bei Patienten mit Nierenerkrankungen hatten wir nämlich nach Aldosteroninjektion keine nennenswerte Vermehrung der Ausscheidung von freiem Aldosteron plus Δ^4-3-Oxo-Konjugat nachweisen können. (KOCZOREK, KH. R. und H. P. WOLFF: Verh. Dtsch. Ges. Inn. Med. **65**, Kongr. 1959, Seite 614; KOCZOREK, KH. R.: Diskussionsbemerkungen in »Diurese und Diuretica. Ein Internationales Symposion«. Springer-Verlag **1959**, Seite **342**, **344** und **345**; KOCZOREK, KH. R. Aldosteron-Metabolismus und Leber. In: Aktuelle Probleme der Hepatologie. Thieme-Verlag, Stuttgart, 1962, Seite 149).

Clinical Application of Diuretics in Cardiac Diseases

Klinische Anwendung der Diuretica bei Erkrankungen des Herzens*)

H. JAHRMÄRKER, Kh. R. KOCZOREK, H. AVENHAUS, H. GROHMANN

Summary: Observations on acute diuresis after a single high dose of a fast acting diuretic (ethacrynic acid or furosemide) are reported on in the following and some problems in diuretic therapy of chronic heart failure are discussed. The therapeutic effect of an acute diuresis in heart failure depends upon loss of volume. Blood volume (J^{131}-albumine-method) was reduced during the first hours of acute diuresis by $^1/_2$ to 1 liter; extravasal volume (calculated from cumulative urine volume and reduction of blood volume) was reduced at the same time by 1 to 2 liters. After 24 hours the blood volume was still reduced compared to the intial value. Simultaneous determinations of blood volume and central venous pressure indicate changes in volume extensibility of the low pressure system. Lowering venous pressure in pulmonary edema is the main objective of an acute diuresis in heart patients. Activation of sodium retention may be an unwanted reaction. Also in acute diuresis the plasma renin activity (PRA) behaved differently depending on whether the patient was in a phase of fluid loss or fluid retention. Lowering of an elevated PRA on one hand and a prolonged increase of PRA on the other has been observed. The relation of sodium- to potassium- and chloride-concentrations in the urine corresponded to the PRA. In the usual diuretic therapy of chronic heart failure, the influence on the electrolyte balance is decisive. Avoidance of electrolyte disturbances, the use of glucocorticoids supplementary to the diuretic therapy and the problem of effects of the diuretic therapy on the heart are briefly discussed.

Die diuretische Therapie bei Ödemkrankheiten und insbesondere bei der chronischen Herzinsuffizienz hat die Aufgabe, die *Elektrolytbilanz* des Organismus so zu verändern, daß retiniertes Salz und Wasser eliminiert und dabei eine Störung der Elektrolytzusammensetzung vermieden oder ggf. korrigiert wird. Bei der akuten Diurese, die insbesondere zur Therapie des Lungenödems in Frage kommt, steht dagegen die *hämodynamische Wirkung des Volumenverlustes* im Vordergrund. Die aderlaßähnliche Wirkung der akuten Diurese ist seit Pugh u. Wyndham (1949) bekannt. Sie ist aktuell geworden, seit mit dem Furosemid und der Etacrynsäure nicht nur besonders *stark*-, sondern auch besonders *rasch*wirkende Diuretica zur Verfügung stehen. In diesem Beitrag sollen einige Gesichtspunkte einerseits der akuten, und andererseits der chronischen Anwendung der Diuretica bei der Herzinsuffizienz besprochen werden.

A. Zur akuten Diurese

1. Methodik. Die Untersuchungen wurden bei Patienten mit chronischer Herzinsuffizienz in verschiedenen Stadien des Ödemzustandes durchgeführt. Es wurde im akuten Versuch

*) Mit Unterstützung der Deutschen Forschungsgemeinschaft.

nach einer Vorbeachtungszeit die Wirkung von Furosemid (40–80 mg i. v., 5 Pat.) bzw. Etacrynsäure (75–100 mg i. v., 2 Pat.) während 24 Std. verfolgt, während der ersten 6 Std. in kurzfristigen zeitlichen Abständen. Dabei wurden simultan bestimmt: Urinvolumen (Blasenkatheter), Elektrolytausscheidung, zentraler Venendruck (Venen- oder Herzkatheter), Blutvolumen (J^{131}-Albumin-Methode, »Volemetron«, Serienbestimmungen mit einer Mischungszeit von 10, 15 und 20 min), Plasma-Renin-Aktivität (nach BOUCHER, VEYRAT, CHAMPLAIN u. GENEST 1964, eigene obere Normgrenze 20 ng/l/min, KOCZOREK u. Mitarb. 1967), Hämatokrit und Serumeiweißkonzentration, Plasma- und Erythrocyten-Elektrolyte (wie in früheren Untersuchungen, JAHRMÄRKER, v. BUBNOFF u. RIECKER 1961), Blutdruck und Herzfrequenz. Die Untersuchungen erfolgten bei unveränderter Basistherapie (Herzglykoside und Natriumrestriktion je nach Lage des Falles, bei allen Patienten unter Antikoagulantien) am horizontal gelagerten Patienten, während der ersten 6 Std. unter Grundumsatzbedingungen (Volumenersatz der abgenommenen Blutproben durch frisches Vollblut und isotone Laevuloselösung). Über einen Teil der Beobachtungen wurde bereits kürzlich berichtet (JAHRMÄRKER, AVENHAUS, GROHMANN u. KOCZOREK 1968).

2. *Volumenveränderungen*. Die Volumenveränderungen der verschiedenen Flüssigkeitsräume des Organismus sollen an einem Beispiel erläutert werden. Abb. 1 zeigt den Verlauf bei einem Patienten (A.F.), bei dem die akute Diurese die Ausschwemmung einleitete. Die große Diurese setzte sich in diesem Fall noch während der nächsten Tage, also über die Diuretica-Wirkung hinaus, weiter fort. In der untersten Spalte der Abbildung ist das *Urinvolumen* angegeben, welches nach Furosemid i. v. innerhalb 5 min stark zunahm und nach 15 min 20 ml/min erreichte, mit einer maximalen Natriurese von 2400 μval/min. In der zweituntersten Spalte ist das kumulative Urinvolumen dargestellt, welches in $3^1/_2$ Std. 2,5 l betrug, begleitet von einer entsprechenden Abnahme des Körpergewichts.

In der gleichen Zeit ($3^1/_2$ Std.) ging das *Blutvolumen* von 6,9 auf 5,95 l zurück. Es handelt sich dabei um die Abnahme des *Plasma*volumens mit entsprechendem Hämatokritanstieg. Diese Blutvolumenabnahme von fast 1 l innerhalb weniger Stunden liegt in der Größenordnung entsprechender Beobachtungen von SCHNEIDER (1966) (kompensierte Hypertoniker, Furosemid), SAMET u. BERNSTEIN (1968) (digitalisbehandelte Herzinsuffizienz, Etacrynsäure) und DAVIDOV, KAKAVIATOS u. FINNERTY (1967) (therapieresistente Herzinsuffizienz, Furosemid). – Nach 24 Std. war das Blutvolumen mit 6,4 l um $^1/_2$ l geringer als der Ausgangswert.

In der Abbildung ist die *Abnahme* des Blutvolumens ($\triangle$ Blutvolumen, dunkel schraffiert) vom kumulativen Urinvolumen abgezogen. Da der Patient während der ersten 6 Std. unter Grundumsatzbedingungen ohne Flüssigkeitszufuhr von außen war, läßt sich überschlagsmäßig sagen, daß die Differenz zwischen kumulativem Urinvolumen und Blutvolumen-Abnahme der *Flüssigkeitsgabe aus dem extravasalen Raum* entspricht, in erster Linie aus dem interstitiellen Raum, aber auch aus dem intrazellulären Raum. Die errechnete Flüssigkeitsabgabe aus dem extravasalen Raum betrug hier nach $3^1/_2$ Std. 1,65 l. (In 24 Std. ergab sich eine Flüssigkeitsbewegung von 5,2 l, die jedoch nicht ausschließlich dem Wasserbestand des Organismus entstammte, sondern nach der 6. Std. zum Teil auch von oraler Flüssigkeitsaufnahme herrührte.) Am *Erythrocyten*-Wassergehalt (am Kopf der Abbildung eingezeichnet) war in allen Versuchen ein prompter Rückgang zu beobachten. Bewegende Kräfte für diese Flüssigkeitsverschiebung sind 1. der onkotische Druck des Plasmas, der mit der Ultrafiltration des Urins etwas ansteigen muß, und 2. der Rückgang des Venen- und Kapillardrucks. Beides führt zum Nachströmen von Flüssigkeit aus dem Interstitium in die Blutbahn. Zum Vergleich sei angeführt, daß KAUFMANN u. MÜLLER (1958) an Gesunden bei Aderlaßversuchen, also ohne primäre Änderung des onkotischen Drucks, einen teilweisen Ausgleich des verlorenen Blutvolumens beobachteten, der in der Größe des Plasmaverlustes lag und bereits innerhalb 20 min beendet war.

3. Hämodynamische Veränderungen. Der *zentrale Venendruck* zeigte regelmäßig einen leichten, bei erhöhten Ausgangswerten meist einen deutlichen Rückgang. Dies steht in

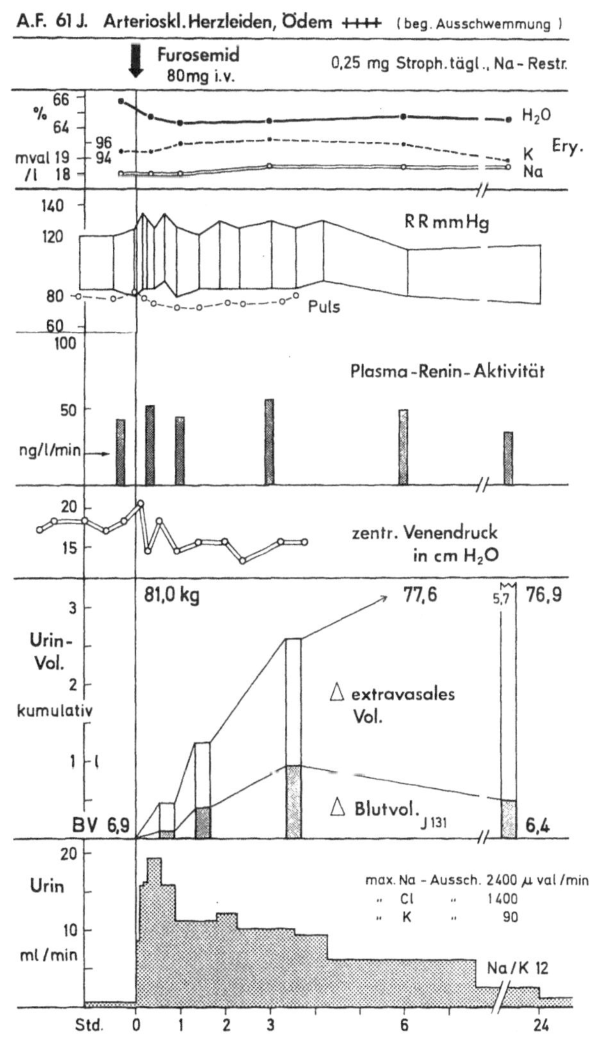

Abb. 1. Synoptische Darstellung der Veränderungen bei akuter Diurese. Pat. A. F., 61 J., arteriosklerotisches Herzleiden, konstante Basistherapie (Bettruhe, Strophanthin, Natriumrestriktion), Ödem ++++, mit der akuten Diurese Beginn der Ausschwemmung. Untersuchung im Liegen, während der ersten 6 Std. unter Grundumsatzbedingungen. Urinvolumen in ml/min sowie kumulativ dargestellt. BV = Blutvolumen (J^{131}-Albuminmethode). △ Blutvolumen = Abnahme des Blutvolumens gegenüber dem Ausgangswert in Liter (hier allein durch Plasmavolumenabnahme bedingt). △ extravasales Volumen = Flüssigkeitseinstrom aus dem extravasalen Raum in die Blutbahn, errechnet als Differenz von kumulativem Urinvolumen und Blutvolumenabnahme. Ery = Erythrocyten; Wassergehalt in Gewichts % und Elektrolytgehalt in mval/l Erythrocytensediment. Auswertung siehe Text. (Erweiterte Darstellung nach JAHRMÄRKER, AVENHAUS, GROHMANN u. KOCZOREK 1968).

Übereinstimmung mit anderen Beobachtungen (NASH, FITZ, WILSON, KIRKENDALL u. KIOSCHOS 1966). Im Fall der Abb. 1 ging der mittlere rechte Vorhofdruck im Mittel von 18 auf 15 cm H_2O zurück. Eine Blutvolumenabnahme betrifft ganz überwiegend das Niederdrucksystem, dessen Volumendehnbarkeit nach GAUER u. HENRY (1956) 7 cm Wasser pro 1000 ml Volumenänderung beträgt. Ein Druckabfall von 3 cm H_2O bei einer Volumenverminderung von fast 1 l liegt unter diesem Wert, während z. B. bei einer anderen Patientin (A.M.) bei einer Blutvolumenabnahme von 8 auf 7 l der Venendruck von 24 auf 15 cm H_2O abfiel. Es ergeben sich also bei einzelnen Herzinsuffizienz-Patienten Hinweise auf eine veränderte Volumendehnbarkeit im Niederdrucksystem.

Das Herzzeitvolumen wurde in den eigenen Untersuchungen nicht bestimmt. PUGH u. WYNDHAM (1949) beobachteten bei einem Patienten mit Diuretica-bedingtem Abfall des stark erhöhten Venendrucks eine gleichzeitige Zunahme der Auswurfleistung. Dieser Effekt ist jedoch nicht regelmäßig zu erwarten und wurde z. B. von FRISK, WERKÖ u. WRANGE (1952, ebenfalls Hg-Diuretica) nicht beobachtet. Ähnliches ist von Orthostase- und Aderlaßversuchen bekannt (OCKENGA, PABST u. STEIN 1968).

Blutdruck und Herzfrequenz zeigten in der Regel keine wesentliche Veränderung oder einen leichten Abfall. Ausnahmsweise war jedoch auch ein abweichendes Verhalten zu beobachten. Bei der in Abb. 2 dargestellten Patientin W.D. kam es zu einem raschen Anstieg besonders des diastolischen Blutdrucks mit Verkleinerung der Blutdruckamplitude. Es liegt nahe, dieses Verhalten als Reaktion der Pressorezeptoren auf Volumenentzug zu deuten. Es handelte sich bei dieser Patientin um eine Herzinsuffizienz, bei der die Ausschwemmung im wesentlichen bereits zuvor erfolgt war; es bestanden noch leichte Ödeme, das Körpergewicht war aber nicht mehr rückläufig. Auf das Verhalten der hormonalen Gegenregulation in diesem Fall wird später eingegangen.

4. Plasma-Renin-Aktivität. Das Verhalten der Plasma-Renin-Aktivität bei akuter Diurese war nicht einheitlich. Im Fall der Abb. 1 war der Ausgangswert infolge Herzinsuffizienz und Natriumrestriktion erhöht. Im Verlauf der akuten Diurese war jedoch *kein* wesentlicher weiterer Anstieg der Plasma-Renin-Aktivität mehr zu beobachten, nach 24 Std. vielmehr ein Abfall. Der Na/K-Quotient im Urin betrug in der Sammelperiode nach 24 Std. 12, so daß man annehmen kann, daß auch kein Aldosteronanstieg erfolgte.

Beim *Gesunden* dagegen ist bei akuter Diureticawirkung ein Anstieg der Plasma-Renin-Aktivität charakteristisch (ROSENTHAL, BOUCHER, NOWACZYNSKI u. GENEST 1968, 10 Fälle, Furosemid; FRAZER, BROWN, ISAAC, LEVER u. ROBERTSON 1965, 2 Fälle, Furosemid; BROWN, DAVIS u. JOHNSTON 1966), der bereits nach einer Stunde maximal ist und von einem Anstieg des Aldosteronspiegels gefolgt wird. Dies Verfahren wird bekanntlich als Provokationstest z. B. bei Verdacht auf renovasculären Hochdruck verwendet. Über den Anstieg der Aldosteronsekretion wurde auch von ESPINER, TUCCI, JAGGER, PAUK u. LAULER (1967) berichtet (Etacrynsäure, 7 Gesunde), wobei Na-Restriktion die Reaktion verstärkte und der Na/K-Quotient im Urin eine gute Übereinstimmung mit der Aldosteronsekretion zeigte. Der Auslösemechanismus des Plasma-Renin-Anstiegs bei akuter Diurese ist strittig oder kann von verschiedenen Punkten ausgehen; so konnten MEYER, MÉNARD, ALEXANDER u. MILLIEZ (1966) den Reninanstieg durch Volumenersatz mittels Periston verhindern (4 Gesunde, Etacrynsäure), während NASH, ROSTORFER, BAILIE, WATHEN u. SCHNEIDER (1968) experimentelle Hinweise für eine Abhängigkeit von der filtrierten Natriummenge fanden. Im übrigen wird auf Übersichten zur Regulation der Reninsekretion verwiesen (KLAUS 1967, GROSS 1968).

5. Abhängigkeit der Reaktionsweise von der Krankheitsphase. Die Abb. 1 und 2 sind Beispiele für ein gegensätzliches Verhalten der Plasma-Renin-Aktivität bei der akuten Diurese. Im ersten Fall handelte es sich um einen schwer ödematösen, aber ausschwemmungsbereiten Patienten, bei dem eine starke Diurese in Gang kam, die Blutdruckamplitude sich nicht wesentlich veränderte und die Plasma-Renin-Aktivität von einem erhöhten Ausgangswert aus eine mehr fallende Tendenz zeigte. Dies Verhalten der Plasma-Renin-Aktivität bzw. der Aldosteronsekretion wird auch im chronischen Verlauf der Herzinsuffizienz bei erfolgreicher Ausschwemmung und Rekompensation beobachtet

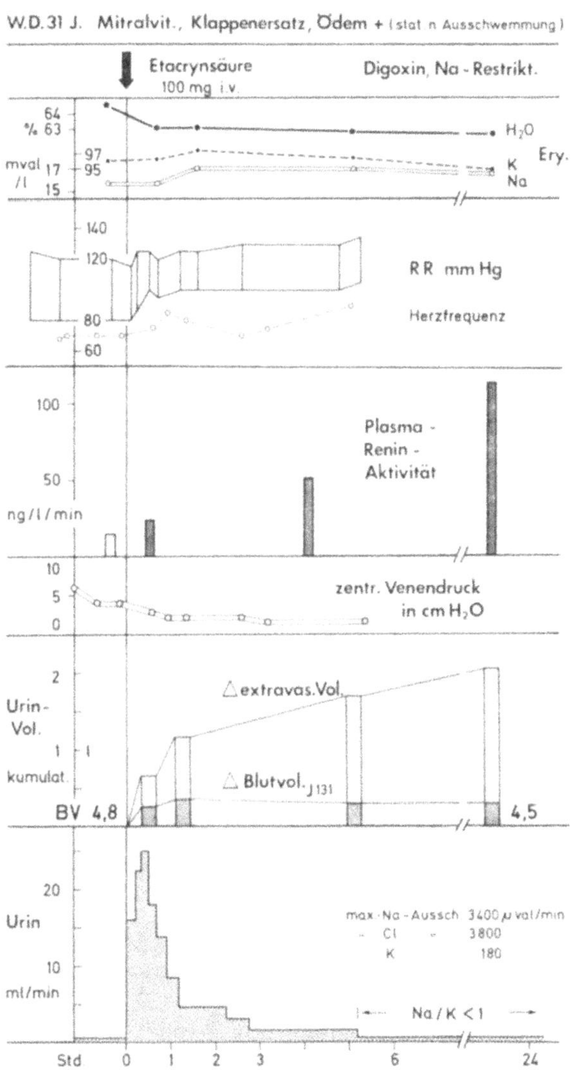

Abb. 2. Patient W. D., 31 J., rheumatisches Herzleiden. Ödem +, stationärer Zustand nach im wesentlichen bereits erfolgter Ausschwemmung, konstante Basistherapie mit Bettruhe, Digoxin, Natriumrestriktion. Darstellung wie Abb. 1, Auswertung siehe Text. (Erweiterte Darstellung nach JAHRMÄRKER, AVENHAUS, GROHMANN u. KOCZOREK 1968)

(Wolff 1968; Truniger u. Siegenthaler 1960; Espiner, Tucci, Lauler u. Jagger 1967). Bei der in Abb. 2 dargestellten Patientin, die sich in relativ stationärem Zustand nach im wesentlichen bereits erfolgter Ausschwemmung befand, war der diuretische Effekt dagegen wesentlich kürzer (was sicherlich nicht auf das verwendete Diureticum zurückzuführen ist), und es kam von einem normalen Ausgangswert aus zu einem Anstieg der Plasma-Renin-Aktivität, der nach 30 min bereits nachweisbar, nach 24 Std. aber besonders stark ausgeprägt war. Durch diesen Spätanstieg unterscheidet sich die Beobachtung auch vom Verhalten des Gesunden. Der gleichzeitige Anstieg besonders des diastolischen Blutdrucks mit Verkleinerung der Blutdruckamplitude läßt daran denken, daß der Anstieg der Plasma-Renin-Aktivität zumindest anfangs auch durch einen Katecholaminanstieg vermittelt wurde (Gordon, Küchel, Liddle u. Island 1967).

6. Elektrolytkonzentrationen. In Abb. 3 ist die Elektrolytausscheidung des in Abb. 2 gezeigten Versuches näher analysiert, und zwar sowohl als *Elektrolytausscheidung* in µval/min als auch als *Elektrolytkonzentrationen im Urin*. Es ergab sich, daß der Na/K-Quotient im Urin vor Gabe des Diureticums mit 0,3 bereits stark erniedrigt war. Unter

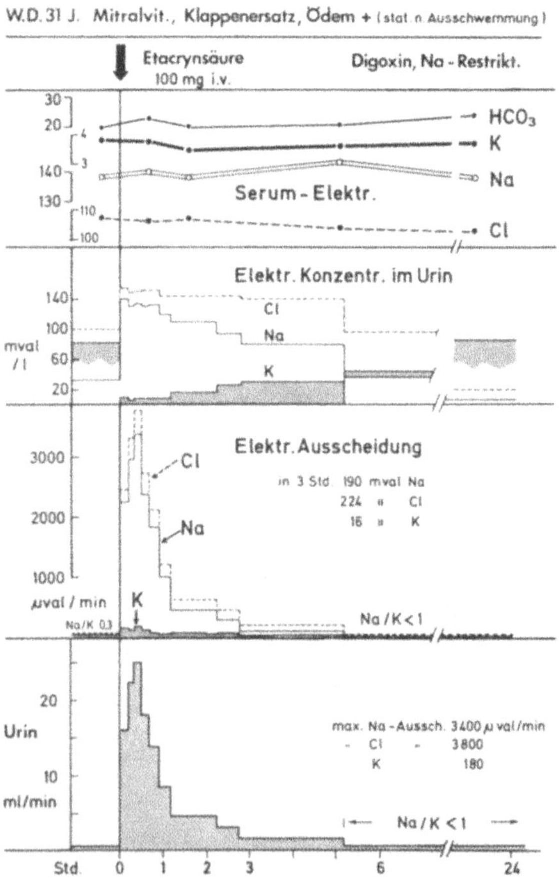

Abb. 3. Erweiterung der Ergebnisse von Abb. 2, hier Darstellung der Elektrolytveränderungen. Elektrolytausscheidung in µval/min, Elektrolytkonzentrationen in mval/l Urin bzw. Plasma. Insbesondere sind die absoluten Elektrolytkonzentrationen im Urin sowie das Verhältnis von Natrium, Kalium und Chlorid zueinander von Interesse.

der akuten Wirkung von Etacrynsäure kam es zu einer starken Natriurese, die allerdings von Anfang an und zunehmend mehr hinter der Chloridausscheidung zurückblieb. Nach 6 Std. sank der Na/K-Quotient wieder unter 1 und war nach 24 Std. kleiner als 0,1. Dies Verhalten läßt auf eine starke Aktivierung der natriumretinierenden Mechanismen schließen und steht in guter Übereinstimmung mit dem starken Anstieg der Plasma-Renin-Aktivität. Ein leichtes Zurückbleiben der Natrium- hinter der Chloridausscheidung war auch bei den anderen Herzkranken die Regel.

Die *Elektrolytkonzentrationen im Plasma* zeigten während der akuten Diurese nur geringe Veränderungen in Form eines leichten Chloridabfalls und Bikarbonatanstiegs bei im wesentlichen unverändertem Natrium- und Kaliumspiegel. Bei der zweiten Patientin war diese Tendenz zur hypochlorämischen Alkalose etwas deutlicher (vgl. Abb. 3). Sie ist nicht nur durch das Zurückbleiben der Natrium- gegenüber der Chloridausscheidung zu erklären – die auf eine Aldosteronwirkung am distalen Tubulus zu beziehen ist –, sondern teilweise auch als Kontraktionsalkalose zu deuten.

7. *Schlußfolgerungen und Indikation der akuten Diurese beim Herzkranken.* Die Beobachtungen lassen sich dahin zusammenfassen, daß es bei der akuten Diurese mit der Flüssigkeitsentnahme aus dem Kreislauf zur Blutvolumenverkleinerung und zum Nachströmen von Flüssigkeit aus dem extravasalen Raum kommt. Diese Vorgänge dauern bei der ödematösen Herzinsuffizienz länger an als beim Gesunden und können zur bleibenden Verkleinerung von Blut- und extravasalem Volumen führen. Die gleichzeitige Beobachtung von Blutvolumen und zentralem Venendruck erlaubt Aussagen über die Volumendehnbarkeit im Niederdrucksystem, die bei hochgradiger Stauungsinsuffizienz herabgesetzt sein kann. Das Verhalten der Plasma-Renin-Aktivität ist auch bei der akuten Diurese unterschiedlich – ähnlich wie im Verlauf der üblichen diuretischen Therapie –, je nachdem, ob sich der Patient in einer Ausschwemmungs- oder Retentionsphase befindet. Sowohl ein Rückgang, als auch ein verzögert verlaufender Anstieg der Plasma-Renin-Aktivität wurde gesehen. Die Beobachtungen lassen auch daran denken, daß dabei eine Pressorezeptorenreaktion mitspielt. Insgesamt ist zu beachten, daß bei Patienten in der Retentionsphase die hormonale Gegenregulation durch eine akute Diurese besonders stark provoziert werden kann.

Für die *Indikation* der akuten Diurese beim Herzkranken ist nicht die Elektrolytausscheidung, sondern der Volumenentzug entscheidend. Er läßt sich vor allem zur Venendrucksenkung beim Lungenödem ausnutzen, und zwar besonders dann, wenn eine Hämokonzentration erlaubt oder erwünscht ist (Anämie, Hypoproteinämie; am sichersten unter Antikoagulantienwirkung). Auch zur akuten Therapie bei pulmonaler Hypertonie bei Mitralstenose ist die akute Diurese geeignet (Levi u. Proto 1966). Die Kenntnis der Vorgänge ist aber auch bei der sonstigen Anwendung größerer Dosen raschwirkender Diuretica wichtig, wie sie z. B. bei therapieresistenten kardialen Ödemen von Davidov, Kakaviatos u. Finnerty (1967) durchgeführt wurde. Die Beobachtungen legen nahe, daß dabei die kleinste ausreichende Dosierung anzuwenden, in der Regel die intermittierende Therapie vorzuziehen ist, da hormonale Gegenregulation und Hämokonzentration nicht beabsichtigt sind. Es ist darauf hinzuweisen, daß die Wirkung von Etacrynsäure und Furosemid auch bei oraler Anwendung fast ebenso rasch erfolgt wie bei intravenöser Applikation (Beyer, Baer, Michaelson u. Russo 1965; Dettli u. Spring 1965; Jahrmärker 1967 u. a.).

B. Zur diuretischen Therapie der chronischen Herzinsuffizienz

Es sollen hier lediglich einige offene Probleme angesprochen werden. Im übrigen wird auf das Symposion: *The Physiology of Diuretic Agents* (SELDIN 1966) und frühere Darstellungen (SCHWIEGK u. JAHRMÄRKER 1960) verwiesen, hinsichtlich der Wirkungsverstärkung durch Diuretica-Kombinationen auf DETTLI u. SPRING (1966) und den Beitrag von KOCZOREK u. Mitarb. (S. 269).

1. Vermeidung von Elektrolytstörungen. Der natriuretische Effekt der Diuretica wird beim Herzkranken durch einen bestehenden, evtl. provozierten Aldosteronismus modifiziert mit dem Ergebnis einer Kaliumverarmung und hypochlorämischen Alkalose (vgl. Teil A Abschnitt 6). Diesem pathogenetischen Mechanismus kann durch gleichzeitige Gabe antikaliuretischer Substanzen (Spironolacton, Triamteren) sowie durch vorsichtige intermittierende Dosierung entgegengewirkt werden (s. Beitrag KOCZOREK u. Mitarb.). Daher spielen diese Elektrolytstörungen heute eher eine geringere Rolle. Das Auftreten einer Hyponatriämie läßt sich nicht durch unmittelbare Diureticawirkung erklären, da im Urin die Natriumkonzentration des Extrazellularraums kaum überschritten wird (vgl. Abb. 3), sondern kommt erst durch Wasserretention trotz Störung der normalen Osmolalität zustande. Die Wasserretention ist bei Mangelhyponatriämie durch zu starke Verkleinerung des Extrazellularvolumens, bei Verdünnungshyponatriämie durch komplexe Vorgänge bedingt, die Züge des Syndroms der inadaequaten ADH-Sekretion (BARTTER u. SCHWARTZ 1967) tragen, jedoch mit dem Unterschied der geringen Natriurese. Die Gabe von Glucocorticoiden kann hier erfahrungsgemäß günstig sein.

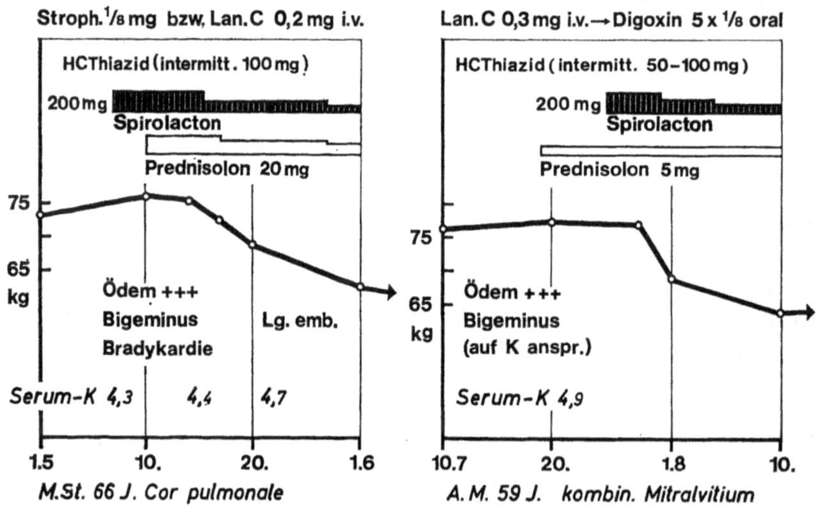

Abb. 4. Schematische Darstellung des Verlaufs bei zwei Patienten mit schwerem kardialem Ödem. Wie die Gewichtskurve zeigt, kam die Ausschwemmung erst in Gang, nachdem außer Herzglykosiden und Hydrochlorothiazid (HCThiazid) auch Spironolacton und Glucocorticoide gegeben wurden (außerdem Bettruhe, Antikoagulantien; zeitweise Antibiotica und Sauerstoff). In beiden Fällen war bei niedriger Glykosiddosierung anfangs auch ein zeitweiser Bigeminus vorhanden.

2. Cortisonanwendung im Rahmen der diuretischen Therapie. HEIDORN u. SCHEMM (1955) beobachteten bei therapieresistenter Herzinsuffizienz eine Besserung nach Zufuhr von ACTH oder Cortison. Seitdem ist wiederholt über einzelne Fälle berichtet worden, in denen die Rekompensation erst nach Cortisongabe in Gang kam. Die Wirkungsweise ist nicht geklärt, wenn man von einer broncholytischen oder entzündungshemmenden Wirkung etwa beim Cor pulmonale absieht. Bei Glucocorticoidmangel, der bei schwerer chronischer Herzinsuffizienz nicht selten ist (KARL 1959, sowie wiederholte eigene Beobachtungen), ist mit einer Verbesserung des Glomerulusfiltrats durch Cortison zu rechnen. Im übrigen scheint das Verhältnis von Mineralo- zu Glucocorticoiden eine Rolle zu spielen (WOLFF, BETTLE, BLAISE u. Mitarb. 1966); so fanden BARGER, BERLIN u. TULENKO (1958) nach Adrenalektomie eine gesteigerte tubuläre Aldosteronwirkung.

In Abb. 4 sind zwei Krankheitsverläufe schematisch dargestellt, in denen anscheinend sowohl Spironolacton als auch Glucocorticoide erforderlich waren, um die Ausschwemmung und Rekompensation der vorher therapieresistenten Fälle einzuleiten. In Übereinstimmung mit JICK (1966) geht das eigene Vorgehen dahin, niedrige oder Substitutionsdosen von Glucocorticoiden zu geben (möglichst unter Antikoagulantienschutz) bei nachgewiesenem Cortisolmangel, bei Therapieresistenz sowie zur Behandlung und Verhütung einer Verdünnungshyponatriämie. Zusätzliche Gesichtspunkte etwa bei entzündlichen Herzleiden oder Cor pulmonale können die Indikation unterstützen oder für etwas höhere Dosen sprechen.

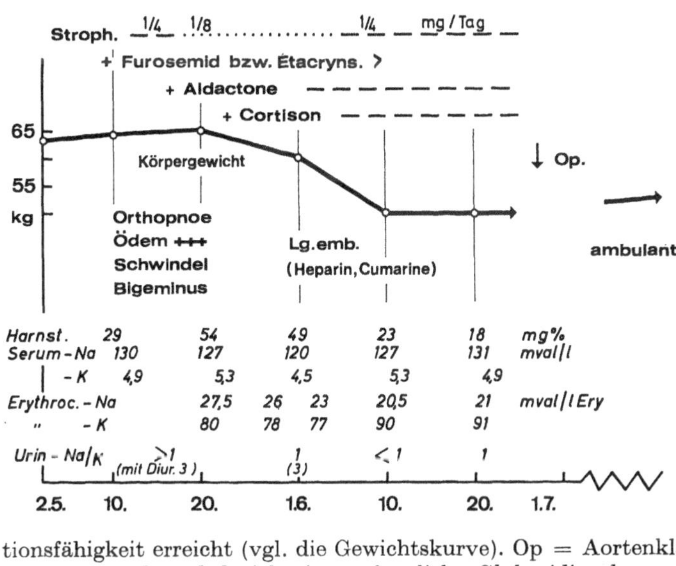

Abb. 5. Schematische Darstellung des klinischen Verlaufs bei einem Pat. mit Aortenklappenstenose und schwerster Herzinsuffizienz (J. K., 44 J.). Nach kombinierter Anwendung von starkwirkenden Diuretica (Furosemid 100–50 mg bzw. Etacrynsäure 100 bis 50 mg intermittierend), Spironolacton (Aldactone 150–100 mg/Tag) und Glucocorticoiden (Prednisolon 10–5 mg/Tag) zusätzlich zur Basistherapie mit Herzglykosiden, Natriumrestriktion und Bettruhe wurden Ausschwemmung und Operationsfähigkeit erreicht (vgl. die Gewichtskurve). Op = Aortenklappenersatz. Es soll hervorgehoben werden, daß sich eine anfängliche Glykosidintoleranz mit zeitweisen Rhythmusstörungen im Verlauf der Behandlung zurückbildete, ohne daß dies durch Veränderungen der extrazellulären Kaliumkonzentration erklärt war. Im Verlauf der Ausschwemmung wurde ein Stadium mit Azotämie und Hyponatriämie durchschritten. Die Erythrozyten-Elektrolyte zeigten eine Tendenz zur Normalisierung. Die Ausscheidung der 17-OH-Corticosteroide betrug vor Beginn der Cortisontherapie 3,5 mg/Tag (Nach JAHRMÄRKER 1968, ergänzt).

3. Rückwirkungen der diuretischen Therapie auf das Herz. Zu diesem Problem liegen bisher kaum Ergebnisse vor. Es ist bekannt, daß Diuretica allein zur Herzverkleinerung führen können (HEDLUND 1952), eine Verbesserung der Kontraktionsleistung kann aber ohne Herzglykoside nicht erwartet werden (vgl. Beitrag SIEGENTHALER, S. 445). Bei schwerer Herzinsuffizienz sind Diuretica ein notwendiger Bestandteil der Therapie, nicht jedoch ihre Basis. Ein gewisser Hinweis auf eine günstige Rückwirkung einer erfolgreichen Ausschwemmungstherapie scheint aus folgenden Beobachtungen hervorzugehen. Wir haben bei Schwerkranken wiederholt beobachtet, daß sich eine herabgesetzte Glykosidtoleranz im Verlauf der Rekompensation wieder besserte, ohne daß dies durch Veränderungen der extrazellulären Kaliumkonzentration zu erklären war. Es scheint sich um einen allgemeinen Effekt der Rekompensation und nicht um eine direkte Wirkung der Diuretica oder anderer einzelner Maßnahmen zu handeln. Die Hypothese scheint möglich, daß eine veränderte Elektrolytzusammensetzung im Myokard gebessert wurde. Abb. 5 gibt den Verlauf eines solchen Falles wieder, bei dem die Strophanthintoleranz zeitweise herabgesetzt war. Im Verlauf der Ödemausschwemmung wurde ein Stadium mit Azotämie und Hyponatriämie durchschritten. Die Erythrocyten-Elektrolyte zeigten eine Tendenz zur Normalisierung. Auch in den Fällen der Abb. 4 kam es zum Verschwinden einer anfänglichen Rhythmusstörung.

Literatur / References

BARGER, A. C., R. D. BERLIN and J. F. TULENKO: Infusion of aldosterone, 9α-fluorohydrocortisone and antidiuretic hormone into the renal artery of normal and adrenalectomized, unanesthetized dogs; effects on electrolyte and water excretion. Endocrinology **62**, 804 (1958).

BARTTER, F. C. and W. B. SCHWARTZ: The syndrome of inappropriate secretion of antidiuretic hormone. Amer. J. Med. **42**, 790 (1967).

BEYER, K. H., J. E. BAER and J. K. MICHAELSON: Renotropic characteristics of ethacrynic acid: a phenoxyacetic saluretic-diuretic agent. J. Pharmacol. Exper. Therapeutics **147**, 1 (1965).

BOUCHER, R. VEYRAT, J. DE CHAMPLAIN and J. GENEST: New procedures for measurement of human plasma Angiotensin and Renin activity levels. Canad. Med. Assoc. J. **90**, 194 (1964).

BROWN, T. C., I. O. DAVIS and C. I. JOHNSTON: Acute response in plane renin and aldosterone secretion to diuretics. Amer. J. Physiol. **211**, 437 (1966).

DAVIDOV, M., N. KAKAVIATOS and F. A. FINNERTY: Intravenous administration of Furosemide in heart failure. J. Amer. Med. Ass. **200**, 824 (1967).

DETTLI, L. und P. SPRING: Pharmakologisch-klinische Prüfung neuer Diuretica. Arzneim.-Forschg. **15**, 1162 (1965).

DETTLI, L. and P. SPRING: Therapy with combination of diuretic agents: Comparative studies. Ann. N. Y. Acad. Sci. **139**, 471 (1966).

ESPINER, E. A., J. R. TUCCI, P. I. JAGGER, G. L. PAUK and D. P. LAULER: The effect of acute diuretic-induced extracellular volume depletion on aldosterone secretion in normal man Clin. Sci. **33**, 125 (1967).

ESPINER, E., J. TUCCI, D. LAULER and P. JAGGER: Absence of an aldosterone response to acute volume depletion in edematous patients. Clin. Res. **15**, 201 (1967).

FRASER, R., V. H. T. JAMES, J. J. BROWN, P. ISAAC, A. F. LEVER and J. I. S. ROBERTSON: Effect of angiotensin and of furosemide on plasma Aldosterone, Corticosterone, Cortisol and Renin in man. Lancet 1965/II, 889.

FRISK, A. R., L. WERKÖ and G. WRANGE: A new mercurial diuretic »diurgin«. Acta med. scand. **144**, 85 (1952).

GAUER, O. H. und J. P. HENRY: Beitrag zur Homöostase des extrazellulären Kreislaufs. Volumenregulation als unabhängiger physiologischer Parameter. Klin. Wschr. **34,** 356 (1956).
GORDON, R. D., O. KÜCHEL, G. W. LIDDLE and D. P. ISLAND: The effect of the sympathic nervous system on the secretion of Renin in man. J. Clin. Invest. **46,** 599 (1967).
GROSS, F.: Physiologie und Pathologie des Renin/Angiotensin-Systems. In: Handb. d. Inn. Med., Band 8/2, 5. Aufl., Springer-Verlag, Berlin-Heidelberg-New York 1968, S.35–168.
HEDLUND, S.: Klinische Untersuchungen mit Cedilanid. Cardiologia (Basel) **20,** Suppl. 3–88 (1952).
HEIDORN, G. H. and F. R. SCHEMM: The clinical use of corticotropin (ACTH) and adrenal corticosteroids in the therapy of intractable edema. Amer. J. med. Sci. **229,** 621 (1955).
JAHRMÄRKER, H.: Die Therapie der akuten Herzinsuffizienz. Dtsch. Med. J. **18,** 178 (1967).
JAHRMÄRKER, H.: Kombinierte Therapie mit Glykosiden und Diuretica. Therapiewoche **18,** 606 (1968).
JAHRMÄRKER, H., H. AVENHAUS, H. GROHMANN und KH. R. KOCZOREK: Hämodynamische Auswirkungen der akuten Diurese bei Herzinsuffizienz. Verh. Dtsch. Ges. Kreislauff. **34,** 374 (1968).
JAHRMÄRKER, H., M. v. BUBNOFF und G. RIECKER: Über Hyponatriämiesyndrome und ihre Analyse durch Elektrolytbestimmung in Erythrozyten. Klin. Wschr. **39,** 317 (1961).
JICK, H.: The use of glucocorticoids for diuresis in patients with fluid retention not resulting from renal disease. Ann. N. Y. Acad. Sci. **139,** 512 (1966).
KARL, H. J.: Untersuchungen über 17-Hydroxycorticosteroide in Plasma und Urin in freier und veresterter Form bei Patienten mit hydropischer Herzinsuffizienz. Klin. Wschr. **37,** 1124 (1959).
KAUFMANN, W. und A. A. MÜLLER: Expansion des Plasmavolumens nach rascher Verminderung der zirkulierenden Blutmenge. Z. Kreislaufforsch. **47,** 719 (1958).
KLAUS, D.: Regulation der Reninsekretion. Dtsch. med. Wschr. **92,** 2128 (1967).
KOCZOREK, KH. R., W. VOGT, P. SCHMIEDECK und H. JOST: Die Auswirkungen von Störungen der Leberfunktion auf das Renin-Angiotensin-System. Dtsch. Ges. Kreislaufforsch. 33. Jahrestagg., Bad Nauheim 1967, Referat: Klin. Wschr. **45,** 896 (1967).
KOCZOREK, KH. R., B. SIMON, P. SCHMIEDECK, W. VOGT und B. LÜDERITZ: Funktionsstörungen des Renin-Angiotensin-Systems bei Leberkrankheiten. V. Lebertagung d. Sozialmediziner, Bad Mergentheim, 13.–15. 10. 67.
LEVI, G. F. et C. PROTO: Effetto ipotensive del furosemide sul circolo polmonare dei mitralici. Minerva Cardioangiologica **14,** 235 (1966).
MEYER, PH., J. MÉNARD, J. M. ALEXANDRE et P. MILLIEZ: Variations de l'activité rénine plasmatique après injection d'acide éthacrynique. J. d'Urol. Nephrol. **72,** 619 (1966).
NASH, H. L., E. A. FITZ, W. R. WILSON, W. M. KIRKENDALL and J. M. KIOSCHOS: Cardiorenal hemodynamic effects of ethacrynic acid. Amer. Heart J. **71,** 153 (1966).
NASH, F. D., H. H. ROSTORFER, M. D. BAILIE, R. L. WATHEN and E. G. SCHNEIDER: Relation to renal sodium load and dissociation from hemodynamic changes.
OCKENGA, TH., K. PABST und U. STEIN: Zentraler Venendruck und Hämodynamik bei Herzinsuffizienten im Lagewechsel- und Aderlaßversuch. Verh. Dtsch. Ges. Kreislaufforsch. **34,** 362 (1968).
PUGH, L. G. C. and C. L. WYNDHAM: The circulatory effects of mercurial diuretics in congestive heart failure. Clin. Sci. **8,** 10 (1949).
ROSENTHAL, J., R. BOUCHER, W. NOWACZYNSKI and J. GENEST: Acute changes in plasma volume, renin activity, and free aldosterone levels in healthy subjects following Furosemide administration. Canad. J. Physiol. Pharmacol. **46,** 85 (1968).
SAMET, P. and W. H. BERNSTEIN: Acute effects of oral ethacrynic acid upon total blood volume. Amer. Heart J. **75,** 288 (1968).
SCHNEIDER, K. W.: Hämodynamische Wirkung von Diuretika. Münch. Med. Wschr. **51,** 2571 (1966).
SCHWIEGK, H. und H. JAHRMÄRKER: Therapie der Herzinsuffizienz. In: Handb. Inn. Med., 4. Aufl., Bd. 9/1, S. 402ff., Springer-Verlag, Berlin-Göttingen-Heidelberg, 1960.

Seldin, D. W. (consulting editor): The physiology of diuretic agents. Ann. N. Y. Acad. Sci. **139**, 273–539 (1966).

Truniger, B. und W. Siegenthaler: Aldosteron und Diuretica. Klin. Wschr. **38**, 133 (1963).

Wolff, H. P.: Das Renin-Aldosteron-System bei hydropischen Erkrankungen. 74. Tagg. dtsch. Ges. Inn. Med., Wiesbaden 1968.

Wolff, H. P., L. Bette, H. Blaise, G. Düsterdieck, J. Jahnecke, T. Kobayashi, F. Krück, D. Lommer and H. Schieffer: Role of aldosterone in edema formation. Ann. N. Y. Acad. Sci. **139**, 285 (1966).

Heidland: Wie verhält sich das Herzminutenvolumen bei hydropischer Herzinsuffizienz nach Diuretica im akuten Versuch?

Jahrmärker: Diese Frage interessiert uns besonders, wir haben jedoch bisher keine einwandfreien Minutenvolumenbestimmungen unter diesen Bedingungen. Man darf aber annehmen, daß nur in Fällen mit besonders hohem Venendruck eine Entlastung auch zu einer Minutenvolumensteigerung führt. Nach Quecksilberdiurese ist nur ausnahmsweise, so von Pugh und Wyndham (Clin. Sci. **8**, 10 [1949]), in der Mehrzahl der Fälle aber keine Minutenvolumenzunahme beobachtet worden (Frisk, Werkö, Wrange, Acta Med. Scand. **44**, 85 [1952]). Ähnliches ist von Aderlaßversuchen bekannt.

On the Use of Diuretics in Congestive Heart Failure

Zur Anwendung der Diuretica bei Herzinsuffizienz

W. SIEGENTHALER

Zusammenfassung: Mit Hilfe der wiederholten Bestimmung verschiedener Kreislaufgrößen kann gezeigt werden, daß unter alleiniger diuretischer Behandlung der Herzinsuffizienz die pathologische Flüssigkeitsansammlung wohl ausgeschwemmt wird, die Kreislaufzeiten als Ausdruck der Myokardfunktion aber nicht unbedingt gebessert werden. Dies hängt in erster Linie damit zusammen, daß das Blutvolumen absinkt, das Herzminutenvolumen jedoch noch stärker gesenkt wird. Erst die kombinierte Behandlung mit Glykosiden und Diuretica vermag auch diese larvierte Herzinsuffizienz zum Verschwinden zu bringen.

Die Herzinsuffizienz ist hämodynamisch einerseits durch das verminderte Herzminutenvolumen und andererseits durch das vergrößerte Blutvolumen charakterisiert. Da die Faktoren Kreislaufzeit, Blutvolumen und Herzminutenvolumen durch die Formel:

$$\text{Kreislaufzeit} = \text{K} \times \frac{\text{Blutvolumen}}{\text{Herzminutenvolumen}}$$

eng miteinander verknüpft sind, stellt die objektive Messung einer Kreislaufzeit (Arm-Ohr-Zeit, Lungen-Ohr-Zeit) eine ausgezeichnete und einfache Methode zur Beurteilung einer Herzinsuffizienz und der dabei verwendeten therapeutischen Maßnahmen dar.

Daraus ergibt sich, daß die Verlängerung der Kreislaufzeiten ein wesentliches Kriterium der mit vermindertem Herzminutenvolumen und vergrößertem Blutvolumen einhergehenden Form der Herzinsuffizienz ist. Aus einer Verkürzung der zuvor verlängerten Kreislaufzeiten nach Therapie darf deshalb auf eine Besserung der Myokardfunktion geschlossen werden.

Es war daher gegeben, bei Patienten mit hämodynamischer Herzinsuffizienz die Kreislaufzeiten zu Beginn der Behandlung zu bestimmen und im Verlauf der Therapie zu kontrollieren. Die Kreislaufzeiten werden stets als Arm-Ohr-Zeit sowie als Lungen-Ohr-Zeit und aus der durch Subtraktion der Lungen-Ohr-Zeit von der Arm-Ohr-Zeit errechneten Arm-Lungen-Zeit mit den von HEGGLIN und Mitarb. angegebenen Methoden berechnet.

a) Die sog. Arm-Ohr-Zeit (AOZ) dauert vom Moment der Farbstoffinjektion in eine Kubitalvene bis zum Erscheinen der ersten Farbstoffpartikel im hyperämisierten Ohr (Norm 8–14 sec).
b) Die sog. Lungen-Ohr-Zeit (LOZ) dauert vom Beginn des ersten Atemzuges nach Apnoe bis zum Wiederanstieg der Sauerstoffsättigung am Ohr (Norm 4–5 sec).
c) Die sog. Arm-Lungen-Zeit (ALZ) kann durch Subtraktion der Lungen-Ohr-Zeit von der Arm-Ohr-Zeit errechnet werden (Norm 4–9 sec).

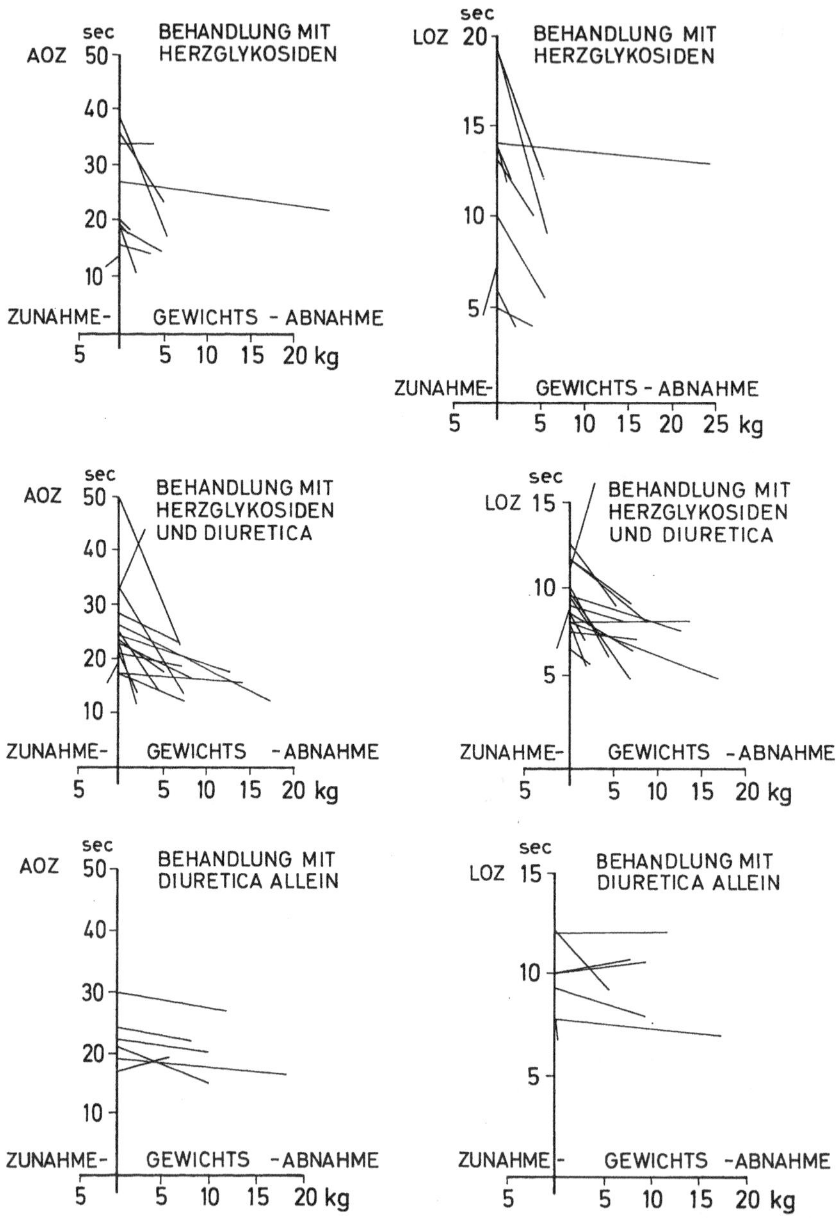

Abb. 1. Kreislaufzeiten (AOZ = Arm-Ohr-Zeit, LOZ = Lungen-Ohr-Zeit) bei Herzinsuffizienz vor und nach Behandlung mit Glykosiden, Glykosiden und Diuretica sowie Diuretica allein.

Fig. 1. Circulation times (AOZ = arm-ear-time, LOZ = lung-ear-time) in congestive heart failure before and after treatment with glycosides, glycosides and diuretics and diuretics alone.

Die Lungen-Ohr-Zeit wird mehr von der Tätigkeit des linken, die Arm-Lungen-Zeit von derjenigen des rechten Ventrikels beeinflußt.

Auf Grund eines an unserer Klinik bei der hämodynamischen Herzinsuffizienz durchgeführten Behandlungsplanes haben wir 3 Gruppen gebildet:

1. Kranke, welche nur Herzglykoside erhielten,
2. Kranke, welche Glykoside und Diuretica erhielten und
3. Kranke, welche Diuretica allein erhalten haben.

Als objektiv erfaßbares Maß für die Schwere der Herzinsuffizienz haben wir das Ausmaß der Ödeme, bestimmt am Körpergewicht, herangezogen und mit den Kreislaufzeiten in Beziehung gesetzt. Nimmt man den Ausgangswert für Gewicht und Kreislaufzeit mit 100% an, so unterscheiden sich die Gruppen der mit Glykosiden oder Glykosiden und Diuretica behandelten Patienten hinsichtlich Verkürzung der Kreislaufzeiten deutlich von der ausschließlich mit Diuretica behandelten Gruppe (Abb. 1).

Bei der ersten Gruppe, welche nur Herzglykoside erhielt, läßt sich bei insgesamt 8 von 10 Fällen eine Übereinstimmung der Kreislaufzeitmessung mit dem klinischen Zustand erkennen, d. h. die Verkürzung der Kreislaufzeiten geht mit der Abnahme des Gewichts und der Abnahme der Lungenstauung parallel (Abb. 1).

Bei der zweiten Gruppe, welche mit Glykosiden und Diuretica behandelt wurde, zeigten 14 Kranke von insgesamt 16 Patienten eine gute Übereinstimmung zwischen Gewichtsabnahme und Verkürzung der Kreislaufzeiten (Abb. 1).

Bei der dritten Gruppe schließlich, die mit oralen Diuretica behandelt wurde und 7 Patienten umfaßt, findet sich im Vergleich zu den beiden ersten Gruppen ein völlig

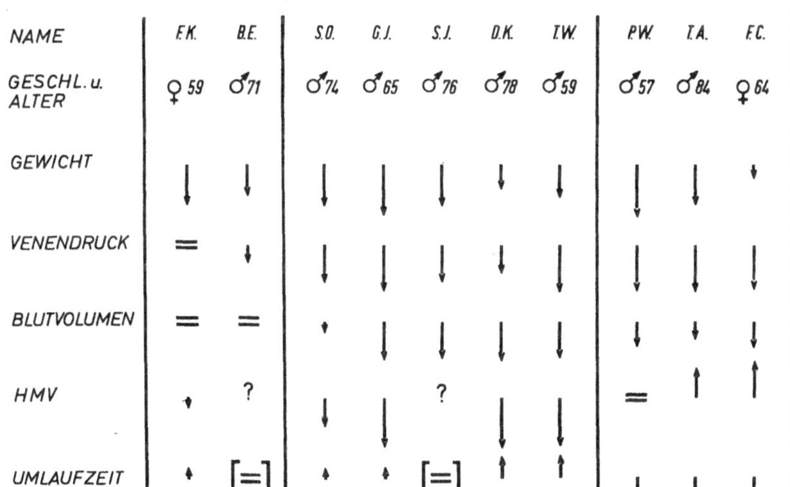

Abb. 2. Verschiedene Kreislaufgrößen bei Herzinsuffizienz nach alleiniger Behandlung mit Diuretica.

Fig. 2. Different circulatory parameters in congestive heart failure after treatment with diuretics alone.

verschiedenes Bild, indem trotz beträchtlicher Gewichtsabnahme die Kreislaufzeiten nur unwesentlich beeinflußt wurden (Abb. 1).

Anhand einer später untersuchten Gruppe von 10 nur mit oralen Diuretica behandelten Patienten war es unter gleichzeitiger Bestimmung weiterer Kreislaufgrößen möglich, die Kreislaufverhältnisse noch eingehender zu analysieren. So konnte durch gleichzeitige Bestimmungen des totalen Blutvolumens und des Herzminutenvolumens gezeigt werden, daß unter der Diureticabehandlung das Blutvolumen vielfach ungefähr entsprechend dem Körpergewicht, das Herzminutenvolumen jedoch noch stärker absinkt. Der massive Rückgang des Herzminutenvolumens hat also trotz gleichzeitig abnehmendem Blutvolumen eine Verlängerung der Kreislaufzeiten zur Folge, weil der Nenner des Bruches in der erwähnten Formel stärker abnimmt als der Zähler (Abb. 2).

Die Reduktion des Blutvolumens führt daher in diesen Fällen nicht, wie man erwarten könnte, zu einer verbesserten Herzleistung. Die Blutmenge sinkt offenbar so stark ab, daß keine genügende diastolische Kammerfüllung bzw. ausreichendes Herzminutenvolumen zustandekommt.

Trotz Normalisierung des Venendrucks bleibt das Myokard also nach wie vor insuffizient. Nur äußert sich diese Art von Dekompensation nicht mehr unter dem Bild der Stauungsinsuffizienz. Die klinischen Zeichen der Lungenstauung wie auch die Ödeme gingen sowohl bei den mit Glykosiden als auch bei ausschließlich mit Diuretica behandelten Fällen in gleicher Weise zurück. Aus dem klinischen Bild allein lassen sich also keine Rückschlüsse auf die Myokardfunktion ziehen. Wir haben es mit einer larvierten Herzinsuffizienz zu tun. Erst die zusätzliche Verabreichung von herzaktiven Glykosiden, welche durch Steigerung der Kontraktionskraft direkt am Myokard angreifen und deshalb das Herzminutenvolumen erhöhen, vermag die verlängerten Kreislaufzeiten gegen die Norm hin zu ändern.

On the Use of Diuretics in Congestive Heart Failure

Summary: With the aid of repeated determinations of various circulatory parameters it could be shown that the treatment of congestive heart failure with diuretics will result only in the elimination of pathological accumulations of fluids, while the circulation times, as an indication of myocardial function do not improve. This is primarily due to the fact that while blood volume falls, cardiac output is reduced still further. Only combined treatment with glycosides and diuretics can bring about the disappearance of this masked type of congestive heart failure.

Congestive heart failure is characterized hemodynamically on the one hand by a diminished cardiac output and on the other by an increased blood volume. As the various factors involed: circulation time, blood volume and heart-minute-volume are closely linked by the formula:

$$\text{circulation time} = K \times \frac{\text{blood volume}}{\text{heart-minute-volume}}$$

the measurement of circulation time (arm to ear or lung to ear time) provides an excellent and simple method for judging the degree of cardiac insufficiency and the success of therapeutic measures.

Since the prolongation of the circulation time is an indication of the type of cardiac insufficiency which is associated with a diminished cardiac output and an increased blood volume, one can, therefore, conclude that myocardial function is improving if previously prolonged circulation times shorten after treatment.

Accordingly, it appeared of interest to determine the circulation times of patients with hemodynamic cardiac insufficiency at the start and during the course of treatment. The circulation times are always expressed as an arm to ear time and as lung to ear time and are also calculated as arm to lung time by deducting the lung to ear time from the arm to ear time. These values were determined with methods described by HEGGLIN and collaborators.

a) The so-called arm to ear time (AET) lasts from the moment the color dye is injected into the cubital vein until the first particles of the dye appear in the hyperaemized ear (normally 8–14 sec).
b) The so-called lung to ear time (LET) lasts from the beginning of the first breath after apnoea until the return of oxygen saturation in the ear (normally 4–5 sec).
c) The so-called arm to lung time (ALT) is calculated by substraction of the lung to ear time from the arm to ear time (normally 4–9 sec).

The lung to ear time is more influenced by the activity of the left ventricle, the arm to lung time by that of the right ventricle. Based on a treatment program which we carried out on patients with hemodynamic cardiac insufficiency in our hospital, we distinguished three groups:

1. patients who were only given cardiac glycosides
2. patients who received glycosides and diuretics
3. patients who received diuretics only.

As an objectively assessable measurement of the degree of cardiac insufficiency, the extent of edema based on the body weight was determined and related to the circulation times. If one assumes the original figure for weight and circulation time to be 100%, the groups treated with glycosides or glycosides and diuretics behave differently with regard to the shortening of the circulation times from the group of patients who were treated exclusively with diuretics (see Fig. 1).

In the first group which was given only cardiac glycosides, in 8 out of 10 cases conformity of circulation time measurements and clinical condition were observed, i. e. the shortening of the circulation times runs parallel to a decrease in body weight and a reduction in the pulmonary congestion (Fig. 1).

In the second group consisting of 16 cases treated with both glycosides and diuretics, 14 of the patients showed a marked correspondence of weight loss with reduction in the circulation times (Fig. 1).

Finally, in the third group comprising 7 patients treated only with oral diuretics, a completely different picture emerges as compared with the two previous groups, since, in spite of a marked loss of weight, the circulation times were affected only slightly.

Based on investigations carried out later on a further group of 10 patients treated with oral diuretics alone, a more detailed analysis of conditions prevailing in the circulation became possible by simultaneous measurement of further circulatory values. In this way, it was possible to demonstrate by the simultaneous determination of the total blood volume and the heart-minute volume that as a result of treatment with diuretics the blood volume diminishes, often corresponding rougly to the decrease in body weight, while the heart-minute volume falls even more drastically. The marked fall of the heart-minute volume results in a prolongation of the circulation time in spite of the simultaneous fall of the blood volume, as the denominator of the fraction is reduced more than the numerator in the formula mentioned above (Fig. 2).

Therefore, in these cases the reduction in blood volume does not lead to an improved cardiac performance as one would otherwise expect. The blood volume obviously falls so drastically that no adequate diastolic filling of the ventricle or a sufficient heart-minute volume is achieved.

Thus, in spite of a normalization of the venous pressure, myocardium activity remains insufficient. Only this type of decompensation does not show the features of congestive failure. The clinical signs of pulmonary congestion, as well as the edema are diminished both in the cases which are treated with glycosides and the ones treated with diuretics alone. The clinical picture by itself, therefore, does not permit any conclusion with regard to myocardial function. We are dealing here with a masked heart failure. Only the additional administration of cardiac glycosides which act directly on the heart muscle and increase the strength of contraction and, therefore, also raise the heart-minute volume will make the prolonged circulation times return to normal.

Literatur / References

HEGGLIN R., F. RHOMBERG und W. RUTISHAUSER: Dtsch. med. Wschr. **85**, 1289 (1960).

HEGGLIN R., W. RUTISHAUSER, G. KAUFMANN, H. SCHEU und E. LÜTHY: In: Kreislaufdiagnostik mit der Farbstoffverdünnungsmethode. Georg Thieme Verlag, Stuttgart 1962.

SIEGENTHALER, W.: Verh. dtsch. Ges. Kreisl. Forsch. **26**, 57 (1960).

SIEGENTHALER, W.: In: Praxis der Herz- und Kreislauferkrankungen. J. F. Lehmanns Verlag München 1963.

The Use of Diuretics in Cardiac Diseases

Zur Anwendung der Diuretica bei Erkrankungen des Herzens

W. KAUFMANN, B. STEINER, F. DÜRR, K. A. MEURER

In Ergänzung zu den Ausführungen von MÜLLER u. JAHRMÄRKER darf auf eigene Untersuchungen über das Verhalten des Aldosteronstoffwechsels unter saluretischer Therapie hingewiesen werden, die unter strengen Bilanzbedingungen durchgeführt wurden. Aldosteron-Sekretionsrate (SR), metabolische Clearance-Rate (MCR) und mittlerer Aldosteron-Plasmaspiegel (MPK = SR/MCR) wurden dabei unter Anwendung der Doppelisotopen-Methode von KLIMAN und PETERSON bestimmt.

Abb. 1 ist hinsichtlich des Aldosteronstoffwechsels bei Herzinsuffizienz weitgehend charakteristisch:

Die Aldosteron-Sekretionsrate (SR) ist im Zustande der kardialen Dekompensation in der Regel im Normbereich (50–250γ/24 Std.). Die Werte liegen nicht selten im unteren Bereich der Norm. Eine Steigerung der Aldosteron-Sekretion erfolgt oft erst unter den Bedingungen der negativen Natriumbilanz, die bei dem hier dargestellten Fall bei diätetischer Natrium-Restriktion (Zufuhr von 30 mval/24 Std.) durch Verabreichung eines Herzglykosids (Digitoxin) und von Saluretica (zunächst Spironolacton, anschl. plus Hydrochlorothiazid bzw. Furosemid) erreicht wurde. Die maximale Natriumexkretion betrug dabei ca. 200 mval/24 Std. Die Aldosteron-Sekretionsrate stieg schließlich auf 1640γ/24 Std. an!

Infolge Leberstauung, d. h. also nur bei kardialer Rechtsinsuffizienz zu erwarten, besteht häufig eine Störung des Aldosteronabbaues, erkennbar an der Verminderung der metabolischen Clearance-Rate (MCR). Diese änderte sich unter den definierten Bedingungen (negative Natriumbilanz) nicht. Trotz mäßiger Verminderung der MCR kann – wie aus der Abb. deutlich wird – der mittlere Aldosteron-Plasmaspiegel im Normbereich liegen. Der Grund hierfür besteht darin, daß die SR – wie bei Herzinsuffizienz nicht selten (s. o.) – im vorliegenden Fall mit 100γ/24 Std. – relativ niedrig ist. Die mittlere Aldosteron-Plasmakonzentration (MPK) reflektiert im weiteren Verlauf der Therapie im wesentlichen die Änderung der adrenalen Aldosteron-Sekretion, da die MCR unverändert bleibt.

Aus der Darstellung folgt, daß die Steigerung der Aldosteron-Sekretion nicht als Ursache der Ödembildung bei Herzinsuffizienz angesehen werden kann, sondern daß es sich dabei um eine Folge der durch die saluretische Therapie erzwungenen negativen Natriumbilanz handelt. Änderungen des Kaliumbestandes scheinen dabei von zusätzlicher Bedeutung zu sein. Ob dieser induzierte Aldosteronismus über das Renin-Angiotensin-System zustande kommt, muß auf Grund der bisher vorliegenden Befunde als fraglich angesehen werden [Lit. b. W. KAUFMANN et al. Klin. Wschr. 47, 16 (1969)].

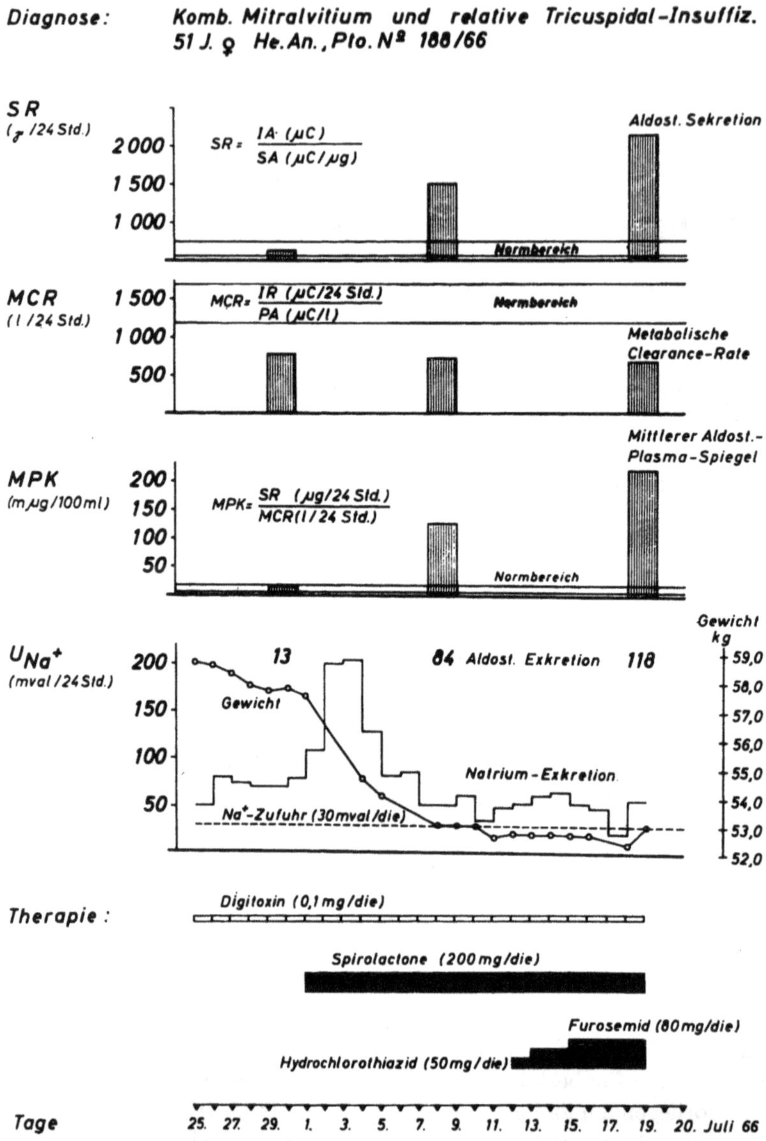

Abb. 1. Verhalten von Aldosteron-Sekretion (SR), metabolischer Clearance Rate (MCR), mittlerer Aldosteron-Plasma-Konzentration (MKP) und Aldosteron-Exkretion (E) bei hydropischer Herzinsuffizienz infolge komb. Mitralvitium und relat. Tricuspidalinsuffizienz unter saluretischer Therapie mit Spironolactone (Aldactone-A), Hydrochlorothiazid (Esidrix) und Furosemid (Lasix) sowie Digitoxin. Durchführung der Untersuchungen unter Elektrolytbilanzbedingungen.

Fig. 1. Behaviour of aldosterone-secretion (SR), of metabolic clearance rate (MCR), mean aldosterone-plasma-concentration (MPK) and aldosterone excretion (E) in hydropic heart failure due to combined mitral vitium and relative tricuspidal insufficiency under saluretic therapy with spironolactone (aldactone), hydrochlorothiazide (esidrix) and furosemide (lasix) and digitoxin. Studies done under electrolyte balance conditions.

The Use of Diuretics in Cardiac Diseases

In addition to the statements of MULLER and JAHRMÄRKER we should like to mention our own results concerning the behaviour of the aldosterone metabolism during saluretic therapy which were carried out under the most stringent balance conditions. Aldosterone secretion rate (SR), metabolic clearance rate (MCR) and mean aldosterone plasma level (MPK = SR/MCR) were determined, using the double-isotope-derivative assay of KLIMAN and PETERSON.

Fig. 1 is characteristic with regard to the aldosterone metabolism in cardiac insufficiency: In cardiac decompensation, the aldosterone secretion rate (SR) is usually within normal limits (50–250 γ/24 hrs). Not seldom, the readings lie within the lower range. A rise of the aldosterone secretion often occurs only under the conditions of a negative sodium balance which in the case presented here was achieved by dietetic sodium restriction (intake of 30 mEq/24 hrs), the administration of a cardiac glycoside (digitoxin) and of saluretics (first spironolactone subsequently together with hydrochlorothiazide resp. furosemide). The maximum sodium excretion then amounted to about 200 mEq/24 hrs. The aldosterone secretion rate ultimately rose to 1640 γ/24 hrs!

As a result of venous congestion of the liver which can only be expected in the presence of rightsided cardiac failure, a disturbance of the aldosterone breakdown usually exists as can be derived from the reduction of the metabolic clearance rate (MCR). MCR did not change under the conditions defined above (a negative sodium balance). In spite of a moderate reduction of the MCR – as can be seen clearly in the illustration – the mean plasma level of aldosterone can remain within normal limits. The reason for this is that the SR in our present case is relatively low at 100 γ/24 hrs, which is not unusual in congestive heart failure (see above). The mean aldosterone-plasma-concentration (MPK) in the further course of treatment essentially reflects the changes in the adrenal secretion of aldosterone since the MCR remains unchanged.

Those findings suggest that the increase of the aldosterone secretion cannot be considered the cause for the edema formation in congestive heart failure, but that they are the consequence of a negative sodium balance resulting from the saluretic therapy. Variations of potassium balance may also be important. Various results suggest that induced hyperaldosteronism in congestive heart failure is not likely to be triggered by increased renin-angiotensin activity [see W. KAUFMANN et al. Klin. Wschr. *47*, 16 (69)].

The Effect of Various Diuretics on Plasma Renin Activity in the Acute Experiment

Die Beeinflussung der Plasmareninaktivität durch verschiedene Diuretica im akuten Versuch

D. KLAUS

Ich möchte über die Beeinflussung der Plasmareninaktivität durch verschiedene Diuretica mit unterschiedlichem Angriffspunkt im Tubulus berichten. Wir haben bei 15 ödemfreien Probanden vergleichend den Anstieg der Plasmareninaktivität nach Furosemid, Hydrochlorothiazid, Azetazolamid und Etacrynsäure, und zwar 3, 8 und 24 Stunden nach intra-

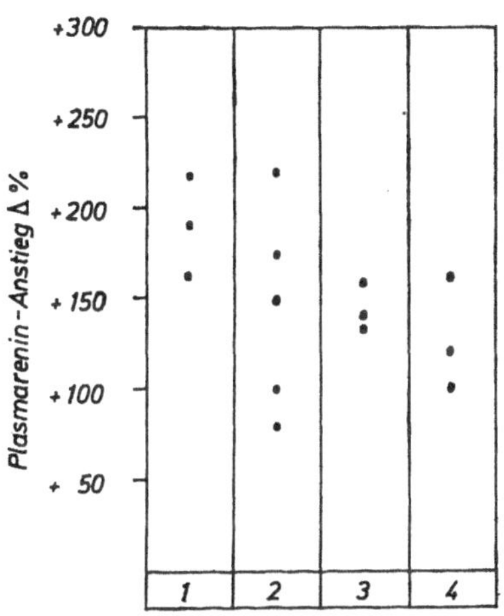

Abb. 1. Prozentualer Anstieg der Plasmareninaktivität 3 Stunden nach Gabe von 500 mg Azetazolamid i. v. (1), 20 mg Furosemid i. v. (2), 20 mg Etacrynsäure oral (3) und 50 mg Hydrochlorothiazid i. v. (4).

Fig. 1. Increase of plasma renin activity (in %) 3 hours after application of 500 mg azetazolamide, i. v. (1), 20 mg furosemide, i. v. (2), 20 mg ethacrynic acid, p. o. (3) and 50 mg hydrochlorothiazide, i. v. (4).

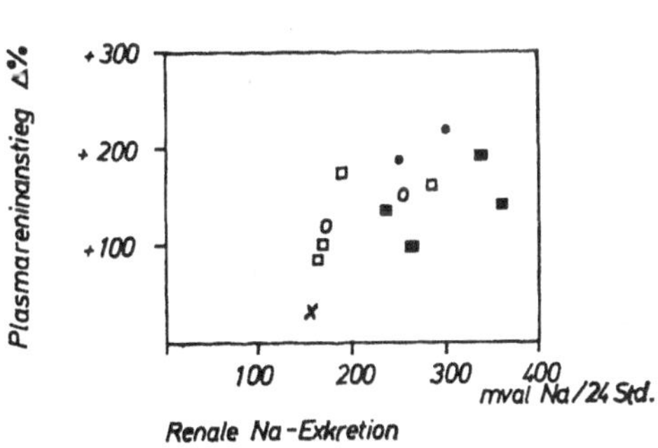

Abb. 2. Beziehung zwischen renaler Natriumexkretion in 24 Stunden und prozentualem Reninanstieg.

Fig. 2. Relation between renal Na-excretion in 24 h and % renin increase.

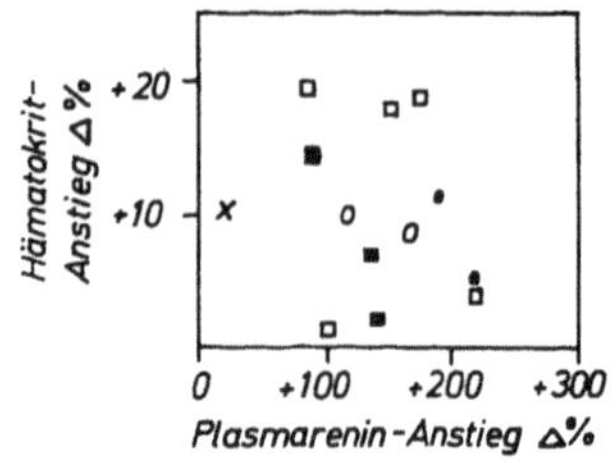

Abb. 3. Beziehungen zwischen prozentualem Reninanstieg im Plasma und Hämatokritanstieg nach Azetazolamid (●), Furosemid (□), Etacrynsäure (■), Hydrochlorothiazid (○) und Amilorid (×).

Fig. 3. Relation between plasma renin rise and increase in hematocrit (%) after azetazolamide (●), furosemide (□), ethacrynic acid (■), hydrochlorothiazide (○) and amiloride (×).

venöser bzw. peroraler Gabe gemessen. Der Anstieg der Plasmareninaktivität ist bei allen untersuchten Diuretica im Mittel nach 3 Stunden gleich hoch und erreicht etwa das Doppelte bis Dreifache der Ausgangswerte (Abb. 1). Setzt man die Größe der renalen Natriumexkretion nach Gabe der Diuretica in Beziehung zum Anstieg der Plasmareninaktivität, so findet sich eine relativ enge Beziehung, allerdings ist die Natriumausscheidung nach Gabe von Etacrynsäure relativ höher als die vergleichsweise Steigerung der Reninsekretion (Abb. 2). Keine Übereinstimmung findet sich zwischen dem Anstieg des Hämatokrits, als Maß der Abnahme des Plasmavolumens, im Vergleich zum Anstieg der Plasmareninwerte nach Gabe der Diuretica (Abb. 3). Dieser Befund entspricht unseren früheren Untersuchungen, nach denen der Plasmareninanstieg nach Furosemid durch gleichzeitige Infusion von salzfreiem Humanalbumin nur partiell, durch die Infusion von

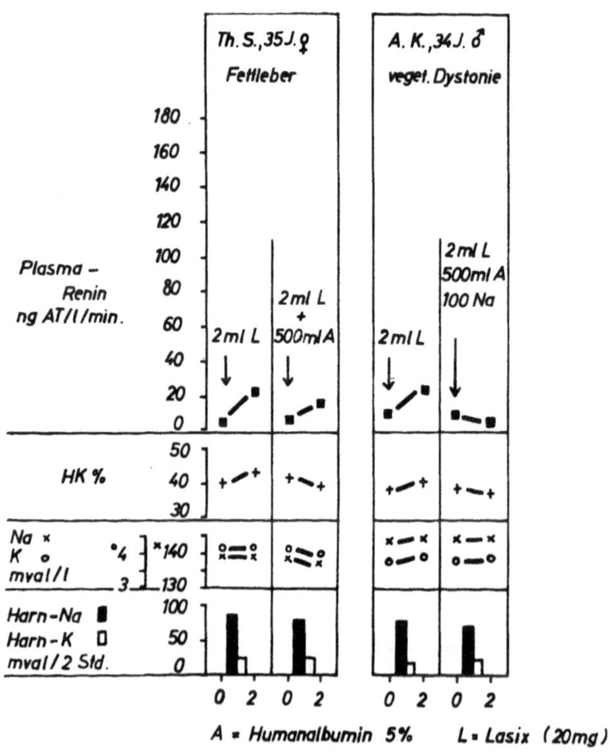

Abb. 4. Beeinflussung des Plasmareninanstiegs nach Furosemid (L) durch salzfreies Humanalbumin (A) und salzhaltiges Humanalbumin beim Gesunden.

Fig. 4. Influence of plasma renin increase after application of furosemide (L) by human albumin (A) without NaCl and human albumin with NaCl in healthy subjects.

salzhaltigem Humanalbumin aber vollständig inhibiert werden konnte (Abb. 4). Für den Anstieg des Plasmarenins nach Diuretica scheint also der renale Natriumverlust über eine noch unbekannte intrarenale Regulation wichtiger zu sein als die Abnahme des Plasmavolumens. Für das Ausmaß der Natriurese und Diurese nach Applikation der Diuretica kommt dem durch den Natriumverlust ausgelösten Anstieg der Plasmareninaktivität und damit auch der Aldosteronsekretion im akuten Versuch keine Bedeutung zu, da die natriuretische Wirkung der untersuchten Diuretica unterschiedlich, ihr Einfluß auf die Plasmareninaktivität aber praktisch gleich ist. Die natriuretische Wirksamkeit der Diuretica ist daher in erster Linie von ihrem tubulären Angriffspunkt und ihren pharmakokinetischen Eigenschaften abhängig. Bei langdauernder Gabe von Diuretica ist aber bei einer Reihe von Patienten, insbesondere solchen mit Herzinsuffizienz, bei denen die Plasmareninaktivität unter der diuretischen Behandlung nicht wie bei der Mehrzahl der Patienten abfällt, sondern ansteigt, die Stimulierung des Renin-Angiotensin-Aldosteron-Systems durch Diuretica zu berücksichtigen, die deren Wirkung limitiert oder abschwächt und die durch Gabe von Aldosteronantagonisten oder anderen Substanzen, die den Natrium-Kalium-Austausch im distalen Tubulus hemmen, aufgehoben werden kann. Amilorid führt im akuten Versuch zu einem Anstieg der Plasmareninaktivität, der nach unseren ersten orientierenden Untersuchungen bei 3 Probanden geringer ist als bei den anderen geprüften Diuretica.

The Effect of Various Diuretics on Plasma Renin Activity in the Acute Test

I am going to report on the effect of various diuretics with different points of attack in the tubules on plasma renin activity. We made comparative tests of the rise of plasma renin activity in 15 edema-free subjects 3, 8 and 24 hours after intravenous or oral administration of furosemide, hydrochlorothiazide, acetazolamide and ethacrynic acid. The rise of plasma renin activity with all the tested diuretics is in the mean the same after 3 hours and reaches about double or treble the initial values (Fig. 1). If the amount of renal sodium excretion after administration of the diuretics is set in relation to the rise of plasma renin activity, a relatively close correlation is found, though admittedly the sodium excretion after ethacrynic acid is relatively higher than the comparatively smaller rise of renin secretion (Fig. 2). There is no correlation between the rise of hematocrit, as a measure of the fall in plasma volume, and the rise in plasma renin values after administration of the diuretics (Fig. 3). This result corresponds to our previous investigations, according to which the rise in plasma renin after furosemide could be inhibited only partially by simultaneous infusion of human albumin without NaCl but completely by infusion of human albumin containing NaCl (Fig. 4). For the rise of plasma renin after diuretics, therefore, the renal sodium loss by way of a still unknown intrarenal regulation seems to be more important than the decrease in plasma volume. For the extent of natriuresis and diuresis after administration of the diuretics no importance attaches to the rise of plasma renin activity due to sodium loss and thus to aldosterone secretion in the acute test, because the natriuretic effect of the tested diuretics varies while their effect on plasma renin activity is practically equal. The natriuretic effectiveness of the diuretics, therefore, depends primarily on their site of action in the tubules and on their pharmacokinetic properties. With prolonged administration of diuretics, however, in a number of patients, especially those with cardiac insufficiency in whom plasma renin activity does not decrease under diuretic treatment as it does in the majority of patients but increases, one must take account of the stimulation of the renin-angiotensin-aldosterone system by diuretics. This stimulation limits or weakens their effect and can be neutralized by the administration of aldosterone antagonists or other substances which inhibit the sodium-potassium exchange in the distal tubules. In the acute test amiloride leads to a rise of plasma renin activity which, according to our first orientating investigations in 3 subjects, is less than with the other tested diuretics.

Clinical Application of Diuretics During and After Heart Surgery

Klinische Anwendung von Diuretica während und nach Herzoperationen

H. OELERT, F. SEBENING

Summary: Operations on the heart with the help of the heart-lung machine create overloads of sodium and water which must be corrected postoperatively by renal activity. The minimal urine flow rate for this purpose should amount to 1.0 ml/min.

Urine secretion was supported in 8 patients who had had atrial septal defects repaired with the aid of the heart-lung machine by spontaneous osmotic diuresis (2) or by administration of mannitol (2) or ethacrynic acid (1) or furosemide (3). Peak osmotic flows amounted to 11–13 ml/min; after furosemide 28 ml/min; and after ethacrynic acid 115 ml/min. It was concluded from measurements of sodium, osmolality and creatinine that during the ethacrynic acid induced diuresis no reabsorption of fluid occurred beyond the proximal tubule.

Furosemide proved to be the most useful diuretic after extracorporeal circulation, since it produced excretion of sodium and water more effectively as compared with mannitol, and a more moderate diuresis as compared with ethacrynic acid. High postoperative potassium loss in the urine occurs with any of these compounds.

Indications for administration of effective diuretics (oral single doses of ethacrynic acid or furosemide) during the remainder of the postoperative course were diminution of the urine flow rate and evidence of congestion of the greater or lesser circulation. Ethacrynic acid proved superior in terms of increased urine volume, diminution of body weight, and reabsorption of pleural effusions. Both compounds counteracted postoperative aldosteronism since the urinary sodium-potassium ratio rose from control values of unity after administration of diuretics to more than 3. Circulatory complications or manifestations of intolerance were not observed.

Die Stadien, die der Kranke im Zusammenhang mit Herzeingriffen durchläuft, können eingeteilt werden in: Operation, Aufenthalt auf der Wachstation und postoperativen Verlauf außerhalb ständiger Beobachtung. Nach dieser Einteilung soll über Indikation und klinische Anwendung diuretisch wirkender Substanzen in der Herzchirurgie berichtet werden. Diuretica, als Einzelgabe verordnet, haben das Ziel, bei Operationen, die mit Hilfe der Herz-Lungenmaschine durchgeführt werden, das akute Nierenversagen zu verhindern und bei im postoperativen Verlauf sich entwickelnder Rechts- bzw. Linksherzinsuffizienz die Flüssigkeitsausscheidung anzuregen.

Intraoperative Beobachtungen

Der Rückgang der Urinausscheidung bei Operationen ist in unterschiedlicher Weise von Flüssigkeitsabgabe an Luft und traumatisiertes Gewebe, erhöhter Ausschüttung von antidiuretischem Hormon (ADH) und gesteigerter Aldosteronaktivität abhängig. Bei

Herzoperationen im extracorporalen Kreislauf bilden außerdem Veränderungen in der Nierenhämodynamik eine besondere Gefahr für das Auftreten des postoperativen Nierenversagens. Nichtpulsatorische Aortenperfusion über die Art. femoralis, Perfusionsmitteldrucke unter 60 mm Hg und verschiedener Abgangswinkel der Nierenarterie von der retrograd durchströmten Aorta können Ursache für Verminderung von Nierendurchblutung und glomerulärer Filtrationsrate (GFR) sein. Die Aufrechterhaltung von Filtration und Urinsekretion ist aber von Bedeutung, damit die Ausscheidung des mit dem Oxygenator dem Körper zugeführten Flüssigkeitsvolumens möglich ist.

An acht, wegen eines Vorhofseptumdefektes mit Hilfe der Herz-Lungenmaschine operierten Kranken, wurde die Zufuhr und Ausscheidung von Wasser und Elektrolyten während und nach extracorporaler Zirkulation untersucht. Das Körpergewicht der Kranken betrug zwischen 58,8 und 75,0 kg, die Perfusionszeiten lagen zwischen 16 und 40 Minuten. Von Beginn der extracorporalen Zirkulation bis zum Abend des Operationstages wurden in Zeitabständen von 10 Minuten bis zu 2 Stunden Blutproben entnommen und die in diesen Zeitabständen ausgeschiedenen Urinmengen gesammelt. In Blut und Urin wurden Na^+-, K^+-, Kreatinin- und Harnstoffkonzentration gemessen, und die Gesamtosmolalität kryoskopisch bestimmt. Die glomeruläre Filtrationsrate wurde aus der Kreatininclearance errechnet.

Das Oxygenatorvolumen der Herz-Lungenmaschine bestand aus 1 400 ml einer Plasmaersatzlösung, die Glucose, Na-Bicarbonat und K-, Mg-Asparaginat in hypertoner Zusammensetzung enthielt. Verbunden mit intravenöser Flüssigkeitszufuhr bekamen die Kranken bis zum Verbringen auf die Wachstation die in Tabelle 1 aufgezeigten Elektrolyt- und Wassermengen intravasal zugeführt. Damit während der Operation eine ausreichende Nierentätigkeit, und postoperativ außerdem stabiler Blutdruck und Blutgerinnung gewährleistet sind, halten wir nach dieser Flüssigkeitsbelastung eine Diurese von 1,0 ml/min für erforderlich.

Tabelle 1. Mittlere Elektrolyt- und Wasserzufuhr bei Herzoperation in extracorporaler Zirkulation.

Wasser	2 100 ml
Glucose	65 g
Natrium	290 meq
Kalium	42 meq
Osmol	1 000 mosmol

Zwei der acht Kranken hatten schon während der Operation auf Grund der Glucosebelastung spontane osmotische Diuresen von mehr als 2 ml/min und benötigten keine zusätzliche Behandlung, um die Harnausscheidung hoch zu halten. Bei den anderen sechs wurden zur Verstärkung der Urinsekretion zweimal 250 ml 20% Mannitollösung, dreimal 40 mg Furosemid und einmal 40 mg Etacrynsäure intravenös infundiert. Grund für die nicht ausreichende Urinsekretion bei diesen Kranken, war eine Verminderung der GFR, die während extracorporaler Zirkulation aufgetreten war und sich nach Abgehen von der Herz-Lungenmaschine nicht selbständig besserte. Mit dem Einsetzen der erhöhten Urinausscheidung nach Mannitol- oder Diureticagabe, erlangte die glomeruläre Filtrationsrate den Ausgangswert von im Mittel 108 ml/min wieder zurück. Auf die Verbesserung eines akut verminderten Glomerulumfiltrats durch Diuretica hat Prof. Reubi bereits hingewiesen (s. Seite 381).

Die Diuresen waren nach Furosemid stärker, dafür kurzfristiger als die nach Mannitol oder als die spontanen osmotischen Diuresen. Sie betrugen nach Furosemid bis zu

28 ml/min und nach Mannitol bzw. ohne Diureticum maximal 11–13 ml/min. Unerwartet stark war der Harnfluß bei einem Kranken nach intravenöser Gabe von 0,5 mg pro kg Körpergewicht Etacrynsäure. Er erreichte innerhalb der ersten 5 Minuten nach Verabreichung 115 ml/min.

Die Kreatininkonzentration dieses Urins lag zwischen 4 und 5 mg% und man kann aus präoperativen Werten und aus Messungen an anderen Kranken unter Perfusionsbedingungen erwarten, daß sie etwa um das 2fache höher war, als die des Plasmas. Ein $\frac{U}{P}$ Kreatinin von 2 entspräche einem Wert, den man als endproximales $\frac{TF}{P}$ Inulin bei starken Diuresen durch Mikropunktion erhalten hat (s. Seite 215). Hierzu paßt, daß die Natriumkonzentration im Endharn mit 114 meq/l ebenfalls der Gleichgewichtskonzentration des proximalen Konvoluts bei osmotischer Diurese entspricht. Die Bedingungen für eine osmotische Diurese bestanden insofern, als durch die zugeführte Glucose der Blutglucosespiegel auf 520 mg% eingestellt war. Diese Betrachtung führt zu dem Schluß,

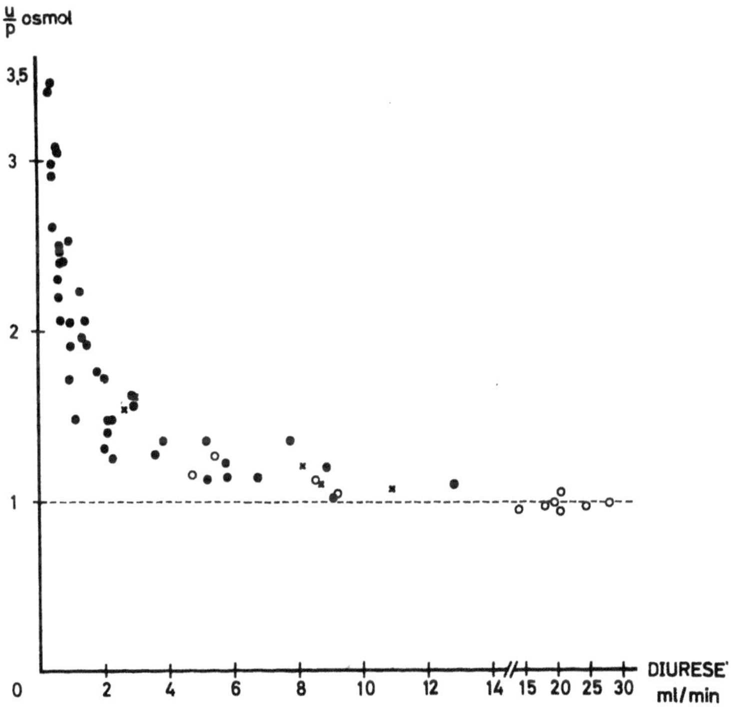

Abb. 1. Abhängigkeit des $\frac{U}{P}$ osmol von der Diurese nach Herzoperation in extracorporaler Zirkulation. Die Symbole bezeichnen die Diuresen nach Gabe von Mannitol (×), Furosemid (○) bzw. ohne Diureticum (●). Auf der Ordinate ist das Verhältnis der $\frac{\text{Urin}}{\text{Plasma}}$-Osmolalität angegeben, auf der Abszisse die Harnflußrate (ml/min). Die unterbrochene Linie bezeichnet Gleichheit der Osmolalität von Urin und Plasma.

Tabelle 2. Mittlere Elektrolytkonzentration und Gesamtosmolalität im 6-Stunden Sammelurin nach Herzoperation in extracorporaler Zirkulation. Anwendung verschiedener Diuretica.

	meq/l		
	Na^+	K^+	mosmol/kg
ohne Diureticum:	97,8	52,4	445
	95,2	56,9	461
bei Mannitol:	40,1	18,8	405
	56,6	42,5	414
bei Furosemid:	97,8	28,6	310
	123,0	44,2	342
	87,6	34,3	362
bei Etacrynsäure:	104,0	23,5	304

daß offenbar nur der proximale Tubulus resorbiert hat, und daß im distalen Tubulus d. h. Henlesche Schleife einschließlich Sammelrohr, keine weitere Resorption stattfand. Das ist ein Befund, wie ihn DEETJEN nach Etacrynsäure bei stark herabgesetzter Filtrationsrate gefunden hat (s. Seite 215). In dem vorliegenden Fall dürfte die GFR indessen nicht mehr als 50% eingeschränkt gewesen sein.

Mit dem Wiedereinsetzen eines Teils der Transportvorgänge im distalen Nephronabschnitt ging die Urinausscheidung deutlich zurück. Der Harnfluß betrug in den nächsten 10 Minuten 34 ml/min, dann 30 ml/min, wobei die Kreatininkonzentration anstieg, die Urinosmolalität dagegen von Plasmaisotonie auf leicht hypotone Werte sank.

In spontaner osmotischer Diurese und Diurese nach Gabe von Mannitol (Abb.1) fiel die Harnosmolalität von stark hypertonen Ausgangswerten nicht unter Plasmaisotonie ab. Nach intravenöser Gabe von Furosemid dagegen, wurde wie nach Etacrynsäure der Harn hypoton gegenüber Plasma, d. h. die Clearance des freien Wassers war positiv. Dieser Befund wurde auch an gesunden Versuchspersonen erhoben, die auf beide Diuretica mit starken Diuresen reagierten (1, 2). Aus ihm erklärt sich (Tab.2), daß die mittlere Osmolalität des postoperativen 6-Stunden Sammelurins bei den mit Furosemid und Etacrynsäure behandelten Kranken zwischen 304 und 362 mosmol/kg betrug, während der Urin ohne Diureticum oder nach Mannitolgabe eine mittlere osmolale Konzentration von mehr als 400 mosmol/kg aufwies.

Der Anteil des Natriums an der Gesamtosmolalität war in den Fällen mit und ohne Diureticum etwa gleich groß, während sich nach intravenöser Gabe von Mannitol eine geringere Natriumkonzentration im Urin einstellte. Die Kaliumkonzentration im Urin war sowohl nach Mannitol als auch nach Furosemid und Etacrynsäure gegenüber den Kontrollen deutlich erniedrigt. Eine Korrelation zwischen der Gesamtosmolalität und der Elektrolytkonzentration in untersuchten Sammelurinen bestand weder für Natrium noch für Kalium; dagegen war eine solche Korrelation für den Harnstoff deutlich nachweisbar (Abb.2). Hieraus geht hervor, daß die Fähigkeit der Niere, Harnstoff zu konzentrieren nach extracorporaler Zirkulation vollständig erhalten ist.

Sechs Stunden nach der Operation waren zugeführte Flüssigkeitsmenge und osmotisch wirksame Substanzen außer bei Etacrynsäure nicht vollständig im Urin wieder ausgeschieden. Tab. 3 zeigt, daß bei den übrigen Diuresen die Wasserretention mit der Natriumretention korrelierte, jedoch die Natriumretention im Überschuß zu Wasser erfolgt ist. Dagegen war die Gesamtkaliumausscheidung stets gleich groß oder größer als die Kaliumzufuhr während der Operation. Die Analyse der Elektrolytausscheidung in den Einzelurinsammelportionen ergab, daß unabhängig von der Diureseart 3 Stunden nach Beendigung der extracorporalen Zirkulation mit Abnahme des Harnflusses die Kaliumkonzentration im Urin anstieg.

Vermehrte Kaliumausscheidung bei Natrium- und Wasserretention kennzeichnen die Auswirkungen des Operationsstresses auf den postoperativen Elektrolyt- und Wasserhaushalt. Die erhöhte distale Natriumrückresorption in der Niere führt zu einer gesteigerten Kaliumsekretion und zu einer Senkung des $\frac{Na^+}{K^+}$ -Quotienten im Urin. Bei der spontanen osmotischen Diurese und der Diurese nach Mannitol sank durch den Abfall der N^+- und den Anstieg der K^+-Konzentration im Urin der $\frac{Na^+}{K^+}$ -Quotient von 2 bis 3 auf Werte kleiner als 1. Bei den Diuresen nach Gabe von Natriuretica nahm der

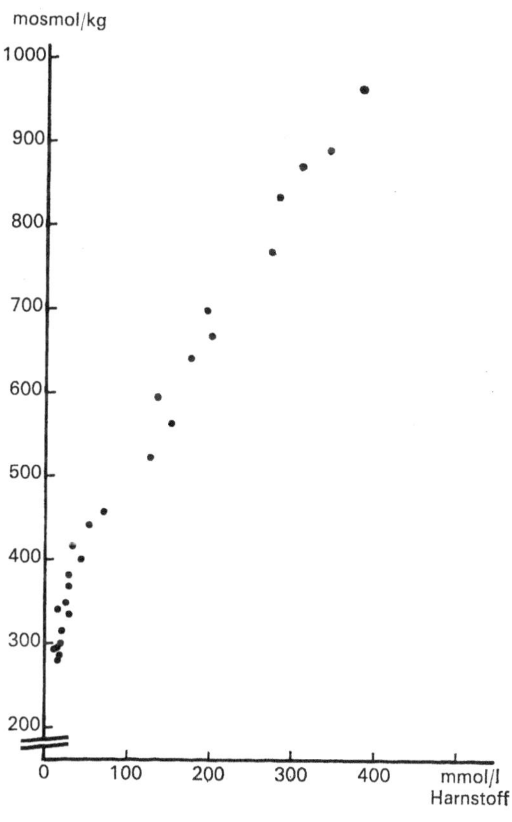

Abb. 2. Beziehung zwischen Osmolalität und Harnstoffkonzentration im Urin nach extracorporaler Zirkulation.

Tabelle 3. Mittlere Ausscheidung von Urinvolumen, Natrium, Kalium und Gesamtsomolalität im 6-Stunden Sammelurin nach Herzoperation in extracorporaler Zirkulation. Anwendung verschiedener Diuretica.

	Volumen (ml)	meq		mosmol
		Na^+	K^+	
ohne Diureticum:	1 552	151,5	81,2	690
	1 298	123,8	73,8	598
bei Mannitol:	1 468	57,3	39,7	583
	1 880	106,1	79,9	779
bei Furosemid:	1 980	193,4	56,4	614
	2 140	262,6	94,5	731
	1 522	133,5	52,2	551
bei Etacrynsäure:	3 094	320,3	72,7	942

Quotient ebenfalls ab, jedoch wurde er nicht kleiner als 1, da sowohl die Kalium-, als auch die Natriumausscheidung im Urin zunahm.

Zusammenfassend kann gesagt werden, daß bei nicht ausreichender Urinsekretion von mehr als 1,0 ml/min nach Herzoperation in extracorporaler Zirkulation diese durch intravenöse Gabe von Mannitol, Furosemid oder Etacrynsäure herbeiführbar ist. Die Zufuhr von Etacrynsäure kann im Einzelfall eine überschießende Diurese mit hoher Natriumausscheidung auslösen. Bei Mannitol-Diurese kommt es trotz Bildung eines hypertonen Urins zu starker Natriumretention; diese ist stärker als die Natriumretention bei Furosemid. Die Kaliumausscheidung ist unabhängig von der Art der Diurese gleich groß. Aus den Befunden kann abgeleitet werden, daß in der saluretischen Wirkung Etacrynsäure und Furosemid dem Mannitol überlegen sind. Furosemid ist der Etacrynsäure vorzuziehen, wenn es sich um Patienten mit starker Natrium- und Wasservorbelastung handelt und eine hohe Urinausscheidung, die mit der Gefahr des akuten Plasmavolumenmangels verbunden ist, sicher vermieden werden soll.

Postoperative Beobachtungen auf der Wachstation

Sechs Stunden nach der Operation ging der Harnfluß regelmäßig zurück auf Werte zwischen 0,4 und 0,6 ml/min. Gesteigerte Aldosteronaktivität, postoperativer Eiweißmangel und Frühinsuffizienz der Ventrikelmuskulatur sind die wesentlichen Faktoren, die zum jetzigen Zeitpunkt Oligurie und Flüssigkeitsretention im Gewebe verursachen.

105 Kranke, die mit Hilfe der Herz-Lungenmaschine operiert worden waren, erhielten zur Aufrechterhaltung der Urinsekretion Diuretica auf der Wachstation. Die Diagnosen der Kranken sind in Tab. 4 in der Reihenfolge der prozentualen Häufigkeit der Diureticagabe zusammengestellt. Bei den angeborenen Vitien bestand eine Beziehung zwischen der Anwendung von Diuretica und der postoperativen Belastung des rechten Ventrikels; bei den erworbenen Klappenerkrankungen ergab sich eine solche zur Leistungsfähigkeit des Myokards. Als Diureticum verwendeten wir Etacrynsäure (Hydromedin®) und im Vergleich dazu Furosemid (Lasix®). Die Dosierung betrug 0,5 mg/kg Körpergewicht für beide Diuretica bei intravenöser und 100 mg für Etacrynsäure bei oraler Verabfolgung.

Tabelle 4. Diagnosen der Kranken.

Angeborene Herzfehler:	Transposition der großen Gefäße Fallot'sche Tetralogie Lungenvenenfehlmündung Totaler A-V Kanal Ventrikelseptumdefekt Vorhofseptumdefekt Pulmonalstenose
Erworbene Herzfehler:	Tricuspidalinsuffizienz Mitralinsuffizienz Komb. Mitralvitium Mitralstenose Aorteninsuffizienz Aortenstenose Mehrklappenvitien

Da postoperative Flüssigkeitszufuhr und Urinausscheidung von der Körperoberfläche der Kranken abhängen, wurde für die Untersuchungen eine Unterteilung in die zwei Altersgruppen über und unter 14 Jahren vorgenommen. 33 Kranke, die unter, und 72, die über 14 Jahre alt waren, erhielten in den ersten 2–4 Tagen nach der Operation im Mittel 889 ml/24 Std. bzw. 1795 ml/24 Std. Flüssigkeit intravenös zugeführt. Die Werte für die Urinausscheidung betrugen in beiden Gruppen im Mittel 597,2 ml/24 Std. und 1056,1 ml/24 Std., ohne Gabe von Diuretica. Nach Diureticagabe war bei denselben Kranken die 24-Stunden Urinausscheidung angestiegen (Tab. 5). Der Anstieg war in beiden Altersgruppen nach Etacrynsäure stärker als nach Furosemid.

Tabelle 5. Mittlere intravenöse Flüssigkeitszufuhr und Urinausscheidung pro 24 Stunden bei 105 Kranken mit und ohne Gabe von Diuretica.

	unter 14 J.	über 14 J.
Flüssigkeitszufuhr	889,0 ml	1 795,0 ml
Urinausscheidung		
ohne Diureticum	597,2 ml	1 056,1 ml
bei Furosemid	865,9 ml	1 728,9 ml
bei Etacrynsäure	946,1 ml	1 955,4 ml

Indikation für die Anwendung von Diuretica waren Abnahme der stündlich gemessenen Urinsekretion sowie klinische und röntgenologische Zeichen der Lungenstauung. Wie Tab. 6 zeigt, betrug die mittlere Urinausscheidung 8 Stunden vor Diureticagabe im Mittel 16,7 ml/Std. bei Kranken unter 14 Jahren und 20,4 ml/Std. bei Kranken über 14 Jahre. Auf Gabe von Etacrynsäure stieg die mittlere Urinausscheidung in einer Sammelzeit von 6 Stunden auf 104,7 ml/Std. bzw. 211,7 ml/Std. an. Danach fiel sie wieder ab, blieb jedoch in den nächsten 10 Stunden weiterhin höher als die Ausgangsdiurese. Eine negative Nachschwankung trat nicht auf.

Tabelle 6. Mittlere Urinausscheidung (ml/Std.) bei 105 Kranken vor, bei und nach oraler Einzelgabe von 100 mg Etacrynsäure.

	Sammelzeit (h)	unter 14 J.	über 14 J.
vor	8	16,7	20,4
bei	6	104,7	211,7
nach	10	25,2	45,5

Zum postoperativen Verlauf außerhalb ständiger Beobachtung

Diureticagaben bei Herzoperierten außerhalb ständiger Beobachtung erfolgten weniger auf Grund einer Abnahme der Urinausscheidung als vielmehr nach klinischen Zeichen der Flüssigkeitsretention und nach dem Thorax-Röntgenbild. Zur Prüfung der diuretischen und elektrolytexcretorischen Wirkung von Etacrynsäure wurde bei 14 Kranken die Urinausscheidung 12 Stunden vor und zweimal 12 Stunden nach einer Einzelgabe von 100 mg Wirksubstanz gemessen und im Sammelurin die Na^+- und K^+-Konzentration bestimmt. Alle Kranken waren digitalisiert, erhielten natriumarme Kost und bekamen nicht mehr als altersentsprechend 900 ml bzw. 1800 ml Flüssigkeit pro Tag oral zugeführt.

Die mittlere 12-Stunden Urinausscheidung (Tab. 7) vor Diureticagabe betrug in den Altersgruppen über und unter 14 Jahren 15,4 ml/Std. bzw. 36,5 ml/Std. In den ersten 12 Stunden nach Verabfolgung von Etacrynsäure stieg die Harnflußrate im Mittel auf das 5- bzw. 3fache des Ausgangswertes an. In den zweiten 12 Stunden sank sie wieder ab, blieb jedoch etwa 20% höher als die Ausgangsdiurese.

Tabelle 7. Mittlere Urinausscheidung und Elektrolytkonzentration im Urin von 6 Kranken unter und 8 Kranken über 14 Jahre jeweils 12 Stunden vor, bei und nach oraler Einzelgabe von 100 mg Etacrynsäure.

	unter 14 J.			über 14 J.		
	ml/h Urin	meq/l Na^+	meq/l K^+	ml/h Urin	meq/l Na^+	meq/l K^+
vor	15,4	55,9	50,7	36,5	41,1	48,4
bei	73,6	108,0	32,4	114,8	87,0	24,6
nach	19,8	42,5	63,5	42,2	63,1	34,7

Die Ausscheidung von Natrium zeigte einen ähnlichen Verlauf. Im ersten 12-Stunden Sammelurin nach Gabe von Etacrynsäure war die Na^+-Konzentration auf etwa das Doppelte des Kontrollwertes erhöht. Die K^+-Konzentration sank dagegen ab. In den zweiten 12 Stunden nach Diureticagabe waren die Veränderungen der Elektrolytkonzentrationen im Urin rückläufig. Die Na^+-Konzentration fiel wieder ab, und die K^+-Konzentration stieg an. Der $\frac{Na^+}{K^+}$-Quotient, der im Kontrollurin Werte um 1 hatte, erhöhte sich nach Diureticagabe auf über 3 und nahm im weiteren Verlauf einen mittleren Wert von 1,2 an. Die Ergebnisse zeigen, daß die wasser- und elektrolytexcretorische Wirkung von

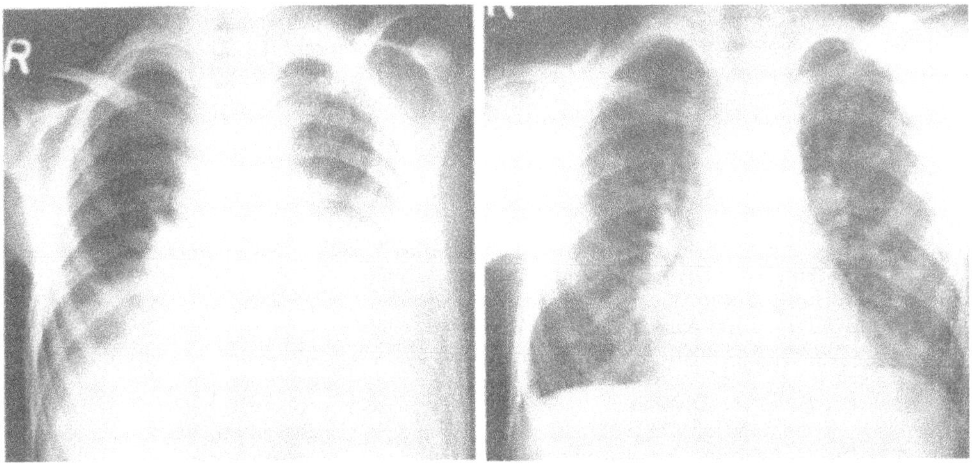

Abb. 3. Thorax-Röntgenbild eines 14 Jahre alten Jungen nach der Operation einer Fallot'schen Tetralogie. Linke Bildhälfte vor, rechte Bildhälfte nach oraler Gabe von 100 mg Etacrynsäure. Man erkennt einen deutlichen Rückgang des Pleuraergusses auf der linken Seite.

Etacrynsäure dem postoperativen Aldosteronismus, der durch Natrium- und Wasserretention bei gesteigerter K-Sekretion gekennzeichnet ist, direkt entgegengesetzt ist.

Alle Kranken, die auf Etacrynsäure mit einer Diuresesteigerung reagierten, zeigten eine deutliche Besserung der Rechtsherzinsuffizienz. Das Körpergewicht nahm bis zu 2 kg ab, die stark vergrößerte Leber wurde wieder kleiner. Besonders gingen Zeichen der Lungenstauung nach Gabe von Etacrynsäure, wenn die Harnflußrate zunahm, deutlich zurück. Kleine bis mittelgradige Stauungsergüsse in den Pleurahöhlen wurden resorbiert und traten später nicht wieder auf. Das Röntgenbild (Abb. 3, linke Bildhälfte) zeigt die Thoraxübersicht eines 14 Jahre alten Jungen am 6. Tag nach der Operation einer Fallot'schen Tetralogie. Man erkennt einen großen Pleuraerguß links und einen kleinen Winkelerguß rechts. Nach einmaliger oraler Gabe von 100 mg Etacrynsäure sind die Ergüsse 4 Tage später (Abb. 3, rechte Bildhälfte) bis auf einen kleinen Rest rechts zurückgebildet; die Gefäßfüllung der Lungen ist jetzt nach der Totalkorrektur deutlich vermehrt.

In der Behandlung der Rechtsherzinsuffizienz nach Herzoperationen hat sich Etacrynsäure als besonders gut wirksames und anderen Diuretica überlegenes Saluretieum erwiesen (Lit. s. bei 3). Trotz ausgeprägter diuretischer Reaktion nach oraler Einzelgabe von 2 bis 3 mg/kg Körpergewicht (3) wurden keine Komplikationen, auch nicht von Seiten des Kreislaufsystems beobachtet. Vermutlich trug eine Abnahme des Plasmavolumens sogar zur Besserung der Rechtsherzinsuffizienz im Anschluß an die Herzoperation bei.

Literatur / References

1. Edel, H. H., J. Eigler und E. Renner: Zum Wirkungsmechanismus der Etacrynsäure, II: Der Einfluß der Etacrynsäure auf das distale Nephron des Menschen. Klin. Wschr. **44**, 421 (1966).

2. Seldin, D. W., G. Eknoyan, W. N. Suki and F. C. Rector: Localisation of diuretic action from the pattern of water and electrolyte excretion. In: The pharmacology of diuretic agents. Ann. New York Acad. Sci. **139,** 328 (1966).
3. Oelert, H. und F. Sebening: Die diuretische Wirkung von Etacrynsäure in der Behandlung der postoperativen Herzinsuffizienz. Dtsch. med. Wschr. **93,** 1550 (1968).

Herms: Sie machen für das Nierenversagen bei einigen Ihrer Patienten nach extrakorporalem Kreislauf den Abfall des Glomerulumfiltrats verantwortlich. Wir haben bei 20 Patienten vor, während und nach Herz-Lungen-Maschinen-Operationen Clearance-Untersuchungen durchgeführt und während der extracorporalen Perfusion regelmäßig einen erheblichen Abfall des Glomerulumfiltrats gefunden. Unter Mannit-Infusion war der Abfall des Glomerulumfiltrates weniger ausgeprägt. Bei mehreren 100 Patienten mit verschiedenen Herzdefekten, die in der Chirurgischen Klinik in Düsseldorf operiert wurden, haben wir außerordentlich selten eine akute Niereninsuffizienz gefunden, und wenn, dann nur bei Patienten, die länger als eine Stunde perfundiert wurden. Sie sagten weiterhin, und das wäre mein zweiter Kommentar, daß Sie ein Diureticum dem Mannit vorzögen wegen der Gefahr einer Natriumretention. Auf unserer chirurgischen Wachstation wurde zeitweise routinemäßig Mannit gegeben, wobei gelegentlich erhebliche Natriumverluste auftraten. Seitdem geben wir Mannit nur noch, wenn die Diurese 24 Std. nach der Operation ohne ersichtlichen Grund nicht in Gang kommt. Wir geben i. a. kein Diureticum, weil man die Diurese mit Mannit besser steuern kann als mit einem Diureticum.

Oelert: Wir geben Mannit oder ein Diureticum nur dann, wenn der Harnfluß nicht von selbst nach der Flüssigkeitsbelastung ansteigt. Im übrigen ist unter Mannit die Natriumretention größer als unter Diuretica, wobei unsere Patienten ja stark natriumvorbelastet sind. Das Auftreten einer Azidose im Blut aus dem peripheren Kreislauf während extracorporaler Zirkulation verlangt, daß intra- und postoperativ Natriumbikarbonat zugeführt wird.

Jahrmärker: Sollte man bei der hohen Kaliumausscheidung antikaliurische Substanzen verwenden?

Oelert: Während und nach der Operation wird Kalium in ausreichenden Mengen substituiert. Wir verwenden dabei K^+-Mg^{++}-Asparaginat, da damit Herzrhythmusstörungen besser verhütet werden als mit Kalium-Chlorid oder Kalium-Lactat. Mit antikaliurischen Substanzen haben wir keine ausreichende Erfahrung. Durch Spironolacton konnte der hohe Kaliumverlust nach extracorporaler Zirkulation nicht verhindert werden.

Koczorek: Kalium ist ein starker Aldosteron-Stimulator. Wenn man schon präoperativ Kalium gibt, müßte man später doch um so mehr mit einer Natriumretention rechnen, sofern der postoperative Aldosteronismus für die starke Natriumretention nach Operationen als Ursache allein angeschuldigt wird.

Kramer: Sie finden bei Ihren Patienten nach Furosemid oder Mannitol eine Steigerung des Glomerulumfiltrates, während man sonst meistens eine Abnahme bekommt. Spielt dabei die Erholung des Patienten mit?

Oelert: Mannitol wird hier bei einem akut erniedrigten Glomerulumfiltrat gegeben. Dabei steigen Nierendurchblutung und Glomerulumfiltrat dann an.

Diuretics in Cerebral Edema

Diuretica beim cerebralen Ödem*)

H. J. REULEN, M. SAMII, KH. R. KOCZOREK, A. BAETHMANN,
K. SCHÜRMANN

Summary: 1. New biochemical results have shown that – in accordance with electron microscopical investigations – the edema of the cerebral cortex is completely different from the edema of the white substance, because of its intracellular localization.

The development of the intracellular edema in the brain cortex is caused by a disturbance of the intra- extracellular ionic distribution, whereas the extracellular edema of the white matter is produced by ultrafiltration into the interstitial space.

2. During the phase of edema accummulation in the brain there is a renal retention of water and sodium which depends of the degree of increase in intracranial pressure. Further, there are data indicating thet there is an increase in tubular aldosterone activity. It is difficult to decide whether an increased aldosterone activity has any pathophysiological relevance, since on the one hand Spironolactone – an aldosterone antagonist – causes an improvement in several forms of brain edema, and on the other hand brain edema is often a consequence of the insufficiency of the adrenals as well as of experimental adrenalectomy – whith can be reversed by application of aldosterone.

3. The effect of ethacrynic acid and spironolactone on the edematous brain tissue of two groups of 5 patients has been observed. The tissue had to be removed as a consequence of neurological operations. In contrast to a untreated group of patients, those treated with ethacrynic acid (75 mg/die) 4 days before surgery revealed a significant decrease of the pathological and water and sodium retention in the cortex and white matter. The urinary volume and the renal sodium excretion increased during treatment with this saluretic. After a 4-day treatment with spironolactone (600 mg/die) the edema in the cortex and the white matter was also reduced, and the renal sodium and water excretion could be increased.

These results make further clinical investigations in a larger group of patients desirable.

I. Zur Pathogenese des cerebralen Ödems

Auf eine Vielfalt von Erkrankungen des Zentralnervensystems reagiert das Gehirn im Experiment und in der Klinik einförmig mit dem Bild des Hirnödems. So sind Hirntumoren, Abszesse, Entzündungen, lokale Läsionen oder Kompressionen des Gehirns ebenso wie z. B. Schädelhirntraumen, Hochdruck, Urämie und Hypoxie häufig vergesellschaftet mit einer pathologischen Ansammlung von Flüssigkeit und Elektrolyten im Hirngewebe. Der Begriff des cerebralen Ödems umreißt damit nicht das ödemauslösende Organ, sondern den Manifestationsort.

*) Mit Unterstützung durch die Deutsche Forschungsgemeinschaft.

1. Die Bedeutung örtlicher Faktoren

Die Bemühungen um die Aufdeckung der pathogenetischen Prinzipien bei der Entstehung des Hirnödems sind erst im letzten Jahrzehnt vorangeschritten, vorwiegend durch die Arbeit mit Modellödemen im Tierexperiment. Als eine der wesentlichsten Erkenntnisse sind die elektronenmikroskopischen Befunde anzusehen, daß die Reaktionsweise des Gehirns auf eine Ödemnoxe beim Menschen und beim Tier konstant durch zwei verschiedene, zum Teil nebeneinander auftretende, morphologische Veränderungen gekennzeichnet ist (Lit. s. 5, 17). So wird beim Ödem der Hirnrinde bzw. der grauen Substanz eine intrazelluläre Flüssigkeitseinlagerung beobachtet. An diesem Zellhydrops sind vornehmlich Gliazellen beteiligt, während Nervenzellen nicht oder nur in sehr späten Stadien schwellen. Der extracelluläre Raum ist in den Anfangsstadien nicht verbreitert. Beim Ödem der weißen Substanz hingegen steht nach den elektronenoptischen Bildern neben der Schwellung der Gliazellen und den Veränderungen an den Markscheiden vor allem eine Erweiterung der extracellulären Räume zwischen den Bündeln von parallel verlaufenden Markfasern im Vordergrund (6, 26). Inzwischen sind Messungen des physiologischen Extracellulärraumes bei verschiedenen Ödemformen mit Indikatoren wie Inulin, Sulfat oder Thiocyanat bekannt geworden, welche die morphologischen Befunde größtenteils bestätigen (1, 5, 16). (Die bisher mit diesen Substanzen am Gehirn ermittelten extracellulären Verteilungsvolumina sind zwar wegen des methodischen Fehlers der sog. »sink-action« (5) zu niedrig, doch erlauben die relativen Unterschiede zwischen dem normalen und dem ödematösen Gehirn eine Aussage.) Ödeme der weißen Substanz zeigen analog den morphologischen Ergebnissen eine Vergrößerung des interstitiellen Raumes; im Gegensatz dazu bleibt der EZR beim generalisierten Ödem der Cortex unverändert. Nur bei einer gewissen Form von Rindenödemen in der unmittelbaren Umgebung von Tumoren oder Läsionen konnten Katzman und Mitarb. (16) eine Zunahme des Verteilungsraumes dieser Indikatoren beobachten, obwohl die elektronenmikroskopischen Bilder nur die geschwollenen Gliazellen zeigen. Es liegen Hinweise vor, daß hier eine Schädigung der Bluthirnschranke und eine Permeation dieser Stoffe in die geschwollenen Astrozyten besteht.

Eine Betrachtung der pathologischen Veränderungen des Wasser- und Kationengehaltes im Hirngewebe vervollständigt dieses Bild unterschiedlicher Reaktionstypen des Ödems in Rinde und Mark (Abb. 1). Im tiefen Marklager ist die Flüssigkeitseinlagerung durchschnittlich $2^1/_2$-fach stärker als in der Cortex, während Natrium in grauer und weißer Substanz in gleichem Ausmaß eingelagert wird. Gleichzeitig findet sich ein Kaliumverlust, der in der Rinde gering stärker ist als im Mark. Die an 32 Patienten mit cerebralem Ödem verschiedener Ätiologie erhobenen Meßwerte stimmen damit prinzipiell mit den bereits bekannten Daten aus dem Tierexperiment überein (2, 4, 9, 10, 16, 20, 22)

Wenn also nach den geschilderten feinstrukturellen und biochemischen Befunden im Marklager eine im üblichen Sinne extracelluläre Ödemansammlung vorliegt, so haben wir es in der Rinde im wesentlichen mit einer intracellulären Variante des Ödems, nämlich einer intra-/extracellulären Verteilungsstörung zu tun. Demnach ist auch zu erwarten, daß die Ödemflüssigkeit in der Rinde und im Marklager eine unterschiedliche Zusammensetzung besitzt. Hierfür sprechen auch eindeutig die am Menschen und Tier erhobenen Befunde. Die pathologische Flüssigkeitseinlagerung im *Mark* entspricht in ihrer Zusammensetzung an Natrium und Chlorid am ehesten dem Serum oder einem Serum-

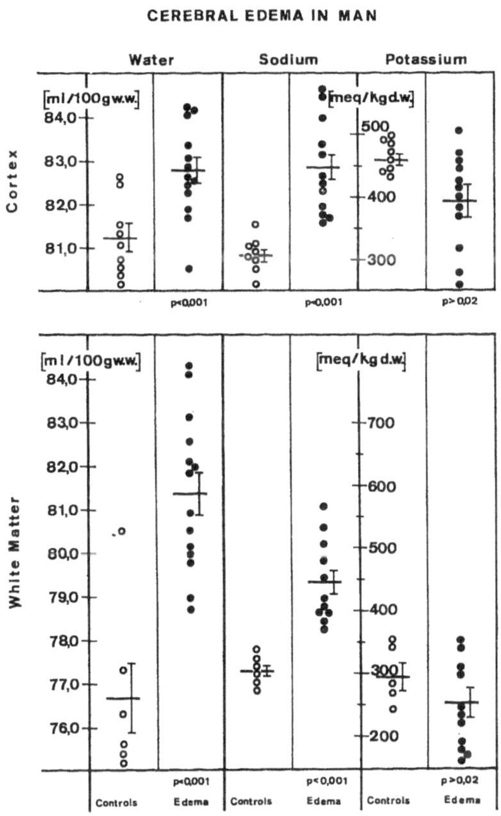

Abb. 1. Der Wasser-, Natrium- und Kalium-Gehalt in normaler und ödematöser Cortex und weißer Substanz beim Menschen. Die Punkte stellen Einzelwerte dar. (w. w. = Feuchtgewicht, d. w. = Trockengewicht). (REULEN, MEDZIHRADSKY und Mitarb. 24).

Ultrafiltrat (Abb. 2) (2, 8, 9, 16). Die meisten dieser Ödemformen zeichnen sich ferner durch einen erhöhten Austritt von J^{131}-markiertem Albumin in das Gewebe aus (1, 16). Man darf daraus schließen, daß dies eine Störung der Kapillarpermeabilität anzeigt, welche für den Austritt von Serumflüssigkeit verantwortlich ist. Beim Menschen und beim Tier zeigen jüngste Ergebnisse von KARCHER und LOWENTHAL (15), CLASEN (10) sowie FRICK (11) mit elektrophoretischen und immunelektrophoretischen Methoden das Vorhandensein von Albumin und bei schwereren Ödemverläufen auch Globulin in der Ödemzone auf. Es hängt wohl im Einzelfall vom Ausmaß der Schädigung der Kapillarwand ab, ob dabei ein Ultrafiltrat oder zusätzlich Albumin oder Globulin in das Gewebe austritt. Der Abstrom von Plasmawasser und Elektrolyten in den interstitiellen Flüssigkeitsraum soll dabei wesentlich von hämodynamischen Faktoren abhängig sein. KLATZO (17) fand experimentell bei Erhöhung des arteriellen Mitteldruckes eine beschleunigte Ausbreitung des Marködems und umgekehrt eine Verlangsamung bei arterieller Hypotension.

Im *Rindengrau* weicht die Natrium- und Chlorid-Konzentration der Ödemflüssigkeit deutlich von der Konzentration der interstitiellen Flüssigkeit ab (Abb. 2) (3, 20, 22, 23). In Verbindung mit dem gleichzeitigen Kaliumverlust, der etwa $^1/_3$ der Natriumzunahme beträgt, sowie dem Fehlen eines Proteinaustrittes bei dieser Ödemform (mit Ausnahme der unmittelbaren Läsionsumgebung, 1, 16) darf man deshalb annehmen, daß die Ödemflüssigkeit intracellulär in den geschwollenen Gliazellen liegt.

Über die Natur dieser Verteilungsstörung an den Zellgrenzflächen der Gliazellen ist bei den klinisch vorliegenden Ödemen wenig bekannt. Im Experiment ließen sich ähnliche Ödeme durch Hemmung des aktiven Ionentransportes (Kälte, Ouabain) oder durch einen Energiemangel durch Störung des Substratstoffwechsels (Hypoxie, Dinitrophenol) nachahmen (4, 22, 23, 30). Wieweit daneben noch eine Beeinflussung passiver, also energieunabhängiger Verteilungsmechanismen oder Änderungen der Membraneigenschaften (Membranpermeabilität) ursächlich beteiligt sind, läßt sich noch nicht übersehen.

2. Die Bedeutung renaler und steroidabhängiger Faktoren

Es stellt sich die Frage, ob bei der Entwicklung des Ödems neben den besprochenen örtlichen Mechanismen renale, steroidabhängige Faktoren im Sinne der Auslösung oder der Unterhaltung des Prozesses beteiligt sein könnten. Vorausgeschickt sei, daß die Rolle des Aldosterons keineswegs geklärt ist, da sich einerseits während der progredienten Ödembildung Hinweise für eine erhöhte renale Aldosteronaktivität ergeben und andererseits durch einen Aldosteronmangel ein Hirnödem ausgelöst werden kann. So war der Gruppe um Brilmayer und Marguth (6) aufgefallen, daß Patienten mit einer akuten Schädelinnendrucksteigerung einen reduzierten, beim Auftreten von Einklemmungserscheinungen einen stark erniedrigten Natrium-/Kalium-Quotienten, bei chronischer Drucksteigerung jedoch einen normalen Na-/K-Quotienten im 24-Stunden-Urin aufwiesen, was als

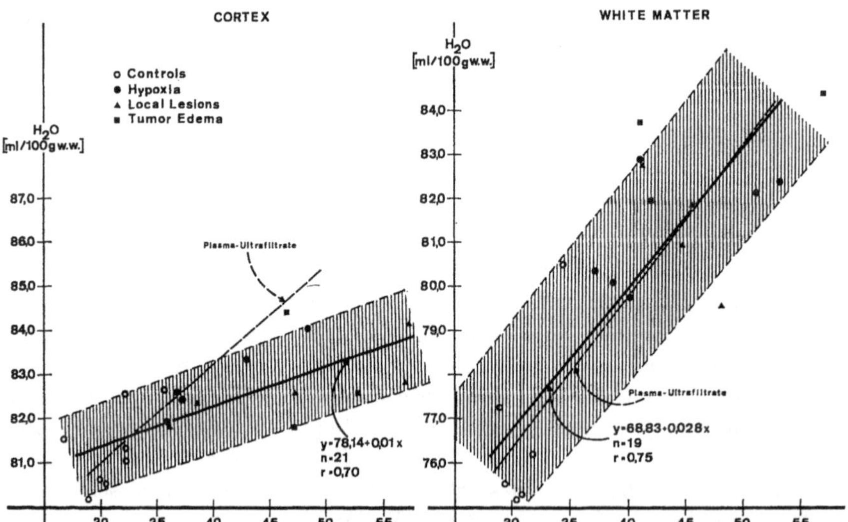

Abb. 2. Die Beziehung zwischen der Zunahme des Natrium- und Wassergehaltes in der ödematösen Cortex und weißen Substanz beim Menschen. Die ausgezogene Gerade gibt die errechnete Regressionsgerade dieser Beziehung an. Zum Vergleich ist als gestrichelte Linie die Beziehung zwischen der Natrium- und Wasserzunahme eines Plasma-Ultrafiltrates angegeben (Reulen, Medzihradsky und Mitarb. 24).

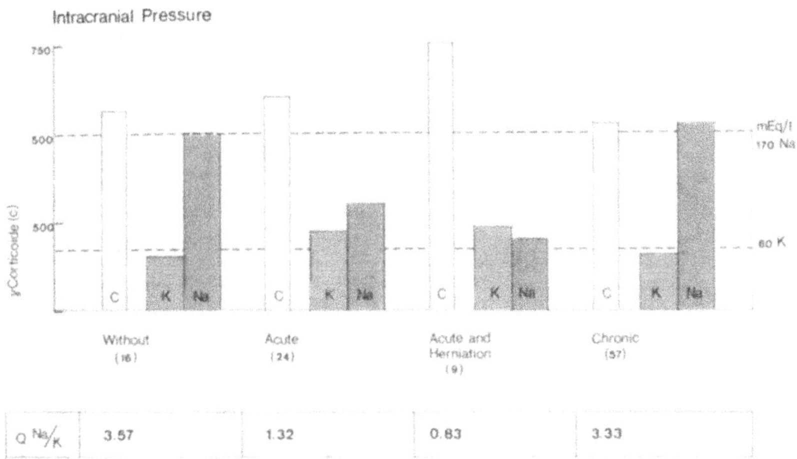

Abb. 3. Corticoid-, Natrium- und Kalium-Ausscheidung bei akuter und chronischer Schädelinnendrucksteigerung (Brilmayer und Marguth, 6).

klinischer Hinweis für eine renal-tubuläre Aldosteronaktivität während der Phase der Ödemeinlagerung aufgefaßt werden darf (Abb. 3). Dieser Befund wird erweitert durch neuere Messungen der Aldosteron-Exkretionsrate beim chronischen Hirnödem durch Koczorek und Mitarbeiter (18). Sieben von zehn untersuchten Patienten wiesen eine erhöhte Aldosteronausscheidung auf, obwohl gleichzeitig das Bild eines renalen Escape-Phänomens vorlag.

Die Bedeutung des Aldosterons als pathophysiologischer Faktor schien sich zunächst durch Beobachtungen bestätigen zu lassen, wonach mit Aldosteron-Antagonisten von Koczorek und Mitarb. (18) beim chronischen Hirnödem, von Buchborn und Hartenbach (8) beim Hirnödem nach schweren Verbrennungen und von Wildhirt (28) beim Hirnödem nach porto-cavalen Shuntoperationen dramatische Besserungen auftraten. Diesen rein klinischen Beobachtungen stehen inzwischen direkte Gewebsanalysen und elektronenoptische Untersuchungen des Gehirns im Tierexperiment zur Seite. Baethmann und Mitarb. (3) konnten beim Hirnödem nach Schädelhirntrauma eine signifikante Ausschwemmung des Ödems nach Verabreichung des Antagonisten und – als interressanter Befund – auch nach Verabreichung von 80 γ Aldosteron pro die nachweisen (Abb. 4). Dies wurde inzwischen von Wesemann und Pia (27) am Modell des Kältetraumas bestätigt, wo sie neben der Ausschwemmung der Natrium- und Wassereinlagerung eine Verminderung der Gliazellschwellung in der ödematösen Cortex beobachten konnten.

Gleichzeitig liegen allerdings viele klinisch und pathologisch gesicherte Berichte vor, wonach unter den Bedingungen des Aldosteronmangels beim Morbus Addison die von Klippel 1899 erstmals beschriebene Addison'sche Encephalopathie mit dem typischen makroskopischen und histologischen Bild des Hirnödems auftreten kann (Lit. s. 13). Gleichsinnig ist wohl das Auftreten eines Hirnödems nach Suppresion der Nebennierenrinden-Funktion durch akutes Absetzen einer chronischen Corticosteroid-Therapie zu werten (Lit. s. 13). Bei der experimentellen Nachprüfung dieser Beobachtung konnten Baethmann und Mitarb. zeigen, daß sich bei der Ratte nach einer bilateralen Adrenal-

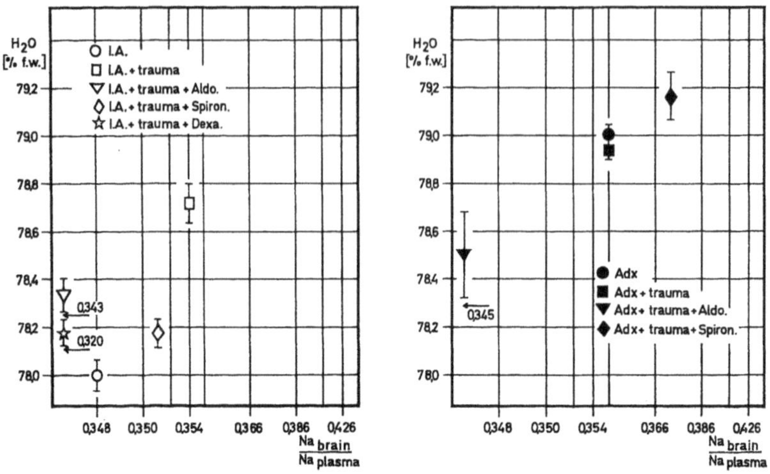

Abb. 4. Die Beziehung zwischen Na-Verteilungsquotient Hirn/Serum und dem Wassergehalt des Gehirns bei Kontrollen (Ko) und bei bilateral adrenalektomierten Tieren (Adx) nach Schädeltrauma (Trauma), nach Trauma unter chronischer Aldosteronsubstitution (Aldo., 14 Tage lang täglich 80 γ/kg KG d-Aldosteron) und nach Trauma und Gabe von Aldadiene-Kalium (MF 465a, 2mal 40 mg/kg innerhalb 27 Std. und nach dem Trauma). Der Anstieg der Na-Verteilungsquotienten beruht bei den Kontrollen auf der Zunahme des Natriumgehaltes im Gehirn, bei den adrenalektomierten Tieren sowohl auf der Zunahme der Na-Konzentration im Hirngewebe, als auch auf der Konzentrationsabnahme im Serum (BAETHMANN, A. und Mitarb., 3).

ektomie ein Hirnödem mit einer Wasser- und Natriumeinlagerung im Hirngewebe entwickelt (Abb. 4), welches dem in der Umgebung von Tumoren oder nach Hypoxie sehr ähnlich ist und welches durch eine ausreichende Substitution der Tiere mit Aldosteron, nicht aber mit dem Antagonisten wieder aufgehoben werden kann.

Nach diesen Befunden fällt es schwer, im Aldosteron weiter einen pathophysiologischen Faktor bei der Ausbildung des cerebralen Ödems zu sehen. Ausgehend von dem Befund, daß das chronische Hirnödem häufig mit einem Aldosteronismus und einem gleichzeitig bestehenden renalen Escape-Phänomen einhergeht, sowie den tierexperimentellen Ergebnissen von BAETHMANN und Mitarb. (3), daß durch exogene Aldosteronzufuhr die pathologische Flüssigkeitseinlagerung sowohl beim traumatischen als auch bei dem durch Adrenalektomie erzeugten Hirnödem vermindert werden kann, hat KOCZOREK folgende Arbeitshypothese zur Deutung dieser zunächst diametralen Befundkonstellation vorgelegt: Der reaktive Aldosteronismus beim chronischen und beim akuten Hirnödem wird durch noch unbekannte Bedingungen des Ödems selbst ausgelöst und stellt einen protektiven Mechanismus gegen das Ödem dar. Da ferner im Tierexperiment sowohl Aldosteron als auch der Antagonist einen gleich günstigen Effekt auf das Hirnödem ausüben, sollte der Antagonist seine therapeutische Wirkung in indirekter Weise auf dem Umweg einer weiteren oder rascheren Steigerung der Aldosteronsekretion ausüben (18). Als weitere Möglichkeit ist eine unterschiedliche Wirkung des Aldosterons auf das Rinden- und das Marködem zu erwägen. Diese interessante Hypothese bedarf allerdings noch einer Erweiterung und Sicherung durch entsprechende Untersuchungen.

II. Zur Therapie des cerebralen Ödems

Bei einem generalisierten schweren Hirnödem kann die im Hirngewebe sequestrierte Menge an Ödemflüssigkeit maximal 150–200 ml und 50–70 mval Natrium betragen. Die Beurteilung des Therapieerfolges durch diuretisch wirkende Maßnahmen läßt sich aus diesem Grunde nicht unmittelbar an der renalen Natrium- und Wasserelimination ersehen. Man ist deshalb auf eine direkte Analyse des ödematösen Hirngewebes vorwiegend im Experiment angewiesen, da eine Beurteilung am Patienten nur in beschränktem Umfang möglich ist. Es soll betont werden, daß die Ödembehandlung mit Saluretica oder hypertonischen Lösungen immer nur ein Teil des Therapieplanes sein kann, der gleichzeitig die Grundkrankheit berücksichtigen muß. Auf die Häufigkeit einer Hypoxie bei bewußtseinsgetrübten Ödempatienten und deren Gefahren hat vor allem die Gruppe um FROWEIN auf Grund ihrer ausgedehnten Untersuchungen hingewiesen (12).

1. Hypertonische Lösungen

Es ist hervorzuheben, daß die Wirkung dieser Substanzen nicht auf der von ihnen induzierten osmotischen Diurese, sondern auf der Erhöhung der Serumosmolalität beruht. JAVID und ANDERSEN konnten nämlich zeigen, daß der Wasserentzug aus dem Gehirn wesentlich ausgeprägter war und länger anhielt, wenn bei den Versuchstieren zuvor eine bilaterale Ureteren-Ligatur vorgenommen worden war. Durch die Erhöhung der extracellulären Osmolalität wird zwischen Plasma und Gehirn bzw. Liquor ein osmotischer Gradient erzeugt, der für den rein osmotischen Entzug der Flüssigkeit aus dem Gehirn und dem Liquorraum verantwortlich ist (Abb. 5), während das pathologisch erhöhte Natrium nicht beeinflußt wird (21). Mannit und Sorbit eignen sich deshalb besonders zur Ausschwemmung des Ödemwassers, weil sie bei intakter Blut-Hirnschranke in das Hirngewebe – im Gegensatz zu anderen Organen wie Herz oder Leber – nicht oder nur äußerst langsam einzudringen vermögen (19, 29). Im Gehirn wird deshalb nicht wie dort ein schneller Konzentrationsausgleich mit dem Serum erreicht, welcher den Wasserentzug begrenzt.

Neuere experimentelle Überprüfungen haben nun Zweifel geweckt, ob die Wirksamkeit der Osmotherapie beim Rinden- und Marködem gleich stark ausgeprägt ist! Die Überprüfung dieser Frage liefert noch kein eindeutiges Bild, es scheint sich aber abzuzeichnen,

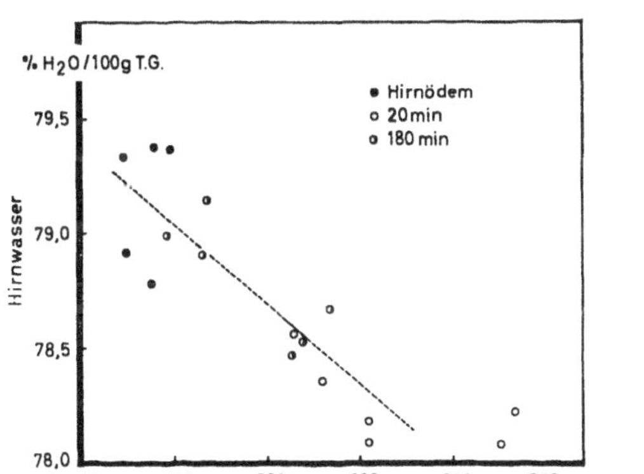

Abb. 5. Die Änderung des Wassergehaltes des ödematösen Rattengehirns 20 und 180 min nach Erhöhung der Serumosmolalität durch akute Infusion von Harnstoff oder Mannitol (REULEN, 21).

daß intracelluläre Rindenödeme und vermutlich auch vorwiegend extracelluläre Marködeme günstig auf die Osmotherapie ansprechen, wobei der oben skizzierte Mechanismus gültig ist (21, 26). Das extracelluläre Marködem mit lokaler Schädigung der Blut-Hirnschranke wird dagegen kaum beeinflußt (9, 20). Vermutlich kann sich bei letzterer Ödemform wegen der aufgehobenen Schranke zwischen Blut und Interstitium kein Osmogradient ausbilden. Wenn sich dabei unter der Osmotherapie trotzdem das Hirnvolumen reduziert, so basiert das auf dem noch vorhandenen Wasserentzug aus den gesunden, nicht veränderten Hirnarealen und aus dem Liquorraum (9, 20).

Nach etwa 8–10 Std. tritt bei beiden Substanzen der sog. Rebound-Effekt auf. Das anfängliche Ödem ist zu diesem Zeitpunkt wieder vorhanden oder hat sogar zugenommen, wobei Messungen des Liquordruckes einen Anstieg über den Ausgangswert vor Beginn der Behandlung zeigen (2, 19, 21, 26, 29). Der Re-Ödematisierung liegt nach der Normalisierung der Serumosmolalität der jetzt in entgegengesetzter Richtung bestehende Osmogradient durch die im Gewebe verbliebenen Elektrolyte (21) und durch den jetzt negativen Mannit- bzw. Sorbitgradienten zwischen Serum und Gehirn bzw. Liquor zugrunde (19, 29), so daß nun entlang diesem Gefälle Flüssigkeit in das Gehirn bzw. auch in den Liquor zurückströmt.

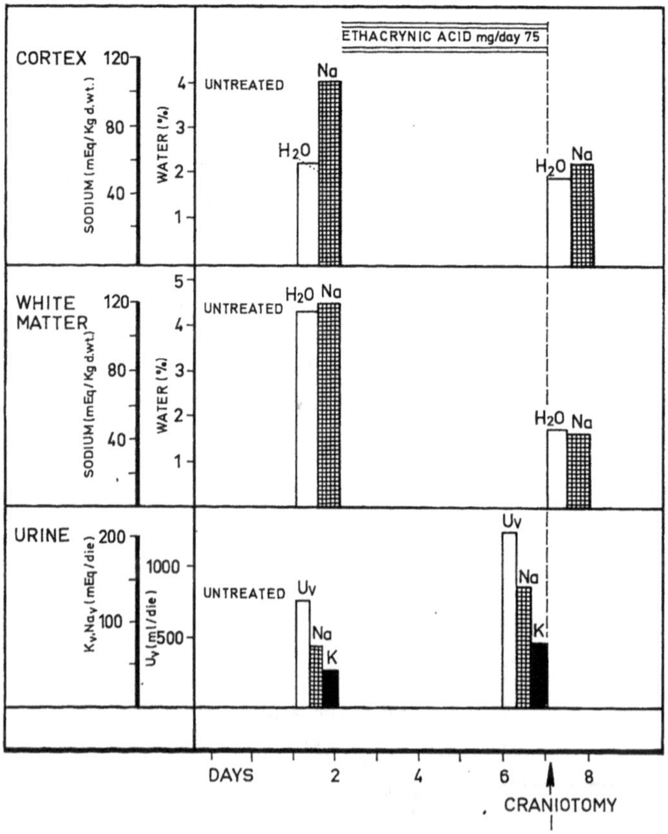

Abb. 6. Das Natrium- und Wassergehalt des ödematösen Gehirns bei 5 unbehandelten Patienten (linke Säulengruppe) und bei 5 Patienten nach 4-tägiger Behandlung mit Etacrynsäure (rechte Säulengruppe). Die Werte sind als relative Veränderungen gegenüber dem Normalwert angegeben. Im unteren Teil der Abb. ist das Urinvolumen und die renale Kationenausscheidung der behandelten Patienten vor Behandlungsbeginn (linke Säulengruppe) und am 4. Behandlungstag (rechte Säulengruppe) wiedergegeben.

Bei diesem Wirkungsmechanismus ist eine Dauertherapie nicht möglich. In der Klinik wird aber die Eigenschaft der passageren Dehydrierung des Gehirns bei Ödemen mit akuter Schädelinnendrucksteigerung mit dem Ziel ausgenützt, in der Phase der starken Volumenvermehrung die intrakranielle Hypertension mit ihren Komplikationen (Einklemmung, Atemlähmung) durch ein- oder mehrmalige Gabe bis zur Remission zu überbrücken, die evtl. bei der verbesserten cerebralen Durchblutung und O_2-Aufnahme (25) früher einsetzt.

2. Saluretica und Aldosteron-Antagonisten

Die Anwendung von Saluretica gründet sich auf die Beobachtung, daß nach schweren Hirntraumen, nach Hirnoperationen und bei Hirntumoren während der Phase der Ödembildung renal Natrium und Wasser retiniert werden. Diese Vorgänge wurden an einem größeren Krankengut von BRILMAYER und FROWEIN (7) und BRILMAYER und MARGUTH (6) dargestellt. Ungeachtet der klinischen Berichte über einen erfolgreichen Einsatz von rasch wirkenden Saluretica (12) als auch Aldosteron-Antagonisten (8, 18, 27, 18) beim Hirnödem ist deren Wirkung durch Gewebsanalysen noch nicht ausreichend untermauert. Unsere bisherigen Untersuchungsergebnisse zusammen mit SAMII, KOCZOREK und SCHÜRMANN beziehen sich auf Beobachtungen an 5 Ödempatienten nach 4-tägiger Vorbehandlung mit Etacrynsäure. Den Patienten wurde während einer Kraniotomie, der sie sich wegen verschiedener cerebraler Läsionen unterziehen mußten, Gewebsproben zur biochemischen Untersuchung aus Arealen entnommen, die später bei der Operation entfernt werden mußten. Gegenüber einer unbehandelten Gruppe von 5 Ödempatienten, die eine deutliche Natrium- und Wassereinlagerung in Cortex und Marklager zeigten, wird nach der Behandlung mit 75 mg Etacrynsäure pro die im Mittel ein wesentlich geringeres Ödem sowohl in der Rinde als auch in der weißen Substanz vorgefunden (Abb. 6). Die Serumnatriumkonzentration veränderte sich innerhalb der Untersuchungsperiode nicht, Kalium fiel gering ab. Das mittlere Urinvolumen vor der Behandlung betrug 810 ml und ist durch eine Einschränkung der Natriumelimination gekennzeichnet. Am letzten Behandlungstag vor der Operation betrug das Urinvolumen im Mittel 1265 ml, die Natriumausscheidung 148 mval/24 Std. Bei einer Vergleichsgruppe von 5 mit einem intravenös verabreichbaren Spirolacton behandelten Patienten wurde eine ähnliche Abnahme des Ödems in grauer und weißer Substanz gefunden. Die Natriumausscheidung nahm dabei gleichzeitig im Mittel auf 162 und das Urinvolumen von 760 auf 1130 ml/ 24 Std. zu (Abb. 7). Bei einem mit Spironolacton behandelten 10-jährigen Mädchen fand sich in der Rinde ein wesentlich stärker ausgeprägtes Ödem als bei unbehandelten Patienten. Ob hier ein therapierefraktäres Verhalten vorliegt läßt sich im einzelnen nicht entscheiden, da uns die Ausgangswerte vor der Behandlung nicht bekannt sind und andererseits der normale Wasser- und Natriumgehalt des Gehirns umgekehrt proportional dem Alter absinkt.

Nach diesen Ergebnissen kann sowohl durch das Saluretícum als auch durch Spironolacton eine Durchbrechung der vorher bestehenden Natrium- und Wasserretention und vor allem eine Ausschwemmung des cerebralen Ödems erreicht werden. Die Kranken befanden sich vor Behandlungsbeginn in verschiedenen Stadien der intrakraniellen Drucksteigerung und retinierten in wechselndem Ausmaß Mengen des täglichen Natriumangebotes. Die geringe Anzahl der bisher untersuchten Fälle erlaubt jedoch nicht, einen

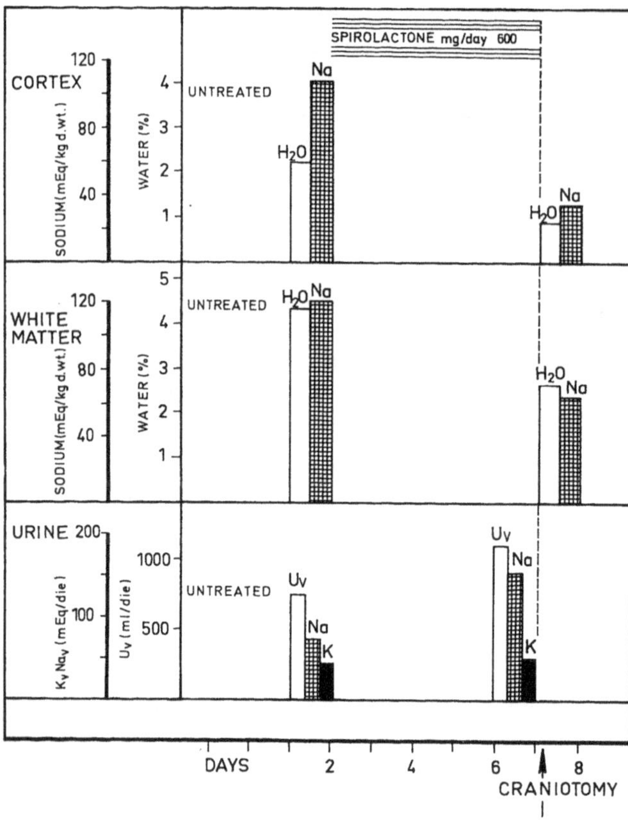

Abb. 7. Der Natrium- und Wassergehalt des ödematösen Gehirns bei 5 unbehandelten Patienten (linke Säulengruppe) und bei 5 Patienten nach 4tägiger Behandlung mit Aldadiene-Kalium (rechte Säulengruppe). Die Werte sind als relative Veränderungen gegenüber dem Normalwert angegeben. Im unteren Teil der Abbildung ist das Urinvolumen und die renale Kationenausscheidung der behandelten Patienten vor Behandlungsbeginn (linke Säulengruppe) und am 4. Behandlungstag (rechte Säulengruppe) wiedergegeben.

Unterschied in dem Wirkungsgrad beider Medikamente abzuleiten. Es scheint sich allerdings abzuzeichnen, daß mit Etacrynsäure eine stärkere Ausschwemmung des Marködems erzielt werden kann, wenn auch diese Aussage noch einer Sicherung an einer größeren Patientengruppe bedarf. Das Ergebnis legt aber doch nahe, die Effekte einer Kombination des Salureticums mit Spironolacton zu überprüfen.

Literatur / References

1. Bakay, L.: Radio-Isotopic studies in brain edema. In: Brain Edema. Springer 1967.
2. Bakay, L. and I. C. Lee: Cerebral edema. Ch. Thomas 1965.
3. Baethmann, A., Kh. R. Koczorek, H. J. Reulen, W. Wesemann, H. F. Hofmann, A. Angstwurm und W. Brendel: Die Beeinflussung des traumatischen Hirnödems durch Aldosteron, Aldosteron-Antagonisten und Dexamethason im Tierexperiment. In: Postop. Störungen des Elektrolyt- und Wasserhaushaltes. Schattauer Verlag 1967, S. 163.
4. Brendel, W. und H. J. Reulen: Die Kälteschwellung des Gehirns. Langenbecks Arch. Klin. Chir. **308**, 903 (1964).
5. Brendel, W. und H. J. Reulen: Die experimentelle Erforschung des Hirnödems. In: Hydrodynamik, Elektrolyt- und Säure-Basen-Haushalt im Liquor und Nervensystem. Thieme 1967.
6. Brilmayer, H. und F. Marguth: Störungen im Zwischenhirn-Hypophysensystem bei Hirntumoren. Dtsch. Z. Nervenhk. **176**, 441 (1957).

7. Brilmayer, H. und R. A. Frowein: Eiweiß- und Elektrolytveränderungen im Blut und Urin während des akuten Stadiums nach Schädel-Hirnverletzungen und nach Hirnoperationen. Langenbecks Arch. Klin. Chir. **294,** 205 (1960).
8. Buchborn, E. und Kh. R. Koczorek: Aldosteronantagonisten und ihre klinische Anwendung. Verhdlg. Ges. Inn. Med. 1962, S. 649.
9. Clasen, R. A., H. H. Sky-Peck, S. Pandolfi, I. Laing and G. M. Hass: The chemistry of isolated edema fluid in experimental cerebral injury. In: Brain Edema. Springer 1967.
10. Clasen, R. A., P. M. Cooke, S. Pandolfi, G. Carnecki and G. Bryar. Hypertonic urea in experimental cerebral edema. Arch. Neurol. **12,** 424 (1965).
11. Frick, E.: Immunhistologische Untersuchungen zum Hirnödem. In: Hydrodynamik, Elektrolyt- und Säure-Basen-Haushalt im Liquor und Nervensystem. Thieme 1967.
12. Frowein, R. A., A. Karimi und K. H. Euler: Hypoxydose nach schweren Hirntraumen. Zbl. Neurochir. **23,** 3 (1963).
13. Glowacki, I., G. C. Guazzi, C. Alvisi, P. P. Gambetti, M. Bonckheer, et C. A. Tassinari: L'oedema cérébral pseudotumoral endocrinien et/ou métabolique. Acta neurol. belg. **65,** 873 (1965).
14. Javid, M. and I. Anderson: The effect of urea on cerebrospinal fluid pressure in monkeys before and after bilateral nephrectomy. J. Lab. Clin. Med. **53,** 484 (1959).
15. Karcher, D. and A. Lowenthal: Hydrosoluble proteins of edematous human nervous tissue. In: Brain Edema. Springer 1967.
16. Katzman, R.: Biochemical correlates of cerebral edema. In: Brain Edema. Springer 1967.
17. Klatzo, I.: Neuropathological aspects of brain edema. J. Neuropath. Exp. Neurol. **26,** 1 (1967).
18. Koczorek, Kh. R., H. Angstwurm, A. Baethmann, D. Engelhardt, H. J. Reulen, P. Schmiedek, W. Vogt, B. Simon, E. Frick und W. Brendel: Aldosteronausscheidung beim Pseudotumor cerebri – einer klinischen Form des Hirnödems unbekannter Ursache. In: Postop. Störungen des Elektrolyt- und Wasserhaushaltes. Schattauer Verlag 1967, S. 177.
19. McQueen, J. D., L. D. Jeanes. Dehydration and rehydration of the brain with hypertonic urea and mannitol. J. Neurosurg. **21,** 118 (1964).
20. Pappius, H. M., L. A. Dayes: Hypertonic urea. Its effect on the distribution of water and electrolytes in normal and edematous brain tissues. Arch. Neurol. **25** (1965).
21. Reulen, H. J.: Vor- und Nachteile der osmotischen Therapie des Hirnödems. Zbl. Neurochir. **26,** 232 (1965).
22. Reulen, H. J.: Energetische Störungen des Kationentransportes als Ursache des intracellulären Hirnödems. Habilschrift, Mainz 1967.
23. Reulen, H. J. und A. Baethmann: Das Dinitrophenol-Ödem. Ein Modell zur Pathophysiologie des Hirnödems. Klin. Wschr. **45,** 149 (1967).
24. Reulen, H. J., F. Medzihradsky, R. Enzenbach, F. Marguth und W. Brendel: Electrolytes, fluids and metabolites of the energy metabolism and glycolysis in human cerebral edema. Im Druck.
25. Schmidt, K.: Zur Wirkung einiger Osmotherapeutica. Anaesthesist **12,** 216 (1963).
26. Struck, G. und W. Umbach: Das elektronenoptische Bild des Hirnödems in Rinde und Mark beim gleichen Patienten vor und nach medikamentöser Dehydrierung. Neurochirurgia **7,** 61 (1964).
27. Wesemann, W. and H. W. Pia: The treatment of the posttraumatic phase after cerebral injury with an aldosterone antagonist. III. Europ. Congr. Exper. Surgery, München 1968.
28. Wildhirt, E. und R. Kreyden: Die Behandlung von Zuständen nach porto-cavalen Shuntoperationen mit Aldactone. In: Klin. Anwendung der Aldosteron-Antagonisten. Thieme 1962.
29. Wise, B. L., R. K. Kerkins, E. Stevenson and K. G. Scott: Penetration of C^{14}-labelled mannitol from serum into cerebrospinal fluid and brain. Exp. Neurol. **10,** 264 (1964).
30. Zadunaisky, J. A., E. Wald and E. D. P. de Robertis: Osmotic behaviour and glial changes in isolated frog brains. In: Biology of Neuroglia, Elsevier 1965.

HERMS: Eine praktisch therapeutische Frage: Meinen Sie, daß man lokale Ödeme mit Diuretica, also auf Kosten der Abnahme des Extracellulärvolumens behandeln sollte, anstatt wie bisher, durch Infusion hochosmolarer Lösungen in die Carotis?

REULEN: Diese Frage ist vorläufig noch schwierig zu beantworten. Die Anwendung von hypertonischen Lösungen – wir ziehen die intravenöse Gabe der Infusion in die Carotis vor – führt nur zu einer kurzfristigen Dehydrierung des Gehirns. Ich möchte das an einer Abbildung demonstrieren (Abb. 8). Sie zeigt den Verlauf eines unbehandelten Hirnödems bis zum Höhepunkt nach 24 Std. und die spontane Rückbildung. Nach Verabreichung von Harnstoff und Mannitol fällt der Wassergehalt des ödematösen Gehirns initial ab und steigt in den folgenden Stunden wieder auf den alten Wert an, da sich die Serumosmolalität wegen der Verteilung des Mannit bzw. des Harnstoffs im gesamten Extrazellulärraum sowie der renalen Ausscheidung wieder normalisiert hat. Der erhöhte Natriumgehalt des Gehirns wird jedoch nicht beeinflußt. Mit diesen Substanzen läßt sich deshalb keine Dauertherapie erzielen. Im Gegensatz dazu scheint es mit dem Salureticum bzw. dem Spironolacton möglich zu sein, sowohl Natrium als auch Wasser aus dem Gehirn zu entfernen. Damit eignen sich letztere Substanzen für eine langfristigere Behandlung des Hirnödems.

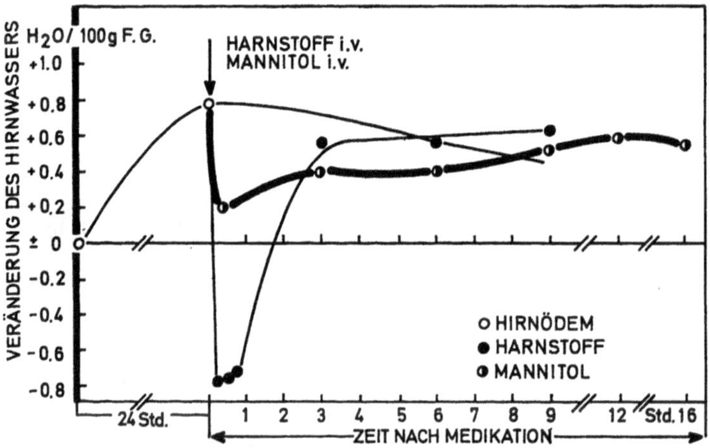

Abb. 8. Verhalten des Hirnwassers nach Gabe von Harnstoff und Mannitol beim Hirnödem. Offene Kreise: Verlauf des unbehandelten Hirnödems. Halbgeschlossene Kreise: Verlauf nach Gabe von 28% Mannit. Geschlossene Kreise: Verlauf nach Gabe von 28% Harnstoff (REULEN, 21).

MÜLLER: Was halten Sie von den ganz hohen Dosen von Cortison, die man neuerdings beim Hirnödem angewandt hat?

REULEN: In der letzten Zeit ist von mehreren Kliniken über gute Erfolge nach Anwendung von Steroiden, meist Dexamethason, beim Ödem in der Umgebung von Hirnmetastasen bzw. Gliomen, beim Pseudotumor cerebri, nach Schädelhirntraumen und vor allem beim postoperativen Hirnödem berichtet worden (s. FRENCH, L. A. BULL N. Y. Acad. Med. **42**, 301 [1966]). Diese Befunde sind durch elektronenmikroskopische Untersuchungen gesichert, die eine deutliche Verminderung der Gliazellschwellung in der Rinde und eine Verkleinerung des EZR im Mark zeigen. Es sind jedoch keine vergleichenden Untersuchungen mit der hypertonischen Therapie oder mit Saluretica bekannt. Wir besitzen an unserer Klinik noch keine größeren Erfahrungen.

BAETHMANN: Im Tierexperiment konnten wir am Beispiel des traumatischen Hirnödems nach Verabreichung von Dexamethason tatsächlich eine Besserung des Ödems, gemessen an der Wasser- und Elektrolyteinlagerung nachweisen.

KRAMER: Ich finde es interessant, daß man eine Differenzierung der Ödembehandlung insofern vornehmen kann, als mit dem Spirolacton bevorzugt die Rinde und mit dem Diureticum das Marklager entwässert wird. Liegen bei solchen Fällen elektroencephalographische oder ähnliche Untersuchungen vor? Es ließe sich damit u. U. klären, ob die cerebralen Funktionsstörungen durch das Mark- oder durch das Rindenödem verursacht werden.

REULEN: Ich möchte noch einmal betonen, daß dieser unterschiedliche Einfluß von Spironolacton und Etacrynsäure auf das Rinden- und Marködem noch an einem größeren Patientengut gesichert werden muß. EEG-Untersuchungen sind m. E. noch nicht durchgeführt worden. Es gibt aber Hinweise, daß die beim Hirnödem auftretenden Störungen der cerebralen Funktion wie Bewußtseinstrübung und Veränderungen im EEG eng mit Änderungen des Stoffwechselumsatzes des Gehirns zusammenhängen, worauf OPITZ und SCHNEIDER 1950 hingewiesen haben. Von BETZ und Mitarbeitern konnte neuerdings eine enge Verknüpfung des energetischen Potentials der Hirnrinde, gemessen am Gehalt an Kreatinphosphat und ATP, mit Änderungen der corticalen elektrischen Aktivität nachgewiesen werden. Auch bei den von uns untersuchten Patienten (24) fand sich in der Hirnrinde ein erheblich reduzierter ATP- bzw. CrP-Gehalt und eine Erhöhung der anaeroben Glykolyserate, was auf einen verminderten Energieumsatz in der Hirnrinde als Ursache des reduzierten Funktionsumfanges hinweisen könnte.

WESSELS: Betrachten Sie eine Diuretica-bedingte Abnahme des Herz-Minuten-Volumens als ein Negativum der Hirnödem-Behandlung?

REULEN: Man sollte vielleicht die Diurese nicht so forcieren, daß es zu einer stärkeren Abnahme des HZV kommt. Es ist bekannt, daß die Autoregulation der Hirndurchblutung in den ödematösen Hirnrealen verringert oder aufgehoben ist und die Durchblutung in der Ödemzone linear, druckabhängig erfolgt. Eine Senkung des Systemdruckes wird sich daher im Ödemgebiet früher ungünstig auf die Durchblutung auswirken als am normalen Gehirn.

HIERHOLZER: Zu der letzten Abbildung möchte ich Sie fragen, über welchen Zeitraum das osmotische Diureticum infundiert wurde? Entspricht das der in der Klinik gebräuchlichen Infusionsdauer? Könnte man die entwässernde Wirkung auf das Gehirn durch längere Infusionsdauer nicht verstärken? Es ist doch zweifelsohne günstig, wenn durch die Ausschwemmung von Wasser Platz im Schädelinnenraum geschaffen wird, selbst wenn durch die Entwässerung vorwiegend die gesunde Hemisphäre an Volumen abnimmt und damit die ödematöse Hemisphäre mehr Platz erhält.

REULEN: Die Infusionsdauer von Mannitol und Harnstoff in den Versuchen betrug 15 Minuten; in der Klinik wird die Lösung innerhalb 30–40 Minuten infundiert. Theoretisch wäre zu erwarten, daß mit einer langsameren Infusionsgeschwindigkeit – nach einem anfänglich raschen Aufbau des osmotischen Gradienten – die entwässernde Wirkung länger aufrecht erhalten werden könnte. Das trifft für Mannitol für einen Zeitraum von ca. 1 Stunde auch zu. Der Nachteil dieser Methode ist aber, daß damit mehr Mannit in das Gehirn eindringt und der spätere negative Osmogradient und damit auch der Reboundeffekt ausgeprägter wird. Bei Verwendung von Sorbit kommt hinzu, daß es in hohem Maße metabolisiert wird, so daß der notwendige osmotische Gradient nur durch große Sorbitmengen aufrecht erhalten werden könnte. Bei der Infusion solch großer Sorbit- bzw. Mannitdosen wäre vermutlich als weiterer Nachteil eine starke Diurese mit einer unerwünschten Einschränkung des EZR zu erwarten.

Index

A

ACETAZOLAMIDE
glomerular filtration rate, 398
proximal tubule, 229
renal clearances, 330
renin, 456
tubular steady state concentration, 231
ACIDOSIS: metabolic, 11, 22
ADENOSINETRIPHOSPHATE, 7
ADRENALECTOMY
cerebral edema, 474
tubular function, 153
ALDACTONE *see* Spironolactone
ALDOSTERONE
AIP, 142
cerebral edema, 473
DNA, 140
escape phenomenon, 427, 430
intracellular action, 139, 146
latent period, 143, 162
metabolism, 379, 423, 431, 451
RNA, 140
toad bladder, 140
ALDOSTERONE ANTAGONISTS
cerebral edema, 473, 477
combined diuretics, 283
heparin, 272
mode of action, 271
progesterone, 273
spirolactones, 281
triamterene and amiloride, 280
ALKALOSIS
hypochloremic, 372
hypokalemic, 367
metabolic, 11, 22
AMILORIDE
aldosterone metabolism, 378
amphibian membrane, 195, 210
electrolytes, 258, 306
ethacrynic acid, 310, 315, 403
excretion, 251, 303
hepatic coma, 373
hypertension, 355
liver cirrhosis, 368
pharmacology, 237, 247, 256
proximal tubule, 217
renin, 456
short circuit current, 198
site of action, 251
sodium transport, erythrocytes, 318
AMPHIBIAN MEMBRANE
aldosterone, 140
amiloride, 210
ethacrynic acid, 211
furosemide, 211
glycolysis, 9
hydrochlorothiazide, 211
oxygen consumption, 209
strophanthin, 210
ANGIOTENSIN
cutaneous reaction, 323
distal tubule, 183
intrarenal action, 173
loop of Henle, 176
proximal tubule, 118, 175
sodium reabsorption, 173
ANGIOTENSINASE
natural angiotensin, 177
synthetical angiotensin, 177
ANTIKALIURETIC SUBSTANCES, 236, 247, 281
chloride excretion, 281
combined diuretics, 283
ASCITES, 366
ATP-ASE
active transport, 67
adrenalectomy, 75
chemical assay, 67
fish kidney, 73, 76
intrarenal distribution, 68
steroid dependency, 75
unilateral nephrectomy, 69
AZOTEMIA
diuretics in cirrhosis, 372
effect of furosemide, 392
ineffectiveness of diuretics, 389

B

BLOOD VOLUME
diuretics, 328, 333, 340, 434
long term diuretic treatment, 331

C

CARBOHYDRATE METABOLISM: diuretics, 344
CARBONIC ANHYDRASE, 190
CATECHOLAMINES: furosemide, 400
CEREBRAL EDEMA
  adrenalectomy, 474
  aldosterone, 473
  aldosterone antagonists, 477
  diuretics, 469, 476, 477
  mannitol, 475
CHLORIDE
  amiloride, 281
  antikaliuretic substances, 281
  ethacrynic acid and amiloride, 373
  intracellular localization, 53
CHLOROTHIAZIDE
  hypertension, 338
  hypokalemia, 371
  renal failure, 383
CIRCULATION TIME, 448
CO_2: renal a.-v. difference, 34
COLLECTING DUCT
  potassium transport, 124, 137
  ultrastructure, 49
COR PULMONALE, 429, 439
COUNTERCURRENT SYSTEM
  bicarbonate, 188
  oxygen, 9
  pCO_2, 187
CREATININE: renal formation, 9
CYCLOPENTHIAZIDE: blood volume, 333

D

DIABETES INSIPIDUS
  diuretics, 409, 412
  sodium restriction, 409
DIAZOXIDE
  hypertension, 329, 346
  potassium excretion, 351
DIFFUSION PERMEABILITY, 105
DISTAL TUBULE
  adrenalectomy, 155
  aldosterone, 153, 160
  amiloride, 207
  angiotensin, 183
  cortisone, 162
  dexamethasone, 163
  diffusion permeability, 105
  electrical potential difference, 131, 134
  filtration permeability, 102
  hydrogen secretion, 129
  potassium transport, 123
  renal hypertension, 183
  sodium concentration, 128
  specific resistance, 135
  ultrastructure, 41, 49
DIURETICS
  aldosterone metabolism, 379
  arterial resistance, 342
  blood volume, 340
  carbohydrate metabolism, 344
  cardiac function, 442, 450
  cerebral edema, 469
  circulation time, 448
  classes, 255
  combined application, 269, 306, 310, 315, 368, 403, 440
  comparative effectiveness, 257
  diabetes insipidus, 409
  extra-intracellular sodium, 341
  and glucocorticoids, 441
  heart failure, 421, 433, 448, 451
  heart surgery, 459
  hypertension
    mode of action, 340, 342
    side effects, 343
    treatment, 321, 337, 355
  hyperurikemia, 345
  intermittant therapy, 293, 421, 440
  liver cirrhosis, 365, 371, 375
  nephrectomy, 351
  pulmonary hypertension, 439
  renal failure, 388

E

ERYTHROCYTES
  amiloride on sodium transport, 318
  diuretics on electrolyte content, 437, 441
ERYTHROPOIETIN, 11
ETHACRYNIC ACID
  and amiloride, 310, 403
  amphibian membrane, 211
  blood volume, 328, 434
  cerebral edema, 476, 477
  effect on hemodynamics, 328, 435
  electrolytes, 306
  extracellular volume, 434
  glomerular filtration rate, 350, 398
  heart failure, 439
  heart surgery, 462
  hepatic coma, 373
  hypochloremic alkalosis, 372
  hypokalemia, 371
  nephrotic syndrome, 389
  pharmacology, 236, 255
  proximal tubule, 217, 226
  pulmonary edema, 439
  renal clearances, 330, 350, 386

renal failure, 383, 393
renin, 436, 456
venous pressure, 434

F

FILTRATION PERMEABILITY, 100, 105
FUROSEMIDE
amphibian membrane, 211
azotemia, 392
blood volume, 434
catecholamines, 400
distal filtration permeability, 103
extracellular volume, 434
glomerular filtration rate, 363, 392, 398
heart failure, 439
heart surgery, 462
hypertension, sodium excretion, 362
hypokalemia, 371
nephrotic syndrome, 389
pharmacology, 236, 255
proximal tubule, 217, 229
pulmonary edema, 439
renal blood flow, 386
renal clearances, 330
renal failure, 383, 393
renin, 277, 436, 456
transplanted kidney, 413
tubular steady state concentration, 231
venous pressure, 434

G

GALL BLADDER
active transport, 78
isotonic fluid reabsorption, 78
ultrastructure, 84
GLOMERULAR FILTRATION RATE
aldosterone, 161
cortisone, 162
diuretics, 36, 383, 398
ethacrynic acid, 350, 386
extracorporeal circulation, 460
furosemide, 383, 392
intrarenal distribution, 180
intrarenal regulation, 180
GLOMERULO-TUBULAR BALANCE
proximal tubule, 111
sodium diet, 176
GLUCOCORTICOIDS
heart failure, 441
hyponatremia, 441
GLUCOSE: renal a.-v. difference, 7
GYNEKOMASTIA, 368, 375

H

HEART FAILURE
aldosterone metabolism, 423, 451
diuretics, 288, 294, 433, 448, 451
electrolytes, 437, 440, 441
ethacrynic acid, 439
furosemide, 439
glucocorticoids, 441
intermittant diuretic therapy, 440
sodium restriction, 421
spirolactones, 440
HEPARIN
aldosterone antagonist, 272
natriuresis, 294
HYDROCHLOROTHIAZIDE
amphibian membrane, 211
electrolytes, 236, 258
glomerular filtration rate, 398
hypertension, 355
proximal tubule, 229
renal clearances, 330
renin, 456
tubular steady state concentration, 231
HYDROGEN SECRETION: distal tubule, 129
HYPERTENSION
diazoxide, 329, 346
diuretics and hypotensive drugs, 342
furosemide, 362
hemodynamics, 324
hydrochlorothiazide, 355
mode of action of diuretics, 332, 340
Na/K-ratio in sweat, 428
side effects of diuretics, 343
sodium restriction, 337
HYPERTENSION, ESSENTIAL
amiloride, 355
angiotensin, 185
diuretics, 323, 338, 355, 362
sodium excretion, 185
HYPERTENSION, MALIGNANT
diuretics, 322, 355
hypotensive treatment, 350
HYPERTENSION, PULMONARY: diuretics, 439
HYPERTENSION, RENAL: distal tubule, 183
HYPERURIKEMIA: diuretics, 345, 351
HYPOKALEMIA: after diuretics, 371
HYPONATREMIA: cirrhosis, 373
glucocorticoids, 441
heart failure, 441
nephrotic syndrome, 389

I

INTRACELLULAR SPACES, 37, 65

J

Juxtaglomerular Apparatus, 178

L

Liver Cirrhosis
aldosterone metabolism, 379
amiloride, 368
azotemia, 372
coma after diuretics, 372, 376
diuretics, 286, 365
hypochloremic alcalosis, 372
hypokalemia, 367, 371
hyponatremia in, 371, 373
prognosis, 375
sodium restriction, 366
spirolactones, 368
triamterene, 368
Loop of Henle
angiotensin, 176
ultrastructure, 49

M

Macula Densa
function, 64, 178, 182
ultrastructure, 49
Mannitol
acute renal failure, 389, 392
cerebral edema, 475
extracorporeal circulation, 462
Medulla
bicarbonate, 187
blood flow, 9
metabolism, 35
oxygen tension, 9
pCO_2, 187
Meralluride: renal failure, 383
Mercurial Diuretics, 255
Metabolism, Renal
alanine, 11
amino acids, 11
ammonia, 11
amphibian membrane, 209
carbohydrate, 3
fatty acids, 3, 9, 35
gluconeogenesis, 1
glucose, 3, 7, 9
glutamine, 11
glycolysis, 5, 7
lactate, 3
renal cortex, 3, 9
renal medulla, 3, 9, 35
Micropinocytosis, 40, 57

N

Nephrotic Syndrome
ethacrynic acid and amiloride, 403
hyponatremia, 389
indication for diuretics, 388
Non-Ionic Diffusion, 27

O

Osmosis: local, 82
Osmotic Flow: standing gradient, 88
Osmotic Gradient: local, 86
Oxygen: renal a.-v. difference, 34
Oxygen Consumption
amphibian membrane, 209
kidney, 1, 9, 29, 36
liver, 2

P

Para-Aminohippuric Acid, 110
Pasteur Effect, 10
pH
distal tubule, 130
tubular fluid, 26
Phosphofructocinase, 7
Potassium
collecting duct, 124
diazoxide, 351
distal tubule, 123
proximal tubule, 123
tissue concentration, cerebral edema, 471
total body content, diuretics, 258
Progesterone
aldosterone antagonist, 273
extrarenal effects, 275
Protein: reabsorption, 57
Proximal Passage Time, 26, 115, 218, 221, 226
adrenalectomy, 157
cortisone, 162
sodium diet, 171, 176
Proximal Tubule
acetazolamide, 229
adrenalectomy, 153
aldosterone, 153, 160
amiloride, 217
ammonia, 25
angiotensin, 118, 175
cortisone, 162
dexamethasone, 163
diffusion permeability, 105
electrical potential difference, 118, 120
ethacrynic acid, 217, 226

filtration permeability, 101
furosemide, 217, 229
glomerulo-tubular balance, 111
hydrochlorothiazide, 229
intratubular pressure, 221, 226
isotonic fluid reabsorption, 97
luminal diameter, 113, 221, 226
para-aminohippuric acid, 110
potassium reabsorption, 123
protein reabsorption, 55
reabsorption rate, 116, 217
sodium permeability, 168
transport characteristics, 109
ultrastructure, 38, 46
PULMONARY EDEMA
ethacrynic acid, 439
furosemide, 439

R

REABSORPTION: isotonic fluid, 77
RENAL BLOOD FLOW, 29
diuretics, 36
ethacrynic acid, 386
furosemide, 386
RENAL FAILURE: diuretics, 381, 383, 388, 395
ethacrynic acid, 393
furosemide, 393
RENAL FAILURE, ACUTE, 179, 184
mannitol, 392
RENAL ISCHEMIA, 179
ultrastructure, 43
RENIN
diuretics, 277, 294, 436, 457
intrarenal distribution, 177, 182
secretion, 178
sodium diet, 180
RESPIRATORY QUOTIENT, 3, 5, 30

S

SODIUM
active transport
aldosterone, 139
amphibian membrane, 195
angiotensin, 173
erythrocytes, 318
kidney, 29
excretion in hypertension, 362
extra-intracellular, diuretics, 341
flux, amphibian membrane, 199
intracellular localization, 53
Na/K ratio in urine and sweat, 426
restriction
cirrhosis, 366
diabetes insipidus, 409
heart failure, 421
hypertension, 337
tissue-concentration, cerebral edema, 471
SODIUM-BALANCE: hypotensive effect of diuretics, 340
SPIRONOLACTONE
aldosterone antagonist, 281
extrarenal effects, 275
gynekomastia, 368, 375
heart failure, 440
heparin, combined action, 294
liver cirrhosis, 368
pharmacology, 256
STROPHANTHIN: amphibian membrane, 210
SWEAT: Na/K ratio, 428

T

TRANSPORT: isotonic fluid, 77, 92, 95
TRIAMTERENE
aldosterone antagonist, 280
liver cirrhosis, 368
pharmacology, 237, 247, 256

U

ULTRASTRUCTURE
collecting duct, 49
distal tubule, 41, 49
gall bladder, 84
loop of Henle, 49
macula densa, 49
proximal tubule, 38, 46
renal ischemia, 43
tubular system, 37

V

VASA RECTA
bicarbonate, 188
glucose, 3, 9
lactate, 3, 9
pCO_2, 188
smooth muscles, 184
VASOPRESSIN
amphibian membrane, 200
gall bladder, 97
VENOUS PRESSURE
ethacrynic acid, 434
furosemide, 434

W

WATER PERMEABILITY, 99

www.ingramcontent.com/pod-product-compliance
Lightning Source LLC
Chambersburg PA
CBHW082005130926
51338CB00021B/44
* 9 7 8 3 6 4 2 8 8 0 9 1 9 *